Pediatric Hematology-Oncology in Countries with Limited Resources

Daniela Cristina Stefan
Carlos Rodriguez-Galindo
Editors

Pediatric Hematology-Oncology in Countries with Limited Resources

A Practical Manual

Springer

Editors
Daniela Cristina Stefan, M.D.
Department of Paediatrics and Child Health
Stellenbosch University
Tygerberg Hospital
Tygerberg, South Africa

Carlos Rodriguez-Galindo, M.D.
Dana-Farber/Boston Children's Cancer and Blood Disorders Center
Harvard Medical School
Boston, MA, USA

ISBN 978-1-4614-3890-8 ISBN 978-1-4614-3891-5 (eBook)
DOI 10.1007/978-1-4614-3891-5
Springer New York Heidelberg Dordrecht London

Library of Congress Control Number: 2013954390

Printed on acid-free paper

Springer is part of Springer Science+Business Media (www.springer.com)

Dedicated to all those looking after children with cancer, whose efforts and hopes never die despite facing challenges in resource limited countries

Dedicated to my husband, Valentin, and my 2 daughters, Dora and Sabina, who are everything to me

Daniela Cristina Stefan

Dedicated to my family, to whom all I owe

Dedicated to all children with cancer and their parents, who continue to inspire all I do

Carlos Rodriguez-Galindo

Foreword

Close to 200,000 children and adolescents are diagnosed with cancer every year worldwide; of those, 80 % live in low- and middle-income countries, which account for 90 % of the deaths. Thus, the burden of pediatric cancer is clearly shifted towards countries with limited resources, making the tragedy of childhood cancer even more unjust.

In September 2000, heads of state and government gathered at the United Nations headquarters for the Millennium Summit and set down the millennium declaration, a series of priorities for peace and security, reduction of poverty, environmental protection, and human rights. This resulted in the Millennium Development Goals; by 2015, with everyone's effort, the world would achieve measurable improvements in those critical areas of human development. Importantly, reduction of child mortality is a Millennium Development Goal, and the world is on its way to fulfilling it. More recently, in September 2011, a high-level meeting of the United Nations General Assembly was dedicated to the prevention and control of noncommunicable diseases, including cancer, thus calling for action by global health agencies and governments. A major challenge is now on the table: cure all children with cancer, wherever they are and build hope and a future for them, whatever it takes.

This will require a tremendous effort on the part of high-, middle-, and low-income countries, if we are all to work together to achieve this goal. Building pediatric cancer programs will become imperative, and developing nations will need guidance on how to develop their capacity, adapt and design treatments, and learn the process. Very tight collaborations between centers in both ends of the spectrum will be needed and examples of very successful twinning partnerships are seen in Latin America and the Caribbean, Africa, the Middle East, and Asia. But documenting what we have learned in this process and how we can provide guidance for those programs under development is key. In this book we have assembled a group of experts in the field to share their knowledge and help us understand the intricacies of diagnosing and treating childhood cancer when so many resources are lacking. We wish there was enough room to share the experiences of so many in the Americas, Europe, Oceania, Asia, and Africa who tirelessly work every day to make a better world for children with cancer and their families. To all of them, and to all the children who suffer every day, this book is dedicated.

Tygerberg, South Africa — Daniela Cristina Stefan, M.D.
Boston, MA, USA — Carlos Rodriguez-Galindo, M.D.

Contents

Contributors

Soad Fuentes Alabí, M.D. Hospital Nacional de Niños Benjamín Bloom, San Salvador, El Salvador

Ana Patricia Alcasabas, M.D. Philippines General Hospital, Manila, Philippines

Nisreen Amayiri, M.D. King Hussein Cancer Center, Amman, Jordan

Federico G. Antillon, M.D. Unidad Nacional de Oncología Pediátrica, Guatemala City, Guatemala

Kalid Asrat, M.D. Department of Paediatrics, School of Medicine, University of Botswana, Gabarone, Botswana

Jean-Jacques Atteby Yao Dépertement of MERE-ENFANT, UFR SM Univresité Cocody/Abidjan RCI, Abidjan, Republique de Cote d'Ivoire

Fulgencio Baez, M.D. Hospital Infantil Manuel de Jesús Rivera "La Mascota," Managua, Nicaragua

Joyce Balagadde-Kambugu, M.B. Ch.B., M.Med(Pead)., M.Phil. Uganda Cancer Institute, Kampala, Uganda

Ronald D. Barr, M.B. Ch.B., M.D. McMaster University, Hamilton, ON, Canada

Eleanor De Beer, R.N. Tygerberg Hospital, Cape Town, South Africa

Wondu Bekele Mathiwos Wondu-YeEthiopia Cancer Society, Addis Ababa, Ethiopia

Miguel Bonilla, M.D. International Outreach Program, St. Jude Children's Research Hospital, Memphis, TN, USA

Eric Bouffet, M.D. Hospital for Sick Children, Toronto, ON, Canada

Erica Brivio, M.D. Pediatric Department, Ospedale San Gerardo, University of Milano Bicocca—Fondazione MBBM, Monza, Italy

Biobele J. Brown, M.D. Department of Paediatrics, College of Medicine, University of Ibadan, Ibadan, Nigeria

Miguela A. Caniza, M.D. Director of the Infectious Diseases—International Outreach Division, Department of Infectious Diseases, St. Jude Children's Research Hospital, Memphis, TN, USA

Julia M. Challinor, Ph.D., R.N., M.A. in Ed, M.Sc. Medical Anthropology School of Nursing, University of California, San Francisco, San Francisco, CA, USA

Guillermo L. Chantada, M.D. Department of Hemato-Oncology, Hospital JP Garrahan, Buenos Aires, Argentina

Chifumbe Chintu, M.D. Division of Haematology and Oncology, Department of Paediatrics and Child Health, School of Medicine, University of Zambia, Lusaka, Zambia

Inam Chitsike, M.D., Ch.B., M.Med. Paeds Department of Paediatrics and Child Health/Consultant Paediatric Oncology Unit, College of Health Sciences, University of Zimbabwe, Harare, Zimbabwe

Valentino Conter, M.D. Pediatric Department, Ospedale San Gerardo—University of Milano Bicocca—Fondazione MBBM, Monza, Italy

International Outreach Program, St. Jude Children's Research Hospital, Memphis, TN, USA

Kenneth Dollman The International Confederation of Childhood Cancer Parent Organizations, CHOC Childhood Cancer Foundation South Africa, Cape Town, South Africa

Agostino Faravelli, M.D. Surgical Pathology, Patologi Oltre Frontiera, Desio, Milan, Italy

Andrea Ferrari, M.D. Pediatric Oncology Unit, Fondazione IRCCS Istituto Nazionale dei Tumori, Milan, Italy

Lindsay Frazier, M.D., M.Sc. Dana-Farber/Boston Children's Center for Cancer, Boston, USA

Blood Disorders and Harvard Medical School, Boston, MA, USA

Paola Friedrich, M.D. Global Health Initiative, Dana-Farber/Boston Children's Cancer and Blood Disorders Center, Boston, MA, USA

Harvard Medical School, Boston, MA, USA

Norbert Graf, M.D. Department of Pediatric Oncology and Oncology, Saarland University, Homburg, Germany

Mhamed Harif, M.D. Centre Hospitalier Universitaire Mohammed VI, Marrakech, Morocco

Scott C. Howard, M.D. Department of Oncology, St. Jude Children's Research Hospital, University of Tennessee Health Science Center, Memphis, TN, USA

Stephen P. Hunger, M.D. Children's Hospital Colorado and the Department of Pediatrics, Center for Cancer and Blood Disorders, University of Colorado School of Medicine, Aurora, CO, USA

David N. Korones, M.D. Department of Pediatrics, Golisano Children's Hospital, University of Rochester Medical Center, Rochester, NY, USA

Tezer Kutluk, M.D., Ph.D. Union for International Cancer Control, Geneva, Switzerland

Department of Pediatric Oncology, Hacettepe University Cancer Institute, Ankara, Turkey

Carlos Leal Leal, M.D. Mexican Retinoblastoma Group, Instituto Nacional de Pediatría, Mexico, DF, Mexico

Giuseppe Masera, M.D. Pediatric Department, Ospedale San Gerardo, University of Milano Bicocca—Fondazione MBBM, Monza, Italy

Gabriela Maron, M.D. Department of Infectious Diseases, St. Jude Children's Research Hospital, Memphis, TN, USA

Natalie McCall, M.D. Associate Professor of Pediatrics, University of Rwanda, College of Medicine and Health Sciences, Kigali, Rwanda

Visiting Associate Professor of Pediatrics at Yale School of Medicine, Kigali University Teaching Hospital, Kigali, Rwanda

Monika Metzger, M.D. Department of Oncology, St Jude Children's Research Hospital, University of Tennessee Health Sciences Center, Memphis, TN, USA

Lisa Morrissey, M.S.N., M.P.H., R.N., CPON® Department of Hematology/Oncology, Boston Children's Hospital, Boston, MA, USA

Colleen Nixon, M.S.N., R.N., CPON® Department of Hematology/Oncology, Boston Children's Hospital, Boston, MA, USA

Jackson Orem, M.B., Ch.B., M.Med(Med). Uganda Cancer Institute, Kampala, Uganda

Roberta Ortiz, M.D. Department of Pediatric Hematology-Oncology, Manuel de Jesus Rivera, La Mascota Hospital, Managua, Nicaragua

Julia Palma, M.D. Bone Marrow Transplant Unit, Hospital Dr. Luis Calvo Mackenna, Providencia, Santiago de Chile, Chile

Nehal S. Parikh, M.D. Connecticut Children's Medical Center, Hartford, CT, USA

Jeannette Parkes, M.D. Department of Radiation Oncology, Groote Schuur and Red Cross Children's Hospitals and University of Cape Town, Cape Town, South Africa

Jan Du Plessis, M.D. Department of Paediatrics and Child Health, Universitas Hospital, University of the Free State, Bloemfontein, Free State, South Africa

Roberto Polillo, M.D. DISCO Department of Informatics, Systems and Communication, University of Milano Bicocca, Milan, Italy

Stelios Poyiadjis, M.D. Chris Hani—Baragwanath Academic Hospital, University of the Witwatersrand, Johannesburg, South Africa

Karina B. Ribeiro, D.D.S., Ph.D. Faculdade de Ciências Médicas da Santa Casa de São Paulo, São Paulo, Brazil

Raul C. Ribeiro, M.D. Department of Oncology, Leukemia and Lymphoma Division and International Outreach Program, St. Jude Children's Research Hospital, Memphis, TN, USA

Carlos Rodriguez-Galindo, M.D. Dana-Farber/Boston Children's Cancer and Blood Disorders Center, Global Health Initiative, Harvard Medical School, Boston, MA, USA

Paul C. Rogers, M.B., Ch.B., F.R.C.P.C., M.B.A. Division of Pediatric Oncology/Hematology/BMT, BC Childrens Hospital & University, Vancouver, BC, Canada

Judy Schoeman, B.Dietetics, B.Compt., M.Sc. Dietetics. Paediatric Oncology Unit, Pretoria, South Africa

Aziza Shad, M.D. Division of Pediatric Hematology Oncology, Blood and Marrow Transplantation, Medstar Georgetown University Hospital, Lombardi Comprehensive Cancer Center, Washington, DC, USA

Furqan Shaikh, M.D., M.Sc. Division of Haematology/Oncology, The Hospital for Sick Children and the University of Toronto, Toronto, ON, Canada

Cristián Sotomayor, M.D. Bone Marrow Transplant Unit, Hospital Dr. Luis Calvo Mackenna, Providencia, Santiago de Chile, Chile

Daniela Cristina Stefan, M.D., Ph.D. Department of Paediatrics and Child Health, Stellenbosch University & Tygerberg Hospital, Tygerberg, South Africa

David K. Stones, M.D. Department of Paediatrics and Child Health, University of the Free State, Bloemfontein, South Africa

Iyad Sultan, M.D. Department of Pediatric Oncology, King Hussein Cancer Center, Amman, Jordan

Julie Torode, Ph.D. Union for International Cancer Control, Geneva, Switzerland

Lisine Tuyisenge, M.D. Kigali University Teaching Hospital, Kigali, Rwanda

Gordan M. Vujanic, M.D. School of Medicine Cardiff University, Cardiff, UK

Kazuyo Watanabe Asian Children's Care League-Japan (ACCL), Tokyo, Japan

Julie Wetter, M.D. Department of Radiation Oncology, Groote Schuur and Red Cross Children's Hospitals and University of Cape Town, Cape Town, South Africa

John T. Wiernikowski, B.Sc. Phm., PharmD Department of Pediatrics, McMaster University, Hamilton, ON, Canada

1 Childhood Cancer in Low-Income and Middle-Income Countries in the Twenty-First Century

Daniela Cristina Stefan

According to the estimations of the International Agency for Research in Cancer (IARC), a little over 175,000 new cases of cancer in children (defined as individuals aged 0–14 years) will appear in the world every year [1]. While these malignancies are mostly not preventable, they are curable. Five-year survival rates as high as 80 % have been achieved in resource-rich countries, where the majority of childhood cancer survivors attain maturity and are productive. In those countries, the emphasis is moving from ensuring survival to minimizing the long-term adverse effects of the therapy. To achieve such percentages of cure, expenditures in the range of USD 100,000 per patient are necessary [2].

This encouraging perspective is only available to 16 % of the children who become ill with cancer. The remaining 84 % or around 147,000 new cases per year, live in low-income or middle-income countries, where their survival chances are much lower since less developed countries account for 94 % of the global mortality from childhood cancer [3, 4]. The striking discrepancy in the above percentages is due mostly to the fact that, out of the seven billion people on our planet, more than 5.8 billion live in limited resource environments [5]. Additionally, the proportion of individuals aged 0–14 years in these populations is around 29 % [6], much higher than the 17 % recorded in the more developed countries.

As the gross national income (GNI) per capita is only USD 1,025 or less in low-income countries and between USD 1,026 and 12,475 in middle-income countries [7], the available funds for health care are limited, with direct consequences on the survival rates. However, very little is known on the real costs of childhood cancer therapy in less developed nations. These may be in fact substantially lower than in the more developed countries. For instance, the average expenditure for treating one case of childhood acute lymphoblastic leukaemia in Shanghai, China, was USD 11,000 in the last decade [8]. Similarly, the cost of treating Stage 2 Hodgkin lymphoma in two South African hospitals, with a cure rate of 80 %, was found to be around USD 6,650 [9].

The burden of disease due to childhood cancer in limited resources countries is gradually increasing. The origin of this increase is multifactorial. Firstly, as the management of childhood infectious diseases and children's nutrition improves, a substantial reduction of the mortality in the 0–5 years age group is seen. However, these children will not be protected from the risk of cancer. Secondly, industrialization and urban living are spreading to the developing world: as was first documented in Europe and the USA, these changes contribute to increasing the incidence of malignancies. Thirdly, a number of widespread infections increase the risk of cancer in children: the Epstein–Barr virus is connected

D.C. Stefan, M.D., Ph.D. (✉)
Department of Paediatrics and Child Health, Stellenbosch University & Tygerberg Hospital, Tygerberg, South Africa
e-mail: cs@sun.ac.za

D.C. Stefan and C. Rodriguez-Galindo (eds.), *Pediatric Hematology-Oncology in Countries with Limited Resources: A Practical Manual*, DOI 10.1007/978-1-4614-3891-5_1,

to Burkitt lymphoma in Central Africa, HIV increases the risk of Kaposi sarcoma and the hepatitis B virus is associated with liver cancer. It is therefore estimated that the number of children with cancer could increase with 30 % by 2020 [10].

A successful strategy for improving the survival rates in children with cancer in limited resource regions should be developed starting from a thorough understanding of the factors which concur to compromise the quality of care. A few insights into the complex difficulties on the path to better cancer care, as they are offered by the studies published to date, are presented below.

Many Children Do Not Access the Cancer Care Facilities

The majority of less developed countries do not have cancer registries and out of the existing registries very few are population-based. In the absence of population-based registries, it is impossible to evaluate not only the incidence of childhood cancer but also the proportion of children who do not access care. Their numbers should be substantial, even in high-medium income countries (i.e. those with GNI's between USD 4,036 and 12,475). South Africa offers an example: according to the GLOBOCAN estimations of an incidence of 85 childhood cancers per million, around 1,300 new cases should appear every year. However, the South African Children's Cancer Registry, which is hospital-based and covers the whole country, only counted between 546 and 723 cases yearly between 1997 and 2007 [11].

Another example originates in Brazil, where in 2009 a number of 234 High Complexity Cancer Care Centers existed, which were equipped and staffed to treat cancer in children and adolescents. In these centres, the mortality from cancer in children, as well as the number of therapeutic procedures, was seen to be much smaller in the northern regions than in the southern ones. At the same time, the proportion of childhood deaths from ill-defined causes, which can be a proxy for the number of children not reaching the health care system, was higher in the north. As the units were planned to cover a roughly similar number of children in the territory, and the incidence of childhood cancer was considered to be generally uniform, the authors concluded that a larger number of children with cancer in the North were never seen at a Cancer Centre before their death [12].

Often There Is a Substantial Delay from the Onset of Symptoms to the Initiation of Treatment

Large time gaps from the clinical onset of the disease to instituting the therapy would allow time for progression of the malignancy towards more advanced and difficult to treat stages. Most of the studies addressing the delay from first symptoms to diagnosis and treatment were done on high-income countries [13, 14]. They present evidence for significant progression of the disease during the time elapsed before the child entered the health care system. Research done in Mexico on the risk factors for delay found that Hodgkin disease, the lower standard of education of the mother, the absence of coverage of the patient by health insurance and the longer distance between home and hospital were correlated with longer delays to the beginning of treatment [15]. Data published from South Africa indicated that in 58 % of cases the initial diagnosis was wrong and the persistence of symptoms in spite of various initial treatments was the most frequent reason to think of malignant disease. In that study, the most important contributor to delay was the physician [16].

Abandonment of Treatment Is Frequent

A recent systematic review and meta-analysis of the literature describing the magnitude of treatment abandonment and its associated factors, in cases of acute leukaemia in children, found that it was vastly different in various studies, from 0 to 74.5 %. The rates were significantly higher in lower-middle income countries (please see definition above), at 29 %, while in higher-middle income countries the figures found were around 2 % ($p<0.0001$).

However, the heterogeneity of the higher rates was interpreted by the authors as an indicator that the abandonment could be reduced, even in restricted resource settings. The analysis could not find clear explanations for the heterogeneity [17].

Another recent, retrospective study, addressing the causes of abandonment of treatment for retinoblastoma in Uttar Pradesh, India, contributes more details to the understanding of the matter: out of 101 children, 50 (49.5 %) defaulted. Around one-third of those families could be traced; the lack of finances and the rejection of enucleation as a means of treatment were the major reasons given for abandonment [18]. A few children returned to complete their treatment, with more advanced disease, which reduced their survival to 50 %, while 75 % of those who never returned died during the monitoring period. Additional statistic data from Delhi, India, this time on a variety of cancers, indicated that the cost of treatment, the great distance to the hospital (over 100 km), the belief that cancer was incurable and the female sex of the child were the reasons given by the parents for discontinuing the therapy [19].

Specialized Care for Children with Cancer Is Not Always Available

While paediatric malignancies are curable to a very large extent, the care required is complex and involves cooperation between several specialties of medicine. A dedicated section in a hospital needs to be reserved for the management of these children; specially trained doctors in paediatric haematology–oncology and specially trained paediatric oncology nurses should ensure the proper medical care; there should be adequate provision of medicines free of charge; access to intensive care units and bone marrow transplant units should be available; a permanent cooperation with pathologists, paediatric surgeons and radiotherapists is necessary; parent support groups and palliative care facilities complete the network of treatment.

What may constitute an ideal availability of specialized physicians for optimal care of children with cancer? The Canadian network of paediatric academic haematology/oncology programmes (C17), after 10 years of surveys and debates, has reached the recommendation that one oncologist is necessary for every 15 newly diagnosed children with cancer, while for every 2.5 oncologists, one haematologist is required. For every 15 bone marrow transplants, one specialized physician should be employed [20].

These ideal standards may not yet exist in Canada and certainly not in the low- and middle-income countries. There is, to these authors' knowledge, no centralized evidence of the number of paediatric oncology units or registered paediatric oncologists in the less developed regions of the world. An approximate estimation of the professional workforce active in the field of paediatric oncology is perhaps offered by the regional distribution of the membership of the International Society of Pediatric Oncology (SIOP): Africa has 93 members, Asia 279, Australia 51, Europe 700, North America 219 and South America 183 [21]. These numbers need to be assessed against the population aged 0–14 of each continent, resulting in an approximate membership per million children of 0.2 in Africa, 0.26 in Asia, 6 in both Europe and Australia–New Zealand–Oceania, 3 in North America and 1 in Latin America [22].

The Chemotherapy Drugs Are Not Always Available or Free of Charge

One of the reasons given for abandonment of therapy, as shown above, is the financial burden created by the need to pay out of pocket for the medication [23]. In some countries, the parents' organizations have succeeded to raise funds for buying the chemotherapy drugs [24]. In the countries or regions where parents' groups exist, they can make a substantial difference in the outcome of childrens' cancer therapy, by educating the parents and raising funds for accomodating the families coming from remote locations and for other forms of support, including covering the cost of treatment. However, in low- and medium-income countries, these organizations are relatively rare. The International Confederation of Childhood Cancer Parent Organizations counts 20 members in Africa, 39 in Asia and 24 in South America, where the majority of low-income populations live [25]. Other solutions were offered by non-governmental organizations or twinning programmes where, besides education and research activities, the partner from a more developed region supplied the medication for the treatment of certain cancers [26].

The interventions required in order to improve the survival of children with cancer in low- and middle-income countries are, considering the facts presented so far, complex and relatively costly. They also need to be sustained in time. Paediatric cancer care cannot be left to be implemented by non-governmental organizations or international academic partnerships. Governments need to develop national cancer control plans where childhood malignancies should be given the attention they deserve. In an attempt to build up the response to the growing burden of cancer, the World Health Assembly adopted, in 2005, the resolution 58.22 [27], which urged member states to create national cancer control programmes, adapted to conditions in each country. From 2006 to 2008, WHO produced a series of six modules addressing all aspects of creating and implementing such programmes [28].

However, in less developed regions of the World, governments were slow to respond to the health care needs of cancer patients, mostly because of more pressing health challenges, such as malaria, AIDS, tuberculosis, malnutrition and trauma. Moreover, children with cancer and their parents cannot institute powerful lobbies: the patients' lives are too short for that. In 2010, WHO organized a survey [29] aimed at evaluating the capacity of response of the World's national health systems to the challenge of non-communicable diseases and found that only 93 countries had policies in place for controlling cancer.

What would be the components of an adequate programme for management of childhood malignancies? A national cancer registry would be necessary in order to evaluate the magnitude of the health problem, the geographic distribution of cancer incidence and the progress made in controlling it. The public should be made aware of the existence of childhood cancer and its early signs. Health care workers at the interface with the public should also be educated about the approach to diagnosis and management of childhood cancer. The need for paediatric haematologists–oncologists should be assessed realistically and training programmes should be funded at the country's academic institutions. In parallel, the training of oncology nurses should be organized. International collaboration may be sought in order to set up these training programmes.

A number of paediatric oncology units should be organized in larger, multidisciplinary hospitals, where the services of paediatric surgeons, radiologists, radiotherapists, bone marrow transplant units, nutritionists and pharmacists would be readily available to the children with cancer. Cytostatic drugs, operating theatres, radiotherapy facilities, antibiotics and analgetics (including opiates) as well as blood for transfusion should be available there, free of charge. These paediatric oncology units would also ensure a qualified and efficient follow-up of patients in remission.

The issues of cost should be addressed by research aimed at establishing simpler, less toxic and less expensive therapy protocols, adapted to the specifics of health care in the low- and middle-income countries while remaining highly effective. Here again, international collaboration may make a substantial contribution, as it was already seen. Further, parent organizations should be supported, as they often contribute funds and educate the parents and the general public. To end with, palliative care units need to be instituted, adequately staffed and funded.

The authors of this book are well aware of the dimensions of the task of establishing an efficient cancer control programme in a country with limited resources. They are also aware of numerous successful programmes across continents, which improved the outcome in paediatric malignancies. Many of the authors have been involved in those programmes. The expertise and the wisdom acquired in decades of activity are now distilled in this volume, to the benefit of all those who work towards preserving the lives and the health of children with cancer.

References

1. GLOBOCAN. Age-specific table of incidence of cancer. http://globocan.iarc.fr. Accessed 6 May 2013.
2. van Litsenburg RR, Uyl-de Groot CA, Raat H, Kaspers GJ, Gemke RJ. Cost-effectiveness of treatment of childhood acute lymphoblastic leukemia with chemotherapy only: the influence of new medication and diagnostic technology. Pediatr Blood Cancer. 2011;57:1005–10.
3. Magrath I, Steliarova-Foucher E, Epelman S, et al. Paediatric cancer in low-income and middle-income countries. Lancet Oncol. 2013;14:e104–16.
4. Pritchard-Jones K, Pieters R, Reaman GH, et al. Sustaining innovation and improvement in the treatment of childhood cancer: lessons from high-income countries. Lancet Oncol. 2013;14:e95–103.
5. Trading Economics. http://www.tradingeconomics.com/low-and-middle-income/population-total-wb-data.html. Accessed 28 May 2013.
6. Trading Economics. http://www.tradingeconomics.com/low-and-middle-income/population-ages-0-14-percent-of-total-wb-data.html. Accessed 28 May 2013.
7. The World Bank. GNI per capita, PPP (current international $). http://data.worldbank.org. Accessed 28 May 2013.
8. Liu Y, Chen J, Tang J, Ni S, Xue H, Pan C. Cost of childhood acute lymphoblastic leukemia care in Shanghai, China. Pediatr Blood Cancer. 2009;53:557–62.
9. Stefan D, Stones D. How much does it cost to treat children with Hodgkin lymphoma in Africa? Leuk Lymphoma. 2009;50:196–9.
10. Kellie SJ, Howard S. Global child health priorities: what role for paediatric oncologists? Eur J Cancer. 2008;44:2388–96.
11. Stefan DC, Stones D. The South African Paediatric Tumour Registry—25 years of activity. S Afr Med J. 2012;102:605–6.
12. Grabois MF, Oliveira EX, Carvalho MS. Childhood cancer and pediatric oncologic care in Brazil: access and equity. Cad Saude Publica. 2011;27:1711–20.
13. Dang-Tan T, Trottier H, Mery LS, et al. Delays in diagnosis and treatment among children and adolescents with cancer in Canada. Pediatr Blood Cancer. 2008;51:468–74.
14. Brasme JF, Morfouace M, Grill J, et al. Delays in diagnosis of paediatric cancers: a systematic review and comparison with expert testimony in lawsuits. Lancet Oncol. 2012;13:e445–59.
15. Fajardo-Gutiérrez A, Sandoval-Mex AM, Mejía-Aranguré JM, Rendón-Macías ME, Martínez-García MC. Clinical and social factors that affect the time to diagnosis of Mexican children with cancer. Med Pediatr Oncol. 2002;39:25–31.
16. Stefan D, Siemonsma F. Delay and causes of delay in the diagnosis of childhood cancer in Africa. Pediatr Blood Cancer. 2011;56:80–5.
17. Gupta S, Yeh S, Martiniuk A, et al. The magnitude and predictors of abandonment of therapy in paediatric acute leukaemia in middle-income countries: a systematic review and meta-analysis. Eur J Cancer. 2013;S0959-8049(13)00258-X. doi:10.1016/j.ejca.2013.03.024.
18. Kumar A, Moulik NR, Mishra RK, Kumar D. Causes, outcome and prevention of abandonment in retinoblastoma in India. Pediatr Blood Cancer. 2013;60:771–5.
19. Ramzan M, Yadav SP, Sachdeva A. Treatment abandonment is a major hurdle to improving survival in childhood cancer in the developing world. Pediatr Blood Cancer. 2013;60:159–60.
20. Halton JM, Hand J, Byron P, Strother D, Blanchette V, C17 Council of Canadian Pediatric Hematology Oncology TD. Establishing physician to patient ratios and predicting workforce needs for Canadian pediatric hematology-oncology programs. Pediatr Blood Cancer. 2013;60:564–9.
21. SIOP Asia. SIOP Members from the 6 continents. http://siop-asia.com/en/information-from-siop/members-and-countries.html. Accessed 28 May 2013.
22. United States Census Bureau. International Data Base (IDB). http://www.census.gov/population/international/data. Accessed 28 May 2013.
23. Mostert S, Gunawan S, Wolters E, et al. Socio-economic status plays important roles in childhood cancer treatment outcome in Indonesia. Asian Pac J Cancer Prev. 2012;13:6491–6.
24. Hessissen L, Madani A. Pediatric oncology in Morocco: achievements and challenges. J Pediatr Hematol Oncol. 2012;34 Suppl 1:S21–2.
25. Member Organisations ICCCPO. International confederation of childhood cancer parent organizations. http://icccpo.org/index.cfm?fuseaction=category&category=16. Accessed 28 May 2013.
26. Groupe Franco-Africain D'oncologie Pédiatrique. http://www.gfaop.org. Accessed 28 May 2013.
27. World Health Organization. Related World Health Assembly Resolutions WHA 58.22. http://www.who.int/ipcs/publications/wha/en/. Accessed 28 May 2013.
28. World Health Organization. Cancer control: knowledge into action, WHO guide for effective programmes. http://www/who.int/cancer/modules/en/. Accessed 28 May 2013.
29. World Health Organization. Assessing national capacity for the prevention and control of noncommunicable diseases. Report of the 2010 global survey. http://www.who.int/cancer/publications/national_capacity_prevention_ncds.pdf. Accessed 28 May 2013.

2 Cancer Registries and the Descriptive Epidemiology of Pediatric Cancer in Low- and Middle-Income Countries

Karina B. Ribeiro and Lindsay Frazier

Introduction

The world population is approaching 7.1 billion people; the vast majority live in low- and middle-income countries (LMIC). Approximately 15 million new cancer cases and nine million cancer deaths will occur in 2015, with 48.2 and 56.5 % of those being observed in low- and middle-income countries, respectively. The growing impact of cancer in the population can be attributed to increased life expectancy, due to better control and treatment of communicable diseases, such as diarrheal diseases and decreased neonatal mortality, thus the consequent emergence of the cancer as a public health problem worldwide.

Cancer in childhood is a rare disease. In developed countries, only about 0.5 % of all cancer occurs in children aged less than 15 years. Yet, LMIC bear a disproportionate burden of this disease in part due to the fact that on average, the proportion of the population under 18 is much higher in LMIC than in high-income countries (HIC). Due to this demographic distribution of the world population, 71.4 % of all childhood cancer cases and 83 % of all childhood cancer deaths occurring worldwide are reported among children living in LMIC [1].

K.B. Ribeiro, D.D.S., Ph.D. (✉)
Faculdade de Ciências Médicas da Santa Casa de São Paulo, São Paulo, Brazil
e-mail: kbribeiro@gmail.com

L. Frazier, M.D., M.Sc.
Dana-Farber/Boston Children's Center for Cancer, Boston, USA

Blood Disorders and Harvard Medical School, Boston, MA, USA

Cancer Registries

For the development of a rational national cancer plan, it is necessary to know the magnitude of the disease in a country, in a region, and in a community. However, cancer is not a single disease; therefore, one must know the distribution of different types in a population, which will illustrate variations in geographic, ethnic, socioeconomic, occupational, and even cultural factors that lead to changes in incidence. The cancer registry is the agency or institution that is dedicated to collect, store, analyze, and interpret data on cancer cases. The cancer registry is a critical component of any cancer control program, and its data can be used in several areas including etiology research, primary and secondary prevention, and health care services planning [2, 3].

There are two different types of cancer registries: the hospital-based cancer registry and the population-based cancer registry. The *hospital-based cancer registry* collects data on all patients treated in a hospital or in a set of hospitals (central hospital-based cancer registry). The main objectives of a hospital-based cancer registry are

D.C. Stefan and C. Rodriguez-Galindo (eds.), *Pediatric Hematology-Oncology in Countries with Limited Resources: A Practical Manual*, DOI 10.1007/978-1-4614-3891-5_2,

to evaluate and improve the quality of patient care, to contribute to professional education, to provide information for hospital administration for planning purposes, and to serve as a basis for clinical research. Furthermore, hospital-based cancer registries can be also responsible for controlling the follow-up of patients treated at a specific hospital. Hospital-based cancer registries cannot be used to calculate incidence [2].

Population-based cancer registries are usually operated by governmental agencies. These registries collect information on all cancer cases occurring in a defined population residing within a specified geographic area. Their main objective is the determination of incidence rates (by sex, age, primary site, stage of disease, etc.). Moreover, the data can also be used to conduct epidemiological studies to evaluate the actions of the cancer control program, as well as to assist in the planning of health services for the prevention, diagnosis, and treatment. If mortality data are also collected (which is not done in all cancer registries), a population-based cancer registry is also able to calculate survival rates (and to estimate prevalence rates) [2, 3].

The value of a cancer registry is entirely dependent on the quality of the data collected. To achieve its objectives, the population-based cancer registry should ensure:

- The inclusion of all new cancer cases in a population (coverage)
- The correct coding and classification of tumors (validity)
- If survival data are also included in the registry, monitoring, and follow-up of patients
- Access to estimates of the population at risk (i.e., census data), preferably stratified by gender and age

The main aspects of data quality of a cancer registry are comparability, coverage, and validity. The coverage can be defined as the proportion of incident cases in a population that is included in the registry. Ideally, this number should be as close to 100 % as possible, so that the comparison of changes over time in the population covered by the registry and the comparison between registries reflect true differences only in cancer risk. However, full coverage is not achievable in most circumstances for the following reasons:

- The patient does not seek or have access to health care and the case is never diagnosed.
- The registry is deficient in their pursuit of cases.
- Underdiagnosis of cancer by the health system leading to selection bias (certain cancers tend to be diagnosed more often) [4, 5].

Several standard metrics have been developed by which the validity of a registry can be judged. The primary measures are (1) the percentage of cases with histological confirmation of the diagnosis (>70 % is the recommended value), (2) the percentage of cases reported by death certificate only (recommended <20 %), (3) percentage of cases reported as unknown primary site (C80.9) or other and unspecified (C26, C39, C48, and C76 (recommended <20 %), and (4) percentage of cases with unknown age (recommended, <20 %) [6].

One of the core functions of The International Agency of Cancer Research (IARC, a unit of the World Health Organization) in Lyon, France, is to support cancer registration worldwide and to make available to the public worldwide statistics on global cancer incidence and mortality. On the IARC website, many useful tools for cancer registration are available, including the monograph "Cancer Registration: Principles and Methods" as well as the free cancer registration software, CanReg 5 (http://www-dep.iarc.fr/CIN_resources.htm), which is available in many languages.

On the IARC website, many databases relevant to global cancer incidence and mortality can also be accessed. The first landmark publication of global cancer incidence, the "Cancer Incidence in Five Continents (CI5)," series was in 1966; eight updates have followed and CI5 has become the gold standard of cancer registry data. The objective was to make comparable data on cancer incidence from as many geographical locations worldwide as possible publicly available. Traditionally, the publication of CI5, containing tabulations of cancer incidence rates, occurs approximately each 5 years. In the last version (volume IX) of the Cancer Incidence in Five Continents, of a total of 225 registries, only 43 registries (from 25 countries) are located in LMIC (19.1 %). However, if we take into consideration the overall childhood population in LMIC (1.67 billion) and the population in the same age group covered by the cancer registries in CI5-volume IX, the percentage of children with cancer captured by cancer registries is only 2 %.

GLOBOCAN is a project aiming to provide up-to-date estimates of the incidence, mortality, prevalence, and disability-adjusted life years (DALYs) from major type of cancers, at national level, for 184 countries of the world. It utilizes a specific methodology to estimate the country-specific burden of cancer, gathering data from population-based cancer registries (national or local), mortality statistics from the WHO, and national population estimates obtained from United Nations population division [1].

Descriptive Epidemiology of Childhood Cancers in LMIC

Childhood cancers, it should be noted, differ from adult cancers—for instance, the most common form of a cancer in adults, carcinoma, which derive from epithelial cells, is extremely rare among children, whereas solid neoplasms occurring in childhood are predominantly embryonal in origin. Therefore, it is more appropriate to classify childhood cancers according to their histology, rather than the site in which the tumor occurs. Kramárová and Stiller published the first edition of the International Classification of Childhood Cancer (ICCC) [7]: the ICCC classifies childhood tumors into 12 major diagnostic groups: leukemias, lymphomas, central nervous system (CNS) tumors, sympathetic nervous system tumors, retinoblastoma, renal tumors, liver tumors, bone tumors, soft tissue sarcomas, germ cell tumors, epithelial tumors, and other and unspecified malignant cancers. In 1988, IARC published the first volume of the series "International Incidence of Childhood Cancer" [8], describing the incidence observed in the 1970s; 10 years later the second volume was published, which was expanded with the inclusion of 15 additional cancer registries [9].

The incidence rates of childhood cancer range between 96 and 138 per million children per year for males and from 70 to 116 per million children for females [6]. Leukemias, CNS tumors, and non-Hodgkin lymphomas (NHL) are the most frequent pediatric cancers in high-income countries, representing 60 % of all cases, whereas in low-income countries NHL are more common than leukemias and brain tumors [1]. Medium-income countries have an intermediate pattern. However, it is important to note that a large heterogeneity is observed across continents.

In the rest of this chapter, we present data from the different regions in the world, highlighting differences in incidence and rates of changes by geographic location, using data derived from GLOBOCAN 2008, which represents the most up-to-date source on cancer incidence globally. One of the limitations in using GLOBOCAN to examine pediatric data is that the childhood specific classification system—the ICCC—is not used; rather, diseases are reported by their ICD-O codes, which report by site but not histology. This limits our understanding of pediatric diseases because, for instance, in adults "liver cancer" would be almost entirely comprised on hepatocellular carcinoma, whereas in children, it would be a combination of both hepatocellular carcinoma and hepatoblastoma. Although hepatoblastoma is the more common histology in children, in regions where hepatitis B/C are endemic, one would expect to see the ratio tip towards hepatocellular carcinoma. Other tumors, such as neuroblastoma and rhabdomyosarcoma, are completely impossible to infer from the GLOBOCAN data. However, this level of detail will be available for analysis when the next edition of International Incidence of Childhood Cancer is published by IARC (expected in 2014).

Childhood Cancer in LMIC from Africa

According to GLOBOCAN, the estimated incidence of all pediatric cancers (0–14 years) in LMIC from Africa is 99 and 73/million for males

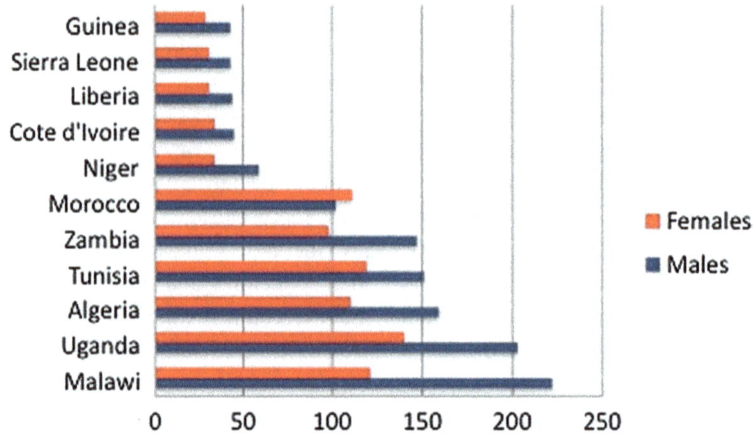

Fig. 2.1 Lowest and highest age-standardized incidence rates for all childhood cancers, LMIC from Africa (Source: GLOBOCAN 2008).

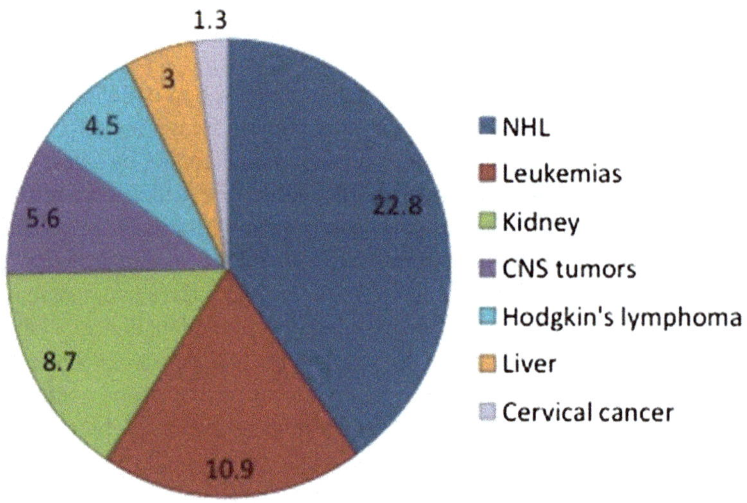

Fig. 2.2 Most frequent cancer types (%) among children 0-14 years in LMIC, Africa (Source: GLOBOCAN 2008).

and females, respectively. There is a wide variation in rates, with the highest rates being recorded in Malawi (220/million for males) and Uganda (140/million among females), while the lowest incidence rates are observed in Guinea (43 and 29/million among males and females, respectively) (Fig. 2.1). Non-Hodgkin lymphoma is the most frequent tumor type, corresponding to 22.8 % of all cancers diagnosed in children living in LMIC from Africa, followed by leukemias and kidney tumors for both sexes (Fig. 2.2).

In Africa, HIV infection is an important cause of childhood cancer. Studies have shown an excess of Kaposi sarcoma and Burkitt lymphoma among HIV-infected children [10–12]. On the other hand, leiomyosarcoma, which is frequently reported among HIV-positive children living in developed countries, is rarely reported in African countries [12]. Of interest, cervical cancer is the seventh most common cancer diagnosis in children less than 14 years of age, probably a reflection of the widespread infection

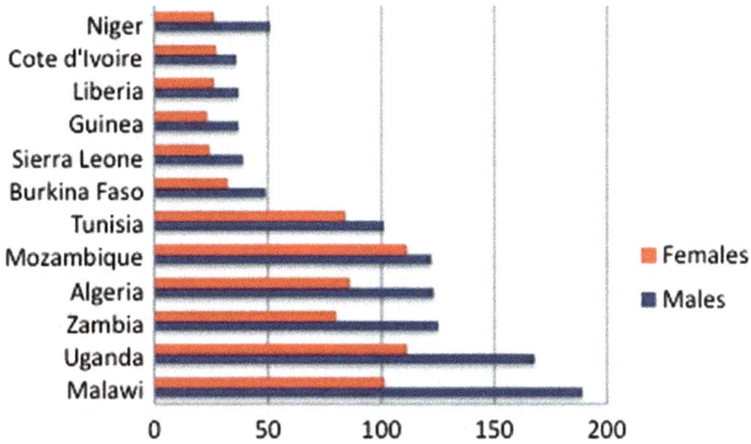

Fig. 2.3 Lowest and highest age-standardized mortality rates for all childhood cancers, LMIC from Africa (Source: GLOBOCAN 2008).

with virulent forms of human papilloma virus as well as the underlying susceptibility due to HIV. Liver cancer is one of the most common cancers in Africa as well, likely due to high prevalence of hepatitis B.

Overall, mortality rates for the group of LMIC from Africa are 80 and 57/million for all cancers for males and females, respectively, ranging from 36 (Cote d'Ivoire) to 189/million (Malawi) for males and between 23 (Guinea) and 111/million (Uganda) for females (Fig. 2.3).

Trends in Childhood Cancer Mortality in LMIC from Africa

According to data available in the WHO Mortality Database, it is possible to obtain a continuous series to assess trends in mortality for only two LMIC from Africa: Egypt (2000–2010) and South Africa (1993–2009). In South Africa, no significant trends were observed in childhood cancer mortality for males (APC = 1.2, 95 % CI −0.1; 2.5), while an increase was observed among females (APC = 1.4, 95 % CI 0.4–2.4). In Egypt, no important changes were observed for both sexes (males, AAPC = 1.2, 95 % CI −3.1; 5.7; females, AAPC = 2.9; 95 % CI −0.2; 6.1).

Childhood Cancer in LMIC from Asia

According to GLOBOCAN estimated incidence of all pediatric cancers (0–14 years) in LMIC from Asia is 96 and 77/million for males and females, respectively. There is a wide variation in rates, with the highest rates being recorded in Kazakhstan (198/million for males) and Sri Lanka (161/million among females), while the lowest incidence rates are observed in North Korea and Tajikistan (51/million among males and females) (Fig. 2.4). Leukemia is the most frequent cancer type, corresponding to more than one third (35.7 %) of all cancers diagnosed in children living in LMIC from Asia, followed by CNS tumors (12.4 %) and non-Hodgkin lymphomas (7.4 %) for both sexes (Fig. 2.5).

Of note, ovarian tumors account for 3.2 % of all pediatric tumors among females, with an age-adjusted incidence rate in the region of 2 new cases/million/year. This is higher than observed in other regions of the world. Liver cancers still remain as one of the most frequent tumor types, for both males (sixth more frequent) and females (seventh more frequent), with incidence rates of 2 and 1/million/year, respectively. Vietnam has the second highest

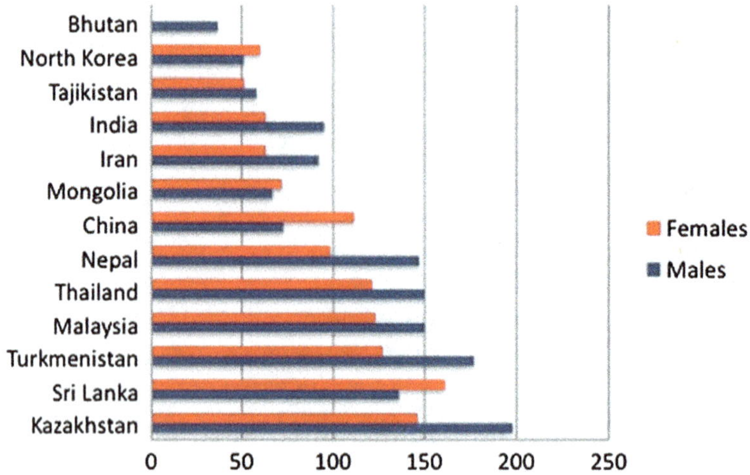

Fig. 2.4 Lowest and highest age-standardized incidence rates for all childhood cancers, LMIC from Asia (Source: GLOBOCAN 2008).

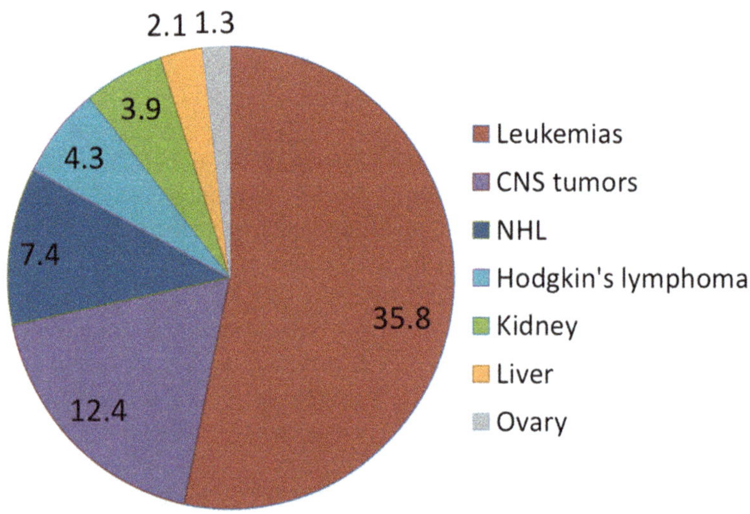

Fig. 2.5 Most frequent cancer types (%) among children 0-14 years in LMIC, Asia (Source: GLOBOCAN 2008).

incidence and mortality rates of liver cancer worldwide (ASIR = 10/million; ASMR = 4/million/year). The association of hepatitis B virus (HBV) infection and liver cancer is well documented in epidemiological studies. The introduction of universal HBV vaccination program for the newborn in endemic regions has started to show a beneficial impact [13]. Vietnam began immunizing newborns in some urban areas against HBV in 1997; however, by 2002, only about 20 % of infants received the hepatitis B vaccine [14]. In addition, the number of mothers who transmit hepatitis B to their newborns during delivery is still very high [15].

Overall, mortality rates for the group of LMIC from Asia are 54 and 45/million for all cancers for males and females, respectively, ranging from 26 (Georgia) to 115/million (Iraq) among males and between 23 (Tajikistan) and 99/million (Myanmar) among females (Fig. 2.6).

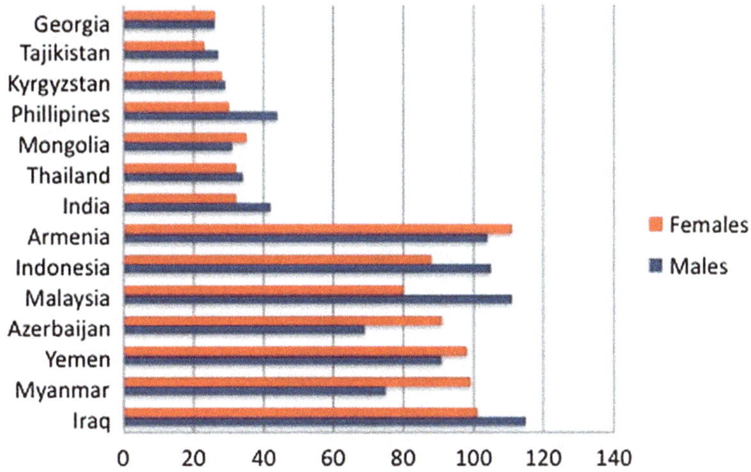

Fig. 2.6 Lowest and highest age-standardized mortality rates for all childhood cancers, LMIC from Asia (Source: GLOBOCAN 2008).

Trends in Childhood Cancer Mortality in LMIC from Asia

According to data available in the WHO Mortality Database, it is possible to assess trends in mortality for only four LMIC from Asia: Azerbaijan (1985–2007), Georgia (1994–2010), Kyrgyzstan (1985–2009), and Russia (1980–2010). In Azerbaijan, among males, a significant decrease in mortality was observed in the period 1985–1992 (APC=−8.4; 95 % CI −14.6; −1.6), followed by a nonsignificant increase in the period 1992–2007 (APC=2.6; 95 % CI −0.3; 5.6), while a significant decrease was observed among females in the period 1985–2007 (AAPC=−4.5, 95 % CI −8.7; −0.2). In Georgia, no significant trends were observed in childhood cancer mortality for both males (APC=−0.4, 95 % CI −4.5; 3.8) and females (AAPC=1.6, 95 % CI −7.9; 12.0). Important declines in childhood cancer mortality rates were observed for both males (APC=−3.7; 95 % CI −4.9; −2.4) and females (APC=−1.7; 95 % CI −3.0; −0.5) in Kyrgyzstan and also in Russia (males, AAPC=−2.1; 95 % CI −2.5; −1.7; females, AAPC=−1.7; 95 % CI −2.7; −0.7).

Childhood Cancer in LMIC from Latin America and the Caribbean

According to GLOBOCAN the estimated incidence of all pediatric cancers (0–14 years) in LMIC from Latin America and the Caribbean is 118 and 94/million for males and females, respectively. There is a wide variation in rates, with the highest ones being recorded in Guyana (171 million for males) and El Salvador (146/million among females), while the lowest incidence rates are observed in Haiti (16 and 12/million among males and females, respectively) (Fig. 2.7). Leukemia is the most frequent cancer type, corresponding to almost 39 % of all cancers diagnosed in children living in LMIC from Latin America and the Caribbean, followed by CNS tumors (13.4 %) and NHL (8.6 %) for both sexes (Fig. 2.8). Renal tumors are the fourth more frequent malignancy among children living in this region, with an annual incidence rate equal to 6 new cases/million. Testicular cancer appears on the list of most frequent cancers for the first time. Testes cancer is more likely in more highly developed countries in general; in this region, countries

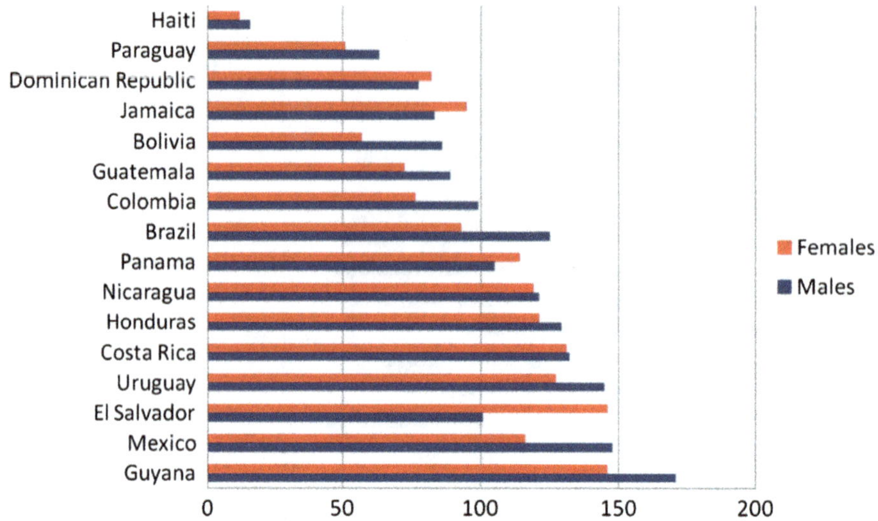

Fig. 2.7 Lowest and highest age-standardized incidence rates for all childhood cancers, LMIC from Latin American & Caribbean (Source: GLOBOCAN 2008).

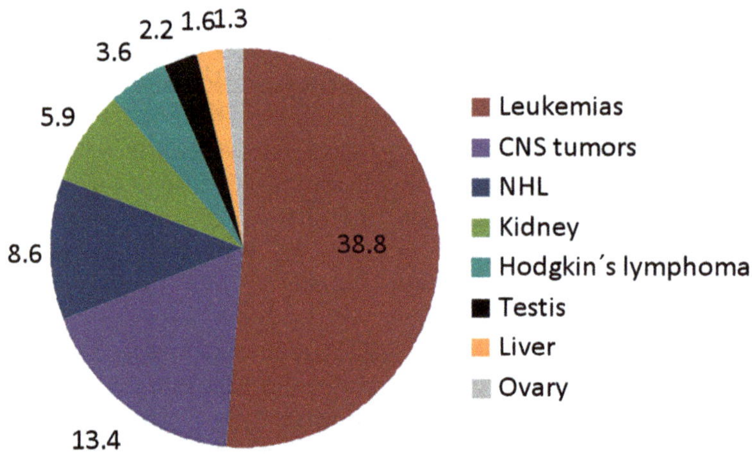

Fig. 2.8 Most frequent cancer types (%) among children 0-14 years in LMIC, Latin America & Caribbean (Source: GLOBOCAN 2008).

like Brazil and Mexico have economic conditions that approach those of HIC.

Overall, mortality rates for the group of LMIC from Latin America and the Caribbean are 54 and 46/million for all cancers for males and females, respectively, ranging from 35 (Chile) to 81/million (Peru) among males and between 26 (Chile) and 71/million (Ecuador) among females (Fig. 2.9). In this region, 43.8 % of all childhood cancer deaths are due to leukemia.

Trends in Childhood Cancer Mortality in LMIC from Latin America and the Caribbean

According to the data available on the last version of WHO Cancer Mortality Database, it is possible to evaluate trends in mortality for several LMIC from Latin America and the Caribbean, including countries with information since 1970s and 1980s: Argentina (1982–2010), Brazil (1979–2010), Chile

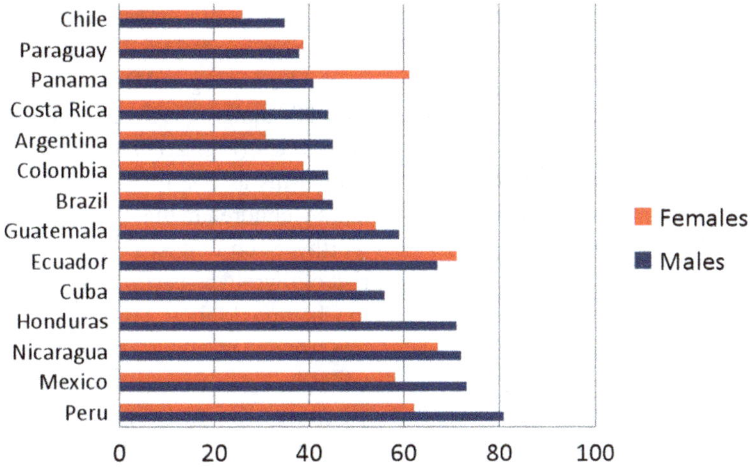

Fig. 2.9 Lowest and highest age-standardized mortality rates for all childhood cancers, LMIC from Latin America & Caribbean (Source: GLOBOCAN 2008).

(1984–2009), Colombia (1984–2009), Costa Rica (1985–2009), Cuba (1970–2010), Ecuador (1977–2010), El Salvador (1995–2009), Guatemala (1986–2008), Mexico (1970–2010), Nicaragua (1996–2010), Panama (1996–2009), Paraguay (1995–2009), Peru (1994–2007), Uruguay (1993–2009), and Venezuela (1996–2007).

Significant decreases in childhood cancer mortality were observed in Chile (males, APC=–2.3, 95 % CI –2.9; –1.7; females, APC=–2.3, 95 % CI –2.9; –1.6), Argentina (males, AAPC=–1.7, 95 % CI –2.4; –1.1; females, AAPC=–2.0, 95 % CI –2.6; –1.3), Costa Rica (males, APC=–2.7, 95 % CI –3.8; –1.6; females, APC=–2.1, 95 % CI –3.4; –0.8), Guatemala (males (2001–2008), APC=–3.6, 95 % CI –6.8; –0.3; females (2000–2008), APC=–3.1, 95 % CI –6.9; 0.9), Cuba (males, APC=–1.0, 95 % CI –1.5; –0.5; females, APC=–1.0, 95 % CI –1.3; –0.7), and Venezuela (males, APC=–1.9, 95 % CI –3.4; –0.3; females, APC=–1.4, 95 % CI –2.7; –0.0), while nonsignificant decreases were noted in Paraguay (males, APC=–0.4, 95 % CI –2.3; 3.2; females, APC=1.9, 95 % CI –1.4; 5.3), Peru (males, APC=–0.1, 95 % CI –1.4; 1.2; females, APC=0.1, 95 % CI –1.3; 1.6), and Uruguay (males, APC=–2.2, 95 % CI –5.8; 1.5; females, APC=–0.6, 95 % CI –4.8; 3.7).

In Ecuador, a significant increase in childhood cancer mortality was noted for both males and females in the period 1977–2010 (males, AAPC=1.4, 95 % CI 0.3; 2.5; females, AAPC=2.2, 95 % CI 0.4; 4.0), while nonsignificant increases in mortality rates were registered in El Salvador (males, APC=1.6, 95 % CI –1.6;4.9; females, APC=2.1, 95 % CI –1.0;5.3), Nicaragua (males, APC=2.0, 95 % CI –0.1;4.1; females, APC=1.6, 95 % CI –0.8; 4.1), Panama (males, APC=0.6, 95 % CI –2.1; 3.3; females, APC=1.4, 95 % CI –3.2; 6.2), and Paraguay (females, APC=1.9, 95 % CI –1.4; 5.3).

In Brazil, for males, a significant decrease in childhood cancer mortality was observed in the period 1984–1992 (APC=–3.3, 95 % CI –4.7; –2.0), followed by a significant increase in the period 1992–1998 (APC=3.4, 95 % CI 1.0; 5.9) and a stabilization between 1998 and 2010 (APC=0.3, 95 % CI –0.3; 0.9). A similar pattern is observed for females, with a significant decrease in mortality rates in the period 1981–1990 (APC=3.0; 95 % CI –4.3; –1.5), followed by a significant increase in the period 1990–2001 (APC=2.3, 95 % CI 1.3; 3.3) and a slight decrease in the years 2001–2010 (APC=–0.6, 95 % CI –1.7; 0.6).

In Mexico, although an overall increase in mortality was observed in the period 1970–2010 among males (AAPC=0.6, 95 % CI –0.3; 1.6), an important decrease in mortality rates has been observed since 2003 (APC=–1.6, 95 % CI –3.1; –0.0). On the other hand, for females no significant change in childhood mortality was observed in the last 40 years (AAPC=0.6, 95 % CI –0.6; 2.0).

Childhood Cancer in LMIC from Europe

According to the World Bank classification, only 14 countries in Europe are middle-income countries (Albania, Belarus, Bosnia, Bulgaria, Kosovo, Latvia, Lithuania, Macedonia, Moldova, Montenegro, Romania, Serbia, Turkey, and Ukraine), and most of them are upper-middle-income countries (10/14).

According to GLOBOCAN, the estimated incidence of all pediatric cancers (0–14 years) in LMIC from Europe is 128 and 109/million for males and females, respectively. There is a wide variation in rates, with the highest ones being recorded in Latvia (169 and 145/million for males and females, respectively), while the lowest incidence rates are observed in Bosnia-Herzegovina (92/million among males) and Moldova (81/million for females) (Fig. 2.10). Leukemia is the most frequent cancer type, corresponding to 31.6 % of all cancers diagnosed in children living in MIC from Europe, followed by CNS tumors (19.3 %) and NHL (8.6 %) for both sexes (Fig. 2.11). The presence of thyroid neoplasms as one of the more frequent cancers among children in this group of countries is noteworthy. Such finding is linked to the increase in risk of thyroid cancer among individuals exposed to Chernobyl fallout [16].

Overall, mortality rates for middle-income countries from Europe are 69 and 63/million for all cancers for males and females, respectively. The lowest mortality rates are observed in Serbia for both males and females (35 and 26/million for males and females, respectively), while highest rates are registered in Turkey (90 and 76/million for males and females, respectively) (Fig. 2.12). In MIC from Europe, the majority of childhood cancer deaths are due to leukemia (39 %), although 20 % are attributed to brain tumors.

Trends in Childhood Cancer Mortality in LMIC from Europe

The evaluation of trends in mortality for some of the middle-income countries from Europe shows an overall significant decrease in childhood cancer mortality, as follows: Bulgaria (1970–2011)

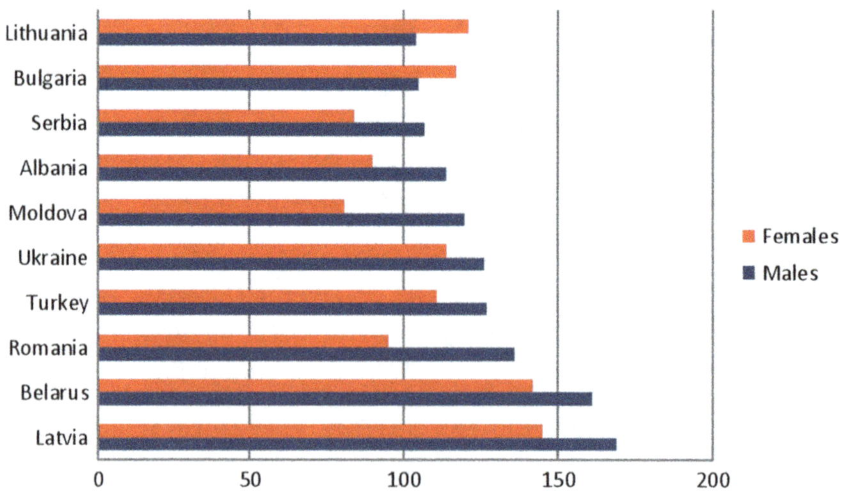

Fig. 2.10 Lowest and highest age-standardized incidence rates for all childhood cancers, LMIC from Europe (Source: GLOBOCAN 2008).

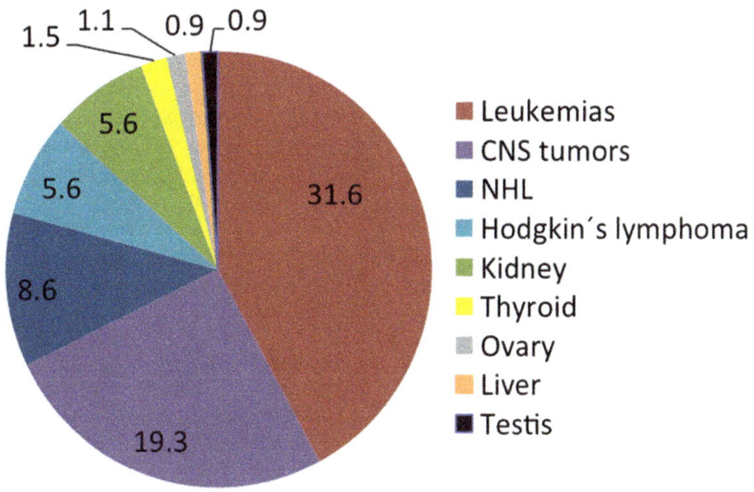

Fig. 2.11 Most frequent cancer types (%) among children 0-14 years in LMIC, Europe (Source: GLOBOCAN 2008).

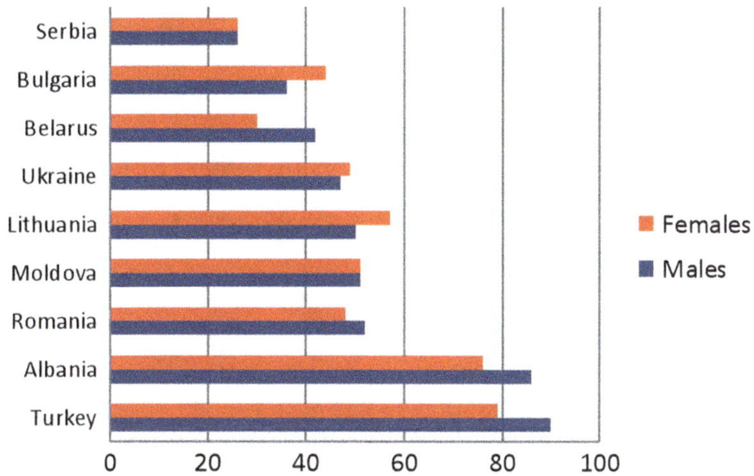

Fig. 2.12 Lowest and highest age-standardized mortality rates for all childhood cancers, LMIC from Europe (Source: GLOBOCAN 2008).

(males, AAPC=−1.8, 95 % CI −2.5; −1.0; females, AAPC=−1.4, 95 % CI −2.4; −0.5), Latvia (1980–2010) (males, APC=−2.7, 95 % CI −3.8; −1.5; females, APC=−3.1, 95 % CI −4.3; −1.8), Lithuania (1985–2010) (males, APC=−3.8, 95 % CI −5.2; −2.4; females, APC=−2.8, 95 % CI −4.2; −1.3), Moldova (1985–2011) (males, APC=−2.2, 95 % CI −3.1; −1.4), Romania (1980–2011) (males, APC=−2.1, 95 % CI −2.9; −1.3; females, APC=−2.4, 95 % CI −3.4; −1.4), and Ukraine (1985–2011) (males, APC=−2.4, 95 % CI −2.8; −2.0; females, APC=−2.3, 95 % CI −2.6; −1.9).

Conclusions

Cancer registries serve as the basis for cancer prevention, cancer planning, cancer treatment, and cancer research. As such, a population-based registry ought to be one of the first priorities of any country once cancer is placed on the public health agenda. In actuality, cancer registries, once the processes are in place, are not an expensive endeavor. Estimates range from US $30 to 50,000 per year, mostly to support key personnel and travel for data collection. However, as can be seen from these analyses, differences in incidence provide an essential basis for cancer planning, such as highlighting high rates of cervical cancer among girls less than 14 in Africa and high rates of thyroid cancer in middle-income countries in Europe. Changes in mortality also provide evidence of either well-working cancer treatment systems or systems in which improvements could be made. Investment in cancer registration is a cost-effective, obligatory element of any rational national cancer strategy.

References

1. Ferlay J, et al. GLOBOCAN 2008 v2.0, cancer incidence and mortality worldwide. IARC CancerBase. Lyon: IARC; 2010. p. 10.
2. Parkin DM. The evolution of the population-based cancer registry. Nat Rev Cancer. 2006;6(8): 603–12.
3. Parkin DM. The role of cancer registries in cancer control. Int J Clin Oncol. 2008;13(2):102–11.
4. Bray F, Parkin DM. Evaluation of data quality in the cancer registry: principles and methods. Part I: comparability, validity and timeliness. Eur J Cancer. 2009;45(5):747–55.
5. Parkin DM, Bray F. Evaluation of data quality in the cancer registry: principles and methods Part II. Completeness. Eur J Cancer. 2009;45(5):756–64.
6. Curado MP, et al. Cancer incidence in five continents, vol. IX. Lyon, France: IARC Scientific Publications; 2007.
7. Kramarova E, Stiller CA. The international classification of childhood cancer. Int J Cancer. 1996;68(6):759–65.
8. Parkin DM, et al. The international incidence of childhood cancer. Int J Cancer. 1988;42(4):511–20.
9. Parkin DM, et al. International incidence of childhood cancer, vol. II. Lyon, France: IARC Scientific Publications; 1998.
10. Mutalima N, et al. Impact of infection with human immunodeficiency virus-1 (HIV) on the risk of cancer among children in Malawi—preliminary findings. Infect Agent Cancer. 2010;5:5.
11. Tukei VJ, Kekitiinwa A, Beasley RP. Prevalence and outcome of HIV-associated malignancies among children. AIDS. 2011;25(14):1789–93.
12. Stefan DC, Stones DK. Children with cancer and HIV infection: what is different about them? J Pediatr Hematol Oncol. 2013.
13. Chang MH, et al. Universal hepatitis B vaccination in Taiwan and the incidence of hepatocellular carcinoma in children. Taiwan Childhood Hepatoma Study Group. N Engl J Med. 1997;336(26):1855–9.
14. WHO. Immunizations, vaccines and biologicals; [cited 2013 May 20, 2013]. Available from: http://www.who.int/immunization/topics/hepatitis_b/en/index.html.
15. PATH. Immunization in Vietnam; [cited 2013 May 12, 2013]. Available from: http://www.path.org/projects/immunization_in_vietnam.php.
16. Demidchik YE, Saenko VA, Yamashita S. Childhood thyroid cancer in Belarus, Russia, and Ukraine after Chernobyl and at present. Arq Bras Endocrinol Metabol. 2007;51(5):748–62.

3 The Role of International Organizations on Collaboration for Global Pediatric Cancer Control

Tezer Kutluk and Julie Torode

Introduction

Despite great progress achieved in improving the survival of children with cancer in developed countries, for the estimated 175,000 newly diagnosed children with cancer and their families in resource-limited settings, the big problem remains the issue of equity of access to diagnosis, treatment, and care of children with cancer [1]. A low survival rate of 10–20 % in some low- and middle-income countries adds to the high number of children who die without being diagnosed at all. In addition 80 % of the 90,000 deaths annually to childhood cancer occur in low- and middle-income settings [2].

In this context many international organizations around the world decided to join forces together to reduce the disparity between HIC and LMIC and improve the survival rate of children diagnosed with cancer. Along the history, the international collaboration based on trust and respect showed the fruitful results of creating partnerships between organizations with the same principles and goals. The defined role of each partner had the potential to contribute in closing the divide in access to diagnosis, treatment, and care and make a significant contribution in the fight against the childhood cancer worldwide [3].

International collaboration on the management of pediatric cancers was initiated in Western Europe and North America and grew from coordinated clinical trials at national level. Large collaborative groups networking across these regions facilitated testing and validation of protocols to establish standards of care and improved and new treatment protocols which have given us these incremental improvements in patient outcomes over past decades. National Wilms tumor study is a good example of the collaboration in early years [4]. Although there are examples of international collaboration reaching out to include sites in other regions of the globe and also to adapt established treatment protocols to make them feasible in low resource settings, these lack in both coverage and scope. Local champions are often fighting to establish childhood cancer units, achieve adequate financing and personnel levels, and battle with lack of continuity in access to even some of the cheapest medicines and technologies on a routine basis.

T. Kutluk, M.D., Ph.D. (✉)
Union for International Cancer Control, Geneva, Switzerland

Department of Pediatric Oncology, Hacettepe University Cancer Institute, Ankara, Turkey
e-mail: tezerkutluk@gmail.com

J. Torode, Ph.D.
Union for International Cancer Control, Geneva, Switzerland

D.C. Stefan and C. Rodriguez-Galindo (eds.), *Pediatric Hematology-Oncology in Countries with Limited Resources: A Practical Manual*, DOI 10.1007/978-1-4614-3891-5_3,

World Cancer Declaration as a Global Tool for Cancer Control

Launched in 2008 by the Union for International Cancer Control (UICC), the World Cancer Declaration is a tool to help bring the growing cancer crisis to the attention of government leaders, health policymakers, and the general public alike. The Declaration outlines 11 aspirational targets and priority actions which together can lead to a reduction in cancer incidence, improved survival, and quality of life for those living with a cancer diagnosis. Other than the risk factor targets, each of them is very much relevant to pediatric cancer, thus providing a framework for decision makers [5].

Despite the clear call to action of the World Cancer Declaration, cancer control advocates were not getting the political attention required to make sustained change at country level. In 2009, UICC took the World Cancer Declaration targets and principles forward to form the basis of a united call to action on noncommunicable diseases (NCDs). The NCD alliance was founded by UICC together with the leading global federations World Heart Federation and International Diabetes Federation and joined 1 year later by the International Union Against Tuberculosis and Lung Disease [6]. NCD alliance unites over 2,000 civil society member organizations from 170 countries through a vision of a future free from preventable suffering and death caused by NCDs. This NCDA global movement has contributed to a shift in global health and development thinking by leveraging a UN High-Level Meeting on NCDs, only the second time in history that Heads of State have engaged at this level on a health topic, bringing world attention to the global NCD epidemic. This NCD movement has influenced governments to commit to unprecedented action and accountability [6–8] and position NCDs as a priority for the successor goals to the current Millennium Development Goals (MDGs), the so-called Post-2015 agenda.

The focus of the global commitments to health promotion, risk factors for cancer and other NCDs, early detection through improved primary care services, and improved access to diagnosis and treatment opens up unprecedented opportunities and political support for cancer control efforts. The "Political Declaration of the High-Level Meeting of the General Assembly on the Prevention and Control of Non-communicable Diseases (NCD)" also calls for whole of government and pan-UN approaches to global health partnerships. Childhood cancer advocates must grasp this opportunity and demonstrate that civil society is ready and prepared to take on a leadership role in such a global health partnership for childhood cancer.

Building on Past Success: Examples of Civil Society Initiatives

UICC and Sanofi Espoir Foundation: My Child Matters Partnership

The My Child Matters partnership was initiated in 2005 by the Sanofi Espoir Foundation and the UICC targeting sustained improvement in awareness, access to diagnosis, and care and childhood cancer survival in developing countries [9–12]. Childhood cancers are mostly curable if they are diagnosed early, properly managed with the right treatment and according to the appropriate protocol. In the period 2006–2012, the partnership invested more than five million Euro and invested in 40 projects in 26 countries. In addition to the financial support, My Child Matters sites benefited from expert advice from a steering committee of the leading and diverse professional organizations in the pediatric oncology field representing both a wide geography and a diversity of discipline ranging from epidemiology and cancer registry through to clinic and public health policy and advocacy. In addition, the sites worked in close collaboration with an assigned individual mentor. Key factors of success in the early projects were (1) improved infrastructure and equipment, (2) targeted training of hospital personnel, (3) focused efforts on building a strong referral network and raising awareness in the catchment community, and (4) focused efforts to work with patients and their families to address the issue of abandonment of treatment. A renewed commitment was announced in 2013 focusing on projects such as early detection as a critical factor in the outcome for patients. One 2013 awardee is WHO/PAHO contributing to their regional efforts to validate and implement the "Module for Early Detection of Childhood Cancers" into the established "Integrated Management of Childhood Cancer" (IMCI) strategy. The module was successfully tested in Brazil and the My Child Matters support will accelerate further validation in four countries. UICC is prepared to work with PAHO to translate this validated model and encourage other WHO regions to adapt and introduce this approach.

Other International Organizations

The International Society of Pediatric Oncology

The International Society of Pediatric Oncology (SIOP) was founded in the late 1960s and is the largest international pediatric oncology society. Through its global members, including all caregivers and annual congress, it has been the major facilitator of sharing knowledge and expertise around the globe. The SIOP network also facilitated the communication among low- and mid-income countries through its PODC (pediatric oncology in developing countries). Additionally, SIOP led research is providing the most updated information for the pediatric oncology community around the world [13].

St. Jude Children's Research Hospital's International Outreach Program

St. Jude Children's Research Hospital's International Outreach Program (IOP) aims to improve survival of children with cancer in resource-poor countries. The goal is to establish partnerships between St. Jude IOP and public pediatric hospitals in poor regions. Building local human capacity, continuing education, training, and financing operations constitute the program's core principles [14].

International Confederation of Childhood Cancer Parent Organizations

The International Confederation of Childhood Cancer Parent Organizations (ICCPO) was founded in 1994 and functions as an umbrella organization for 158 parent organizations from 85 countries. With a mission of "to share information and experiences in order to improve access to the best possible treatment & care for children with cancer everywhere in the world," it also offers practical assistance and guidance in the establishment of new support groups. ICCCPO representatives sit on committees that determine cancer policy globally, as well as at local and regional government level [15].

The International Network for Cancer Treatment and Research

The International Network for Cancer Treatment and Research (INCTR) is an international not-for-profit, nongovernmental organization established to address a neglected health problem—cancer in developing countries. INCTR is aiming to build capacity for cancer treatment and research in countries with limited resources through long-term collaborative projects coupled to training and educational programs and to promote international collaboration directed towards cancer control between technologically advanced countries and countries with limited resources [16].

French African Pediatric Oncology Group Initiative

Groupe Franco-Africain d'Oncologie Pédiatrique (GFAOP) was founded in 2000 by Prof Jean Lemerle. The aim was to initiate a collaborative program to develop pediatric cancer care in Africa. Six countries were initially involved including Algeria, Cameroon, Madagascar, Morocco, Senegal, and Tunisia. They were subsequently joined by Burkina Faso, Cote d'Ivoire, Mali, Mauritania, Republic Democratic du Congo, and Togo. Support is provided to local teams regarding education, medication, and medical supplies [17]. At the moment there are 12 African Francophone units working together and more than 4,500 children with cancer have been treated.

African Organization for Research and Training in Cancer

African Organization for Research and Training in Cancer (AORTIC) was formed in 1983 by expatriate African cancer care workers, scientists, and their friends and is dedicated to the promotion of cancer control in Africa.

AORTIC's key objectives are to further the research relating to cancers prevalent in Africa, support the management of training programs in oncology for health care workers, deal with the challenges of creating cancer control and prevention programs, and raise public awareness of cancer in Africa. The pediatric oncology group was formed in 2011 and includes all involved in the care of children with cancer in Africa (pediatric oncologists, pediatricians, radiotherapists, pharmacists, nurses, social workers, dieticians, etc.). The group is involved in adapting protocols to the local conditions, involved in different clinical trials and with the research of the main pediatric cancers on the continent. It has also a very active component in the education, teaching, and training of the health professionals in the field of cancer on the African continent.

Association of Pediatric Hematology Oncology of Central America

Association of Pediatric Hematology Oncology of Central America (AHOPCA) is a collaboration between children's oncology groups in the Central American, Spanish speaking countries of Guatemala, El Salvador, Nicaragua, Honduras, Costa Rica, Panama, and Dominican Republic. Founded in 1998 as a result of interaction fostered by Monza International School of Pediatric Hematology/Oncology (MISPHO) to promote twinning in centers of Latin America, they aim to provide treatment protocols for common childhood cancers. In each of these countries, there is only one tertiary care center for treating pediatric cancer, and the total number of new cases of childhood cancer in the seven AHOPCA countries exceeds 1,000 cases per year. The mission of the group is to increase the survival in children with cancer. AHOPCA meets annually to promote the establishment of common protocols in the region. AHOPCA receives support from the IOP of St. Jude Children's Research Hospital (SJCRH) [18, 19].

What Are the Factors for Success?

The above examples illustrate that there are many experienced civil society organizations from the academic, health professional, and NGO sectors have been collaborating on international work for several years. New players such as Global Task Force on Expanded Access to Cancer Care and Control in Developing Countries (GTF.CCC) [20] and NCD illustrate the readiness to explore new approaches and reach out to build on existing health services at country level. These model projects and success stories provide evidence that a global partnership for childhood cancer has great potential and demonstrates that civil society is ready to join governments, intergovernmental agencies, and the private sector to scale up efforts for sustained impact in both access and patient outcomes. Key drivers to gaining support and focusing efforts are:

- Making the financial case for a comprehensive childhood cancer plan as part of national cancer control plan to support advocacy
- Innovative approaches to procurement and financing of childhood cancer medicines and technologies
- Coordinated and targeted international training efforts to build capacity to drive cancer plans and build the skilled health workforce dedicated to pediatric oncology

- Reaching out to existing child and adolescent health service providers working in the community with the goal building on infrastructure and harnessing expertise in both communicable and NCDs improved early detection and efficient referral
- Strong building of awareness of signs and symptoms of childhood cancer with health professions, particularly at community level, supported by public awareness campaigns in partnership with survivor and parent groups

The pediatric oncology community is ready for the challenge of new and innovative ways of collaboration to accelerate to the progress on reaching the best available cancer care for children in all regions of the world. A well-orchestrated global health partnership, with each of the partners having a defined role, has the potential to harness the expertise and proven tools we have now to close the divide in access to diagnosis, treatment, and care to make a significant contribution to the fight against pediatric cancer.

References

1. Ferlay J, Shin HR, Bray F, Forman D, Mathers C, Parkin DM. GLOBOCAN 2008, cancer incidence and mortality worldwide: IARC CancerBase No. 10 [Internet]. Lyon, France: International Agency for Research on Cancer; 2010. Available from: http://globocan.iarc.fr.
2. Ribeiro RC, Steliarova-Foucher E, Magrath I, Lemerle J, Eden T, Forget C, Mortara I, Tabah-Fisch I, Divino JJ, Miklavec T, Howard S, Cavalli F. Baseline status of paediatric oncology care in ten low-income or mid-income countries receiving My Child Matters support: a descriptive study. Lancet Oncol. 2008;9(8):721–9. doi:10.1016/S1470-2045(08)70194-3.
3. Working toward transformational health partnerships in low and middle income countries. [Internet]; September 2012 [cited 2013 March 24]. Available from: www.bsr.org/reports/BR_Working_Toward_Transformational_Health_Partnerships.pdf.
4. History of the national Wilms tumor study. [Internet]; 2013 [cited 2013 March 24]. Available from: www.nwtsg.org/about/history.html.
5. World cancer declaration [Internet]; 2013 [cited 2013 March 03]. Available from: http://www.uicc.org/world-cancer-declaration.
6. Non-communicable disease alliance [Internet]; 2013 [cited 2013 March 03]. Available from: www.ncdalliance.org.
7. WHO report: draft action plan for the prevention and control of noncommunicable diseases 2013–2020. Executive Board 132nd session. EB132/7; 11 Jan 2013.
8. Updated revised draft. Global Action Plan for the prevention and control of noncommunicable diseases 2013–2020. [Internet]; 2013 [cited 2013 March 24]. Available from: www.who.int/cardiovascular_diseases/15March2013UpdatedRevisedDraftActionPlan.pdf.
9. Childhood Cancer (ChiCa) [Internet]; 2013 [cited 2013 March 03]. Available from: http://www.uicc.org/programmes/chica/issue.
10. My Child Matters: fighting chilhood cancers in developing countries. [Internet]; 2013 [cited 2013 March 03]. Available from: http://www.fondation-sanofi-espoir.com/en/ngo_child-matters.php.
11. Adams C, Boniface C, Ribeiro R. My Child Matters: fighting against childhood cancer in low and middle-income countries. Geneva Health Forum at 18–20 April, 2012 [Internet]; [updated 2012 March 27; cited 2013 March 03]. Available from: http://www.ghf12.org/?p=5619.
12. Ribeiro RC, Eden T, Hartford J, Lemerle J, Magrath I, Sancho-Garnier H, Steliarova-Foucher E, Thaxter G, Tabah-Fisch IM, Cavalli F. My child matters program: a UICC-sanofi-aventis partnership to improve pediatric cancer care in developing countries. J Clin Oncol. 2007 ASCO Annual Meeting Proceedings;2007;25(18S):9526.
13. International Society of Pedaitric Oncology [Internet]; 2013 [cited 2013 March 03]. Available from: http://www.siop-online.org.
14. Guide to establishing a Pediatric Oncology Twinning Program [Internet]; 2013 [cited 2013 March 03]. Available from: http://www.stjude.org/stjude/v/index.jsp?vgnextoid=3443ab6717440210VgnVCM1000001e0215acRCRD&vgnextchannel=3332ab6717440210VgnVCM1000001e0215acRCRD.
15. International Confederation of Childhood Cancer Parent Organizations [Internet]; 2013 [cited 2013 March 03]. Available from: http://icccpo.org/index.cfm?fuseaction=category&category=29&subcategory=30.
16. International network for cancer treatment and research [Internet]; 2013 [cited 2013 March 03]. Available from: http://www.inctr.org/about-inctr/.
17. Groupe Franco-Africain d'Oncologie Pediatrique (GFAOP). [Internet]; 2013 [cited 2013 March 03]. Available from: http://www.gfaop.fr/.
18. Howard S, Marinoni M, Castillo L, Meeting Report. Improving outcomes for children with cancer in low-income countries in Latin America: a report on the recent meetings of the Monza International School of Pediatric Hematology/Oncology (MISPHO)-Part 1
19. Sala A, Antillon F, Meeting Report. Nutritional status in children with cancer: a report from the AHOPCA Workshop, Guatemala City, 31 Aug–5 Sept 2004.
20. Global Task Force on expanded access to cancer care and control in developing countries. [Internet]; [cited 2013 March 24]. Available from: http://gtfccc.harvard.edu.

4 The Role of Twinning Programs and Telemedicine in Pediatric Oncology

Valentino Conter, Roberto Polillo, Erica Brivio, Agostino Faravelli, and Giuseppe Masera

Introduction

Most children diagnosed with cancer live in low- and middle-income countries (LMIC), where unfortunately they receive poor or no therapy [1–3]. As countries develop and infectious diseases are increasingly well controlled, noncommunicable diseases (including cancer) take on increasing importance, providing ample justification for directing more resources into pediatric cancer in developing countries [4–7].

V. Conter, M.D. (✉)
Pediatric Department, Ospedale San Gerardo, University of Milano Bicocca—Fondazione MBBM, Monza, Italy

International Outreach Program, St. Jude Children's Research Hospital, Memphis, TN, USA
e-mail: v.conter@hsgerardo.org

R. Polillo, M.D.
DISCO Department of Informatics, Systems and Communication, University of Milano Bicocca, Milan, Italy
e-mail: roberto.polillo@unimib.it

E. Brivio, M.D. • G. Masera, M.D.
Pediatric Department, Ospedale San Gerardo, University of Milano Bicocca—Fondazione MBBM, Monza, Italy
e-mail: g.masera@hsgerardo.org

A. Faravelli, M.D.
Surgical Pathology, Patologi Oltre Frontiera, Desio, Milan, Italy
e-mail: faravelli50@gmaill.com

There has been much debate regarding the most appropriate strategy for promoting the progress of pediatric oncology in LMIC. In this context two major problems can be spotted. On one side, programs needed to fill the large gap between the North and the South of the world have been rarely translated into national programs capable to assure the continuity of the initially supported intervention. On the other side, many cooperation projects have preferably reported the short–medium-term results, with less information on the attributable medium–long-term outcomes [8, 9].

Many questions can thus be raised. Is it possible to draw resources for pediatric oncology programs in LMIC without competing with programs of primary care? How can therapeutic strategies developed in economically developed countries (EDC) be applied in LMIC? Do all LIC qualify for cooperative projects in childhood oncology or only those who can afford a minimum standard of care? Should these programs be offered to all children or only to families which may be reliable for treatment compliance? Should these programs take care of all neoplastic diseases or only of those characterized by low treatment burden and favorable outcome? How should these cooperative projects be conducted to prevent the risk of being considered a sort of new colonialism? How relevant is the local governmental authorities commitment and the involvement of local solidarity associations to raise public and private resources?

D.C. Stefan and C. Rodriguez-Galindo (eds.), *Pediatric Hematology-Oncology in Countries with Limited Resources: A Practical Manual*, DOI 10.1007/978-1-4614-3891-5_4,

Which impact on socioeconomical and cultural aspects could have these programs in LMIC? Which role can telemedicine play in the development of pediatric oncology and in the management of patients in LIC? What are the challenges in starting a twinning program? What is required to create such a program?

In this chapter we will discuss these issues and some initiatives which may serve as examples of practical application. The chapter will include also guidelines on the establishment of a twinning program.

The "La Mascota" Twinning Program

In 1986, pediatric oncologists in Monza (Italy) had the opportunity to initiate a long-term twinning program with the La Mascota Pediatric Hospital in Managua, Nicaragua ("La Mascota Program"), which, later on, involved also hospitals of Milan (Istituto Nazionale dei Tumori) and Bellinzona (Switzerland). Due to this program, it was possible to train progressively a full team of pediatric oncologists, nurses, technicians, one surgeon, and one pathologist. In addition, and emphasizing the holistic approach taken at La Mascota, the team included two psychologists and one social worker who provided noteworthy support.

At the beginning it was chosen to treat some solid tumors, lymphomas, and ALL. Other diseases, such as AML or brain tumors, were considered too difficult to be managed for the available structures, services, and local expertise. The experience with diseases such as Hodgkin's disease or Wilms' tumor was found quite successful [10–12]. Treatment of ALL was problematic. Treatment protocols for ALL have been derived mainly from schedules commonly used in developed countries. Their intensity has been reduced however, since the beginning, to cope with needs and constraints and later on continuously modify on the base of the local experience and results. The first ALL treatment protocols (Managua 1988 and 1993) allowed testing the feasibility of a reduced intensity BFM-oriented chemotherapeutic regimen in a country with limited supportive care. This experience clearly showed that major drawbacks were early deaths and "abandon of treatment" (total patients 110: early deaths 7.2 %, abandon of treatment 27.0 %, relapse rate 30 %, deaths in continuous complete remission 3.6 %, 5-year event free survival 29.0 %) [13], which in part were due to the absence of minimum structures for provision of adequate stay in hospital, for lodging the parents of children, and for outpatient care. The construction of two new pavilions (ten beds each for hematological diseases and for solid tumors), of an outpatient clinic, and of a parent house was made possible through the support from Italy and Switzerland, which allowed to benefit from additional funds beyond what had been planned for the provision of drugs, laboratory facilities, and family needs.

The results of subsequent ALL protocols (ALL Managua 1995 and 2000) showed an overall EFS of 38.1 % (2.1) and survival of 48.0% (2.2) at 5 years from diagnosis, with rates for abandon of treatment of 9.4 % and for early deaths of 7 % [14]. From these experiences it became also evident that peripheral units were needed to improve treatment compliance. Thus, a short training was offered to physicians working in provinces far from the capital city to get them used to deliver basic treatments in outpatient's clinics, closer to patients' home.

Much progress has been made. Between 1990 and 2012, approximately 3,500 children with cancer have been treated at La Mascota Hospital, and all diagnostic procedures and treatments have been provided to patients free of charge. The overall survival rate has steadily and rapidly increased: from 10 % in the 1980s, before La Mascota Project activation, to 60 % 20 years thereafter and continues to rise [15–17].

Extended Benefits of the "La Mascota Project"

The "La Mascota" program has had a major impact also on other services, involving in the cooperation other hospitals or solidarity groups from EDC. Services which benefited mostly were neonatology, infectious diseases, the emergency department, and nephrology. The cooperative project between the pediatric nephrology units of Milan and Managua started in 2000 and led the development of a specialized unit and personnel for pediatric nephrology and urology, to offer since the beginning basic clinical care free of charge to children referred to the hospital. Shared protocols, renovation of infrastructure, and an information technology (IT) program were implemented, and in 2003 dialysis and kidney transplant for selected children were initiated along with a network of peripheral department hospitals and health units to prevent chronic kidney disease. The clinical activities of Managua department in 2008 are similar to those of pediatric nephrology units worldwide and depict the level of clinical autonomy achieved [18].

The positive results of the "La Mascota" program have been extended also to other Latin America countries with the collaboration and activation of other twinning programs. Monza's International School for Pediatric Hematology/Oncology (MISPHO) was created in 1996 and organized different meetings and training courses with the participation of pediatric hemato-oncologists of many countries of Central and South America [19–22]. These meetings were functional to merge other international cooperation activities in the area, namely, those of St. Jude Children's Research Hospital (SJCRH) and Pediatric Oncology Group of Ontario (POGO), to promote intercountry cooperative efforts and the development of a pediatric oncology group in Central America (Associaciòn de Hemto-Oncologìa Pediatrica de Centro America, AHOPCA). In this context it has been possible to design and conduct many collaborative studies, to institute a retrospective tumor registry and a prospective clinical registry, and to adopt psychosocial care guidelines (derived from the SIOP guidelines) [15, 23, 24]. The Web-based resource "Cure4Kids" (www.cure4kids.org created by SJCRH, Memphis, USA), described in the telemedicine section, allows participants in LMIC to interact by systematic online live conferences for each relevant disease to discuss patients and protocols [25].

Development of Pediatric Oncology in LMIC

It is clear that the overall picture can hardly be seen as fully satisfactory, despite the positivity of some relevant achievements. It is important therefore to explore more closely the findings in order to identify the determinants of the less favorable results, and to assess the conditions, which could allow better outcomes of the patients.

The challenges faced in developing a twinning program in LMIC include the late and incorrect diagnosis, shortage of skilled staff, lack of financial resources, inappropriate supportive care, and treatment abandonment (Table 4.1).

The key factors which appear to impact more profoundly on the outcomes do not coincide with clinical but with logistical, cultural, socioeconomic variables like the geographical distance from treatment centers, which end up conditioning survival and compliance profile and suggesting need of more targeted caring and supportive strategies [26, 27].

The investment of a twinning program for pediatric oncology into the more directly clinical aspects (e.g., by assuring free access to drugs and monitoring inhospital complications) must therefore be matched by an equally intensive activation and support of peripheral monitoring, with a participation of the personnel of the health care system. It is clear that an effective continuity of integrated supportive networks can hardly be guaranteed by a sum of interventions organized and financed by external collaborations. The important clinical and human results obtained by a twinning program must be integrated into a fully shared national responsibility.

It is vital to establish a long-term commitment to a comprehensive and holistic strategy that incorporates supply of drugs, training and supervision of health professionals, and the care of the children and their parents. A long-term program should be based on a bilateral agreement, with periodic reassessments and adjustments of strategies and needs. Management responsibilities should be given to local professionals, with respect for local culture and traditions, to increase

Table 4.1 Common challenges faced in developing a twinning program

Challenge	Ways to overcome challenge
Treatment abandonment	Provide guest housing for patients and parents
	Provide food for patients and parents
	Organize parent support groups
	Assist with cost of transportation
	Set up satellite clinics to facilitate access to treatment
	Organize patient follow-up procedures
	Provide aggressive patient and parent education
	Provide aggressive community education
	Encourage community involvement
Shortage of trained nurses	Provide continuing education and training for nurses
	Provide salary supplements for key trained nurses
	Encourage the local foundation to provide incentives to current nursing staff
	Encourage active participation of nurses in multidisciplinary team activities
Suboptimal infection control	Provide continuing education and training on infection-control practices
	Encourage the establishment of infection-control policies and procedures
	Provide salary supplements for infection-control professionals
	Encourage local foundation to provide continual supply of hand hygiene products and facilities when not available
Insufficient funds	Help local foundation strengthen local fundraising capabilities
	Encourage local foundation and medical team to obtain for additional government funding
	Encourage applications to international funding agencies
Cost and availability of medication	Encourage local foundation to seek bulk purchases either with regional foundations or through WHO's Pan American Health Organization (PAHO)
	Use services provided by the Global Outreach Program of the National Children's Cancer Society
Late diagnosis	Develop local community education campaigns
	Develop educational materials for community health workers and general pediatricians
Incorrect diagnosis	Provide local professionals access to consult from experts in sponsor hospital
	Cover costs for immunophenotyping

self-confidence and progressive autonomy; this may be crucial to avoid the risk for a project to be considered a sort of new colonialism.

A program for childhood cancer should trigger also the development of similar programs in other medical fields and should promote a closer relationship between specialized centers and peripheral hospitals. A local training of medical, nursing, and technical staff can encourage specialists to develop subspecialty practices in their national communities. It can also stimulate awareness about health care needs, highlighting poor governance and poor planning into health outcomes in LMIC, so that, instead of diverting resources from basic health care services, international partnerships to treat children with cancer may increase resources available to the local health care system. A "therapeutic alliance" should be established among local health professionals, parents, and volunteers in order to sensitize institutions and health authorities, mobilize resources, and effectively identify needs and priorities [28].

Protocols for diagnosis and therapy should be tailored to the local situation and extended progressively from cancers with more favorable results to the other common pediatric tumors [29]. Particular attention should be given to the problem of refusal or early abandonment of treatment, which may be a relevant cause of failure in childhood cancer treatment in LMIC [30–32]. These programs however can be hardly successful in countries with extreme poverty; additional resources are needed also to support very poor families to treat all children.

The challenges related to the beginning of a twinning program are summarized in Table 4.1.

Formal research projects should be promoted too. Priority should be given to topics of interest for LMIC centers, and the visibility of their contribution (e.g., in publications) must be assured. The role of telemedicine may be crucial as detailed below.

The components for establishing a twinning program include the following steps:

- Initial assessment
- Identification of local leaders (the local champion)

- Establishment of an initial 5-year plan
- Establishment of a formal memorandum of understanding
- Establishment of a hospital cancer registry
- Financial assistance
- Targeted education and training
- Follow-up visits
- Continuous communication[1]

Telemedicine in Low-Income Countries

Telemedicine (which literally means "healing at distance") is the use of medical information exchanged from one site to another via electronic communications to improve patients' health. A closely related but broader term is "tele-health," which is used to denote remote health care, which does not necessarily involve clinical services.[2] Telemedicine can be used in many medical specialties and is classified according to its area of application: teleradiology (actually the most widespread), telecardiology, telepathology, teledermatology, teledentistry, teleaudiology, telepsychology, etc.

Despite the fact that research and developments in telemedicine have been carried on since the 1970s, it is only the recent evolution of the Internet that allows easy and affordable applications of telemedicine and—more generally—tele-health. Indeed, broadband Internet with the related software technologies and the new paradigms of cloud and mobile computing are important enablers of telemedicine applications.

In 2009, WHO carried out a global survey to obtain general information about the state of telemedicine in member states and, in particular, in developing countries. The report clearly expressed the potential large benefits of telemedicine in general and for low-income countries in particular: "it could be even more beneficial for underserved and developing countries where access to basic care is of primary concern. One of the biggest opportunities telemedicine presents is increased access to health care. Providing populations in these underserved countries with the means to access health care has the potential to help meet previously unmet needs and positively impact health services. Telemedicine applications have successfully improved the quality and accessibility of medical care by allowing distant providers to evaluate, diagnose, treat, and provide follow-up care to patients in less economically developed countries" [33].

Nevertheless, the WHO report describes a number of "barriers," which can be of obstacle to the widespread adoption of telemedicine. While developed countries expressed concerns about legal issues surrounding patient privacy and confidentiality, competing health system priorities, and a perceived lack of demand, developing countries considered resource issues such as high costs, underdeveloped infrastructure, and lack of technical expertise as the main barriers. For these countries, substantial difficulties are still related to the availability and maintenance of the technical infrastructures necessary to implement telemedicine solutions and in particular instability of electric power supply, unavailability of Internet connectivity beyond large cities, unreliable connectivity, computer viruses, limited bandwidth, and limited local skills and resources.

We suggest a more optimistic view, based on the belief that—at least—the costs and difficulties connected with the technology infrastructures are often overemphasized. This view is supported by the following considerations:

1. Internet connectivity (access availability, quality, and costs) is improving, or will improve in the near future, even in low-income countries. There are already many countries in which connectivity is widespread and reasonably priced. At end 2011, Internet user penetration stood at 24 % in developing countries

[1] Guidelines adapted from St Jude: International Outreach Program—Guide to Establishing a Pediatric Oncology Twinning Program.

[2] Many different definitions are used in the literature. WHO [1] adopts a broader definition, encompassing general eHealth: telemedicine is "the delivery of health care services, where distance is a critical factor, by all health care professionals using information and communication technologies for the exchange of valid information for diagnosis, treatment and prevention of disease and injuries, research and evaluation, and for the continuing education of health care providers, all in the interest of advancing the health of individuals and their communities."

and 15 % in LIC. This is still low compared to developed countries (70 %), but steadily growing [34].

2. The incredibly rapid evolution of the software technologies connected with the Internet allows now—and will increasingly allow in the future—the implementation of software applications accessible from the Internet at a fraction of the costs necessary only a few years ago. As a matter of fact, the costs of developing and setting up these applications have been considerably lowered in recent years and will continue to decrease. In some Web applications, cost reductions obtained in the last decade are of an order of magnitude or even more. This is mainly a consequence of the developments of important open-source software platforms and the growing availability of ready-made software components and services that can be easily integrated and mixed up to create applications that, only a decade ago, would have required long and expensive development efforts.
3. Cloud computing solutions—and in particular "software as a service" (SaaS) solutions, where a software application is hosted and managed by an online service provider—can reduce drastically the upfront investments necessary to implement a telemedicine application. In some cases there will be no capital expenses ("capex") to set up the application, but only operation expenses ("opex"), consisting in the monthly fees paid to the service provider, on a "per use" pricing. This is particularly true for the software applications in the areas of communication, collaboration, and social networking, which can be most useful in the area of telemedicine.
4. The penetration of mobile cellular subscriptions in the developing world has undergone an exceptional growth in the last few years, and reached 78 % at end of 2011, the level reached by the developed world only 6–7 years before [34]. This exceptional growth continues at 2-digit increase every year. There are now more than six billion mobile telephone subscriptions worldwide. Ultra-low-cost mobile telephones are becoming available and will be more and more in the next future. British carrier Vodafone has recently announced ultra-cheap mobile devices, starting at below $15, specifically addressed to low-income markets. These are still bare boned on the feature side (voice calls, SMS and mobile payments, and in the upper model FM radio), but a high growth in smartphones and (affordable) tablets is to be expected within the next couple of years. These will allow mobile access to the Internet and to all online applications from the "cloud" from low-cost mobile devices.

ICTs (Information and Communication Technologies) have substantially changed in the last decade, and will continue to evolve, at a pace that would have been unthinkable only a few years ago. This should be always considered when planning any cooperation project aimed at improving health in low-income countries. Some solutions, which are impractical or even technically unfeasible in the project planning phase, may become easily implementable and cost-effective before the end of the project execution.

Affordable Telemedicine

In the following, we mention a few examples of telemedicine solutions that can be affordable and can be implemented without technical difficulties even in poorly served countries. Some programs connect local to remote health care professionals (HCP) (HCP2HCP); others directly connect a patient to an HCP (P2HCP). Some programs involve synchronous, real-time communication while others asynchronous communication.

Store-and-Forward Telemedicine (HCP2HCP, Asynchronous)

In this case, medical data from a certain patient are collected by a local professional and transmitted to a remote specialist for assessment offline at a convenient time. It does not require the presence of both parties at the same time, and it does not require the presence of the patient.

The data are usually produced by diagnostic instruments and may be complemented by additional patient medical data (in electronic form). So the specialist does not perform any direct examination of the patient, with which he/she has no direct contact, but relies only on registered reports, which may include, in particular cases, audio or video records. When a local specialist is available, the remote specialist may be involved for a second opinion.

This is the application requiring the simplest technological infrastructure. In its basic implementation, only an Internet connection of both communicating parties is required, and the communication may be done using email or simple file transfer protocols. An appropriate data format must be defined, to provide an information readable and understandable by both parties.

Teleradiology, teledermatology, and telepathology are common specialties that can be performed with these arrangements. The network bandwidth requirements may be significantly different. For example, scans of histological slides may be extremely large (some gigabytes) and may require a large bandwidth or suitable data compression techniques in order to be practically manageable. Other specialties may have much less demanding requirements.

In many situations, even the availability of an Internet connection is not necessary. As an example, a study carried out in Uganda, Afghanistan, and Bangladesh showed that mobile phones can be easily used, without any adaptor or device, to photograph and send images from a microscope to reference. During the study period, the peri pheral health centers in the rural areas were not equipped with Internet connection, while health workers diffusely owned mobile phones, including models with a built-in camera. The availability, but not the use, of MMS (Multimedia Messaging System) was widespread in the three countries, and the possibility of combining the use of mobile phones and a microscope for diagnostic purposes was easily and enthusiastically learned by local health workers. This process allowed microscopic diagnoses thanks to the high interactivity provided by the sharing of microscopic fields among peers and with referent expert. This methodology may be used also in areas where more efficient and currently available technologies are not in place [35, 36].

Shared Database Applications of Telemedicine (HCP2HCP, Asynchronous)

In this case, local medical personnel and remote specialists access a common server containing a properly structured database of medical data, which are loaded locally in the patient database and accessed by remote HCPs. The physical location of the server is immaterial and can be suitably chosen when technical conditions and support are adequate. It may even be located at the premises of a hosting service provider, if privacy of medical data is properly assured.

This is obviously a more structured setup and from a technical point of view can be implemented in different ways, depending on privacy and level-of-service requirements. In the simplest way, the medical database is contained in a Web site accessible from the Internet with proper credentials. More sophisticated implementations would put the database server in a virtual private network (VPN), in order to be visible only by the involved personnel. In any case, even this system would be easily implementable with open-source software components, either available freely or at low cost. Technology would not be a problem, but, again, a fundamental issue would be the quality, speed, and cost of the Internet connection.

Of course, these solutions would be more organizationally demanding than the elementary, store-and-forward arrangement, because it would require the definition of common procedures to manage and access the database in an ordered way. This architecture is particularly suited to support twinning programs between geographically remote institutions. With the help of proper organizational procedures and protocols, this architecture may support different applications, according to the kind of data which are shared. They may be simply statistical data regarding the performances of shared clinical protocols or even data allowing the remote monitoring of patients for a certain period of time (e.g., during the admission in a local hospital), implementing, so to speak, a kind of "geographically distributed medical service." Some experiences in the area of telepathology are described below.

Patient Remote Monitoring (P2HCP, Asynchronous)

This solution enables HCPs to monitor a patient remotely using various technological devices. This is different from the previous solutions, in which there is no direct interaction between patient and the remote consultant, which is only involved through the mediation of the local medical personnel. This method is primarily used to monitor chronic diseases or specific conditions, such as heart disease, diabetes mellitus, or asthma.

Some solutions may use simple and low-cost devices, such as, typically, cell phones. As mentioned before, low-end cell phones are nowadays available almost to everybody on the planet, even in the poorest countries. Smartphones, which allow more sophisticated applications, are still expensive, but their cost is declining, and we can expect that in a few years they will be affordable for the large majority of the inhabitants of the world. Specific government policies can further accelerate this process. For example, the Indian government has recently released a new tablet computer, Aakash, at a cost of $35 with government subsidies for students or $60 in stores.

In the meanwhile, simple solutions based on SMS may strongly improve health conditions of the poorest. For example, FrontlineSMS is a free, open-source software platform, developed from 2005, and largely used, for example, in sub-Saharan Africa. It allows HCPs to text message with large groups of people anywhere there is a mobile signal. This software allows a laptop, plugged into a cell phone, to become a low-cost communication hub, to be used in a wide range of health care applications, without necessity of any Internet connection, e.g., collecting sanitary data from patients, managing medical visits follow-ups, supplying remote assistance in emergencies, announcing vaccination campaigns, and sending information on medicine availability and dosage and appointment reminders [37]. Similar services may be set up using Twitter—which also may be used through SMS without any Internet access and which is already used, e.g., in emergencies. When an Internet connection with a smartphone is available, for example, through Wi-Fi, new smartphone applications such as WhatsApp can exchange SMSs at no charge, bypassing the telephone operator [38].

Interactive Telemedicine (P2HCP, Synchronous)

These solutions allow direct, real-time interaction between patient and remote HCP and may be implemented using a variety of real-time communications technology, either text based (e.g., Internet chats) or—preferably—voice and video based (e.g., phone, Skype, or other Internet videoconferencing services). Most of these services—which were unthinkable only a decade ago—are now free and largely available. Skype has an extremely large user base in every country (more 700 millions user accounts in 2011): a quarter of all world international phone calls passed through it in the same year, according to Skype data. It can be easily used at no cost from any computer and from many smartphones, provided that an Internet connection is available (e.g., through Wi-Fi).

Many activities such as history review, physical examination, psychiatric evaluations, and some ophthalmology assessments can be conducted comparably to those done in traditional face-to-face visits.

As a more sophisticated example, E Health Points are public health units, owned and operated by Healthpoint Services India (HSI), a for-profit company launched in 2009. These units provide families in rural villages with clean drinking water, medicines, comprehensive diagnostic tools, and advanced tele-medical services that "bring" a remote doctor to their community. They provide the remote doctor with the patient's more important data—including digital stethoscope, noninvasive blood pressure monitor, and electrocardiogram (ECG)—and offer more than 70 additional diagnostic tests covering all major infectious diseases and many chronic conditions, including malnutrition, heart disease, and diabetes [39].

Tele-health Applications

Closely related to the above applications are the many applications in the broader area of telehealth, which also largely benefits from the availability of Internet connectivity, and software technologies and services in the area of communication and cooperation, either open source or proprietary. They can be extremely useful to improve health care in LIC, possibly in connection with telemedicine applications. They may use social media, collaboration, and communications software platforms to implement Web sites supporting the worldwide distribution of online webinars or offline courses on medical issues, collect and maintain repository of medical information, allow real-time interaction among medical personnel in different countries to exchange experiences or discuss specific technical issues, allow people with specific diseases to create online communities to discuss their specific problems, and so on. Some applications are oriented to the HCPs, other are oriented to all people in need of medical counseling.

An important example of a large-scale Web application directed to HCPs is www.cure4kids.org, a Web site managed from St. Jude Children's Research Hospital in Memphis (USA), with the mission of improving health care for children with cancer or other catastrophic diseases in all countries. Started in 2002, it provides continuing medical education focusing on cancer, pediatric oncology, and global communication tools to HCPs and scientists worldwide. The site can be used at no charge by the registered users and allows access to online seminars and conferences, a digital library, self-instruction courses, recent research results, case studies, best practices and analysis of specific treatments, online meetings, and much more. At mid-2012, cure4kids had more than 31,000 registered users in 183 countries. Over 300 international groups meet online in cure4kids Web conferencing rooms to discuss clinical cases and share knowledge. In 2007 cure4kids launched Oncopedia, compiled using online submissions from registered users [40].

Other examples, specifically directed to people affected by specific diseases, are www.tudiabetes.org and www.estudiabetes.org, two large online social networks for people touched by diabetes, managed since 2007 from the California-based nonprofit Diabetes Hands Foundation. These social networks (in English and Spanish respectively) have more than 45,000 registered members from all countries and are visited by over 200,000 people per month. Members can discuss problems related to their disease in online forums, thematic groups, and blogs [41]. They are implemented using Ning, an (proprietary) online service allowing to easily set up a private social network, supporting a rich set of communication functions [42].

Telepathology: The Experience of POF

Scientific information on cancer epidemiology in many LIC is still largely inadequate. In 2008 WHO focused the attention on the real emergency of cancer in countries of sub-Saharan Africa. In this context, a small Italian NGO, called "Patologi Oltre Frontiera" (POF: Pathologists Across Borders), had already been operating since 1999, having as a main goal the institution of surgical pathology labs or the improvement of those already available. About 300 Italian pathologists, biologists, and technicians have registered in POF and 40 of them are really engaged as volunteers in projects that span from Cuba to Palestine, to Africa (Tanzania, Zambia, Madagascar, Republic of Djibouti, DR Congo, Uganda, Nigeria, and Mauritania).

Since 2007, with projects in Zambia first and then in Madagascar, POF have included telepathology in their operational techniques, in order to try and improve their efficacy. It has to be considered to this purpose that very few pathologists are available in these areas; for example, there are only ten pathologists in Kinshasa for 90 million inhabitants in an area of 2,500,000 km^2 in DR Congo (versus 2,500 pathologists for 60 million people in Italy). Furthermore, it takes many years to provide adequate pathologist training.

In 2009 POF contributed to the development of a new association of European pathologists called "APOF, Pathologists Beyond Borders Association" (http://esphumanitarian.wordpress.com/). This association is still growing being recognized and acknowledged by WHO.

Telemedicine Perspectives

The Internet in the last decade has undergone a dramatic transformation. From its original nature of an information network, it has evolved into a powerful tool to support communication and collaboration (both asynchronous and synchronous) between individuals and organizations, regardless of their physical location. Some of these transformations would have been considered, only 15 years ago, science fiction even by the ICT insiders. And this transformation continues. In a few years from now, access to the Internet will be mainly through mobile, portable devices, either tablet or new generation smartphones.

Through these devices, we can already use a large number of online services supporting communication and collaboration, essentially at no cost. The only requirement is the availability of an Internet connection, preferably broadband (otherwise we would be severely limited in many online activities, especially when voice or video is involved).

The digital divide between the developed and developing world is still significant. Nevertheless, as we have already seen, in the last decade exceptional progresses have been made, especially in the area of mobile telephony. We may expect, in a future not too far from now, a world substantially connected—in mobility. The Broadband Commission for Digital Development jointly launched in 2010 from ITU and UNESCO set up as a target for 2015, "ambitious but achievable" a 50 % Internet penetration in developing countries and 15 % in less developed countries [34]. Availability of mobile broadband is still very limited and expensive, but steady progress is being made globally. Telemedicine shall thus be implemented more and more in the development of pediatric hemato-oncology in LIC.

Acknowledgments We would like to thank the following for their contribution to the project "La Mascota": Fondazione CARIPLO, Comitato Maria Letizia Verga, Fondazione Tettamanti, Fondazione Zegna, AMCA (Bellinzona, Switzerland), CONANCA and MAPANICA (Nicaragua), the HMJR "La Mascota" Hospital (Managua), St. Jude Children's Research Hospital (SJCRH, Memphis, USA), and the Pediatric Oncology Group of Ontario (POGO).

References

1. Wilimas JA, Ribeiro RC. Pediatric hematology-oncology outreach for developing countries. Hematol Oncol Clin North Am. 2001;15(4):775–87, x.
2. Howard SC, Metzger ML, Wilimas JA, Quintana Y, Pui CH, Robison LL, Ribeiro RC. Childhood cancer epidemiology in low-income countries. Cancer. 2008; 112(3):461–72.
3. Magrath I, et al. Pediatric oncology in less developed countries. In: Pizzo PA, Poplack DG, editors. Principles and practice of pediatric oncology. Philadelphia, PA: Lippincott; 1993. p. 1225–51.
4. Ribeiro RC, Pui CH. Saving the children–improving childhood cancer treatment in developing countries. N Engl J Med. 2005;352(21):2158–60.
5. Kellie SJ, Howard SC. Global child health priorities: what role for paediatric oncologists? Eur J Cancer. 2008;44:2388–96.
6. Wagner HP, Antic V. The problem of pediatric malignancies in the developing world. Ann N Y Acad Sci. 1997;824:193–204.
7. Masera G, Baez F, Biondi A, et al. Bridging the childhood cancer mortality gap between economically developed and low income countries: lessons from the MISPHO experience. In: Tannenberg S, Cavalli F, Pannuti F, editors. Cancer in developing countries. The great challenge for oncology in the 21st century. Muenchen: Zuckschwerdt; 2004. p. 42–60.
8. Wagner H. Alliances in pediatric oncology: where do we go from here? Med Pediatr Oncol. 2001;36(2):310–1.
9. The Montevideo Document. SIOP News. 1997;17:32.
10. Baez F, Ocampo E, Conter V, et al. Treatment of childhood Hodgkin's disease with COPP or COPP-ABV (hybrid) without radiotherapy in Nicaragua. Ann Oncol. 1997;8:247–50.
11. Baez F, Pillon M, Manfredini L, et al. Treatment of pediatric non-Hodgkin lymphomas in a country with limited resources: results of the first national protocol in Nicaragua. Pediatr Blood Cancer. 2008;50:148–52.

12. Baez F, Fossati Bellani F, Ocampo E, et al. Treatment of childhood Wilms' tumor without radiotherapy in Nicaragua. Ann Oncol. 2002;13:944–8.
13. Masera G, Baez Lacayo F, Malta Corea A, et al. Pediatric oncology in developing countries: a cooperative program in Nicaragua. Ann Oncol. 1993;4:37–40.
14. SIOP. 43rd Congress of the International Society of Paediatric Oncology (SIOP) 2011, Auckland, New Zealand, 28th–30th October 2011. Abstracts Pediatr Blood Cancer. 2011;57(5):705–897. doi:10.1002/pbc.23299.
15. Masera G, Baez F, et al. North–south twinning in paediatric haemato-oncology: the La Mascota programme, Nicaragua. Lancet. 1998;352(9144):1923–6.
16. D'Angio GJ. The La Mascota project. J Pediatr Hematol Oncol. 2009;31(10):709.
17. Masera G. Bridging the childhood cancer mortality gap between economically developed and low-income countries. J Pediatr Hematol Oncol. 2009;31(10):710–2.
18. Edefonti A, Montini G, Castellon M; for the Nicaraguan Network of Pediatric Nephrology—NINEPEN. Comprehensive cooperative project for children with renal disease in Nicaragua. Clin Nephrol. 2010;74 Suppl. 1:S119–25.
19. Sala A, Barr RD, Masera G, MISPHO Consortium. A survey of resources and activities in the MISPHO family of institutions in Latin America: a comparison of two eras. Pediatr Blood Cancer. 2004;43(7):758–64.
20. Howard SC, Marinoni M, Castillo L, Bonilla M, Tognoni G, Luna-Fineman S, Antillon F, Valsecchi MG, Pui CH, Ribeiro RC, Sala A, Barr RD, Masera G, MISPHO Consortium Writing Committee. Improving outcomes for children with cancer in low-income countries in Latin America: a report on the recent meetings of the Monza International School of Pediatric Hematology/Oncology (MISPHO)-Part I. Pediatr Blood Cancer. 2007;48(3):364–9.
21. Howard SC, Ortiz R, Baez LF, Cabanas R, Barrantes J, Fu L, Peña A, Samudio A, Vizcaino M, Rodríguez-Galindo C, Barr RD, Conter V, Biondi A, Masera G, MISPHO Consortium Writing Committee. Protocol-based treatment for children with cancer in low income countries in Latin America: a report on the recent meetings of the Monza International School of Pediatric Hematology/Oncology (MISPHO)—part I. Pediatr Blood Cancer. 2007;48(4):486–90.
22. Valsecchi MG, Tognoni G, Bonilla M, Moreno N, Baez F, Pacheco C, Hernandez AP, Antillon-Klussmann F, Machin S, Cabanas R, Navarrete M, Nieves R, De Lorenzo P, Masera G, Monza's International School of Paediatric Hematology-Oncology. Clinical epidemiology of childhood cancer in Central America and Caribbean countries. Ann Oncol. 2004;15(4):680–5.
23. Rohatiner A. Keynote comment: not just an exercise in solidarity. Lancet Oncol. 2005;6(11):818–9.
24. Antillon F, Baez FL, Barr R, Barrantes Zamorra JC, Carrasco LF, Moreno B, Bonilla MM, Tognoni G, Valsecch MG, Howard S, Ribeiro RC, Masera G. AMOR: a proposed cooperative effort to improve outcomes of childhood cancer in Central America. Pediatr Blood Cancer. 2005;45(2):107–10.
25. Quintana Y, Nambayan A, Ribeiro R, et al. Cure4Kids—building online learning and collaboration networks. AMIA Annu Symp Proc. 2003;2003:978.
26. Israëls T, Chirambo C, Caron H, de Kraker J, Molyneux E, Reis R. The guardians' perspective on paediatric cancer treatment in Malawi and factors affecting adherence. Pediatr Blood Cancer. 2008;51: 639–42.
27. Hesseling PB, Broadhead R, Molyneux E, Borgstein E, Schneider JW, Louw M, Mansvelt EP, Wessels G. Malawi pilot study of Burkitt lymphoma treatment. Med Pediatr Oncol. 2003;41:532–40.
28. Mostert S, Sitaresmi M, Gundy C. PK020 influence of socioeconomic status on childhood acute lymphoblastic leukaemia treatment in Indonesia [abstract]. Pediatr Blood Cancer. 2006;47:489.
29. Hunger SP, Sung L, Howard SC. Treatment strategies and regimens of graduated intensity for childhood acute lymphoblastic leukemia in low-income countries: a proposal. Pediatr Blood Cancer. 2009;52(5):559–65. doi:10.1002/pbc.21889.
30. Arora RS, Eden T, Pizer B. The problem of treatment abandonment in children from developing countries with cancer. Pediatr Blood Cancer. 2007;49(7):941–6.
31. Sitaresmi MN, Mostert S, Schook RM, Sutaryo, Veerman AJ. Treatment refusal and abandonment in childhood acute lymphoblastic leukemia in Indonesia: an analysis of causes and consequences. Psychooncology. 2010;19(4):361–7. doi:10.1002/pon.1578.
32. Spinetta JJ, Masera G, Eden T, et al. Refusal, non-compliance, and abandonment of treatment in children and adolescents with cancer: a report of the SIOP Working Committee on Psychosocial Issues in Paediatric Oncology. Med Pediatr Oncol. 2002;38: 114–7.
33. World Health Organization, Telemedicine: opportunities and developments in member states; report on the Second Survey on eHealth, 2010 (Global Observatory for eHealth Series 2). Available from http://www.who.int/goe/publications/goe_telemedicine_2010.pdf
34. ITU. Measuring the information society; 2012. Available from http://www.itu.int/ITU-D/ict/publications/idi/material/2012/MIS2012_without_Annex_4.pdf
35. Bellina L, Missoni E. Mobile cell-phones (M-phones) in telemicroscopy: increasing connectivity of isolated laboratories. Diagn Pathol. 2009;4:19.
36. Bellina L, Missoni E. M-learning: mobile phones' appropriateness and potential for the training of laboratory technicians in limited-resource settings. Health Technol. 2011;1:93–97
37. http://en.wikipedia.org/wiki/FrontlineSMS
38. http://en.wikipedia.org/wiki/WhatsApp
39. http://en.wikipedia.org/wiki/E_Health_Point
40. http://en.wikipedia.org/wiki/Cure4Kids
41. http://en.wikipedia.org/wiki/Diabetes_Hands_Foundation
42. http://en.wikipedia.org/wiki/Ning_(website)

Pediatric Cancer Units and Optimization of Resources

5

Paola Friedrich, Natalie McCall, and Aziza Shad

What Is a Pediatric Cancer Unit?

A pediatric cancer unit (PCU) can assume a variety of shapes and forms. A standard definition does not exist, but in general, the term PCU is used to represent the assembly of dedicated resources and staff invested in the provision of coordinated inpatient and outpatient pediatric cancer care.

Sometimes the physical layout of a PCU is a few beds in a general or pediatric ward or in an adult oncology service. Other times, the PCU is one of several wards in a general, pediatric, or adult oncology hospital. Some countries have a physically separate pediatric oncology wing, building, or area that functions semi-independently from the general hospital but requests most consultative services from the adjacent primary institution. Finally, sometimes the PCU is a freestanding or independent institution. Thus, the PCUs' human resources, financial supports, and collaborations vary accordingly. In high-income countries, PCUs are often dedicated wards within a large tertiary- or quaternary-level pediatric hospital and are often called "centers." Examples of PCUs in low- and middle-income countries (LMC) are shown in Table 5.1. The variety and lack of one-size-fits-all definition is evident. Therefore, the first step in conceptualizing and building a PCU is to realize that what makes a PCU is not the space it occupies, but the conscious decision by a team of providers to make the effective addressing of pediatric cancer a priority.

What Are the Benefits to Building Pediatric Cancer Units?

In low-income countries (LIC) when children with cancer are referred to tertiary institutions, they are often grouped with children with other diagnoses, amidst adults with cancer, or both; wards may be overcrowded and/or have substandard hygienic facilities (lacking hand washing stations, hand sanitizers, individual toilets, etc.). Knowing that in the absence of reliable and accessible laboratory services most children with

P. Friedrich, M.D. (✉)
Global Health Initiative, Dana-Farber/Boston Children's Cancer and Blood Disorders Center, 450 Brookline Avenue, D-3123, Boston, MA 02115, USA

Harvard Medical School, Boston, MA, USA
e-mail: paola_friedrich-medina@dfci.harvard.edu

N. McCall, M.D.
Associate Professor of Pediatrics, University of Rwanda, College of Medicine and Health Sciences, Kigali, Rwanda

Visiting Associate Professor of Pediatrics at Yale School of Medicine, Kigali University Teaching Hospital, 1024 rue de la Paix, Kigali, Rwanda

A. Shad, M.D.
Division of Pediatric Hematology Oncology, Blood and Marrow Transplantation, Medstar Georgetown University Hospital, Lombardi Comprehensive Cancer Center, Washington, DC, USA

D.C. Stefan and C. Rodriguez-Galindo (eds.), *Pediatric Hematology-Oncology in Countries with Limited Resources: A Practical Manual*, DOI 10.1007/978-1-4614-3891-5_5,

Table 5.1 Examples from pediatric cancer units (PCU) across the world and income economy classification

Country	Physical layout	Human resources	Financial support	Collaborations
Ethiopia (sub-Saharan Africa) (low-income economy)	Dedicated ward in the pediatric unit of a general hospital, largest referral hospital in country for all pediatric cancer cases	Few pediatricians, no oncologist. Nurses not trained in pediatrics or oncology. Pathology poorly developed	Government hospital with minimal outside financial support	International: INCTR/Georgetown twinning program. Fellowship in pediatric oncology started 2013. Training for pediatric oncology nurses and pharmacists started
Rwanda (sub-Saharan Africa) (low-income economy) (two examples)	1. A separate wing in the pediatric department of the main referral hospital where patients are hospitalized for diagnosis, surgeries, and if there are any complications during chemotherapy 2. A hospitalization ward within a district hospital supported by an NGO 2.5 h away from the central hospital where patients receive chemotherapy and are seen for follow-up	Nurses with no specific training in pediatrics or oncology General nurses with some training in oncology	Government hospital with no external financial support	International: unofficial consultations obtained with pediatric oncologists in the USA, South Africa International: consultations with a US institution
Pakistan (South Asia) (lower-middle-income economy) (four examples)	1. Freestanding children's cancer hospital in a major city (1 of 3 pediatric cancer units in the city). Most consultative services available in the community 2. Large pediatric unit in government hospital 3. Separate wing in the pediatric department of University Teaching Hospital with well-developed adult cancer program. Research facilities available 4. Pediatric unit in the only comprehensive cancer center in the country. Subspecialty support at the cancer center and in the community. Research facilities available	Trained pediatric oncologists, pediatric nurses, pharmacist Trained pediatricians and nurses Trained pediatric oncologists, nurses, and pharmacists. All subspecialty support including radiation oncology on-site available Trained pediatric oncologist, nurses, pharmacists	Totally financed by philanthropy Government hospital with local philanthropic support Fee for service Philanthropy and fee for service	Several international affiliations, local network through Pakistan Society of Pediatric Oncology (PSPO) Local support from PSPO International and local collaborations International and local collaborations

Guatemala (Latin America and Caribbean) (lower-middle-income economy)	Independent 3-story building adjacent and connecting to a general pediatrics hospital The unit has dedicated intensive care, procedure area, urgent/emergent care area, pharmacy, data management, inpatient and outpatient pediatric oncology areas	Pediatric oncology trained physicians and nurse educators Began a fellowship program in 2004 Some services (pathology, radiology, surgery, etc.) are contracted out to general pediatrics hospital or other institutions	Not-for-profit organization and public partnership (the organization fundraises for the PCU and the ministry of health provides an annual sum for care of oncology patients)	Regional: collaboration with 6 other countries in the region for development and monitoring of standardized treatment guidelines by disease (AHOPCA—Association of Central American Pediatric Hematologists and Oncologists) International: twinning with St. Jude Children's Research Hospital International Outreach Program
Costa Rica (Latin America and Caribbean) (upper-middle-income economy)	Pediatric oncology ward in a general pediatrics hospital Has dedicated inpatient and outpatient pediatric oncology areas, others shared with pediatric hospital	Pediatric oncology trained physicians and nurse educators All other services are provided through the general pediatric hospital	Universal coverage for children National healthcare system absorbs all treatment costs A non-for-profit organization supports the hospital	Regional: collaboration with AHOPCA as detailed for Guatemala International: support from St. Jude Children's Research Hospital International Outreach Program
Colombia (Latin America and Caribbean) (upper-middle-income economy)	Pediatric oncology ward in a national cancer institute (primarily an adult cancer institute) The unit has dedicated inpatient and outpatients pediatric oncology area, others shared with adult institute	Pediatric oncology trained physicians and nurse educators Most ancillary services are provided through the cancer institute, some are subcontracted to neighboring pediatric hospitals	Universal coverage for children Ministry subcontracts with private insurances to serve as intermediaries with contributive and subsidized policies	International: twinning with Dana-Farber/Boston Children's Global Health Initiative

Based on World Bank Country and Lending Groups (available at http://data.worldbank.org/about/country-classifications/country-and-lending-groups)

leukemia will die of infection before leukemia is diagnosed and that in the absence of chemotherapy or radiotherapy, solid tumors are exclusively surgical diseases, the absence of separate pediatric oncology wards in some LIC is no surprise. Furthermore, when standards of living are poor and health systems are fragmented or inadequate, pediatric cancer may either not seem to occur (because they are not diagnosed), present to medical attention for surgical interventions only (due to presence of a mass), or present to medical attention severely ill (due to advanced disease or sepsis). The reasons overcrowded settings prevail in LIC are likely multifactorial and variable from one place to another. Lack of space, staff, drugs, or expertise, as well as fatalism or a sense of futility of treatment, among others, may serve as explanations. It is through improvement of standards of living and health care infrastructure that children with cancer are able to reach medical care, be diagnosed with cancer, and stimulate the mobilization of resources towards the offering of cancer-directed therapy. Once the need to address pediatric cancer is acknowledged and more patients are diagnosed, expertise is built, and fundamental barriers to oncology care such as access to chemotherapy and safe handling of chemotherapy are addressed, clinicians building a PCU and looking to improve pediatric cancer outcomes must devise strategies for expanding towards the effective delivery of multimodal therapy (treatment that incorporates medical, psychosocial, supportive, surgical, and/or radiation oncology services).

PCUs often aim to cohort children with cancer. The justification for grouping children with cancer together and separating them from patients with other diagnoses, stems primarily from the desire to protect them [1]. However, this practice also creates several important opportunities that deserve to emphasized. From an organizational stand point, the introduction of chemotherapy, the infectious risks imposed by it, the need for close monitoring of toxicities, and the need for safe handling of chemotherapy and waste products often triggers the desire to separate cancer patients from others. Therefore, chemotherapy availability and administration can become the catalyst for physical creation of pediatric oncology wards. However, as mentioned before, a PCU is more than its infrastructure or physical space and can look differently in different parts of the world. Therefore, conceptualizing, creating, restructuring, or building a PCU creates opportunities for development of expertise by nurses, physicians, and surgeons (among other staff); standardization of care; education of dedicated staff in safe handling of chemotherapy; tracking of outcomes; prevention of infections; prevention or early management of toxicity; building of care teams; and provision of multidisciplinary patient-centered care (Fig. 5.1).

Opportunities provided by the development of a PCU:

- Development of expertise by nurses, physicians, surgeons and other staff
- Standardization of care
- Education of dedicated staff in safe handling of chemotherapy
- Tracking of outcomes
- Prevention of infections
- Prevention and early management of toxicity
- Building of care teams
- Provision of multidisciplinary patient-centered care

Fig. 5.1 Opportunities provided with the development of pediatric cancer units

In the absence of dedicated space and staff, the quality of care provided to children with cancer can suffer [1, 2]. Some practical examples include the following. Without specialized PCUs, general physicians and nurses may not be able to build the expertise to guide development and implementation of treatment guidelines (or protocols). Without standardization of care, outcomes cannot be reliably measured and the need or areas to improve may be overlooked or neglected. When cancer patients need to share rooms or beds with other patients, they may be exposed to infectious diseases (respiratory, diarrheal, or other) that are mild to moderate in the normal host but can lead to death in them due to their immunosuppressed status. Without specialized nursing (generated by experience or formal curriculum), toxic effects of chemotherapy and complications may not be recognized and managed promptly, leading to morbidity or death. Furthermore, if standard procedures to protect staff during administration of chemotherapy and to handle and dispose of potentially dangerous materials are not developed, health professionals and family members are unnecessarily exposed to potentially toxic substances. Finally, in the absence of a sense of unity, respect, and common purpose among providers, decision making about care and communication with patients and families can be heavily fragmented.

What Are the Key Components of a Pediatric Cancer Unit?

Key Components, Human Resources: The spectrum of human resources needed at the PCU depends on the diagnoses being treated, the volume of patients seen at the center, and its economic supports. As adapted from the St. Jude Children's Research Hospital International Outreach Program in their "Guide to Establishing a Pediatric Oncology Twinning Program" [3], ideally human resources at the PCU include a medical director, other physicians (generalists, pediatricians, pediatric oncologists) trained and designated to care of children with cancer, nurses and nurse educator, data managers, and administrators, along with specialists in infectious disease and infection control, pathology, radiology, radiation oncology, surgery (general or pediatric oncologic, orthopedic, and neurologic), pharmacy, pain, palliative and psychosocial services, child life, nutrition, and rehabilitation. Some staff, such as physicians and nurses, are ideally dedicated to the PCU and do not work at other locations. Other staff is likely shared with other departments or institutions depending on the volume of patients at the PCU.

Key Components, Other: In conceptualizing a PCU, the natural reaction is to focus on diagnostics, therapeutics, and supportive care. However, a multitude of biologic `and nonbiologic factors likely influence pediatric cancer outcomes at the PCU (see Fig. 5.2). Biologic factors include genetics, exposures, clinical characteristics, and

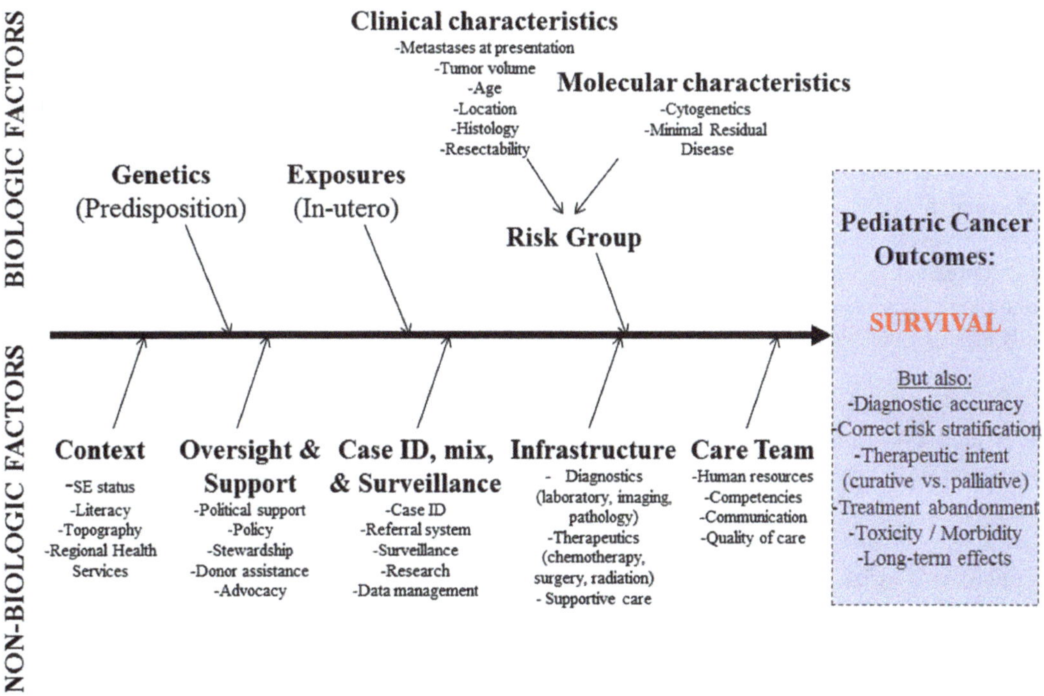

Fig. 5.2 Development of a pediatric cancer unit—conceptual model of factors that influence pediatric cancer outcomes

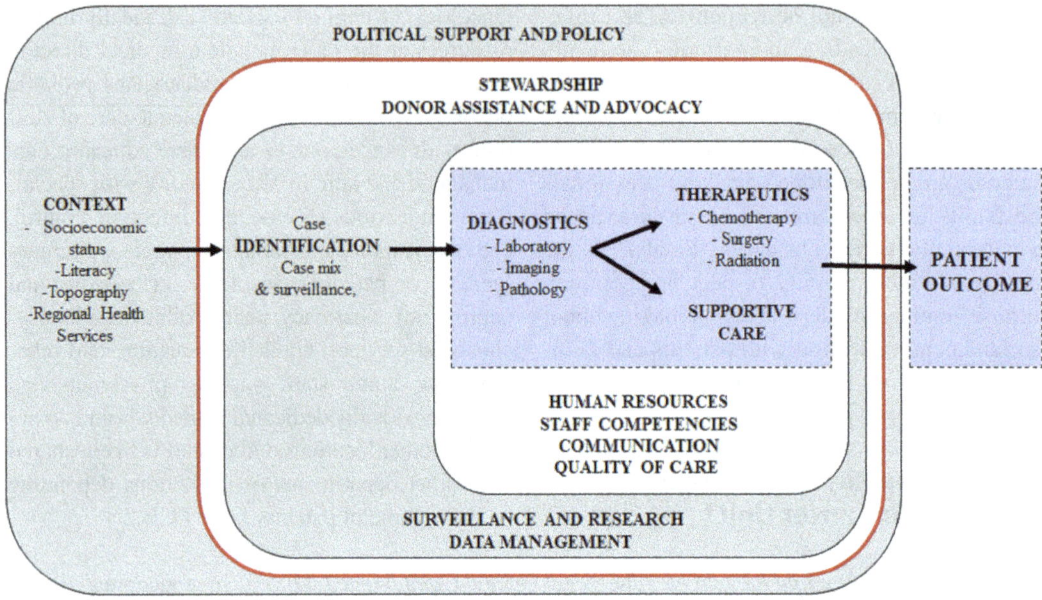

Fig. 5.3 Development of a pediatric cancer unit—linear and ecological conceptual model of nonbiologic factors that influence pediatric cancer outcomes

molecular characteristics of the cancer. However, by the time the patient arrives to the PCU and is diagnosed, biologic factors are for the most part not modifiable. Nonbiologic factors include social and economic context, oversight and support, referral and surveillance capacities, infrastructure availability, and the functionality of the care team at the PCU. In LMC, nonbiologic factors and their influence on outcomes need to be studied in more detail because nonbiologic factors are likely most influential, prevalent, and actionable among barriers to improvement of pediatric cancer outcomes. A comprehensive linear and ecologic model of nonbiologic factors that influence pediatric cancer outcomes in a PCU is presented in Fig. 5.3.

International Society of Pediatric Oncology and International Network for Cancer Treatment and Research (SIOP and INCTR) Recommendations: In 1991, the SIOP Working Committee on Standards of Care and Training and Working Committee on Psychosocial Issues in Pediatric Oncology put forward recommendations for the organization of a PCU [4]. This consensus document recommended that all children with cancer should be offered child-oriented diagnosis, treatment, aftercare, and follow-up and gave basic guidelines for the development of PCUs. With progressive improvement in the standard of care in many countries resulting in improved survival, it was recognized that the guidelines for development of a PCU needed to be updated. In 2008, the first revised document was presented at the SIOP Pediatric Oncology in Developing Countries (PODC) meeting, which was further revised at consecutive meetings, and consensus was obtained. In 2010 the SIOP guidelines were further modified by the members of the INCTR Pediatric Oncology Working Group, many of whom were active SIOP PODC members. Table 5.2 shows the joint SIOP/INCTR recommendations for the development of a PCU [58].

Certification or Needs Assessment Program for PCUs: No consensus exists regarding the need for certification or periodic assessment of a PCU. In the SIOP/INCTR recommendations, it was suggested that programs that had international collaborations or twinning programs could use those resources for guidance and improvement. However, there was consensus that a process of certification, though voluntary, could be used to obtain support and additional services from governmental agencies or supporting NGOs.

Table 5.2 SIOP/INCTR recommendations for the development of a PCU

Introduction		
1. All children, adolescents, and young adults deserve age-appropriate diagnosis, treatment, aftercare, and long-term follow-up. This is best offered in a dedicated pediatric cancer unit (PCU)		
2. A PCU should be situated in or have an affiliation with a general hospital, pediatric departments, or cancer center		
3. Depending on the extent of services offered, all PCUs can be divided into Level I, II, or III		
General guidelines for all levels of PCUs		
1. The age range of patients served in a PCU can range from infancy through adolescence or even early adulthood (i.e., up until the age of 21 years)		
2. Basic infection control practices (e.g., good hand-washing policies, isolation of infectious cases) should be incorporated into all levels of PCUs		
3. All PCUs should be staffed by pediatric oncologists or pediatricians who have had some formal training in pediatric oncology		
4. All physicians involved in the diagnosis and care of cancer patients should have a working knowledge of palliative care including pain management		
Level I PCU	Level II PCU	Level III PCU or center of excellence
Definition		
1. A Level I PCU is defined as a unit capable of diagnosing and delivering care for the most curable and least complicated pediatric oncology diagnoses (i.e., Hodgkin's disease, non-Hodgkin's lymphoma, ALL, and Wilms' tumor)	1. Level II PCUs should be able to provide all the services of a Level I PCU and most/many of the services of a Level III PCU	1. A Level III PCU should be a special unit within a large general hospital, cancer center, pediatric department, or children's hospital capable of treating all forms of pediatric cancers
2. This PCU should also have the capability of diagnosing and stabilizing patients with more complicated cancer diagnoses prior to transfer to a higher level PCU	2. Level II PCUs should work in close collaboration with a Level III PCU locally or nationally	2. Should have a minimum of 50 or more new diagnoses of pediatric cancer/year
	3. Level II PCUs could be involved in the training of pediatric oncology specialists, but the main responsibility/direction of such training efforts would remain with the Level III units	
	4. Under the direction of the Level III PCUs, these units could participate in clinical trials and research	
Facility and infrastructure		
1. Level I PCUs could be located in large cities (as one of several units) or small cities and towns (outside major metropolitan areas) where the PCU might be the only center for treatment for noncomplicated cancers	1. Level II PCUs should be able to provide all the services of a Level I PCU and most/many of the services of a Level III PCU	1. Inpatient facilities in an advanced PCU should include a dedicated pediatric cancer unit with isolation rooms, some hepa-filtered rooms, and a separate procedure room

(continued)

Table 5.2 (continued)

2. Be located within or associated with a general hospital	2. Level II PCUs should work in close collaboration with a Level III PCU locally or nationally	2. Outpatient facilities should include the following
		Day clinic or infusion center (for short-term infusion chemotherapy and blood products)
		Area for routine chemotherapy (i.e., vincristine by IV push) and antibiotics
		Procedure area with capacity for conscious sedation
		Rooms for physical exam
		Designated areas for blood draws, including management of central lines
		Chemotherapy safety protocol and procedures to avoid chemotherapy errors and to manage chemotherapy accidents (i.e., spills)
3. Have capacity for both inpatient and outpatient care (ability to deliver chemotherapy for abovementioned tumors, provide antibiotics for fever and neutropenia, and transfusions)		3. Have at least a hospital-based tumor registry
4. Have the ability to communicate with all ancillary services (e.g., telephone or pager)		4. Have the resources and capability to be the training center for pediatric oncology specialists (including, but not limited to, doctors, nurses, advanced practice nurses and/or physician assistants, pharmacists, and social workers)
5. Have a chemotherapy safety protocol and procedures to avoid chemotherapy errors and manage chemotherapy accidents (i.e., spills)		5. Have an organized medical record keeping system in place with data managers
6. Have a hospital policy for the procurement, storage and accountability of drugs (usage, expiration dates, availability of stock), and other essential supplies needed for chemotherapy preparation and administration. A link with a central procurement agency may be needed in some countries		6. Have multidisciplinary clinics for bone tumors, brain tumors, and retinoblastoma
		7. Pediatric ICU capable of taking care of all oncological emergencies
		8. Access to an accredited blood bank with capability to supply all components of blood (PRBC, platelets, plasma, cryoprecipitate, factor concentrates)
		9. A hospital infection control team
		10. Hand-washing facilities on all inpatient and outpatient units, dirty and clean utility areas, and a waste disposal system
		11. Have a hospital policy for the procurement, storage and accountability of drugs (usage, expiration dates, availability of stock), and other essential supplies needed for chemotherapy preparation and administration
		12. A link with a central procurement agency may be needed in some countries
		All drugs listed in the WHO Essential Drug List should ideally be available in the hospital pharmacy
		13. All chemotherapy drugs and antibiotics needed for the execution of treatment protocols should be available in the hospital pharmacy

Staff		
1. Pediatric oncologists or pediatricians with basic training in pediatric oncology	1. Level II PCUs should be able to provide all the services of a Level I PCU and most/many of the services of a Level III PCU	1. Medical personnel who have specialized training in pediatric oncology (pediatric oncologists, pediatric oncology nurses, pediatric oncology pharmacists, pediatric oncology social workers and/or psychologists, etc.)
2. Nurses trained in basic pediatric care and care of the immunocompromised patient	2. Level II PCUs should work in close collaboration with a Level III PCU locally or nationally	2. "Round the clock" access to a pediatric oncologist/pediatrician, nursing, social worker, and chaplain should be available 7 days a week
3. Availability of a pathologist or interventional radiologist for fine needle aspirate/biopsy		3. Dedicated oncology pharmacy with laminar hoods. An oncology pharmacist would be ideal; however, a pharmacist trained in oncology, working within a general pharmacy setting would be acceptable
4. Availability of a surgeon—preferably pediatric surgeon		4. Availability and access to other essential subspecialty services
		Pediatric surgery, neurosurgery, orthopedic surgery, and ophthalmology
		Radiation oncology
5. Nursing staff should have a working knowledge of chemotherapy administration, i.e., placement of IVs, administration of fluids, and basic chemotherapy (i.e., vincristine, cyclophosphamide)		Cardiology, renal (dialysis), infectious diseases, gastroenterology
6. Pediatricians should have a basic, working knowledge of chemotherapy; its administration; and side effects. This includes intrathecal chemotherapy		
7. Pediatricians should be trained to do procedures (bone marrow aspiration/biopsy, spinal taps with intrathecal chemotherapy) and the interpretation of the results		
8. "Round the clock" access to a pediatric oncologist/pediatrician and nursing should be available 7 days a week		
Diagnostic facilities		
1. Access to a basic laboratory (crossmatch, basic chemistry, bone marrow stain, and CBC)	1. Level II PCUs should be able to provide all the services of a Level I PCU and most/many of the services of a Level III PCU	1. Radiology services should include availability of CT, MRI, nuclear medicine services including PET, MIBG, and bone scan
2. Plain X-ray facility—optimally ultrasound capability	2. Level II PCUs should work in close collaboration with a Level III PCU locally or nationally	2. Availability or access to pathology services, including hematopathology, flow cytometry, cytogenetics, and molecular genetics
3. Have a close link to a higher level PCU which could accept patients with more advanced disease, confirm diagnoses, and recommend treatment		3. Specialized laboratory services with the ability to do all chemistries, special tests, and microbiology
4. Availability of pathology services for diagnosis		
5. Access to an accredited blood bank		

(continued)

Table 5.2 (continued)

Support services		
1. Emergency transportation for patients between institutions or for home	1. Level II PCUs should be able to provide all the services of a Level I PCU and most/many of the services of a Level III PCU	1. Nutrition
		Availability of a dietitian or nutritionist
2. Basic resuscitation equipment on-site including wall or portable oxygen	2. Level II PCUs should work in close collaboration with a Level III PCU locally or nationally	2. Rehabilitation services
		Occupational therapy, physical therapy, speech therapy
3. Adequate hand-washing facilities and sinks		3. Psychosocial services for patient and families
		Social work, child life, pediatric psychology/psychiatry, pastoral care, and teachers
		Neuropsychologist—if possible
4. Transportation for patient-related activities		4. Resources for placement and maintenance of central lines, administration of high-dose chemotherapy, and management of anticipated complications
		5. Long-term follow-up/cancer survivorship program
		6. Palliative care program
		Inpatient and outpatient services with access to home care and hospice
		Staffed by dedicated personnel familiar with pain and symptom management and end-of-life care
		7. Bone marrow/stem cell transplantation program
		Advanced PCUs may, but would not, necessarily need to have an "on-site" BMT/Stem Cell Transplant Program
		8. Parent support group
		9. Availability of a guest house, food, subsidized payment structure, transportation, and housing
Academic activities		
1. Have a close link to a higher level PCU, which could accept patients with more advanced disease, confirm diagnoses, and recommend treatment	1. Level II PCUs should be able to provide all the services of a Level I PCU and most/many of the services of a Level III PCU	1. All Level III PCUs should be linked to a national and/or international multidisciplinary pediatric oncology organization
2. Have the ability to follow simple therapeutic protocols	2. Level II PCUs could be involved in the training of pediatric oncology specialists, but the main responsibility/direction of such training efforts would remain with the Level III units	2. Academic affiliation

3. Continuing education for all physicians and, as appropriate, for other members of the pediatric oncology team. Must attend at least one local/national/international conference or formal meeting devoted to pediatric oncology annually		3. Academic activities
		IRB, Ethics Committee
		Tumor board
		Multidisciplinary conferences
		Participate in a "twinning program" with another center of excellence
		Be directly involved in or have the ability to conduct clinical trials and research
		Be the center for CME conferences, training of residents, fellows, nurses, pharmacists, and social workers
Additional recommendations		
1. Access to microbiology facilities		
2. Only utilize established treatment protocols		

Can We Address Pediatric Cancer in Resource-Limited Settings?

Eighty percent (80 %) of the children with cancer live in low- and middle-income (LMC) [5]. Although regional variations in the incidence of childhood cancers have been reported [6, 7], the high proportion of pediatric cancer in LMC stems primarily from the fact that most of the world's population under 18 years of age lives in LMC [8]. The etiology of childhood cancers remains predominantly unknown [6, 7] and increases in incidence of childhood cancer in LMC are usually a reflection of improved detection rates [2, 5]. Mortality from childhood cancer on the other hand is significantly higher in LMC compared to HIC, with a survival gap >50 % between some LMC and HIC [2]. Therefore, the highest burden of pediatric cancer in LMC and the centerpiece of cancer disparities between HIC and LMC does not result from high or changing incidence, but from differences in cancer-related mortality. In order to address this burden, PCUs in LMC can focus on reducing the risk of cancer-related death by promoting early diagnosis, delivering effective care, reducing the risk of treatment-related death, and reducing treatment abandonment (Fig. 5.4).

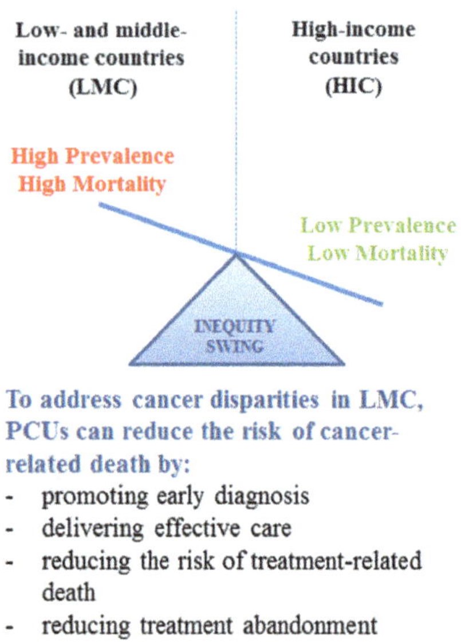

Fig. 5.4 Cancer disparities inequity swing

What about LIC or extreme resource-limited settings (ERLS)? What can clinicians do to address pediatric cancer in these settings? While providing an answer, experts in HIC sometimes struggle with envisioning pediatric cancer care without the full spectrum of technologies routinely used for diagnosis, monitoring, and treatment. In contrast, clinicians in LIC or ERLS struggle with how not to address pediatric cancer despite known human resource scarcity, equipment shortages, and high workloads. Clinicians in LMC are witnesses to how, as standards of living improve and health systems are strengthened, the burden of cancer becomes more noticeable and the need to address it imperative [9].

When addressing pediatric cancer in LMC, clinicians should keep in mind pediatric cancer is a heterogeneous group of diseases. Therefore centers in LMC, even those in ERLS, can make valuable contributions to the burden of childhood cancer in their settings. In this section we summarize four key examples of optimization of resources: the case-by-case approach; protocol development and prioritization; comprehensive integration of pain, palliative, and psychosocial services; and capacity building and education through twinning.

The Case-by-Case Approach: Epidemiologists seek to understand patterns, causes, and consequences of childhood cancer; pediatric oncology collaborative groups seek to standardize care and study and compare best strategies; and public health departments seek to address prevention, screening, and delivery of care at the population level. However, ultimately, cancer occurs at the level of the individual and must be addressed case by case. Even in pediatric oncology centers of excellence in HIC where access and standardization are the norm, the fit between open collaborative trials, standards of care, patient and family's goals of therapy, and the patient's diagnosis and clinical situation is made case by case. When making decisions about pediatric oncology treatment, centers in LMC, including ERLS, must consider factors such as the patient's status,

Table 5.3 Factors to consider when making decisions about pediatric oncology treatment using the case-by-case approach

Patient	Therapeutic plan	Resources	Nonbiologic factors
Diagnosis	Goals of therapy	Chemotherapy safety	Direct and indirect costs of therapy
Extent of disease	Expected toxicity	Supportive care	Transportation, housing, income
Nutritional status	Expected morbidity (from treatment, surgery, or radiation)	Surgical equipment and postoperative care	Culture and values
Comorbidities	Resectability (upfront surgery vs. delayed)	Radiation therapy access, planning, and toxicity	Family's goals and understanding
	Radiation therapy (upfront vs. delayed)	Rehabilitation services	

proposed therapeutic plan, resources available, and nonbiologic factors (see Table 5.3).

Regarding the development and implementation of protocols in LMC, experience tells us that the most intense and aggressive regimen is not always the best answer [10]. This occurs because high therapeutic intensity must be matched by highly skilled and resourceful supportive care in order to prevent toxic and septic deaths [11, 12]. However, for most localized childhood cancers, a curative strategy can be identified and attempted upfront; even lower-resource settings (see chapters by disease for details on recommended strategies by setting). Once treatment is initiated, if the biology of the cancer proves to be more aggressive than the therapy that can be safely delivered (which would be evidenced by disease progression, early relapse, or refractoriness), the goals of therapy can be reassessed and intensification of palliative care services strongly considered or pursued. This action would be supported by ethical principles of beneficence and non-maleficence.

Regarding nonbiologic factors, these are important for the comprehensive assessment of each case and for advanced planning (examples listed in Table 5.3). However, although nonbiologic factors such as socioeconomic status have been associated with treatment abandonment [13, 14], PCUs should aim to address barriers to care rather than incorporate them into their triage criteria. Resource limitations at the patient level should not be the cornerstone used to guide decisions about curative vs. palliative upfront therapeutic intent. Case studies from World Child Cancer foundation [15] and Partners in Health [16] serve as evidence of how the case-by-case approach can change and save lives in LIC and ELRS. Even in the most extreme situations, sometimes, cure can be achieved.

Protocol Development and Prioritization: Based on the great improvements in survival for children with cancer in HIC over the past 50 years [17, 18], childhood cancer is often portrayed as "highly curable" and efforts in HIC are increasingly funneled to address long-term effects or survivorship [19]. However, pediatric cancer is heterogeneous and wide variation in outcomes exists between diagnoses and between subgroups of diagnoses. This is the case for example in standard and refractory childhood leukemia [20], favorable and unfavorable histology Wilms' tumor [21], low- and high-risk pediatric sarcomas [22], and *N-MYC*-amplified and non-*N-MYC*-amplified neuroblastoma [23]. In each instance there are both highly favorable and highly refractory disease groups, some of which are resistant to even the most technologically advanced oncologic care. Therefore, PCUs in LMC must critically assess their capacities and resources, develop or implement protocols based on their setting, adjust intensity to match supportive care capabilities, and track outcomes. It is often necessary to start with diagnoses for which all components of treatment can be secured and that offer a high survival probability, then gradually expand and intensify therapy while remaining watchful to ensure a favorable balance between the toxicity profile, supportive care

Table 5.4 Common childhood cancers by 5-year survival in HIC

>75 % survival	50–75 % survival	30–50 % survival	<30 % survival
Standard-risk B-ALL High-risk B-ALL	T-ALL (high risk) High-stage ALCL	Very-high-risk ALL Diffuse anaplasia stage IV, stage V Wilms' Tumor	Infant ALL Metastatic osteosarcoma
Low-risk AML	Stage III Wilms' tumor with diffuse anaplasia	High-risk NB	Metastatic Ewing sarcoma
Low-stage NHL	Localized osteosarcoma	High-risk RMS (one adverse factor)	High-risk RMS (>1 adverse factor)
High-stage B-NHL Stage I–IV HL Stage I and II Wilms' tumor Stage III–V Wilms' tumor with FH Low- and intermediate-risk NB Low-risk RMS Intraocular RB Standard-risk MB CML (with imatinib) Nasopharyngeal carcinoma	Localized Ewing sarcoma Intermediate-risk RMS Extraocular RB Soft tissue sarcomas	High-risk AML Metastatic RB	Brainstem and high-grade gliomas

Based on data reported at National Cancer Institute PDQ Cancer Topics by Disease (available at http://www.cancer.gov/cancertopics/types/alphalist)

B-ALL B-cell acute lymphoblastic leukemia, *T-ALL* T-cell acute lymphoblastic leukemia, *ALL* acute lymphoblastic leukemia, *AML* acute myeloid leukemia, *NHL* non-Hodgkin's lymphoma, *B-NHL* B-cell non-Hodgkin's lymphoma, *HL* Hodgkin's lymphoma, *FH* favorable histology, *NB* neuroblastoma, *RMS* rhabdomyosarcoma, *RB* retinoblastoma, *ALCL* anaplastic large cell lymphoma, *MB* medulloblastoma

capabilities, and outcomes. Table 5.4 summarizes common childhood cancers by prognosis and risk group.

Common reaction to implementing a prioritization strategy include ethical and human rights concerns. Prioritization of one disease over another may be perceived as unfair and difficult to apply at the bedside. Reductions in treatment intensity may be perceived to equal the provision of suboptimal care.

Prioritization is a strategic process that does necessarily appeal naturally to clinicians but is increasingly applied in healthcare, even in HIC [24]. In countries with limited resources, which diagnostic groups are systematically approached with curative intent and which are approached with palliative intent is ideally not for one clinician to decide. Ideally, prioritization is based on consensus, recognition of the described heterogeneity of childhood cancers, and a critical assessment of strengths, weaknesses, resources, and experience at the PCU and decisions stem from agreement between providers and review of evidence-based literature. The discussion integrates the ministry of health and supporting national and international organizations. Importantly, prioritization does not contradict clinical judgment and therefore, the case-by-case approach. The benefit of a prioritization strategy is that it can pool and streamline resources, improve transparency, and help relieve the bedside clinician in ERLS from the burden of ad hoc prioritization based on day-to-day adequacy of resources and shortages.

Regarding concerns about reductions in therapeutic intensity, the experience gained from treatment of low-stage Burkitt lymphoma in Africa documents how standardization of care and implementation of dose reductions can increase rather than decrease survival compared to higher intensity regimens in ERLS [25]. Similar positive balances have been documented for leukemia [26], Wilms' tumor [27], and rhabdomyosarcoma [28] in other continents with the use of reduced intensity regimens. This counterintuitive outcome results from reduction of treatment-related mortality (toxic deaths) when supportive care is suboptimal. Therefore, in the development and strengthening of PCUs, intensity reductions are not only ethically justified but imperative. Finally, PCUs should not be perceived as static; as improvements in diagnostics, therapeutics, and supportive care occur, centers in LMC can provide more intensive and complex therapies and achieve results comparable to HIC [29–31].

Comprehensive Integration of Pain, Palliative and Psychosocial Services: Two-thirds of patients with advanced cancer have pain [32]. However, although the burden of cancer is highest in LMC [5], access to pain and palliative care services in LMC is considerably limited [33], including for children with cancer [34]. Furthermore, little is known about the quality of hospice and palliative care that is actually provided in most LMC [33]. Therefore, among the largest impact a PCU can have on the burden of pediatric cancer to patient and families, from the lowest to the highest resource level, is the development of comprehensive and well-integrated pain, palliative, and psychosocial teams. Detailed strategies for the implementation of palliative and supportive care in pediatric oncology settings are available in Chap. 11. Definitions and psychosocial strategies to address treatment abandonment in LMC are addressed in Chap. 12.

The World Health Organization (WHO) also advocates for palliative care service integration into the development of national cancer programs [35]. WHO defines palliative care as an approach that improves the quality of life of patients and their families facing the problems associated with life-threatening illness, through the prevention and relief of suffering by means of early identification and impeccable assessment and treatment of pain and other problems—physical, psychosocial, and spiritual [36].

As PCUs are conceptualized and built, its leadership must recognize that integration of these services into existing medical care or health systems is not necessarily easy. Described barriers for the implementation of pain and palliative care programs in LMC include financial and material resources, problems relating to opioid availability, problems with regulations surrounding the prescription of opioids, lack of public awareness, lack of government recognition of palliative care as a field of specialization, and lack of pain and palliative care education and training programs [33, 37, 38]. In the case of children, palliative care is further complicated by the need to support both the patient and the parents [36]. Furthermore, effective pain management is complicated by misconceptions about pain in this age group, variability in practice, and active or passive denial (Fig. 5.5) [39]. However, reports from LMC working to address these barriers show that they can be surpassed [40–42].

The palliative care field has seen a paradigm shift in recent years [43], which may improve receptivity of palliative care services in LMC. In the past, palliative care services were incorporated into cancer care as a sudden transition from curative therapy to end-of-life care (Fig. 5.6a). More recently, the early and consonant integration of pain and palliative care services has been advocated, with focus given to pain management, quality of life, advanced directives, etc., rather than exclusively to "end-of-life" issues (Fig. 5.6b). In this revised framework, palliative care is integrated into the comprehensive care of the patient and provided along with disease-modifying or curative therapy. This paradigm shift is important because not all patients facing a life-threatening illness will ultimately die from the illness, yet all patients need support in facing the enormous challenge. In PCUs in countries with limited resources, this paradigm shift may positively impact receptivity by fostering the building of integrated teams for pain, palliative, and psychosocial services (Fig. 5.6c). In LMC, human resources are often scarce; therefore, having a team that will have a role for all children with cancer at the PCU and able to offer care throughout the course of treatment is a strong motivator for building a robust and dedicated pediatric integrated pain, palliative, and psychosocial team. Of particular interest are teams apt to respond to the particular needs of a child, rather than relying in a general or adult palliative care service. Figure 5.7 shows suggestions for an integrative team at the PCU.

Fig. 5.5 Barriers to effective pain management in children

Barriers to effective pain management in children and adolescents:

- Outmoded beliefs:
    - Newborn infants do not experience pain
    - Children rarely require analgesia
    - Pain is merely a symptom and not necessarily harmful in itself
    - Effective analgesia is dangerous, makes diagnosis difficult or impossible, delays discharge
- Variability in practice:
    - Postoperative analgesia not prescribed
    - Analgesia is prescribed, but doses are too low or too infrequent
- Active or passive denial:
    - Analgesia not administered because pain not assessed
    - Pain denied by children due to fear of intramuscular injection

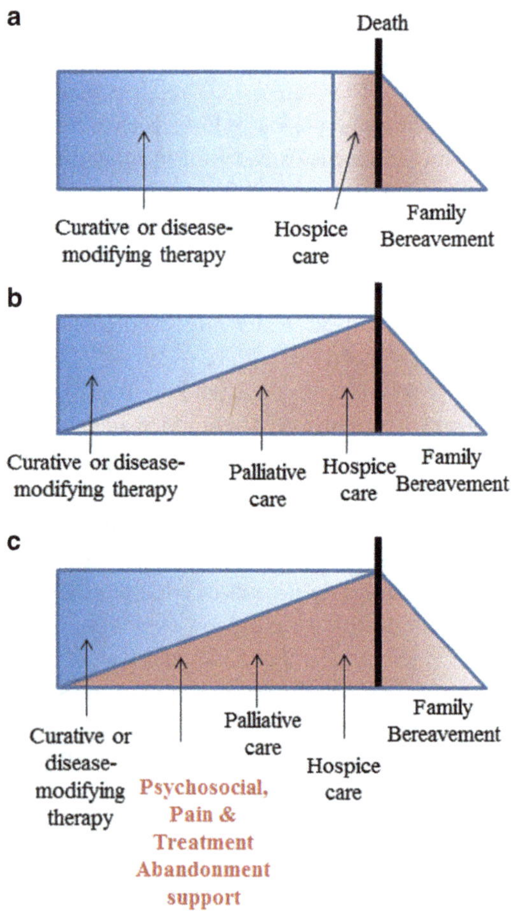

Fig. 5.6 Paradigm shifts in palliative care (**a**, **b**) and recommended paradigm for implementation in LMC (**c**)

Building an integrative pain, palliative care, and psychosocial team:

- Visibility: Build one strong team that knows the patients throughout treatment and positively interacts with the oncology team and ancillary staff
- Timing: Encourage clinicians to involve the team early even if cure is likely (for emotional support, quality of life concerns, and for the prevention of treatment abandonment)
- Pain: Train the team to be vigilant and avid about pain assessment and management
- Narcotics: As a start, focus on oral formulations (they are highly effective, more accessible than intravenous formulations, and can address pain at home)
- Awareness: Raise awareness regarding pain assessment and management, quality of life, and palliative care among patients, families, nursing staff, and trainees
- Education: Continuously educate staff and trainees on frameworks, strategies, and algorithms used at the center and the vocabulary to use with patients when addressing psychosocial, pain & palliative care concerns
- Regulations: Liaison with others to revise national drug legislation and facilitate the availability of analgesic drugs for patients
- Governmental commitment: Liaison with others to seek governmental commitment for the provision of pain and palliative care services to cancer patients

Fig. 5.7 Suggestions for building an integrative pain, palliative care, and psychosocial team in the pediatric cancer units

Capacity Building and Education Through "Twinning": The fourth and last strategy discussed in this chapter to address pediatric cancer in LMC is perhaps the best described [3] and studied [1, 44–47]. The concept of twinning entails a long-term commitment between two partners, usually one from a resource-rich and one from a resource-poor environment. Sharing of knowledge, capacity building, education, and training are cornerstones of the process. See Chap. 4 for examples and more information.

In brief, through twinning programs, PCUs receive technical and financial support to improve clinical practice, build multidisciplinary care teams, access expert opinion, escalate staff education, guide strategic planning, increase accountability, and diversify funding sources, among others [3], and most importantly, decrease treatment abandonment, decrease toxic deaths, and improve survival for children with cancer [1]. Challenges for development of twinning programs include treatment abandonment and the socioeconomic supports needed to address it, shortage of trained nurses, suboptimal infection control, insufficient funds, cost and availability of medications, late diagnosis, and incorrect diagnosis [3].

However, the benefits of twinning programs are not unidirectional, as summarized by the World Child Cancer Foundation in their online resources about twinning [48] (Fig. 5.8). Twinning programs can be of benefit to centers and hospitals in both lower- as well as higher-income countries. The number of twinning programs has risen over the past decade and a survey of all twinning programs is not currently available. However, as of 2013, the authors estimate over 30 twinning programs to exist worldwide.

The collaborations below are only a few examples of twinning programs, all of which have shown how development or upgrading PCUs through the twinning model can foster capacity building, improvements in care, and clinical research. The cost-benefit of these programs has not been studied, but most would agree the benefits are substantial for their relatively low cost.

1. St Jude Children's Research Hospital's International Outreach Program long-standing partnership with the Association of Central American Pediatric Hematologists and Oncologists (AHOPCA) in Latin America for

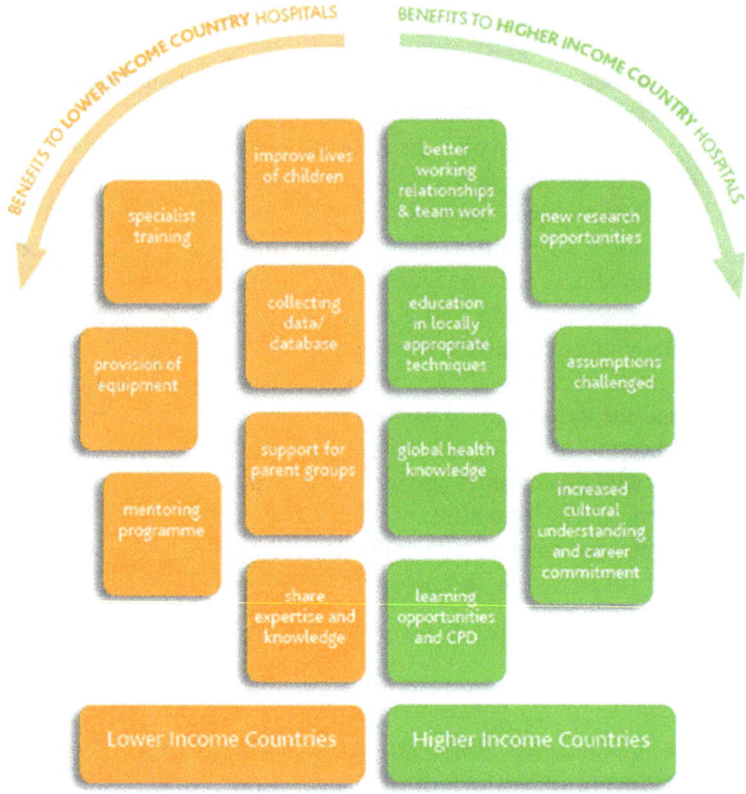

Fig. 5.8 Benefits of twinning for lower- and higher-income countries

twinning, clinical research support, and development of a pediatric oncology fellowship program in Guatemala [12, 49–52]
2. Monza's International School of Pediatric Hematology-Oncology (MISPHO) in Milan, Italy, partnership for twinning, training, and clinical research support with "La Mascota" Hospital in Nicaragua and other Central American countries [53–55]
3. Dana-Farber/Boston Children's Global Health Initiative twinning with the National Cancer Institute in Bogota, Colombia, Collaboration for improved pediatric sarcoma care in Central America, and partnership with Children's Cancer Hospital Egypt 57357 for development of a pediatric oncology fellowship program [52, 56, 57]
4. International Network for Cancer Research and Treatment (INCTR)/Georgetown University partnership with Tikur Anbessa Hospital in Ethiopia for twinning and development of a pediatric oncology fellowship program [58].

PCUs from LMC at any stage in their development, new or established, big or small, can benefit from establishing twining relationships with international partners and cooperative relationships with regional partners. This is detailed in the suggested steps to implementation of national pediatric oncology programs in resource-poor countries originally proposed by Howard et al. [54] and included in St. Jude Children's Research Hospital International Outreach Program in their "Guide to Establishing a Pediatric Oncology Twinning Program" [3] (Table 5.5).

In summary, this section described four strategies to address pediatric oncology in countries with limited resources: the case-by-case approach; protocol development and prioritization; comprehensive integration of pain, palliative care, and psychosocial services; and capacity building and education through twinning. Hopefully, clinical and nonclinical readers feel more apt to answering questions on what clinicians and staff at PCUs

Table 5.5 Suggested steps for the implementation of national pediatric oncology programs in LMC

Phase	Purpose	Requirements	Role of outsiders	Examples
Demonstration project	A successful pilot project demonstrates that childhood cancer can be cured in the local setting	A dedicated local leader and a twinning relationship with a center of excellence in a resource-rich country	Provide essential technical support in protocol selection and monitoring, safety measures, nursing education, and organizational structure	Lilongwe Central Hospital, Malawi
			Provide essential financial support for staff retention, education, and needs otherwise unmet	
Pediatric cancer unit	Centralizes resources devoted to the treatment of childhood cancer to improve efficiency and the quality of care	Cooperation of a variety of pediatric specialists and support of the hospital administration	Provide essential technical support in clinical care, capacity building, education and training, nursing, strategic planning, and clinical research	La Mascota Children's Hospital, Managua, Nicaragua
			Provide financial support for staff retention, education, innovative projects, and clinical research	
Multidisciplinary program	Expansion of the pediatric cancer unit to offer broad range of activities	Mobilization of patients, parents, the government, and nongovernmental organizations	Modest technical support in multidisciplinary care, patient-centered care, education, and training	Instituto Materno Infantil de Pernambuco, Recife, Brazil
			Modest financial support for staff retention, education, and innovative projects	
Decentralization projects	Extend the benefits to a wider geographical area and reduce the burden of travel on families from distant areas	Training and supervision of satellite-center personnel by the center of excellence with increased governmental support	Modest technical and financial support for design, monitoring, and evaluation of outcome for specific projects	Hospital Materno Infantil, Tegucigalpa, Honduras
Regional program	Increased quality of care and independence of centers of excellence and satellite centers with coverage of a wide geographic area (province, state, or adjacent small countries)	The regional government takes responsibility for treatment of all children with cancer as a regional priority	Minor technical and financial support for educational meetings, knowledge-sharing, data management and sharing, communication tools, and clinical research	AHOPCA (Association of Central American Pediatric Hematologists and Oncologists), Central America
National program	Nationwide network of pediatric oncology units. National pediatric oncology association for protocol design, continuing education, and advocacy activities	The national government takes responsibility for treatment of all children with cancer as a national priority	Advisory only	PINDA (National Program for access to chemotherapy for children), Chile

Adapted from the St. Jude Children's Research Hospital International Outreach Program in their "Guide to Establishing a Pediatric Oncology Twinning Program." Column titled "Role of Outsiders" expanded to include examples of technical and financial support can do to address pediatric cancer in LIC and ERLS. Furthermore, they are hopefully able to recognize that PCUs from all levels in the resource spectrum can make valuable contributions to the burden of childhood cancer in their settings.

What Can We Learn from Other Experiences? Why and How Is the Approach to Pediatric Cancer Different from Other Diseases?

What Can We Learn from the HIV Experience? The global response to the HIV/AIDS epidemic was unprecedented. The HIV/AIDS experience taught the international community that known socioeconomic disparities should not be allowed to promote disparities in care [59]. At the start of the HIV global epidemic, the goal of making highly active antiretroviral therapy (HAART) accessible to HIV-infected persons living in LIC was met with skepticism, primarily due to economic reasons (i.e., the high cost of ARVs, lack of adequate medical infrastructure, and difficulties with adherence) [59, 60]. For years the international response to HIV/AIDS in poor countries emphasized HIV prevention over treatment [60], which sent the message that across-the-board palliation was appropriate in LMC. However, human rights advocates, clinicians on the ground, and patients, among others, made a strong ethical, social, and economic case against this approach [60]. By confronting a double standard that justified action for the rich and inaction for the poor, HIV/AIDS advocates were able to foster the development of a more integral approach combining prevention, treatment, and palliation along with strengthening of healthcare delivery systems. Although perhaps not all programs and interventions have proved to be successful [61], most would agree that the act of action has been a positive one for individuals and the health systems in which they receive care.

Pediatric cancers and HIV/AIDS are very different diseases. One is a noncommunicable disease (NCD) that arises from heterogeneous defects in cell-cycle regulatory mechanisms, leads to broad manifestations of disease (depending on cell type, location, and aggressiveness), and requires meticulous selection of a therapeutic plan. The second is a communicable disease with an identified vector, transmission pattern, measurable impact in the host's immune system, and narrower compendium of drugs and therapeutic strategies needed to treat patients. Despite their differences, another lesson to be learned from the HIV epidemic resides in the debate it generated regarding the funding and promotion of "vertical" vs. "horizontal" vs. "diagonal" healthcare programs and interventions (see Table 5.6) [62–64].

The initial response to HIV was primarily "vertical" with creation of stand-alone programs for delivery of antiretroviral therapy (ART) [62]. However, over time the evaluation of ART impact on population health and the shifting of funding priorities led to interesting debates among public policy and public health researchers [62, 64]. In pediatric oncology, leukemia and/or lymphoma demonstration projects more closely resemble vertical programs, even under the twinning framework [1, 25]. However, as the PCU expands services to diagnosis and treatment of solid tumors, vertical approaches may fall short in the provision of multimodal and multidisciplinary care due to infrastructure, human resource, and organizational deficits and improvements in outcomes lag behind those achieved for leukemia and/or lymphoma [52]. National cancer programs are of value, but in LMC they are often primarily focused on provision of screening and preventive adult cancer care [35]. Therefore, as PCUs grow, diagonal strategies may be of most short- and long-term value. For example, in the development of solid tumor programs and interventions to improve and strengthen pathology, radiology, and surgery services, leaders should not assume that a positive "spillover" effect will occur and be of value to other services. Instead, leaders should be explicit regarding the design of how interventions will improve the general status of health systems in the hospital, city, or country.

Table 5.6 Vertical vs. horizontal vs. diagonal interventions

Vertical	Horizontal	Diagonal
Disease specific	Integrated, generalized, comprehensive intervention	Mixed approach
Single-purpose machinery	Usually public	Aims for disease-specific results through improved health systems
Intervention focused	Tackle problems on a wide-front and on a long-term basis	Uses explicit intervention priorities to drive required improvements into health systems
Freestanding	Create permanent institutions	
Often transient/temporary	Include a variety of managerial and operational changes to health systems	
Rapid responses are possible		
Attractive for donors		
Easier to manage		
Spillover to more generalized healthcare system is expected		
Illustrative metaphor		
Fragile, islands of sufficiency in seas of under provision	Generalized insufficiency	Broad-based islands of sufficiency in a swamp of insufficiency

Sources: Atun et al., Ooms et al., and Msuya et al. Illustrative metaphors in Ooms et al. (see references)

What Can We Apply from WHO Strategies to Address Adult Cancers? The World Health Organization (WHO) Cancer Control Knowledge into Action Guides for Effective Programs address planning, palliative care, diagnosis and treatment, advocacy, early detection, and prevention. These guides and other WHO guides and resources are available online free of charge [65]. WHO and the International Union against Cancer (IUAC) encourage clinicians and policy-makers to focus on four broad approaches to cancer: prevent, cure, care, and manage. In pediatric oncology, prevention and screening are of little or no value, but timely and accurate diagnosis and prompt initiation of treatment are key for reducing morbidity and mortality from disease and its stage-dependent interventions [66]. In countries with limited resources, PCUs can study reasons for lag time and determine their origin, establish education campaigns in the community, document impact, and positively improve pediatric cancer outcomes in their settings [66–68].

Can We Address the "Natural" Conflict Between Pediatric Cancer and Other Pediatric Diseases in Public LMC Hospitals? Pediatric oncology care is demanding, complex, time-consuming, and sometimes expensive. Furthermore, it requires multi and interdisciplinary interventions. As described in Table 5.1, many PCUs are in or adjacent to a general pediatric public hospital. Therefore, the goals, mandates, and needs of the pediatric hospital must be taken into account. As PCUs are developed, tension is often noticeable between the goals and needs of the PCU and the priorities of the pediatric hospital. PCUs and more general institutions may appear to be working under opposing rather than consonant frameworks. As shown in Fig. 5.9, this tension can occur because public tertiary pediatric hospitals are often dealing with high-volume, population changes; increased burden of other NCDs; political changes; budgetary constraints; fragmentation concerns; and accountability issues. Recognizing and understanding the contextual reality, leadership at the PCU must work to identify "triggers" that can help the two "systems" function in more consonant ways. Possible triggers include twinning programs, education and training of staff, building of dedicated teams, projects in common, implementation of diagonal interventions, sharing of outcomes, and incentives (Fig. 5.10).

The twinning literature evidences that these triggers work and can have long-term measurable

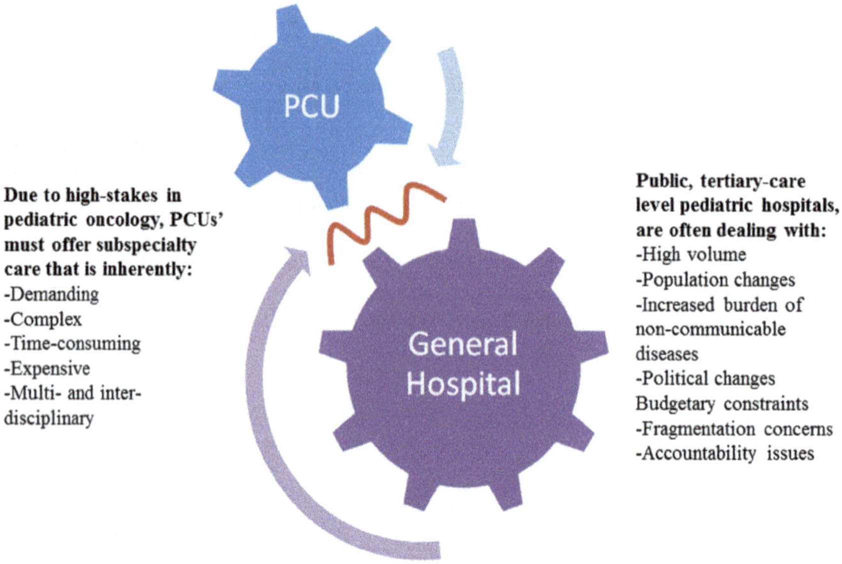

Fig. 5.9 The "natural conflict": PCUs and general pediatric hospitals can often appear to be working in opposite directions

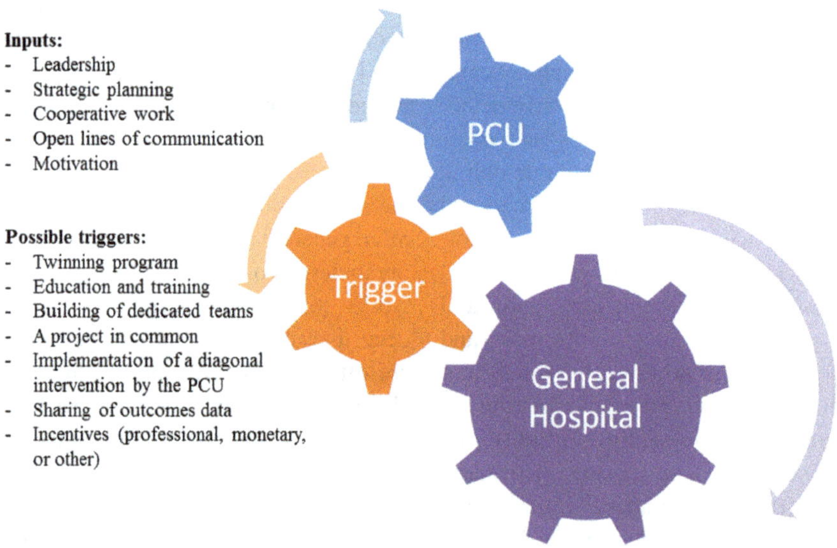

Fig. 5.10 The solution: leadership in the PCU must work to identify the common triggers that can help the systems work in a consonant way

benefits [1, 45–47, 69]. However, experience tells us that these triggers (external interventions) can also transiently put more pressure in the system than was originally intended. With good strategic planning, cooperative work, open lines of communication, and motivation, PCUs can overcome these "growing pains" and the system can positively "reset" into more consonant motion.

What Are Some Assumptions That Can Discourage Staff and Set the PCU Back?

In building and developing a PCU in countries with limited resources, four assumptions need to be explicitly addressed by the PCU leadership:

Pediatric Cancer Is Incurable in Countries with Limited Resources: In countries with limited resources where little or no treatment is available for children with cancer, a diagnosis of cancer can be perceived to carry a sentence for painful death. Healthcare workers can become discouraged from caring for these patients; withdrawal or neglect can result as a coping strategy. Furthermore, although some healthcare workers are aware of the high rate of cure of cancer in the high-income countries, they strongly believe cure of a patient with pediatric cancer cannot be achieved in their setting. Treatment of cancer is known to be expensive, and healthcare workers know that when little resources exist, countries will often prioritize using resources to address other major public health issues that can be treated at lower cost and/or with simpler measures (e.g., infectious diseases, malnutrition, neonatal mortality). Leadership at the PCU must address these notions and apprehensions explicitly. Demonstration projects at PCUs can show staff, supporters, and society that childhood cancer can be cured and kindly and effectively cared for in their setting.

Pediatric Cancer Is Always Curable: Improvements in outcome for children with cancer in HIC from survival of less than 30 % to more than 80 % in 6 decades allow talking of pediatric cancer as a "curable" disease. However, these outcomes must be interpreted in the context they occurred: long, systematic, and dedicated commitment to improve outcomes by cooperative groups and efficient provision of multimodal therapy and multidisciplinary care. Although rapid improvement in outcomes can be achieved in countries with limited resources for specific diseases with high cure rates [1], the cure rate for pediatric cancers needing more advanced or complex care can lag behind [52] and discourage staff. Leadership at the PCU must be explicit with staff and supporters about short- and long-term expectations from the interventions implemented. Also, help them recognize that maximal cure rates are achieved through dedicated, long-term, strategic commitment to improving outcomes (a "marathon") rather than quick or improvised interventions (a "sprint").

Pediatric Cancer = Leukemia: Acute leukemia is the most common pediatric cancer. In countries with limited resources, this often results in the focus of clinical, educational, and research to begin with addressing leukemia. However, pediatric cancer is heterogeneous and interventions that work for patients with leukemia cannot be assumed to work and have similar impact or magnitude in other pediatric cancers, particularly extracranial solid tumors and brain tumors. Leadership at PCUs needs to recognize the specific needs for each disease group and be explicit with staff and supporters about how and why interventions should be implemented differently for different groups.

Cure Is the Only Measure of Success: As discussed in this and other chapters, leadership at PCUs should work with staff and supporters to shift from a focus on "cure" to a focus on "care." This mind-set is not a way to justify disparities in access or delivery of curative therapy in countries with limited resources, but a way to change focus from the goal outcome (cure) to the process (care). This shift in mind-set would help the PCU create a culture focused on improving, for example, (a) supportive, multidisciplinary, and palliative care; (b) safety, quality, early diagnosis, treatment abandonment, and psychosocial interventions; and (c) fragmentations in health delivery systems. Each time a child with cancer passes away, the staff can feel discouraged and lose motivation. However, a culture that validates the value of all interventions performed in the process of providing care can help staff validate their work and cope with loss.

How Can We Optimize Resources? Final Recommendations

As described throughout the chapter, LMC differ greatly from each other in availability of resources, economic growth, social and political structure, and current status of healthcare services and infrastructure. All these factors play a role in what a PCU in a particular country looks like. "No one prescription works for all." However, to establish, maintain and expand services in a PCU, it is essential that resources are optimized and shared to achieve maximal success.

Identifying Strengths and Weaknesses of the PCU: Site visits, needs assessment, and studies of the healthcare system and current available resources are essential prior to setting up a new PCU and periodically thereafter. This helps greatly in identifying resources, deciding protocols and treatment strategies by disease, potential sources of funding, and potential partners.

Establishing a Twinning Program: Using the "twinning" model, partnerships between institutions in high- and low- resource settings have been particularly effective in pediatric cancer treatment. More than 30 programs are estimated to exist as of 2013 and as described in this chapter and Chap. 4, the benefits are substantial for both the lower- and higher-income partner.

Maximizing Distance Learning and Collaboration: Probably the most important element of a successful PCU is capacity building—training the doctors, nurses, and other personnel involved in a PCU. It can be a very costly venture, whether it is done through visiting faculty, short-term exchanges, or hiring of qualified pediatric oncologists on the site. Informal case-based learning can be achieved for low cost through discussion of cases with international collaborators using telemedicine. A successful example of more formal distance learning is the Cure4Kids website [44] (www.cure4kids.org)—an internet-based distance-learning program provided free to physicians, nurses, scientists, and healthcare workers who treat children with cancer. The site is used by almost 8,400 professionals in over 155 countries and has been extremely effective in the growth of PCUs in LMC. The internet tools include:

1. Online education on cancer and other catastrophic illnesses
2. Work space for online meetings and conferences
3. Technology and training for better management of patient information
4. Access to digital material, articles, and online seminars and courses

Building of regional and international collaborations and initiatives:

1. More efforts are being devoted to the development of regional programs, which include joint seminars, workshops, training, and research collaboration.
2. Successful examples are those established by the AHOPCA and the INCTR Pathology Program in East Africa, among others.
3. An effort is currently in the preliminary stages to pool orders for chemotherapy agents for several countries in one region of Africa, in order to negotiate better prices from pharmaceutical companies.

Monitoring of progress and outcomes:

1. Incorporating clinical research into clinical practice and studying resource optimization through cost-benefit research are vital to the success of a PCU.
2. This is best done through collaboration with a partner in an HIC, twinning, and research grants.
3. "My Child Matters," Jiv Daya Foundation, and more recently the NIH offer competitive grants for projects in developing countries.

References

1. Howard SC, Pedrosa M, Lins M, et al. Establishment of a pediatric oncology program and outcomes of childhood acute lymphoblastic leukemia in a resource-poor area. JAMA. 2004;291(20):2471–5.
2. Ribeiro RC, Steliarova-Foucher E, Magrath I, et al. Baseline status of paediatric oncology care in ten low-income or mid-income countries receiving My Child Matters support: a descriptive study. Lancet Oncol. 2008;9(8):721–9.

3. St. Jude Children's Research Hospital. International Outreach Program: guide to establishing a Pediatric Oncology Twinning Program. Available at: http://www.stjude.org/SJFile/IOP_Twinning_Manual_082908.pdf. Accessed 10 July 2013.
4. International Society of Paediatric Oncology (SIOP). Standards of care and training 1991 document. Available at: http://www.siop-online.org/page/standards-care-and-training-1991-document. Accessed 12 July 2013.
5. Howard SC, Metzger ML, Wilimas JA, et al. Childhood cancer epidemiology in low-income countries. Cancer. 2008;112(3):461–72.
6. Bunin GR. Nongenetic causes of childhood cancers: evidence from international variation, time trends, and risk factor studies. Toxicol Appl Pharmacol. 2004;199(2):91–103.
7. Stiller CA, Parkin DM. Geographic and ethnic variations in the incidence of childhood cancer. Br Med Bull. 1996;52(4):682–703.
8. Polulation Reference Bureau—2012 World population data sheet. Available at: http://www.prb.org/pdf12/2012-population-data-sheet_eng.pdf. Accessed 27 May 2013.
9. 2008–2013 Action Plan for the global strategy for the prevention and control of noncommunicable diseases. Geneva Switzerland: WHO Press. Available at: http://www.who.int/cancer/en/. Accessed 30 Jan 2012. (Printed by WHO Document Production Services, Geneva, Switzerland).
10. Israels T, Chagaluka G, Pidini D, et al. The efficacy and toxicity of SIOP preoperative chemotherapy in Malawian children with a Wilms tumour. Pediatr Blood Cancer. 2012;59(4):636–41.
11. Gupta S, Bonilla M, Fuentes SL, et al. Incidence and predictors of treatment-related mortality in paediatric acute leukaemia in El Salvador. Br J Cancer. 2009;100(7):1026–31.
12. Gupta S, Bonilla M, Valverde P, et al. Treatment-related mortality in children with acute myeloid leukaemia in Central America: incidence, timing and predictors. Eur J Cancer. 2012;48(9):1363–9.
13. Sweet-Cordero A, Antillon F, Baez F, et al. Factors that influence abandonment of care among children with cancer in Guatemala [abstract]. Med Pediatr Oncol. 1999;33:151.
14. Bonilla M, Rossell N, Salaverria C, et al. Prevalence and predictors of abandonment of therapy among children with cancer in El Salvador. Int J Cancer. 2009;125(9):2144–6.
15. World Child Cancer. Case studies—our patients. Available at: http://www.worldchildcancer.org/what-we-do/case-studies/patient-case-studies/. Accessed 24 May 2013.
16. Partners in Health. Revolutionary cancer care in Rwanda. Available at: http://www.pih.org/blog/revolutionary-cancer-care-in-rwanda. Accessed 24 May 2013.
17. Smith MA, Seibel NL, Altekruse SF, et al. Outcomes for children and adolescents with cancer: challenges for the twenty-first century. J Clin Oncol. 2010;28(15):2625–34.
18. Kaatsch P. Epidemiology of childhood cancer. Cancer Treat Rev. 2010;36(4):277–85.
19. Rowland JH. Foreword: looking beyond cure: pediatric cancer as a model. J Pediatr Psychol. 2005;30(1):1–3.
20. August KJ, Narendran A, Neville KA. Pediatric relapsed or refractory leukemia: new pharmacotherapeutic developments and future directions. Drugs. 2013;73(5):439–61.
21. Davidoff AM. Wilms' tumor. Curr Opin Pediatr. 2009;21(3):357–64.
22. Hawkins DS, Spunt SL, Skapek SX. Children's Oncology Group's 2013 blueprint for research: soft tissue sarcomas. Pediatr Blood Cancer. 2013;60(6):1001–8.
23. Zage PE, Louis CU, Cohn SL. New aspects of neuroblastoma treatment: ASPHO 2011 symposium review. Pediatr Blood Cancer. 2012;58(7):1099–105.
24. Kenny N. Uncharted territory: Hippocratic ethics and health systems. CMAJ. 2006;174(10):1385; 1387.
25. Hesseling PB, Molyneux E, Tchintseme F, et al. Treating Burkitt's lymphoma in Malawi, Cameroon, and Ghana. Lancet Oncol. 2008;9(6):512–3.
26. Luo XQ, Ke ZY, Guan XQ, Zhang YC, Huang LB, Zhu J. The comparison of outcome and cost of three protocols for childhood non-high risk acute lymphoblastic leukemia in China. Pediatr Blood Cancer. 2008;51(2):204–9.
27. Trehan A, Chowdhary SK, Marwaha RK. Wilms tumor: five-year tumor-free survival on a modified SIOP protocol from an Indian university hospital. J Pediatr Hematol Oncol. 2012;34(1):57–62.
28. Al-Jumaily U, Ayyad O, Masarweh M, et al. Improved care of rhabdomyosarcoma in Jordan using less intensive therapy. Pediatr Blood Cancer. 2013;60(1):53–8.
29. Muwakkit S, Al-Aridi C, Samra A, et al. Implementation of an intensive risk-stratified treatment protocol for children and adolescents with acute lymphoblastic leukemia in Lebanon. Am J Hematol. 2012;87(7):678–83.
30. Rivera GK, Quintana J, Villarroel M, et al. Transfer of complex frontline anticancer therapy to a developing country: the St. Jude osteosarcoma experience in Chile. Pediatr Blood Cancer. 2008;50(6):1143–6.
31. Villarroel M, Tordecilla J, Salgado C, et al. Multimodal therapy for children and adolescents with Ewing sarcoma: results of the First National Chilean Trial (1986–1991). Med Pediatr Oncol. 1997;29(3):190–6.
32. Cancer pain relief and palliative care. Report of a WHO Expert Committee. World Health Organ Tech Rep Ser 1990;804: 1–75.
33. Webster R, Lacey J, Quine S. Palliative care: a public health priority in developing countries. J Public Health Policy. 2007;28(1):28–39.
34. Delgado E, Barfield RC, Baker JN, et al. Availability of palliative care services for children with cancer in economically diverse regions of the world. Eur J Cancer. 2010;46(12):2260–6.
35. World Health Organization. National cancer control programmes : policies and managerial guidelines. 2nd ed. Geneva: World Health Organization; 2002.

36. World Health Organization website. Definition of palliative care. Available at: http://www.who.int/cancer/palliative/definition/en/. Accessed 10 July 2013.
37. Lynch T, Clark D, Centeno C, et al. Barriers to the development of palliative care in the countries of Central and Eastern Europe and the Commonwealth of Independent States. J Pain Symptom Manage. 2009;37(3):305–15.
38. Mathew PJ, Mathew JL, Singhi S. Knowledge, attitude and practice of pediatric critical care nurses towards pain: survey in a developing country setting. J Postgrad Med. 2011;57(3):196–200.
39. Kost-Byerly S, Chalkiadis G. Developing a pediatric pain service. Paediatr Anaesth. 2012;22(10):1016–24.
40. Laudico AV. Development of cancer pain relief and palliative care in the Philippines. Ann Acad Med Singapore. 1994;23(2):292–5.
41. Engel L, Love R. Safe patient handling education in Nepal: a Canadian perspective in creating and conducting training in a developing country. J Palliat Med. 2013;16(3):295–300.
42. Downing JD, Marston J, Selwyn C, Ross-Gakava L. Developing children's palliative care in Africa through beacon centres: lessons learnt. BMC Palliat Care. 2013;12:8.
43. Pastrana T, Junger S, Ostgathe C, Elsner F, Radbruch L. A matter of definition–key elements identified in a discourse analysis of definitions of palliative care. Palliat Med. 2008;22(3):222–32.
44. Ribeiro RC. Improving survival of children with cancer worldwide: the St. Jude International Outreach Program approach. Stud Health Technol Inform. 2012;172:9–13.
45. Qaddoumi I, Musharbash A, Elayyan M, et al. Closing the survival gap: implementation of medulloblastoma protocols in a low-income country through a twinning program. Int J Cancer. 2008;122(6):1203–6.
46. Qaddoumi I, Mansour A, Musharbash A, et al. Impact of telemedicine on pediatric neuro-oncology in a developing country: the Jordanian-Canadian experience. Pediatr Blood Cancer. 2007;48(1):39–43.
47. Wilimas JA, Wilson MW, Haik BG, et al. Development of retinoblastoma programs in Central America. Pediatr Blood Cancer. 2009;53(1):42–6.
48. World Child Cancer Foundation. What we do. Twinning. Available at: http://www.worldchildcancer.org/what-we-do/twinning/. Accessed 12 July 2013.
49. Luna-Fineman S, Barnoya M, Bonilla M, Fu L, Baez F, Rodriguez-Galindo C. Retinoblastoma in Central America: report from the Central American Association of Pediatric Hematology Oncology (AHOPCA). Pediatr Blood Cancer. 2012;58(4):545–50.
50. Sala A, Rossi E, Antillon F, et al. Nutritional status at diagnosis is related to clinical outcomes in children and adolescents with cancer: a perspective from Central America. Eur J Cancer. 2012;48(2):243–52.
51. Antillon F, Castellanos M, Valverde P, et al. Treating pediatric soft tissue sarcomas in a country with limited resources: the experience of the Unidad Nacional de Oncologia Pediatrica in Guatemala. Pediatr Blood Cancer. 2008;51(6):760–4.
52. Friedrich P, Ortiz R, Strait K, et al. Pediatric sarcoma in Central America: outcomes, challenges, and plans for improvement. Cancer. 2013;119:871–9.
53. Masera G, Sala A, Locati MG, Bonanomi S, Chiesa R, Marinoni M. [A report on the international cooperative network for paediatric hemato-oncology: the MASCOTA-MISPHO program]. Assist Inferm Ric. 2004;23(3):186–95.
54. Howard SC, Marinoni M, Castillo L, et al. Improving outcomes for children with cancer in low-income countries in Latin America: a report on the recent meetings of the Monza International School of Pediatric Hematology/Oncology (MISPHO)-part I. Pediatr Blood Cancer. 2007;48(3):364–9.
55. Howard SC, Ortiz R, Baez LF, et al. Protocol-based treatment for children with cancer in low income countries in Latin America: a report on the recent meetings of the Monza International School of Pediatric Hematology/Oncology (MISPHO)—part I. Pediatr Blood Cancer. 2007;48(4):486–90.
56. Dana-Farber Cancer Institute. Insight. Teaching Egyptian doctors to care for young cancer patients. Available at: http://blog.dana-farber.org/insight/2012/10/teaching-egyptian-doctors-to-care-for-young-cancer-patients/. Accessed 10 July 2013.
57. World Child Cancer Foundation. Project factsheet: Colombia. Available at: http://www.worldchildcancer.org/wp-content/uploads/Colombia1.pdf. Accessed 12 July 2013.
58. Shad A, Challinor J, Cohen M. Pediatric oncology in Ethiopia: an INCTR USA and Georgetown University Hospital Twinning Initiative with Tikur Anbessa Specialized Hospital. Cancer Control 2013: Cancer Care in Emerging Health Systems. 2013. p. 108–12. Available at: http://globalhealthdynamics.co.uk/cc2013/wp-content/uploads/2013/04/108-112-Ethiopia-PEDIATRIC-ONCOLOGY-NEW_2012.pdf. Accessed 12 July 2013.
59. Piot P, Russell S, Larson H. Good politics, bad politics: the experience of AIDS. Am J Public Health. 2007;97(11):1934–6.
60. Individual Members of the Faculty of Harvard University. Special contribution: consensus statement on antiretroviral for AIDS in poor countries. International AIDS Society—USA: topics in HIV medicine. 2001;9(2). Available at: https://www.iasusa.org/sites/default/files/tam/9-2-14.pdf. Accessed 14 July 2013.
61. Twenty-five years of AIDS: unhappy anniversary. Economist 2006:24–5. Available at: http://www.economist.com/node/7001554. Accessed 7 October 2013.
62. Atun RA, Bennett S, Duran A. Policy brief: when do vertical (stand-alone) programmes have a place in health systems? Health Systems and Policy Analysis. World Health Organization 2008 and World Health Organization, on behalf of the European Observatory on Health Systems and Policies; 2008.

63. Msuya J. Horizontal and vertical delivery of health services: what are the tradeoffs? Washington, DC: World Bank; 2005.
64. Ooms G, Van Damme W, Baker BK, Zeitz P, Schrecker T. The 'diagonal' approach to Global Fund financing: a cure for the broader malaise of health systems? Global Health. 2008;4:6.
65. WHO Cancer control: knowledge into action. WHO guide for effective programmes. Available at: http://www.who.int/cancer/modules/en/. Accessed 7 October 2013.
66. Dang-Tan T, Franco EL. Diagnosis delays in childhood cancer: a review. Cancer. 2007;110(4):703–13.
67. De Angelis C, Pacheco C, Lucchini G, et al. The experience in nicaragua: childhood leukemia in low income countries-the main cause of late diagnosis may be "medical delay". Int J Pediatr. 2012;2012:129707.
68. Leander C, Fu LC, Pena A, et al. Impact of an education program on late diagnosis of retinoblastoma in Honduras. Pediatr Blood Cancer. 2007;49(6):817–9.
69. Al-Qudimat MR, Day S, Almomani T, Odeh D, Qaddoumi I. Clinical nurse coordinators: a new generation of highly specialized oncology nursing in Jordan. J Pediatr Hematol Oncol. 2009;31(1):38–41.

6 Early Warning Signs of Cancer in Children/Models for Early Diagnosis

Stelios Poyiadjis and Lisine Tuyisenge

Introduction

Childhood cancer despite being a rare disease is highly curable, especially if diagnosed early. It is estimated that worldwide there are about 200,000 new cases diagnosed each year [1] and the biggest burden of disease is expected in developing countries. Most cases diagnosed in low- and middle-income countries (LMICs) present late with advanced disease, contributing to the challenges of treatment and reducing the chances of survival.

The 5-year overall survival rate for all cancers in high-income countries is currently approximately 80 %, but survival rates in LMICs are far below that, since more than 70 % of children do not have access to modern treatment regimens [1]. There is a marked discrepancy between the expected number of paediatric cancers in the developing world (if extrapolated from population-based data) and those that are actually identified by health care providers [2]. This fact emphasizes the importance of fostering and reinforcing an awareness of early childhood cancer warning signs among health care workers, parents and the community.

One effective way to improve childhood cancer survival in developing countries is to identify the disease as early as possible. Early stage diseases are associated with less intense treatment regimens, shorter duration of treatment, less side effects, reduced cost, less complications and a better prognosis. An awareness of early warning signs would avoid inappropriate medical interventions that could further delay the diagnosis [1]. As soon as the suspicion of cancer arises, the child should be referred to an appropriate specialized centre where further investigations can be performed.

Awareness campaigns are required in order to increase the level of education and knowledge in the general population and to strengthen continuous medical professional education. In Brazil in 2007, a prospective study of community health workers was performed to assess the knowledge related to early warning signs in childhood cancer [3]. It was shown that overall knowledge was poor, with 63 % being the highest score obtained on a questionnaire among all participants. This is closely related to limited formal education on this topic among health care workers.

Time delay in reaching a final diagnosis of cancer inevitably lead to advanced stage presentation of the disease and a negative effect on the long-term disease-free survival. Stefan et al. found a considerable delay in making the diagnosis of childhood cancer, mostly due to failure of

S. Poyiadjis, M.D. (✉)
Chris Hani—Baragwanath Academic Hospital, University of the Witwatersrand, Johannesburg, South Africa
e-mail: poyiadji@mweb.co.za

L. Tuyisenge, M.D.
Kigali University Teaching Hospital, Kigali, Rwanda

D.C. Stefan and C. Rodriguez-Galindo (eds.), *Pediatric Hematology-Oncology in Countries with Limited Resources: A Practical Manual*, DOI 10.1007/978-1-4614-3891-5_6,

health care professionals to recognize the symptoms and signs [4]. A malignancy was correctly diagnosed on a first visit in only 34 % of cases. This study found no correlation between the type of tumour and the delay, while in most previous studies such a correlation could be demonstrated [5–7]. The median delay before patients attended a health care facility was 5 days, whereas the median physician delay was 20 days. In a similar study by Wainwright and Poyiadjis et al. at Baragwanath hospital in Johannesburg, South Africa, an average delay of 10 months was found in establishing the diagnosis of retinoblastoma [8]. The major part of this delay was attributed to clinicians, with misinterpretation of symptoms and delay in referring children.

Despite the fact that in the developed world the management of patients with advanced disease, especially those with solid tumours, often remains a challenge, the number of such cases is far less than those in developing countries. In low-income countries, paediatric cancer has its own unique problems, including the tumour load at the primary site which is often massive, multiple sites of metastatic disease, genetic and other factors.

Increased awareness and more efficient referral systems in developing countries will result in less patients presenting with advanced disease.

Awareness of Early Warning Signs of Childhood Cancer

Early diagnosis of cancer is reliant on three pillars: a high index of suspicion, the recognition of groups with an increased risk of developing cancer and the recognition of the "red flag signs" of childhood cancer [1].

High Index of Suspicion

Because current priorities in reducing childhood mortality worldwide are focused on infectious diseases (as reflected by WHO health strategies for children), the emphasis is not being placed on paediatric cancer. In the developing world, the extra burden of childhood malnutrition further divides already stretched resources. Unless a suspicion of childhood cancer is raised with each patient seen, such a diagnosis is never going to be made. Common sites to be aware of include bone marrow, bone, lymph nodes and abdominal and soft tissue tumours [1]. The seemingly simple complaint of bone pain can easily be attributed to non-malignant causes, but this may mask a much more sinister diagnosis of leukaemia.

Recognition of High-Risk Groups

It is well known that certain disease types and chromosomal disorders have a strong correlation with development of childhood cancer (Table 6.1.). Of note is a study in Great Britain by Narod et al., where it was found that the types of cancer with the highest rates of associated anomalies were Wilms tumour, Ewing sarcoma, hepatoblastoma and gonadal and germ cell tumours [9]. In this study, cases of spina bifida and abnormalities of the eye, ribs and spine were more common in children with cancer compared to the rest of the population. The overgrowth conditions of Beckwith-Wiedemann syndrome and Sotos syndrome both have an increased risk of childhood cancers [10]. Children with a previous malignant disease that required treatment with chemotherapy and/or radiotherapy have an increased risk of developing a second malignancy.

Recognizing the "Red Flag Signs" of Childhood Cancer

The majority of childhood cancers present with some distinguishing signs that can alert the clinician to such a diagnosis. Although many of these signs and symptoms are not exclusive to childhood cancer, it is still essential to consider malignancy in the differential diagnosis. Symptoms that should raise suspicion are summarized in Table 6.2.

Table 6.1 Conditions associated with a higher risk of malignancy

Condition	Association
Genetic abnormalities, including:	
Down syndrome	Acute myeloblastic leukaemia
Beckwith-Wiedemann	Wilms tumour, hepatoblastoma
Fanconi anaemia	Acute myeloblastic leukaemia
Immunodeficiency, including:	
All conditions (congenital and acquired)	Lymphoma
HIV	Non-Hodgkin's lymphoma, Kaposi sarcoma
Congenital malformations, including:	
Aniridia (absent iris), hemi-hypertrophy	Wilms tumour
Neurocutaneous syndromes, including Neurofibromatosis	Benign and malignant tumours, e.g. sarcoma, optic glioma and other brain tumours
Previous malignancy and treatment with chemotherapy and radiotherapy	Osteogenic sarcoma, leukaemia, brain tumour, etc.
Sibling with a malignancy	e.g. retinoblastoma
Cirrhosis	Hepatocellular carcinoma
Cryptorchidism	Testicular germ cell tumour

Campaigns Targeting Early Warning Signs of Cancer in Children

Many international organizations promote awareness of childhood cancer. The International Confederation of Childhood Cancer Parent Organizations (ICCCPO) and the International Society of Paediatric Oncology (SIOP) raised awareness in 2013 through the campaign and slogan: "Early detection…making a difference". These and other campaigns have led to many checklists or awareness acronyms being designed to assist in recognizing early warning signs. One example is "CHILD CANCER" which is endorsed by the Union for International Cancer Control (UICC) and the SIOP (Table 6.3).

Table 6.2 Symptoms and signs raising suspicion of childhood cancer

General symptoms	Unexplained fever, fatigue, listlessness, nausea, loss of appetite, weight loss, night sweats
Haematological malignancies	Pallor, fatigue, fever, recurrent infections, bone pain, refusal to walk, epistaxis, easy bruising, petechiae, lymphadenopathy, abdominal distension, mass at any site
Abdominal solid tumours	Change in bowel habits (often constipation), vomiting, hypertension, abdominal pain, abdominal distension, abdominal mass, haematuria
Neurological malignancies	Change in temperament, regression of milestones, abnormal balance (ataxia), signs of raised intracranial pressure (progressive headache, vomiting (especially early morning), altered level of consciousness, bulging fontanelle, increasing head circumference), double vision, new-onset squint, convulsions, focal neurological abnormality
Ophthalmological malignancy	Leukocoria, new-onset squint, proptosis, visual disturbance
Bone tumours	Swelling or mass, persistent pain, pathological fracture
Soft tissue tumours	Masses at any site
Neuroblastoma	Pallor, hypertension, lymphadenopathy, Horner syndrome, raccoon eyes, bony masses, abdominal mass, petechiae, ecchymoses, opsoclonus myoclonus, watery diarrhoea

Another example is the Saint Siluan warning signs list used in South Africa [11, 12] (Table 6.4). The list consists of easily recognizable symptoms and signs arranged according to the mnemonic: SILUAN after Saint Silouan the Athonite, a Russian Orthodox monk.

Saint Siluan warning signs were adopted by ICCCPO and SIOP-PODC.

Table 6.3 Child cancer (acronym)

C	Continued, unexplained weight loss
H	Headaches, often with early morning vomiting
I	Increased swelling or persistent pain in the bones, joints, back or legs
L	Lump or mass, especially in the abdomen, neck, chest, pelvis or armpits
D	Development of excessive bruising, bleeding or rash
C	Constant infections
A	A whitish colour behind the pupil
N	Nausea that persists or vomiting without nausea
C	Constant tiredness or noticeable paleness
E	Eye or vision changes that occur suddenly and persist
R	Recurring or persistent fevers of unknown origin

Table 6.4 Saint Siluan warning signs

S	Seek medical help early for persistent symptoms
I	Eye: white spot in the eye (leukocoria), new squint, new blindness, bulging eyeball
L	Lump: abdomen and pelvis, head and neck, limbs, testes, glands
U	Unexplained: prolonged fever over 2 weeks, loss of weight, pallor, fatigue, easy bruising or bleeding
A	Aching: bones, joints and back and easy fracture
N	Neurological signs: change or deterioration in walk, balance or speech, regression of milestones, headache for more than a week with or without vomiting, enlarging head

A Practical Guide to the Saint Siluan Warning Signs of Cancer in Children [13]

S: Seek Medical Help Early for Persistent Symptoms

A child with any one of the warning signs of cancer, as mentioned in the list, needs to be closely monitored; if the symptoms persist for more than a week or 10 days, despite the conservative treatment given by the family and by the active treatment of a local clinic or hospital, the patient needs to be referred to a tertiary centre. Cancer does not respond either to conventional first-line medications or to local treatment with physiotherapy, massage, ointments and various types of liquids.

Classical examples of events which are experienced in developing countries and are implicated in misdiagnosis and mismanagement and consequently in late referral to specialist centres are:

- The use of eye drops or ointments for leukocoria in retinoblastoma. When the symptoms persist, often health workers change eye drops on the same patient for prolonged periods of time.
- The bulging eyeball is often confused with injury of the eye. When there is an associated sepsis, local treatment and oral antibiotics are often prescribed.
- Cultural beliefs of bewitchment.
- Ointments with or without oral antibiotics are often given to patients with a mass or masses anywhere on the body.
- "Red herrings" such as injury from falling, sports trauma, teacher corporal punishment or "someone hitting the child", subsequently "resulting" in a mass starting to grow.
- Long history of "growing pains". The patient attends physiotherapy or receives various other types of therapy provided by practical healers.
- Constipation and chronic "worm" problems are often thought to be the causes of abdominal swellings and masses.
- Haematological malignancies like leukaemias are often confused with HIV disease, malaria or other infections, mainly viral.
- Abnormal neurological signs are often attributed to psychological problems; for example, the child does not like the teacher or the school and for this reason he/she has morning vomiting or other strange neurological behaviour and headache.

The important point from *S* of the "Saint Siluan warning signs" is that a strict follow-up visit is mandatory for patients with unusual symptoms. The persistence of these symptoms requires referral to a specialist centre.

I, Eye: White Spot in the Eye (Leukocoria), New Squint, New Blindness, Bulging Eyeball

These signs refer mainly to the most common eye cancer of childhood which is retinoblastoma. Leukocoria is probably the most common early

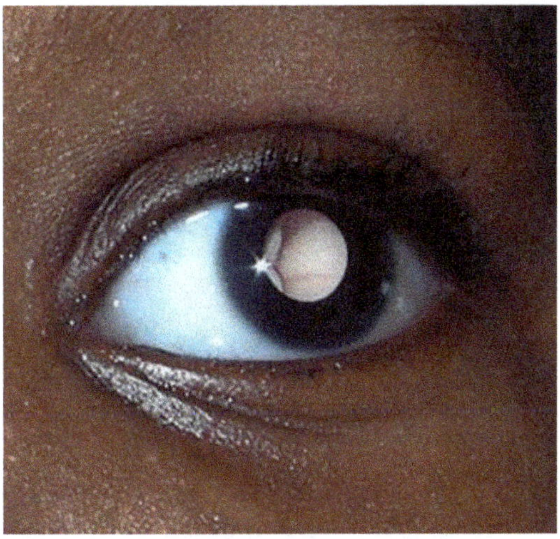

Fig. 6.1 Leukocoria

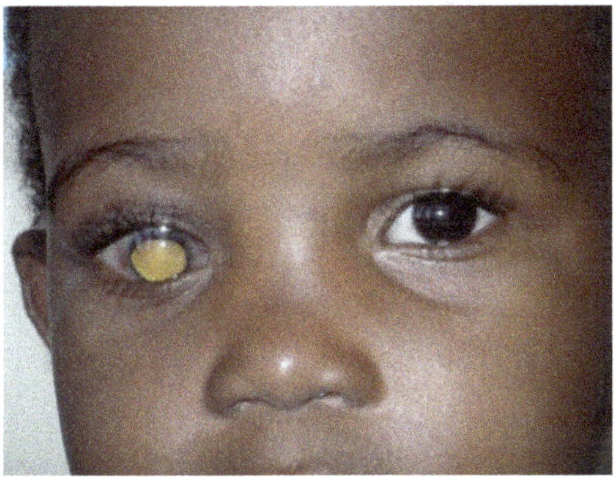

Fig. 6.2 Leukocoria

warning sign of retinoblastoma. Leukocoria is an abnormal white pupillary reflex from the retina of the eye (Figs. 6.1 and 6.2). The mother often is the first person to notice this sign and she needs to be educated to report it to the health care provider. Retinoblastoma is a disease of young children and can be unilateral or bilateral in a third of the patients. The median age of diagnosis of bilateral retinoblastoma is 14 months, while for unilateral disease, it is 23 months [14]. In developing countries, a bulging eyeball due to the mass effect of a retro-orbital mass is common. New squint and new blindness might also be early signs of retinoblastoma. Squint at birth needs to be distinguished from a physiological one.

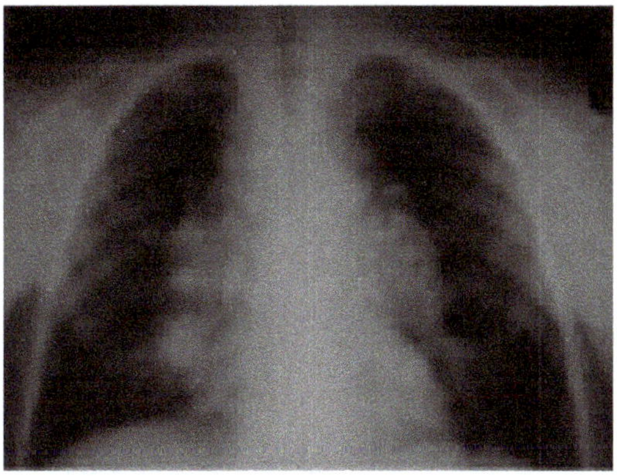

Fig. 6.3 X-rays (Hodgkin's disease)

L, Lump: Abdomen and Pelvis, Head and Neck, Limbs, Testes, Glands

A lump, i.e. a mass, anywhere in the body can be an early presentation of a childhood cancer. Visceromegaly, hepatomegaly or splenomegaly can be early signs of a malignancy. Lymphadenopathy is often slightly difficult to interpret especially in a developing country with an HIV epidemic and high prevalence of TB. It is accepted that a patient with lymph nodes larger than 2 cm × 2 cm that is not responding to an oral broad spectrum antibiotic needs to be referred to a specialist centre. Fine needle aspiration or an open biopsy is recommended, depending on the available expertise. It is of note that in developing countries where the prevalence of TB is high, patients with adenopathy due to Hodgkin's disease have often been treated empirically for TB prior to the final diagnosis (Fig. 6.3).

An abdominal or pelvic mass—often reported by a parent—has to be considered as malignant until it is proven otherwise. The patient needs immediate referral (Fig. 6.4).

U, Unexplained: Prolonged Fever over 2 Weeks, Loss of Weight, Pallor, Fatigue, Easy Bruising or Bleeding

Childhood cancer can often present with non-specific symptoms. Pyrexia of unknown origin persisting for more than 10–14 days and unexplained constitutional symptoms of loss of weight and loss of appetite can be early signs of a malignancy.

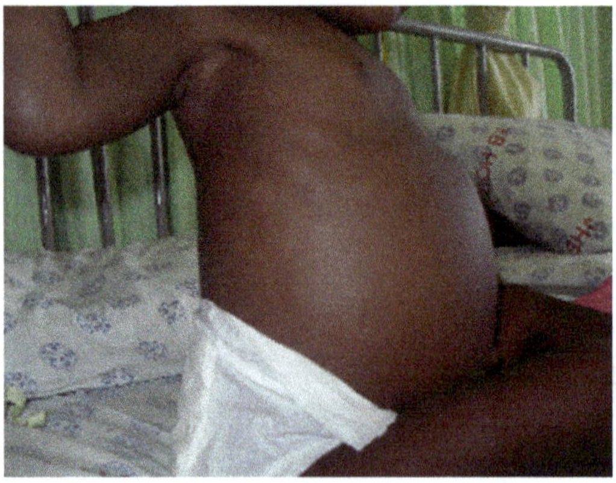

Fig. 6.4 Distended abdomen

Evidence of blood loss (active or occult) with pallor and/or petechiae, gum bleeding, persistent epistaxis, vaginal or rectal bleeding and easy bruising might all be evidence of a haematological malignancy, but of a solid tumour as well. A patient with the above symptoms needs to be referred to a specialist centre even if these symptoms are not due to a malignancy.

A, Aching: Bones, Joints and Back and Easy Fracture

Haematological malignancies (leukaemias and lymphomas) often present with bone and joint pain and often with back pain. Primary bone tumours, e.g. osteosarcoma and Ewing sarcoma, and other solid tumours with bone metastases can present with bone pain.

A common problem is the so-called growing pains of the knee joint or femur in adolescent children which delays presentation to a specialist centre. Pain is also often attributed to a traumatic incident and treated as an injury. Patients with osteogenic sarcoma often attend physiotherapy for months or they are managed conservatively by other practitioners. Sudden onset of limping or inability to perform usual physical activities due to bone pain needs to be investigated.

Sometimes the incorrect diagnosis of juvenile rheumatoid arthritis (JRA) in children with joint pains leads to a resistant disease of leukaemia or other haematological malignancy if the patient is treated with steroids. A patient with suspected JRA needs to have a bone marrow aspiration for cytological investigation before being initiated on steroids (Figs. 6.5 and 6.6).

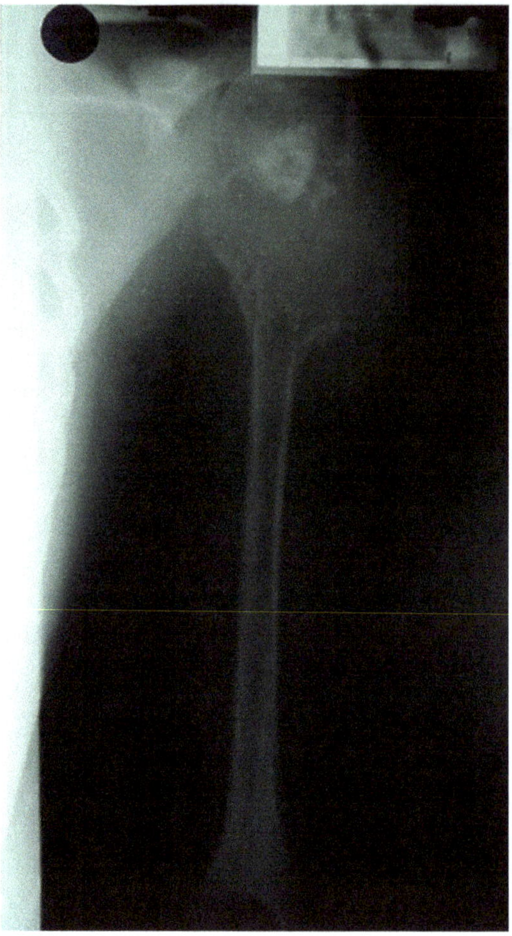

Fig. 6.5 X-rays (osteosarcoma)

N, Neurological Signs: Change or Deterioration in Walk, Balance or Speech, Regression of Milestones, Headache for More Than a Week with or Without Vomiting and Enlarging Head

Any new abnormal neurological symptoms and signs in children of any age can be due to a brain tumour, benign or malignant. A brain scan is always recommended when such symptoms appear. A common problem with space-occupying lesions of the brain is that the early morning vomiting with or without headache is often attributed to psychological reasons, such as

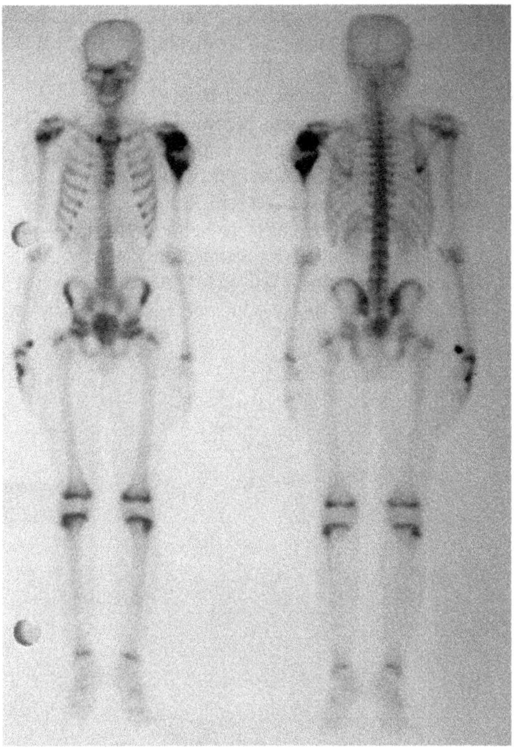

Fig. 6.6 Bone scan (osteosarcoma)

school avoidance. Unexplained headaches or sudden onset of migraines need to be investigated, especially if other symptoms and signs of raised intracranial pressure, including progressive headache, vomiting (especially early morning), altered level of consciousness, bulging fontanelle and an increasing head circumference are found. Cerebellar signs (ataxia, nystagmus, etc.) can be the first signs of posterior fossa tumours. Regression of milestones is often found in children with brain tumours.

Although the Saint Siluan system is comprehensive, it is not all inclusive. In 2007, the "One World, One Vision" symposium was organized as a collaboration between developed and developing countries. Whereas developed countries can focus on salvaging eye surgery, in the developing world, the high mortality of retinoblastoma is still the major issue. The focus of this collaboration was on developing strategies for early diagnosis and improved outcome of retinoblastoma in children [15].

Conclusion

The majority of children with cancer in developing countries are diagnosed late and subsequently their advanced stages of disease contribute to poor survival rates. One way of improving the outcome of childhood cancer is to diagnose the disease as early as possible. This can be attained by means of far-reaching awareness campaigns among parents and communities in order to make them aware of when a child should be taken to a health care facility as cancer is suspected. The campaigns should also reach health care providers of all levels in order to increase the number of cases identified, as well as to facilitate early recognition of childhood cancer warning signs.

Early signs and symptoms of childhood cancers are not specific to cancer. Each country should adopt a recognized awareness checklist or design their own according to local requirements and use it in awareness campaigns. Once a child with early warning signs of cancer has been identified, an effective referral system should be in place to prevent a delay in the confirmation of the diagnosis.

References

1. Stones DK. Childhood cancer: early warning signs. CME. 2010;28(7):314–6.
2. Ribeiro R, Steliarova-Foucher E, Magrath I, et al. Baseline status of paediatric oncology care in ten low-income or mid-income countries receiving My Child Matters support: a descriptive study. Lancet Oncol. 2008;9:721–9.
3. Workman GM, Ribeiro R, Rai SN, Pedrosa A, Workman DE, Pedrosa F. Pediatric cancer knowledge: assessment of knowledge of warning signs and symptoms for pediatric cancer among Brazilian community health workers. J Cancer Educ. 2007;22:181–5.
4. Stefan D, Siemonsma F. Delay and causes of delay in the diagnosis of childhood cancer in Africa. Pediatr Blood Cancer. 2011;56:80–5.
5. Loh AH, Aung L, Ha C, Tan AM, Quah TC, Chui CH. Diagnostic delay in pediatric solid tumors: a population based study on determinants and impact on outcomes. Pediatr Blood Cancer. 2012;58:561–5.
6. Dang-Tan T, Trottier H, Mery LS, et al. Delays in diagnosis and treatment among children and adolescents with cancer in Canada. Pediatr Blood Cancer. 2008;51:468–74.

7. Dang-Tan T, Trottier H, Mery LS, et al. Determinants of delays in treatment initiation in children and adolescents diagnosed with leukemia or lymphoma in Canada. Int J Cancer. 2010;126:1936–43.
8. Poyiadjis S, Wainwright L, Naidu G. Time delay in the presentation of solid tumours in developing countries. Pediatr Blood Cancer. 2004;43:342.
9. Narod SA, Hawkins MM, Robertson CM, Stiller CA. Congenital anomalies and childhood cancer in Great Britain. Am J Hum Genet. 1997;60:474–85.
10. Rahman N. Mechanisms predisposing to childhood overgrowth and cancer. Curr Opin Genet Dev. 2005; 15:227–33.
11. Poyiadjis S, Wainwright L, Naidu G. Warning signs for cancer in children in a developing country. MPO. 2000;324:414.
12. SIOP News; December 2000. p. 21.
13. Poyiadjis S, Wainwright L, Naidu G, Mackinnon D, Poole J. The Saint Siluan warning signs of cancer in children: impact of education in rural South Africa. Pediatr Blood Cancer. 2011;56:314–6.
14. Lanzkowsky P. Manual of pediatric hematology and oncology. Burlington: Academic; 2005. p. 856.
15. Rodriguez-Galindo C, Wilson MW, Chantada G, et al. Retinoblastoma: one world, one vision. Pediatrics. 2008;122:e763–70.

Care and Prevention of Infection 7

Miguela A. Caniza and Gabriela Maron

Abbreviations

AFB	Acid fast bacilli
AmB	Amphotericin B
ANC	Absolute neutrophil count
APIC	Association for Professionals in Infection Control and Epidemiology
CDC	Centers for Disease Control
CMV	Cytomegalic virus
CRBI	Catheter-related blood stream infection
CT	Computed tomography
CVC	Central venous catheter
FN	Fever and neutropenia
GI	Gastrointestinal
HAI	Healthcare-associated infection
HCI	High-income country
HCP	Healthcare providers
HEPA	High-efficiency particulate air
HSCT	Hematopoietic stem cell transplantation
HSV	Herpes simplex virus
ICP	Infection prevention control
ICU	Intensive care unit
ID	Infectious disease
IFD	Invasive fungal disease
IGRA	Interferon gamma release assays
IV	Intravenous
L-AmB	Liposomal amphotericin B
LMCI	Low- and middle-income countries
NCI	National Cancer Institute
NGO	Nongovernmental organization
PCC	Pediatric cancer center
PV	Peripheral vein
SENIC	Study of the Efficacy of Nosocomial Infection Control
SP	Subcutaneous port
TB	Tuberculosis
TD	Time to detection
TMP-SMX	Trimethoprim—sulfamethoxazole
TST	Tuberculin skin test
WHO	World Health Organization

M.A. Caniza, M.D. (✉)
Director of the Infectious Diseases—International Outreach Division, Department of Infectious Diseases, St. Jude Children's Research Hospital, 262 Danny Thomas Place, Memphis, TN 38105, USA
e-mail: Miguela.caniza@stjude.org

G. Maron, M.D.
Department of Infectious Diseases, St. Jude Children's Research Hospital, 262 Danny Thomas Place, Memphis, TN 38105, USA
e-mail: Gabriela.maron@stjude.org

Care and Prevention of Infection in Developing Countries

Children with cancer are at increased risk for developing infections caused by pathogens that range from those circulating in the community [1] to multidrug-resistant, opportunistic microorganisms

D.C. Stefan and C. Rodriguez-Galindo (eds.), *Pediatric Hematology-Oncology in Countries with Limited Resources: A Practical Manual*, DOI 10.1007/978-1-4614-3891-5_7,

[2]. In most low- and middle-income countries (LMICs), childhood cancer treatment is often suboptimal and survival rates are lower than those in high-income countries (HIC) [3]. After access to appropriate anticancer medications, support to prevent and manage infectious complications is the most important factor to improve survival of these patients [4]. In this chapter, we address key points in the care and prevention of infections during the treatment of children with cancer. We also share our experience of working on infection care and prevention with pediatric cancer care centers in LMICs. In the first section, we discuss the management of the most frequent infectious syndromes in children with cancer. In the second section, we review important concepts in infection prevention in general and in children with cancer, especially in LMICs.

Infection Care

1. Fever and neutropenia
2. Central venous catheter infections
3. Respiratory infections
4. Fungal infections
5. Gastrointestinal infections

General Concepts

Infections in cancer patients should receive prompt and adequate treatment to increase survival. Many pediatric centers in LMICs face challenges related to infection care. These challenges fall into five major categories: (1) lack of qualified healthcare personnel trained in infection care and prevention of children with cancer; (2) insufficient or poor infrastructure of healthcare facilities; (3) insufficient or inconsistent availability of supplies (antimicrobials, catheters, syringes, antiseptics, bandages, tubing system, flushes, etc.); (4) suboptimal microbiological diagnosis due to insufficient supplies, equipment and trained personnel; and (5) lack of institutional policies and procedures and organizational structure for quality of care. We address some of these challenges in the care of the various infectious syndromes. Ideally, standardized, evidence-based, institutional guidelines informed by local infectious epidemiology should be used. However, the concepts behind the treatment of infections in cancer patients are universal and applicable in any setting. In this section, we base our recommendations in currently published guidelines and our experiences in caring for sick children in LMICs.

Table 7.1 Common bacterial pathogens in fever and neutropenia

Common gram-positive pathogens
Coagulase-negative *staphylococci*
Staphylococcus aureus, including methicillin-resistant strains
Enterococcus species, including vancomycin-resistant strains
Viridans group streptococci
Streptococcus pneumoniae
Streptococcus pyogenes
Common gram-negative pathogens
Escherichia coli
Klebsiella spp.
Enterobacter spp.
Pseudomonas aeruginosa
Citrobacter spp.
Acinetobacter spp.
Stenotrophomonas maltophilia

Adapted with permission from Freifeld AG et al. *Clin Infect Dis*. 2011;52:e56–93 [5]

Fever and Neutropenia

The most common reason for seeking care in children with cancer is febrile neutropenia (FN). Fever is defined as a single oral temperature measurement of ≥38.3 °C (101 °F) or a temperature of ≥38.0 °C (100.4 °F) sustained over a period of 1 h. Neutropenia is defined as an absolute neutrophil count (ANC) (including band cells) of less than 0.5×10^9/L (500 cells/μL) or a count of 1.0×10^9/L (1,000 cells/μL) predicted to decrease below 0.5×10^9/L [5].

Etiology. Table 7.1 lists the bacterial pathogens that cause most bloodstream infections in FN. Drug-resistant organisms such as extended-spectrum β-lactamase (ESBL)-producing gram-negative bacteria and carbapenmase-producing strains are being increasingly reported as the cause of infections in FN. Resistant gram-positive organisms, particularly methicillin-resistant *S. aureus* (MRSA) and vancomycin-resistant enterococci (VRE) are gaining prevalence in some centers [6]. Invasive fungal disease (IFD) is rarely identified as the cause of infection early in the course of FN [7].

Initial management. Fever in patients with neutropenia should be considered as a manifestation of infection, and patients should promptly receive empirical antibiotic therapy, ideally within an hour of onset, as infection may progress rapidly. This may be difficult in many LMCIs, where access to care may delay initiation of antibiotics. The management of FN is influenced by patient characteristics, drug availability and cost, and local epidemiology. The management principles presented in this section are based on published guidelines [5, 7], but institution-specific guidelines need to be developed based on the antibiotic susceptibility pattern of organisms commonly isolated at a healthcare center.

The current tendency for the treatment of FN in many pediatric cancer centers (PCC) is the use of risk-stratification schemas. These schemas are based on factors related to patients (including age, type of malignancy, disease status), the type and timing of chemotherapy, and both clinical and laboratory characteristics of the specific FN episode, such as height of fever, hypotension, mucositis, blood counts, and C-reactive protein levels [7]. Patients at risk for invasive bacterial infection and clinical complications are those with anticipated prolonged and profound neutropenia (>7 days duration) following chemotherapy (ANC <100 cells/μL), and important comorbid conditions, including unstable vital signs, pneumonia, abdominal pain, and mental status changes [5, 7]. Validated stratification schemas in pediatrics exist, but none have been validated across various geographic locations. However, it is recommended that each institution use and keep a record of performance of a validated risk-stratification schema [7].

Laboratory and imaging studies. If the patient has no central venous catheter (CVC), ideally two sets of peripheral blood cultures should be obtained. If the patient has a CVC, blood specimens from each lumen should be obtained. Obtaining a peripheral blood culture in patients with CVCs is recommended. Chest radiographs are required only if there are pulmonary signs or symptoms.

Antibiotic treatment. Empiric antibiotic therapy for patients with FN needs to provide coverage for gram-negative organisms, including *P. aeruginosa.* Monotherapy regimens evaluated in children include antipseudomonal penicillins (piperacillin-tazobactam and ticarcillin-clavulanic acid), antipseudomonal cephalosporins (cefepime), and carbapenems (meropenem or imipenem). Antipseudomonal penicillins are an excellent option for initial monotherapy if cefepime is not available. Carbapenems should be conserved for broadening antibiotic spectrum and for intrabdominal process (see section on typhlitis). Ceftazidime or aminoglycosides are not sufficient as monotherapy because of intrinsic and acquired resistance among gram-negative organisms [8]. Aminoglycosides and/or fluoroquinolones may be added to the initial regimen to manage complications (evidence of sepsis or pneumonia) or if antimicrobial resistance is suspected [5]. Vancomycin is not recommended as part of the initial antibiotic regimen for FN, unless there are specific clinical indications (Table 7.2) or the center reports a high rate of resistant pathogens [5].

Empiric antifungal treatment can be initiated in children at high risk for IFD who have persistent fever despite prolonged (>96 h) broad-spectrum antibiotic therapy. Currently, caspofungin or liposomal amphotericin B (L-AmB) is recommended for empiric antifungal therapy [9]. If these compounds are not available, amphotericin B (AmB) deoxycholate is equally effective. Close monitoring of renal and hepatic function is recommended to avoid toxicity.

Ongoing management. Initial antibacterials should be modified only if clinical, microbiological,

Table 7.2 Indications for addition of antibiotics active against gram-positive organisms to the empirical regimen for fever and neutropenia

Hemodynamic instability or other evidence of severe sepsis
Pneumonia documented radiographically
Positive blood culture for gram-positive bacteria, before final identification and susceptibility testing is available
Clinically suspected serious catheter-related infection (e.g., chills or rigors with infusion through catheter and cellulitis around the catheter entry/exit site)
Skin or soft-tissue infection at any site
Colonization with methicillin-resistant *Staphylococcus aureus*, vancomycin-resistant enterococcus, or penicillin-resistant *Streptococcus pneumoniae*
Severe mucositis, if fluoroquinolone prophylaxis has been given and ceftazidime is employed as empirical therapy

Adapted with permission from Freifeld AG et al. *Clin Infect Dis*. 2011;52:e56–93 [5]

or imaging changes indicate a new infection. In patients who respond to initial empiric antibiotic therapy, double coverage for gram-negative infection and glycopeptides can discontinued after 24–72 h if susceptible bacteria are not recovered in cultures. In children with persistent fever who become clinically unstable, the initial empiric antibacterial regimen can be escalated to include coverage for resistant gram-negative, gram-positive, and anaerobic bacteria, particularly if blood culture results are indicative of resistant bacteria [7].

Duration of antibiotic treatment. Empiric antibiotics can be discontinued in patients with negative blood cultures at 48 h, who have been afebrile for at least 24 h, and who have evidence of marrow recovery (increasing ANC >500 cells/μL). Empiric antibiotics may be discontinued at 72 h for low-risk patients who have negative blood cultures and have been afebrile for at least 24 h, irrespective of marrow recovery status, only if close follow up is possible [7].

In patients with clinically or microbiologically documented infections, the duration of therapy is dictated by the particular organism and site. Appropriate antibiotics should be continued for at least the duration of neutropenia (until ANC is >500 cells/μL) or longer if clinically necessary. Alternatively, if an appropriate treatment course has been completed and all signs and symptoms of a documented infection have resolved, oral fluoroquinolone can be administered until marrow recovery in patients who remain neutropenic [5] (Table 7.3).

Central Venous Catheter Infections

Classification. CVC infections are classified according to the primary site of infection. An exit-site infection is a superficial infection at the site of insertion with erythema, tenderness, induration, or purulence within 2 cm of the exit of the CVC or edge of the subcutaneous port (SP). Tunnel tract infections affect the subcutaneous tissue surrounding the CVC or SP at a distance greater than 2 cm from the skin exit. An infection of the subcutaneous tissue surrounding a SP is referred to as a pocket infection. A catheter-related bloodstream infection (CRBI) is a laboratory-confirmed bacteremia or fungemia arising from microbial colonization of a CVC or SP, which may be associated with systemic symptoms. Septic thrombosis can occur as a complication of CVC infections [10].

Etiology. The most frequently isolated organisms are Gram-positive bacteria, the most common being coagulase-negative *Staphylococcus*. Other organisms include *S. aureus*, *Streptococcus viridans*, enterococcus, gram-negative organisms (*E. coli*, *Klebsiella* spp., or *Enterobacter* spp.), and *Pseudomonas aeruginosa*. *Bacillus* species, *Mycobacterium chelonae*, and *Mycobacterium fortuitum* are less frequent. *Candida* spp. are the most commonly isolated fungal organism [10].

Diagnosis. For exit-site infections, culture of discharge or wound aspirate is recommended. A swab specimen from the exit site is acceptable, but may be contaminated with skin flora. Gram staining, staining for fungal organisms and acid-fast bacilli (AFB), and routine bacterial and fungal cultures should be performed. AFB culture should be ordered if there is no improvement after 48–72 h of therapy. Diagnosis of CRBI is best made by collecting paired CVC and peripheral

Table 7.3 Suggested empiric antibiotic therapy for patients with febrile neutropenia

Suggested first line therapy needs to provide coverage for gram-negative organisms including *P. aeruginosa*	Piperacillin-tazobactam or Cefepime +/- Aminoglycosides*
Fever persists after 48-h of treatment/suspected Staphylococcal infection	↓ Vancomycin
Persistent fever beyond 96-h, add empiric antifungal treatment	↓ Antifungal treatment (amphotericin B, echinocandins, triazoles)**
No improvement/suspected hospital-acquired infection/ neutropenic colitis	↓ Meropenem***

*Aminoglycosides should be added for severe infections or suspected resistance. Ceftazidime or aminoglycosides are not sufficient as monotherapy due to resistance

**Empiric antifungal therapy will depend on previous exposure and local epidemiology

***Carbapenems should be conserved for broadening antibiotic spectrum and for intra-abdominal process

vein (PV) blood cultures. All lumens of all indwelling intravenous catheters should be cultured simultaneously. A diagnosis of CRBI can be made by comparing the time to detection (TD) [11] of paired CVC and PV cultures. If the TD of blood cultures drawn through the suspected CVC is at least 120 min less than the TD of PV drawn at the same time, a CRBI is likely [11]. If only paired cultures from two lumens of a CVC are available, a CRBI is likely if TD of Lumen 1 is 120 min or more of the TD of Lumen 2 [12].

Indications for removal of catheters. The CVC or SP should be removed if no longer needed. Catheters should be also removed if (1) the patient's clinical condition deteriorates, (2) there are signs of sepsis, (3) blood cultures remain positive after 48–72 h of effective therapy, and (4) if CRBI relapses. Infections by *S. aureus*, *Candida* spp., and *Malassezia* spp., also require catheter removal. Removal should be strongly considered in bacteremia caused by *Bacillus* spp., rapidly growing *Mycobacterium* spp., and Gram-negative bacilli, as infection may be very difficult to eradicate without line removal [10]. Catheters should also be removed if septic thrombosis is present.

Management. Most exit-site infections can be managed with local care and topical antibiotics in non-neutropenic patients. Patients with mild to moderate signs and symptoms, but without fever, may be treated with oral antibiotics such as dicloxacillin, amoxicillin/clavulanic acid, or oral cephalosporin. Clindamycin may be used if MRSA is suspected. All patients with fever or rapidly progressing infections should be treated with parenteral antibiotics. Initial antibiotic therapy should include a broad-spectrum antipseudomonal penicillin or cephalosporin plus vancomycin. If infection with gram-negative bacteria is suspected, an aminoglycoside should be added. If the patient has severe abdominal pain or clinical symptoms of sepsis, the antipseudomonal β-lactams can be substituted with carbapenems. Definitive antibiotic therapy should be based on susceptibility testing of isolated pathogens.

Exit-site infections that improve promptly should be treated for 5–7 days. Infections of the tunnel tract or pocket of the SP usually require removal of the CVC or SP and at least 7–10 days of appropriate antimicrobial therapy. Patients with CRBI who respond promptly to therapy and have no complications should receive 10–14 days of antibiotic therapy. For infections due to yeasts, antifungals should be given for 14 days after the last positive blood culture after removal of catheter. In local peripheral vein thrombosis with purulent collection, surgical debridement might be needed. For a central blood vessel thrombosis, an anticoagulant is recommended in addition to antibiotics. For septic embolism, antibiotic therapy may be continued for 4–6 weeks. The CVC or SP should not be reinserted until effective parenteral antibiotic therapy is begun and repeat blood cultures yield negative results [13].

Antibiotic dwell therapy consists in instilling the lumen of the infected catheter with a high concentration (1–5 mg/mL) of an antibiotic surpassing the minimal inhibitory concentration to which the isolated microorganism is susceptible and closing the lumen for 8–12 h. In patients with a single lumen catheter for which sufficient dwell time cannot be arranged, a peripheral IV to administer other medications should be considered. Dwell therapy is recommended for as much of the 10- to 14-day treatment course as possible [13].

Respiratory Infections

Cancer patients are at increased risk for respiratory infections. The diagnosis of pulmonary infections in immunocompromised patients can be challenging because of atypical presentations and the absence of localizing signs and symptoms, particularly during severe neutropenia. Most patients present with nonspecific symptoms such as cough and fever, which may be accompanied by tachypnea and dyspnea in more severe cases. Local epidemiology, the setting from which the patient presents (community vs. hospital), and seasonality of viral infections may also aid in the etiological diagnosis.

Diagnosis. Nasopharyngeal washings or swabs are useful to diagnose viral infection. Polymerase chain reaction methods are currently the gold standard for diagnosis of respiratory viruses. If not available, samples may be sent for direct fluorescent antibody analysis and viral culture [14]. Serologic studies may be performed to identify organisms producing atypical pneumonia and other organisms (cytomegalovirus, *Cryptococcus*, *Aspergillus*). If tuberculosis is suspected, sputum or gastric aspirates for acid fast stain and culture should be obtained. A tuberculin skin test (TST) may aid in the diagnosis; however, a negative test does not rule out tuberculosis. Interferon-gamma release assays (IGRAs) indicate the immune response to *Mycobacterium tuberculosis* but does not differentiate between active and latent infections. Similarly to TST, a negative result of IGRA may not rule out active tuberculosis. Access to this type of study is still limited in most LMICs. Urinary antigen tests can be used to diagnose *Legionella pneumophila* and *Histoplasma capsulatum*. Blood cultures should be obtained from all immunosuppressed patients with pneumonia [15].

Etiological diagnosis of respiratory infections may be a challenge in most LMCIs, particularly if microbiological tests are not available. In this scenario, imaging studies may provide additional clues to the etiology of infection. A radiologic pattern of lobar or segmental pneumonia with reactive pleural effusion is indicative of bacterial organisms. In hospital-acquired pneumonia, infiltrates can be bilateral with diffuse or multilobar consolidation and pleural effusions. Atypical pneumonia may present with unilateral or bilateral infiltrates with a segmental distribution or as a diffuse bilateral reticular nodular infiltrate. In viral pneumonia, a radiologic pattern of poorly defined nodules and patchy areas of peribronchial ground glass opacity is seen. A diffuse pattern of pulmonary infiltrates may also suggest infection with *Legionella* spp., fungi, or parasites. The presence of nodules, with or without cavitations, suggests infection by molds or mycobacteria. Miliary lesions suggest tuberculosis, histoplasmosis, or coccidiomycosis. Radiologic findings of pneumocystis pneumonia reveal diffuse, bilateral, interstitial, or alveolar infiltrates [15, 16]. In patients with neutropenia, radiographic evidence of pneumonia may appear only with immune reconstitution. Computed tomography, if available, is more sensitive and specific than chest radiography in these patients [16].

Bronchoscopy is suggested if persistent infiltrate, nodules, or masses are present and to obtain specimens for microbiological analysis. Patients with an endotracheal tube in place may require flexible bronchoscopy for bronchoalveolar lavage for cultures. Lung biopsy is used to obtain a definitive diagnosis of pneumonia in immunosuppressed patients with a pulmonary infiltrate. A previous nondiagnostic bronchoscopy or the need for larger specimens of tissue for diagnosis may support the need for thoracoscopic or open lung biopsy [15].

Management. Empiric therapy may be guided by local epidemiology and imaging. If the radiographic image shows focal lesions suggestive of bacterial infection, broad-spectrum antibiotics against gram-positive and gram-negative organisms should be given and the response evaluated after 48–72 h. If there is good response to antibiotics, treatment can be continued for at least 2 weeks if etiological diagnosis is not available. If broad-spectrum antibiotics are not effective, empiric treatment for organisms such as *Pneumocystis carinii* (using TMP-SMX), *Legionella* spp., or *Mycoplasma* spp. (using macrolides), and viruses (i.e., influenza virus) should be initiated. Frequently, susceptibility testing for influenza is not available in LMICs. Empiric treatment using oseltamivir may be initiated. Tuberculosis should be treated with a four-drug regimen, determined by local epidemiology. Empiric antifungal treatment can be given to patients with pulmonary nodules or cavitation or who develop new pulmonary infiltrates while receiving broad-spectrum antibiotics. Pulmonary fungal infections, particularly molds, may require longer therapy (up to months), which should be continued through periods of immunosuppression, until resolution of clinical findings and improvement of lesions in imaging studies [15].

Fungal Infections

Patients with acute myeloid leukemia or relapsed acute leukemia, patients receiving highly myelosuppressive chemotherapy for other malignancies, and allogeneic HSCT recipients who are expected to present with prolonged neutropenia (>10 days) are at high risk for IFD [7].

Candida species can cause bloodstream infection and disseminated disease such as hepatosplenic candidiasis. Mold infections, including aspergillosis, zygomycosis, and fusariosis, occur in patients with profound (<100 cells/μL) and prolonged (>10 days) neutropenia, and may affect lungs, sinuses, and soft tissues [16].

Early diagnosis is difficult due to nonspecific signs and symptoms; in early stages, persistent or recurrent fever may be the only sign of infection. In advanced infection, organ system involvement may be evident. Blood cultures are useful for the diagnosis of yeast infections, but not usually for mold infections. Galactomannan antigens have been validated as a surrogate marker for detection of invasive aspergillosis in patients with hematological malignancy [16]. Tissue obtained from lesions should be sent for fungal stains, culture, and histopathology.

Radiographic imaging such as CT may reveal abnormalities in either the lungs or sinuses. Pulmonary macronodules with or without a halo sign are the most typical findings associated with invasive aspergillosis and are evident during neutropenia. Other manifestations include nodular, wedge-shaped, peripheral, multiple, or cavitary lesions. In hepatosplenic candidemia, ultrasonography will reveal characteristic "bull's-eye" or "target" lesion with a hypoechoic mass containing a hyperechoic center. CT images may reveal areas of low density in the liver, spleen, and, sometimes, the kidney. A radiologic abnormality is more obvious after the resolution of neutropenia [16].

Empirical antifungal therapy is indicated in patients with persistent or recrudescent FN. The choice of empirical antifungal agent depends upon the likely fungal pathogens, toxicities, and cost. Prophylaxis with fluconazole reduces the incidence of invasive *Candida* infections but has no activity against molds. In patients who have not received antifungal prophylaxis, candidemia is initially the greatest concern. For patients receiving prophylaxis, infections by fluconazole-resistant strains or molds are more likely [9]. AmB desoxycholate has been the standard empirical choice. Empiric therapy with other antifungal agents, including alternate formulations of AmB, azoles with mold activity (itraconazole or voriconazole), and echinocandins (caspofungin) have been described. None have proven to have greater efficacy, but are generally less toxic than AmB [16]. For patients already receiving mold-active prophylaxis, switching to an IV anti-mold agent within a different antifungal class is recommended. Therapy should be continued until lesions have resolved (usually months) and through periods of immunosuppression (e.g., chemotherapy and transplantation) [9]. If culture of lesions is obtained, susceptibility testing should guide treatment.

Gastrointestinal Infections

Chemotherapy leads to mucositis, characterized by atrophy of the gastrointestinal (GI) mucosa, degeneration of the connective tissue, and ulceration. It is frequent among patients receiving high-dose methotrexate, cyclophosphamide and cytarabine, or anthracyclines.

Oral mucositis. Oral mucositis can be a port of entry for infectious agents, which may predispose the patient to local and severe systemic infections. Infections generally reflect the oral microbiome, such as viridans group of streptococci. Reactivation of herpetic lesions is common. Other contributing factors are periodontal disease, inadequate oral hygiene, xerostomia, and poor nutritional status. The severity of oral mucositis is assessed by the Common Toxicity Criteria for Oral Mucositis by the National Cancer Institute (NCI) and the Oral Toxicity Score of the World Health Organization (WHO) (Table 7.4).

The management of mild, uncomplicated oral mucositis is through oral hygiene and antibacterial mouthwashes. No antibiotic therapy is recommended. For infection associated with fever, localized ulceration, or lymphadenitis in patients with neutropenia, broad-spectrum antibiotic therapy is recommended. In patients with grade 3 or greater mucositis, vancomycin should be added for coverage against viridans streptococci and intravenous clindamycin for empiric coverage against *Capnocytophaga* spp. [17]. In patients who have tender cervical lymphadenopathy while receiving broad-spectrum antibiotics, antifungal agents should be considered for lymphadenitis due to *Candida* spp. [18]. For herpetic lesions, acyclovir should be given.

Table 7.4 Scales for assessment of chemotherapy-induced mucositis

World Health Organization Mucositis Toxicity Scale
0 = None
1 = Soreness ± erythema
2 = Erythema, ulcers, patient can swallow food
3 = Ulcers with extensive erythema, patient cannot swallow solid food
4 = Alimentation is not possible
National Cancer Institute Common Toxicity Criteria for Oral Mucositis
Appearance score
0 = None
1 = Erythema of the mucosa
2 = Patchy ulcerations or pseudomembranes
3 = Confluent ulcerations or pseudomembranes, bleeding with minor trauma
4 = Tissue necrosis, significant spontaneous bleeding, life-threatening consequences
Functional/symptomatic score
1 = Ability to eat solids
2 = Requires liquid diet
3 = Not able to tolerate a solid or liquid diet
4 = Symptoms associated with life-threatening consequences

Source: http://painconsortium.nih.gov/symptomresearch/chapter_17/sec7/cghs7table71pop1.htm

Enteric infections. Enteric infections are common public health issues in many LMCIs. Infections in children with cancer can be produced by community-acquired pathogens, including bacteria, viruses, and parasites. Other microorganisms (*Aeromonas* spp., *Listeria monocytogenes*, *Salmonella* spp., *Clostridium difficile*, cytomegalovirus, adenovirus, *Candida* spp., *Strongyloides stercoralis*, and *Cryptosporidium* spp.) are also known to cause enteric infection in immunocompromised hosts [19]. Most enteric pathogens are transmitted by the oral–fecal route. Risk factors include contaminated food or water, and contact with animals. Prolonged hospitalization and exposure to other infected patients can put cancer patients at risk for hospital-acquired enteritis. In patients receiving broad-spectrum antibiotics, *Clostridium difficile* may cause watery diarrhea, pseudomembranous colitis, or toxic megacolon.

For the diagnosis, stool samples should be sent for white blood cell smear, routine microscopy (ova and parasites) modified acid fast stains

Table 7.5 Treatment of bacterial infections in the child with cancer and infectious diarrhea

Organism	Antibiotic	Alternative antibiotic	Duration of treatment
Aeromonas spp.	Azithromycin (10–12 mg/kg/day daily) Ceftriaxone (50 mg/kg/day daily)	TMP-SMZ (8–12 mg/kg/day ÷ 2 TMP)	3–5 days
Campylobacter jejuni	Azithromycin (10–12 mg/kg/day daily) Erythromycin (40 mg/kg/day ÷ 4)	Ciprofloxacin** (20 mg/kg/day ÷ 2)	5–7 days
Clostridium difficile	Metronidazole (30 mg/kg//day ÷ 3 IV/oral)	Vancomycin (oral) (40 mg/kg/day ÷ 4)	10–14 days
E. coli	Ciprofloxacin** (20 mg/kg/day ÷ 2)	Azithromycin (10–12 mg/kg/day daily)	3–5 days
Plesiomonas shigelloides	TMP-SMZ (8–12 mg/kg/day ÷ 2 TMP)	Ciprofloxacin** (20 mg/kg/day ÷ 2)	3–5 days
Salmonella (colitis)	Cefotaxime (150 mg/kg/day ÷ 3) Ceftriaxone (50 mg/kg/day daily)	Ciprofloxacin** (20 mg/kg/day ÷ 2) Azithromycin (10–12 mg/kg/day daily)	7–10 days
Shigella spp.	Ceftriaxone (50 mg/kg/day daily) Ciprofloxacin** (20–30 mg/kg/day ÷ 2)	Azithromycin (12 mg/kg/day daily)	5 days
Vibrio cholerae	Doxycycline (2–4 mg/kg/day ÷ 2) Tetracycline* (25–50 mg/kg/day ÷ 4)	Azithromycin (12 mg/kg/day daily) Ciprofloxacin** for resistant strains	3 days
Vibrio vulnificus	Ceftriaxone (50 mg/kg/day daily) plus Doxycycline (2–4 mg/kg/day ÷ 2)	TMP-SMX plus aminoglycoside	Until clinical resolution
Yersinia enterocolitica	TMP-SMX (8–12 mg/kg/day ÷ 2 TMP)	Cefotaxime Aminoglycosides Fluoroquinolones** Doxycycline/tetracycline*	–

Treatment recommendations based on *Red Book: 2012 Report of the Committee on Infectious Diseases*
TMP-SMX trimethoprim/sulfamethoxazole
*Stains developing teeth; use only in children > 8 years of age
**Use of fluoroquinolones in children is indicated when no safe and effective alternative exists and clinicians should be cognizant of fluroquinolones specific adverse reactions

(coccidian protozoa), antigen testing (rotavirus), *C. difficile* toxins, and cultures for enteric bacteria. If the patient with enteric symptoms has fever, blood cultures should be obtained.

Patients with enteritis should receive replacement therapy for lost fluids and electrolytes, with the goal of maintaining appropriate levels of fluids and electrolytes and promptly reintroducing feeding. Table 7.5 outlines the treatment of common bacterial processes, and Table 7.6 gives the treatment of parasitic enteric pathogens [19, 20]. If tests for *C. difficile* toxins are unavailable, empiric therapy should be considered in patients with compatible clinical symptoms and in whom other etiology has been ruled out.

Esophagitis. Symptoms of esophagitis include odynophagia, dysphagia, retrosternal pain, and upper GI tract bleeding. Common etiological agents in immunocompromised patients are *Candida* spp., herpesviruses, and cytomegalovirus [21]. Definitive diagnosis is established using endoscopy. If not available, clinical findings may provide etiological clues for empiric therapy. The presence of oral thrush in patients with cancer is a reliable clinical marker of esophageal candidiasis [22]. Patients with herpes esophagitis typically have an acute onset of severe odynophagia and lesions in the oral mucosa. Although less specific, cytomegalovirus esophagitis can be associated with adenopathy and an erythematous or ulcerated oropharynx.

Candida and herpes esophagitis can often be diagnosed on double-contrast studies, obviating endoscopy. If radiographic findings are equivocal or if response to treatment is inadequate, endoscopy should be performed for a more definitive diagnosis. Material for culture and histological

Table 7.6 Treatment of selected parasitic enteric pathogens in immunocompromised children with infectious diarrhea

Organism	Antiparasitic	Alternative
Blastocystis hominis	Metronidazole (30–50 mg/kg/day ÷ 3 PO × 10 days) followed by Iodoquinol (30–40 mg/kg/day ÷ 3 × 20 days)	Nitazoxanide × 3 days
		(1–3 years: 200 mg/day ÷ 2)
		(4–11 years: 400 mg/day ÷ 2) (>12 years: 500 mg oral twice daily) TMP-SMX (160/800) 1 tab BID × 7 days
Cryptosporidium parvum	Nitazoxanide × 3 days	Paromomycin (25–35 mg/kg/day ÷ 3)
	(1–3 years: 200 mg/day ÷ 2)	plus
	(4–11 years: 400 mg/day ÷ 2) (>12 years: 500 mg oral twice daily)	Azithromycin (12 mg/kg/day daily)
Cyclospora cayetanensis	Trimethoprim/Sulfamethoxazole (8–12 mg/kg/day ÷ 2 TMP × 7–10 days)	Ciprofloxacin (500 mg PO BID × 7 days)
Cystoisospora belli (formerly known as Isospora)	Trimethoprim/sulfamethoxazole (8–12 mg/kg/day ÷ 2 TMP × 10 days)	
Entamoeba histolytica	Metronidazole (30–50 mg/kg/day ÷ 3 PO × 10 days) followed by iodoquinol (×20 days) or paromomycin (×7 days)	Tinidazole (50 mg/kg/day daily; above 3 years) followed by iodoquinol or paromomycin
		Nitazoxanide
Giardia lamblia	Metronidazole (15 mg/kg/day ÷ 3PO × 5–7 days)	Paromomycin × 5–10 days
	Tinidazole (50 mg/kg/day daily, once; above 3 years)	
	Nitazoxanide × 3 days	
Microsporidia	Albendazole (15 mg/kg/day ÷ 2 doses, max 400 mg/dose)	Nitazoxanide
Strongyloides	Ivermectin (200 μg/kg/day PO × 2 days)	Albendazole (400 mg PO BID × 7 days)

Treatment recommendations based on *Red Book*: *2012 Report of the Committee on Infectious Diseases*

examination may be obtained during the endoscopic examination.

Candida esophagitis can be treated with fluconazole in stable patients. Seriously ill patients should be given an echinocandin or AmB formulation. Definitive treatment should be guided by using susceptibility testing. Duration of treatment is 14–21 days [9]. Esophagitis caused by herpes simplex virus (HSV) should be treated with acyclovir for 14–21 days or if resistant with foscarnet for 7–14 days. Patients with cytomegalic virus (CMV) esophagitis should receive ganciclovir or foscarnet for 14–21 days [21].

Typhlitis. Typhlitis (also called neutropenic enterocolitis, neutropenic colitis, or cecitis) is characterized by fever and abdominal pain in cancer patients with neutropenia. Common signs and symptoms include nausea, vomiting, diarrhea (bloody in 54 %), decreased bowel sounds, abdominal distension, rebound and guarding, and right lower quadrant fullness or mass. In the early stages, typhlitis is difficult to differentiate from the effects of chemotherapy, especially if fever is absent [23, 24]. In patients with bacteremia, isolates commonly correspond to colonic flora.

Abdominal ultrasound or CT is useful to confirm the diagnosis. Radiological findings include thickening of the intestinal mucosa, decreased diameter of the intestinal lumen, inflammatory changes around the cecum, and the presence of intraperitoneal fluid. Imaging results do not alter management unless bowel perforation is suspected. In such cases, CT is the preferred imaging modality [24]. All cancer patients with diarrhea or suspected typhlitis should have a stool test for the *Clostridium difficile* toxin if available.

Antibiotics need not be given if no specific or significant signs and symptoms are present. Stable patients with fever and GI signs and symptoms of typhlitis can be managed with carbapenem monotherapy. In toxic or ill-appearing patients with clinical evidence of sepsis, vancomycin and an aminoglycoside should be administered in addition to carbapenems. Vancomycin can also be considered in patients who have recently received high-dose Ara-C or those who received quinolones before the onset of symptoms. Narcotics enhance stasis of bacterial and fungal organism in the cecum and should be avoided. If the patient does not improve within 72–96 h or has been on broad-spectrum antibiotic therapy in the week before onset, empiric antifungal therapy can be initiated [23, 24]. Intravenous antimicrobials should be continued until neutropenia and abdominal symptoms resolve, or until the diagnosis of typhlitis is excluded. Indications for surgical treatment are persistent GI bleeding and intestinal perforation; worsening clinical status suggesting an uncontrolled sepsis; and the presence of symptoms of a surgical intra-abdominal process.

Conclusion

Infections in children with cancer should be appropriately treated to increase survival. Although LMCIs are faced with limitations, some practices are cost-effective and can decrease morbidity and mortality. These practices are: (1) expeditious clinical evaluation, including the collection of microbiology samples and initiation of therapy in children with febrile neutropenia; (2) adapting published guidelines to local epidemiology for initial empiric management of common infections; (3) reserving local supplies of broad-spectrum antibiotics for use in patients with febrile neutropenia and severe infections; and (4) treating seriously ill children with unstable vital signs with intravenous broad-spectrum antimicrobials effective against pathogens associated with high morbimortality (e.g., gram-negative or multidrug resistant pathogens).

Infection Prevention

General Concepts

Prevention of infection, both in the home environment and in the hospital, is very important in the management of an immunosuppressed child receiving cancer treatment. In the mid-1970s, the Study on the Efficacy of Nosocomial Infection Control (SENIC Project) in hospitals across the USA found that healthcare-associated infections (HAI) rates were reduced by 32 % in hospitals that implemented infection prevention control (IPC) programs [25]. The main goal of an IPC program is to establish strategies to protect patients, staff, and visitors from infection and to achieve this goal in the most economical manner possible [26]. A collaborative effort by the St. Jude Children's Research Hospital (St. Jude) focuses on improving the capacity for care and prevention of infections among children at pediatric cancer centers (PCCs) in Latin America, Morocco, and the Philippines [27]. Interventions in the care and prevention of infections at PCCs are carried out in collaboration with local clinicians at partner and non-partner sites.

Challenges to Implementing Infection Prevention and Control in Low- and Middle-Income Countries

Structure of IPC programs. Structured institutional programs as recommended by leading organizations [26, 28–30] do not yet exist in many hospitals in LMICs. Appropriate legislation of IPC programs in conjunction with education of healthcare workers, surveillance of HAI, and consistent implementation of basic IPC measures are essential elements to sustain such programs [31]. Most Latin American countries [27], by promulgating a legislation for IPC programs, have established a legal accountability of healthcare institutions in implementing IPC programs.

Competent and certified personnel in IPC programs. Qualified team members (e.g., infection preventionist, program director, and data manager or statistician) are essential. Despite the presence of legislation in some Latin American countries that require the training of preventionists [27], this requirement is not enforced in most cases. Individual efforts, such as those by St. Jude [32], have filled the void of trained preventionists via structured IPC training since 2005. The requirement for qualified preventionists is part of the core standard for IPC recommended by the International Joint Commission's international accreditation standards for hospitals [33]. Only a few hospitals outside the USA, including those in LMICs, have received this accreditation [34, 35].

Role and number of preventionists. The role of preventionists includes infection prevention, as well as studying risks for healthcare personnel, evaluating the physical environment, and laying out contingency plans [35]. However, in LMICs, basic concerns such as the number of preventionists and their availability continue to exist. Low standards of healthcare delivery, lack of institutional resources, insufficient training of healthcare providers (HCP), and limited institutional support for IPC programs add a burden on preventionists. Thus the newer recommendations of 1 preventionist per 100 beds continue to be highly inappropriate for institutions in LMICs.

Administrative and financial support to IPC programs. Investing in IPC programs by assigning a budget for essential activities leads to important cost saving by preventing HAIs and their associated problems. For a strong IPC program, training support from experts (e.g., microbiologists), support for obtaining and managing data, training of hospital staff, and feedback on their performance and participation in purchasing essential supplies for patient care are recommended [26]. Healthcare institutions at LMICs are beginning to recognize the impact of the cost savings and the quality of healthcare provided by the IPC programs [36].

Human and nonhuman institutional resources. Scarcity of healthcare personnel and lack of training are significant obstacles to IPC procedures. The absence of basic infrastructure (e.g., sinks, safe water, physical space), lack of basic supplies (e.g., antiseptics, cleaning products), and the lack of standardized procedure can also impede IPC initiatives [37]. Prioritizing areas for IPC investment will ensure that the program integrates into the organizational structure, thereby allowing sustainability. A good example for this type of investment is hand hygiene and safe vascular access [38, 39].

Monitoring the composition and functioning of the IPC program. A periodic review of the composition and performance of the IPC program is essential to enforce the standards of quality care delivery.

Access to data on HAIs for primary healthcare providers and patients. Surveillance of infections and their risk factors is scarce in most institutions in LMICs, and in those where surveillance has been implemented the quality of the data is poor, unreliable, and inconsistent. Our experience with some of the St. Jude international partner sites shows that surveillance data are not standardized, definitions are not used consistently, and quality of data is not checked. To improve IPC programs, good quality surveillance provides a tool for initial and ongoing reference for interventions to improve IPC.

Challenges to Infection Prevention and Control in Children with Cancer

To protect immunocompromised patients from infections, a safe environment of care is required in which infection prevention measures are enforced.

Diagnosis of HAIs in children with cancer and the source of infecting pathogens. Children with cancer are susceptible to common community-acquired pathogens as well as to rarer opportunistic pathogens. The causative microorganisms can be part of the skin, respiratory, gastrointestinal, or genitourinary flora, and during prolonged hospital stays some microorganisms can be acquired from the hospital environment. Infecting pathogens acquired either at home or at the hospital can be similar because these microorganisms can become part of the resident microbial flora in the patients due to multiple hospitalizations; therefore, ascertaining where the patients acquired the infection can be difficult. Moreover, in many cases the standard incubation period cannot be used to determine the relationship between the onset of acute infection and the time of hospital admission because of the lack of protective immunity. If a patient with cancer shows signs and symptoms of infection while hospitalized, the causative microorganism might have been acquired before admission, during a previous hospitalization, or after a current admission to the hospital.

A complicating factor in ascertaining whether an infection is hospital acquired is that latent infections acquired early in life may become activated during immunosuppression. Reactivation of those infections must be differentiated from acute primary infections caused by the same microorganism, which could have been acquired during or after hospitalization. These infections could include those from the herpes family group, pneumocystis, mycobacteria, parasites, and fungi. Thus, the interpretation of pathogens isolated in an immunocompromised host is different from that in a healthy host. Also, the recognition of an infected site may be difficult, as the signs of infection may be blunted in patients with neutropenia or anemia because of lack of inflammatory response. Patients with neutropenia and anemia might show mild or no clinical evidence of infections of the skin and subcutaneous tissues, urinary tract and meninges, or in the case of pneumonia, radiographic findings might be subtle or absent.

Establishing the source of infection may be difficult because the patient might have had multiple hospitalizations or required multiple, often multidisciplinary, sites for care during a hospitalization. When assessing HAIs in cancer patients, the surveillance must include infection rates based on the number of patient-days at risk (defined as a period of neutropenia), antimicrobial prophylaxis, and the diagnostic resources to track potential pathogens.

Host risk factors. Mucositis, antimicrobials, low stomach acidity, impaired intestinal motility, presence of vascular catheters, and deficient humoral and cellular immunity are risk factors for infection in children with cancer. Infecting pathogens can be part of patients' own flora that translocate into the blood stream to produce bacteremia and sepsis. Microorganisms in the blood stream, unchallenged by phagocytes, can multiply exponentially and quickly kill the host when the burden of the pathogens' metabolic needs and toxic waste cannot be borne by the infected host [40]. In LMICs, lack of hygiene can facilitate more frequent exposure to foodborne pathogens, for which children with cancer are at increased risk. In addition to these inherent problems in children with cancer, endemic infections, parasitosis, frequent insect bites, and malnutrition can be frequently encountered in low-income countries [41, 42]. These health problems tend to exacerbate when cancer treatments are administered.

Environment of care. Care of children with cancer requires a multispecialty team, and multiple hospital admissions are often the norm. This increases the risk for exposure to cross-transmitted pathogens, especially when compliance with procedures for infection preventions is suboptimal.

In most LMICs, PCCs function within large healthcare institutions, most of them public hospitals supported by the government and associated with teaching institutions. These hospitals are referral hospitals, and in some countries the only hospital for specialized pediatric care. As these hospitals provide care free-of-charge or with minimum payment, they are overcrowded with indigent patients and are understaffed. Frequently, targeted training of HCPs happens only periodically. This lack of standard is more pronounced in teaching hospitals, where undergraduate medical and nursing students and other health-related professionals care for children with cancer with limited supervision. In addition, in many PCCs in LMICs, pediatric residents are the only care providers for these children after hours with oncologists usually available only telephonically. Because of the limited availability of pediatric oncologists, exclusive care by them can rarely be provided round the clock. Furthermore, pediatric infectious disease (ID) specialists and preventionists in many PCCs do not actively participate in the care of children with cancer. If the PCC has access to ID physicians, they are consulted only when the child has a severe infection, a rare pathogen needs to be isolated, or during the emergence of an infectious outbreak. Most ID physicians and preventionists are also not well prepared to care for children with cancer who have infections. Usually, these professionals have not had sufficient exposure to cancer care or been trained in care and prevention of infections in cancer during their studies. Therefore, they lack an understanding of the complexity and the urgency of care during infections. Moreover, healthcare employees in public hospitals are not paid well and work in multiple healthcare sites to supplement their income. Some hospitals function with minimum personnel and IPC standards are poor or nonexistent, increasing the risk of infections in children with cancer during critical times of immunosuppression.

In most hospitals that have a PCC, the multiple needs of children with other pathologies compete with the needs of children with cancer. The lack or absence of essential antimicrobials, forcing HPCs to use less optimal treatment, is a major concern. During times of critical shortage, family members or NGOs need to purchase antimicrobials and supplies.

Essential Areas of Engagement to Improve Care and Prevention of Infections

Patient hygiene and safe food. The mechanical removal of dirt and bacteria can be achieved through careful body washing. Recent reports show that a chlorhexidine wash decreases the incidence of infections in patients in the intensive care unit (ICU) [43]. Meticulous and frequent mouth care during chemotherapy can decrease the complications of mucositis and ventilator-associated pneumonias (Joanna Acebo, 2012, personal communication).

The CDC recommends a low-bacteria diet for 3 months after autologous hematopoietic stem cell transplantation (HSCT) and until all immunosuppressive drugs are discontinued for allogeneic recipients [44]. In low-bacteria diets, consumption of raw fruits and vegetables is restricted because of concerns of contamination with Gram-negative bacilli. Guidelines for safe food preparation should be followed in the hospital's kitchen as well as at home. Strategies for safe food preparation include good hand hygiene, clean utensils and food preparation surfaces, and cooking at recommended temperatures. Other strategies include choosing packed food, drinking boiled or bottled water, and avoiding traditional foods that do not comply with safety regulations. Supplemental feeding, such as enteral feeding, can become contaminated with *S. epidermidis*, *S. aureus*, and Gram-negative bacilli during preparation and administration of products and systems. Colony counts in enteral feedings increase with the hang time of the product and the administration set. Therefore, it is recommended [35] that high-risk patients receive ready-to-feed enteral feeding via closed systems and that administration sets be changed every 24 h.

Hand hygiene and safe vascular access. The WHO *Clean Care is Safer Care* focuses on the aspects of hand hygiene and safe injections [45]. The first step is to improve hand hygiene by improving access to essential infrastructure (sinks) and supplies (soaps, towels, alcohol gel), awareness (through health education and promotion), policies and procedures, and working on the institution buy-in by providing feedback on hand hygiene procedures to hospital leaders [46]. After hand hygiene practices have been instated, the focus should be on other key practices such as vascular access. Important components of safe vascular access include trained HCP, access to all the supplies at the point of care, careful site location, skin asepsis, and catheter securing. After catheter insertion, careful hand hygiene and frequent site evaluation, cleaning of the catheter every time it is accessed, and flushing the catheter after use prevent infections-related complications and clotting [47].

Safe blood. The Pan American Health Organization Blood Transfusion Safety program encourages four main strategies to manage a safe blood service: (1) planning and managing a national integrated system for blood banks, (2) promoting the voluntary donation of blood, (3) guaranteeing the quality of blood, and (4) appropriately using blood and its components.

Modern chemotherapy relies on highly myelosuppressive treatment; thus blood and blood products are essential for supportive care. However, blood-transmitted diseases are a major concern. Therefore, a local institutional or country-wide program based on careful screening of donors, safe storage and use of blood can decrease the risk of transmitting infections.

Safe environment of care. A safe environment can be provided by closely monitoring the cleaning and disinfection process and using appropriate cleaning supplies and methods. The goal of environmental cleaning is to remove organisms that survive in the environment and to prevent dust dispersal [48]. To achieve this goal, written environmental services policies must be in place; cleaning must be performed by trained and reliable personnel; dust accumulation should be prevented by daily cleaning of frequently touched areas; and damp dusting and mopping should be done by using hospital high-grade disinfectants and high-efficiency particulate vacuum cleaners in carpeted areas or by avoiding carpeting all together. Rooms of patients infected with *C. difficile* should be cleaned carefully and disinfected with hypochlorite cleaning solutions [49]. It is important to de-clutter the patient's room by providing lockers to families for storage. Linens must be handled by standard methods. Linens washed and dried per standard hospital protocol contain very few pathogenic organisms, and sterile linens are therefore not needed. Vase water from fresh flowers can harbor Gram-negative bacilli such as *Pseudomonas aeruginosa* and dried and fresh flowers and potted plants can harbor fungi such as *Aspergillus* and *Fusarium* spp. Hence, both fresh and dried plants and flowers should be avoided in units that house immunocompromised patients.

The goal of management of air and ventilation is to minimize the risk of transmission of airborne pathogens such as *Aspergillus*. Hospital ventilation systems can facilitate the dissemination of *Aspergillus* spores; therefore incoming air should ideally be high-efficiency particulate air (HEPA) filtered, which can remove up to 99.97 % of spores as small as 0.3 μm from the air. Laminar air flow allows air to move through a bank of HEPA filters, thereby providing optimal airflow with minimal turbulence. Air quality for immunocompromised patients can be improved by maintaining positive room air pressure relative to the corridor, well-sealed rooms to prevent flow of air from the outside, and ventilation to provide more than 12 air changes per hour. Air sampling needs to be performed when HEPA filters are changed, before opening areas that have undergone construction and when investigating outbreaks of invasive *Aspergillus* infection. Construction and renovations require careful planning to protect patients from the risk associated with fungal infections, especially molds. Containment measures include adequate barriers and negative pressure inside the construction site. Barriers required include plastic for low-risk areas (offices) and hard-wall barriers with sealed joints in most areas delivering healthcare adjacent to the demolition and/or removal of large numbers of ceiling tiles. If flooding occurs during construction due to broken pipes or obstructed drains, the source of water must be identified, the problem fixed as soon as possible, and patients immediately evacuated from the exposed area. If the water is clean and the structural material can be dried within 72 h, no removal or replacement of contaminated materials may be necessary. If drying cannot be accomplished in a timely manner or if dirty water or sewage is involved in the flooding, removal of contaminated materials and disinfection of the area with germicide is required. Water damage remediation plans must be available to reference in case such events occur.

Isolation measures to prevent dissemination of pathogens are a frequent problem, especially during limited space availability. Maintaining a minimum distance of at least 1 m between beds; providing essential needs to each patient and educating parents on avoiding sharing; frequent cleaning of beds and beds rails; access to alcohol gel at the beds; and categorizing patients by the type of pathogen infection are some strategies to reduce the dissemination of pathogens.

Access to diagnostic laboratories and essential antibiotics and administration supplies. The expedited initiation of antimicrobials improves survival and decreases the spread of contagious pathogens [50]. Access to microbiology laboratories can allow pathogens to be identified and isolated so that timely treatment can be initiated [51]. Publication and hospital-wide distribution of the yearly summary of pathogens isolated in the microbiology laboratories with the corresponding antibiogram will allow the HCP to make an educated guess while choosing empiric antimicrobial regimens.

Conclusion

The treatment of children with cancer is expensive and prolonged and requires a broad range of critical resources in the already overburdened healthcare institutions in the developing world. As described herein, investment in an IPC program for PCCs is cost-effective, considering the heavy cost of care of children with cancer imposed on the institution.

Infections can be prevented by using simple procedures such as hand hygiene, patient hygiene, complete and frequent evaluation of patients to identify the risk for infection or early infection, safe food preparation, and using barriers during invasive activities. Procedures of medium complexity require isolation and might need special infrastructure and supplies, whereas procedures of high complexity require special ventilation and other technologies for improving air quality.

To build onsite infection care prevention capacity for PCCs in LMICs, it is important to address the financial aspects and gain support from medical and administrative leaders. The long-term support for infection care and prevention programs will depend on demonstrating a financial benefit of providing better quality healthcare for children with cancer via the structured and organized activities of ICP programs.

References

1. Watson RS, Carcillo JA, Linde-Zwirble WT, Clermont G, Lidicker J, Angus DC. The epidemiology of severe sepsis in children in the United States. Am J Respir Crit Care Med. 2003;167(5):695–701.
2. Pizzo PA, Rubin M, Freifeld A, Walsh TJ. The child with cancer and infection. I. Empiric therapy for fever and neutropenia, and preventive strategies. J Pediatr. 1991;119(5):679–94.
3. Ribeiro RC, Steliarova-Foucher E, Magrath I, Lemerle J, Eden T, Forget C, et al. Baseline status of paediatric oncology care in ten low-income or mid-income countries receiving My Child Matters support: a descriptive study. Lancet Oncol. 2008;9(8):721–9.
4. Tamburro R. Pediatric cancer patients in clinical trials of sepsis: factors that predispose to sepsis and stratify outcome. Pediatr Crit Care Med. 2005;6(3 Suppl): S87–91.
5. Freifeld AG, Bow EJ, Sepkowitz KA, Boeckh MJ, Ito JI, Mullen CA, et al. Clinical practice guideline for the use of antimicrobial agents in neutropenic patients with cancer: 2010 update by the infectious diseases society of America. Clin Infect Dis. 2011;52(4):e56–93.
6. Ramphal R. Changes in the etiology of bacteremia in febrile neutropenic patients and the susceptibilities of the currently isolated pathogens. Clin Infect Dis. 2004;39 Suppl 1:S25–31.
7. Lehrnbecher T, Phillips R, Alexander S, Alvaro F, Carlesse F, Fisher B, et al. Guideline for the management of fever and neutropenia in children with cancer and/or undergoing hematopoietic stem-cell transplantation. J Clin Oncol. 2012;30(35):4427–38.
8. Furno P, Bucaneve G, Del FA. Monotherapy or aminoglycoside-containing combinations for empirical antibiotic treatment of febrile neutropenic patients: a meta-analysis. Lancet Infect Dis. 2002;2(4): 231–42.
9. Pappas PG, Kauffman CA, Andes D, Benjamin Jr DK, Calandra TF, Edwards Jr JE, et al. Clinical practice guidelines for the management of candidiasis: 2009 update by the Infectious Diseases Society of America. Clin Infect Dis. 2009;48(5):503–35.
10. Raad I, Hanna H, Maki D. Intravascular catheter-related infections: advances in diagnosis, prevention, and management. Lancet Infect Dis. 2007;7(10): 645–57.
11. Gaur AH, Flynn PM, Giannini MA, Shenep JL, Hayden RT. Difference in time to detection: a simple method to differentiate catheter-related from non-catheter-related bloodstream infection in immunocompromised pediatric patients. Clin Infect Dis. 2003;37(4):469–75.

12. Gaur AH, Flynn PM, Heine DJ, Giannini MA, Shenep JL, Hayden RT. Diagnosis of catheter-related bloodstream infections among pediatric oncology patients lacking a peripheral culture, using differential time to detection. Pediatr Infect Dis J. 2005;24(5):445–9.
13. Mermel LA, Allon M, Bouza E, Craven DE, Flynn P, O'Grady NP, et al. Clinical practice guidelines for the diagnosis and management of intravascular catheter-related infection: 2009 Update by the Infectious Diseases Society of America. Clin Infect Dis. 2009; 49(1):1–45.
14. Hirsch HH, Martino R, Ward KN, Boeckh M, Einsele H, Ljungman P. Fourth European Conference on Infections in Leukaemia (ECIL-4): guidelines for diagnosis and treatment of human respiratory syncytial virus, parainfluenza virus, metapneumovirus, rhinovirus, and coronavirus. Clin Infect Dis. 2013; 56(2):258–66.
15. Stokes DC. Sinopulmonary infections in immunocompromised infants and children. In: Patrick CC, editor. Clinical management of infections in immunocomprised infants and children. Philadelphia: Lippincott Williams & Wilkins; 2001. p. 353–87.
16. Kaste SC. Infeciton imaging of children and adolescent undergoing cancer therapy: a review of modalities and an organ system approach. Semin Pediatr infect Dis. 2000;11:122–41.
17. Shenep JL. Combination and single-agent empirical antibacterial therapy for febrile cancer patients with neutropenia and mucositis. Natl Cancer Inst Mongr. 1990;9:117–22.
18. Shenep JL, Kalwinsky DK, Feldman S, Pearson TA. Mycotic cervical lymphadenitis following oral mucositis in children with leukemia. J Pediatr. 1985;106(2):243–6.
19. Mitchell DK, Pickering LK. Enteric infections. In: Patrick CC, editor. Clinical management of Infections in Immunocompromised Infants and Children. 2nd ed. Philadelphia: Lippincott Williams & Wilkins; 2001. p. 413–49.
20. Pickering LK, Baker CJ, Kimberlin DW, Long SS. Red Book: 2012 report of the Committee on Infectious Diseases. 29th ed. Elk Grove Village, IL: American Academy of Pediatrics; 2012.
21. McDonald GB, Sharma P, Hackman RC, Meyers JD, Thomas ED. Esophageal infections in immunosuppressed patients after marrow transplantation. Gastroenterology. 1985;88(5 Pt. 1):1111–7.
22. Samonis G, Skordilis P, Maraki S, Datseris G, Toloudis P, Chatzinikolaou I, et al. Oropharyngeal candidiasis as a marker for esophageal candidiasis in patients with cancer. Clin Infect Dis. 1998;27(2):283–6.
23. McCarville MB, Adelman CS, Li C, Xiong X, Furman WL, Razzouk BI, et al. Typhlitis in childhood cancer. Cancer. 2005;104(2):380–7.
24. Sloas MM, Flynn PM, Kaste SC, Patrick CC. Typhlitis in children with cancer: a 30-year experience. Clin Infect Dis. 1993;17(3):484–90.
25. Haley RW, Culver DH, White JW, Morgan WM, Emori TG, Munn VP, et al. The efficacy of infection surveillance and control programs in preventing nosocomial infections in US hospitals. Am J Epidemiol. 1985;121(2):182–205.
26. Scheckler WE, Brimhall D, Buck AS, Farr BM, Friedman C, Garibaldi RA, et al. Requirements for infrastructure and essential activities of infection control and epidemiology in hospitals: a consensus panel report. Society for Healthcare Epidemiology of America. Am J Infect Control. 1998;26(1):47–60.
27. Ade y Torrent MP, Bolis M. Infecciones Hospitalarias: Legislacion en America Latina. internet 2007 [cited 2011 Dec 19]. www.who.int/csr/resources/.../WHO.../index.html.
28. World Health Organization. Prevencion de las infecciones nosocomiales. 2nd ed. Geneva, Switzerland: World Health Organization; 2003.
29. World Health Organization. Componentes basicos para los programas de prevencion y control de infecciones. Internet 2008 June 26 [cited 2011 Dec 19]. www.who.int/csr/resources/.../WHO.../index.html
30. Freidman C. Infection prevention and control programs. In: APIC, editor. APIC text of infection control and epidemiology. 3rd ed. Washington, DC: Association for Professionals in Infection Control and Epidemiology, Inc.; 2009.
31. Pittet D, Allegranzi B, Storr J, Donaldson L. 'Clean care is safer care': the global patient safety challenge 2005–2006. Int J Infect Dis. 2006;10(6):419–24.
32. Caniza MA, Maron G, McCullers J, Clara WA, Cedillos R, Duenas L, et al. Planning and implementation of an infection control training program for healthcare providers in Latin America. Infect Control Hosp Epidemiol. 2007;28(12):1328–33.
33. Joint Commission International. Joint Commission International Accreditation Standards for hospitals. 4th ed. Oakbrook Terrace, IL: Department of Publications, Joint Commission Resources; 2010.
34. JCI Accredited Organizations. Internet. 2012. www.who.int/csr/resources/.../WHO.../index.html. Accessed 31 Dec 2012.
35. Association for Professionals in Infection Control and Epidemiology, Joint Commission on Accreditation of Healthcare Organizations. The APIC/JCR infection prevention and control workbook. 2nd ed. Oakbrook Terrace, IL: Department of Publications Joint Commission Resources; 2010.
36. Higuera F, Rangel-Frausto MS, Rosenthal VD, Soto JM, Castanon J, Franco G, et al. Attributable cost and length of stay for patients with central venous catheter-associated bloodstream infection in Mexico City intensive care units: a prospective, matched analysis. Infect Control Hosp Epidemiol. 2007;28(1):31–5.
37. Huskins WC, O'Rourke EJ, Hrinehart E, Goldmann DA. Infection control in countries with limited resources. In: Mayhall CG, editor. Hospital epidemiology and infection control. 3rd ed. Philadelphia, PA: Lippincott Williams & Wilkins; 2004. p. 1889–917.
38. Cummings KL, Anderson DJ, Kaye KS. Hand hygiene noncompliance and the cost of hospital-acquired methicillin-resistant Staphylococcus aureus infection. Infect Control Hosp Epidemiol. 2010;31(4):357–64.

39. Duda CR, Spergel LM, Holland J, Tucker CT, Bander SJ, Bosch JP. How a multidisciplinary vascular access care program enables implementation of the DOQI guidelines. Part I. Nephrol News Issues. 2000; 14(5):13–7.
40. Rubin LG. Comparison of in vivo and in vitro multiplication rates of Haemophilus influenzae type b. Infect Immun. 1986;52(3):911–3.
41. Martinez PA, Justiniani Cedeno NE. [Incidence of intestinal parasites in pediatric patients with hematologic neoplasms from 1 to 15 years of age]. Rev Alerg Mex. 1999;46(1):26–9.
42. Antillon F, Rossi E, Molina AL, Sala A, Pencharz P, Valsecchi MG, et al. Nutritional status of children during treatment for acute lymphoblastic leukemia in Guatemala. Pediatr Blood Cancer. 2013;60: 911–5.
43. Derde LP, Dautzenberg MJ, Bonten MJ. Chlorhexidine body washing to control antimicrobial-resistant bacteria in intensive care units: a systematic review. Intensive Care Med. 2012;38(6):931–9.
44. Centers for Disease Control and Prevention; Infectious Disease Society of America; American Society of Blood and Marrow Transplantation. Guidelines for preventing opportunistic infections among hematopoietic stem cell transplant recipients. MMWR Recomm Rep. 2000;49(RR-10):1–7.
45. World Health Organization. Clean care is safer care; internet 2012 [cited 2012 Nov 7]. http://www.who.int.
46. Haas JP, Larson EL. Compliance with hand hygiene guidelines: where are we in 2008? Am J Nurs. 2008;108(8):40–4.
47. Pronovost P, Needham D, Berenholtz S, Sinopoli D, Chu H, Cosgrove S, et al. An intervention to decrease catheter-related bloodstream infections in the ICU. N Engl J Med. 2006;355(26):2725–32.
48. Association for Professionals in Infection Control and Epidemiology I. APIC text of infection control & epidemiology. 2nd ed. Washington, DC: Association for Professionals in Infection Control and Epidemiology, Inc.; 2005.
49. Cohen SH, Gerding DN, Johnson S, Kelly CP, Loo VG, McDonald LC, et al. Clinical practice guidelines for Clostridium difficile infection in adults: 2010 update by the society for healthcare epidemiology of America (SHEA) and the infectious diseases society of America (IDSA). Infect Control Hosp Epidemiol. 2010;31(5):431–55.
50. Gavidia R, Fuentes SL, Vasquez R, Bonilla M, Ethier MC, Diorio C, et al. Low socioeconomic status is associated with prolonged times to assessment and treatment, sepsis and infectious death in pediatric fever in El Salvador. PLoS One. 2012;7(8):e43639.
51. Stratton CW, Greene JN. Role of the microbiology laboratory in hospital epidemiology and infection control. In: Mayhall CG, editor. Hospital epidemiology and infection control. 2nd ed. Philadelphia: Lippincott Williams & Wilkins; 1999. p. 1423–35.

Nutritional Assessment and Intervention

8

Paul C. Rogers and Judy Schoeman

Introduction

Adequate nutrition is a fundamental necessity to ensure adequate growth and development during infancy, childhood and adolescence. Disease processes are well described in children who have inadequate or inappropriate nutrition of calories, protein, vitamins, essential fatty acids and trace elements [1]. In the presence of an additional disease, such as cancer, poor nutrition may exacerbate the state of the child's ill health and increase the morbidity and mortality associated with the cancer and malnutrition [2–4].

Malnutrition has two ends of the spectrum, the one side is undernutrition with protein energy malnutrition (PEM) and the other end of the spectrum malnutrition is due to excess calorie consumption leading to overweight or morbid obesity. Although undernutrition is far more common in low income countries (LIC), the problems of obesity are increasing due to adaptation of a western diet and easy access to fast food vendors. The risk for developing PEM depends on the type of cancer, the stage and treatment regimens [5–10].

P.C. Rogers, M.B., Ch.B., F.R.C.P.C., M.B.A.
Division of Pediatric Oncology/Hematology/BMT, BC Childrens Hospital & University of BC, 4480 Oak Street, Vancouver, BC, Canada V6H 3V4

J. Schoeman, B.Dietetics, B.Compt., M.Sc. Dietetics (✉)
Paediatric Oncology Unit, Oncology Complex 4th Floor, Steve Biko Academic Hospital, Private Bag X139, Pretoria 0001, South Africa
e-mail: judy.schoeman@gmail.com

Effects of Malnutrition on Patients

It is reported that 5–50 % of patients are undernourished at diagnosis of their cancer and is definitely more frequently reported in LIC [5, 8, 9]. During treatment patients may become undernourished as well [6]. Cancer cachexia is multifactorial and can be due to an interaction of the host, the disease, treatment and psychosocial or central nervous system factors [4, 7, 10]. Lists of these interactive causes are noted in Table 8.1. The pathogenesis of energy imbalance in Table 8.1 shows the relationship between increased needs, increase losses and decreased intake which will result in an energy deficit and potential organ dysfunction.

At the other end of the malnutrition spectrum is obesity. Obesity has been shown to be related to increased toxicity of treatment in acute myeloblastic leukaemia and an increase relapse rate in acute lymphoblastic leukaemia [11–13]. It has been documented that undernutrition, overweight and obesity are associated with a change in pharmacokinetics of drugs as seen in Table 8.2, which may result in inappropriate dosing by either inadequate- or overdosing [14–17]. For example, drugs such as *Methotrexate* have delayed clearance in the underweight patient, especially when

D.C. Stefan and C. Rodriguez-Galindo (eds.), *Pediatric Hematology-Oncology in Countries with Limited Resources: A Practical Manual*, DOI 10.1007/978-1-4614-3891-5_8,

Table 8.1 Multifactorial causes of cancer cachexia

Cancer cachexia	
Multifactorial	
• Disease	
• Host	
• Socio-economic	
• Treatment	
Interactive tumour and host-related effects	• Socio-economic, inadequate supply of nutrients • Anorexia • Bowel obstruction • Malabsorption • Pain • Metastatic disease • Metabolic effects (*Paraneoplastic*) • Altered metabolism of protein, fat and carbohydrate • Increased resting energy expenditure (*REE*)
Therapy related effects	• Multimodal treatments (*chemotherapy, radiation and surgery*) • GI: nausea and vomiting, mucositis, impaired digestion, diarrhoea, ileus, morphological changes to gut mucosa, decrease appetite • Infection and antibiotics • Other drugs • Other organ toxicities
CNS/psychosocial	• Anorexia • Food aversion • Anticipatory vomiting • Depression/anxiety • Body image • Loss of control by the patient of their environment • Parental influence and perceptions • Changes in taste and smell

Source: Sala et al. [4]

high doses are being utilised, this may result in prolonged toxicity such as mucositis or renal damage [17].

Not only does decreased protein and/or energy intake result in increased morbidity of cancer but also deficiency of micronutrients (*both vitamins and trace elements*) can exacerbate the co-morbidities associated with cancer and its treatment [18, 19]. Some of the co-morbidities related to vitamin and trace element deficiency are listed in Table 8.3.

Table 8.2 Alterations of drug disposition in severely underweight patients

Absorption	Decreased rate and possibly extent of absorption
Distribution	Decreased serum proteins (*albumin an α-1 acid glycoprotein*) • May increase free active drug, but may increase clearance of some drugs
Metabolism	Reduced oxidative and conjunctive reactions • Decreases terminal clearance of metabolised drugs, but may also increase oral absorption of drugs with extensive presystemic metabolism in the gut or liver
Renal excretion	Glomerular filtration rate and possibly tubular secretion are reduced

Source: Krishnaswamy [14], Murry [15]

Increased Risk of Infection

It has been well documented in children without cancer that undernutrition will result in increased risk of variety of infections [7–9, 20, 21]. These infections themselves can exacerbate the malnourished state in the cancer patient and is most apparent in infections such as tuberculosis or HIV. The presence of parasitic disease is ubiquitous, especially in African countries, and will also add to the degree of undernutrition. Bacterial and viral infections are frequent occurrences during treatment of patients with cancer. The inability to ward off such infections during treatment is impaired by the presence of undernutrition [1, 7, 20].

Chronic diarrhoea, due to a multitude of causes, is a frequent problem in developing countries. In countries such as Bangladesh, chronic diarrhoea patients are often zinc depleted and zinc substitution benefits these patients [22].

An important aspect that needs reiterating is the need to maintain or improve the quality of life for our patients that we treat for cancer, the sense

Table 8.3 Clinical findings associated with nutritional inadequacies

Area of examination	Findings	Considered **nutritional** inadequacy
General	Underweight; short stature	↓Calories
	Oedematous; decreased activity level	↓Protein
	Overweight	↓Calories
Hair	Ease of pluckability; sparse, depigmented; lack of curl; dull, altered texture; flag sign	↓Protein
Skin (general)	Xerosis, follicular keratosis	↓Vitamin A
	Symmetric dermatitis of skin exposed to sunlight, pressure, trauma	↓Niacin
	Oedema	↓Protein
	Petechiae, purpura	↓Ascorbic acid
	Scrotal, vulval dermatitis	↓Riboflavin
	Generalised dermatitis	↓Zinc, essential fatty acids
	Erythematous rash around mouth and perianal area	↓Zinc
Skin (face)	Seborrheic dermatitis in nasolabial folds	↓Riboflavin
	Moon face; diffuse depigmentation	↓Protein
Subcutaneous tissue	Decreased	↓Calories
	Increased	↓Calories
Nails	Spoon-shaped; koilonychia	↓Iron
Eyes	Dry conjunctiva; keratomalacia; Bitot's spots	↓Vitamin A
	Circumcorneal injection	↓Riboflavin
Lips	Angular stomatitis	↓Riboflavin, Iron
	Cheilosis	↓B-complex vitamins
Gums	Swollen, bleeding	↓Vitamin C
	Reddened gingiva	↓Vitamin A
Teeth	Caries	↓Fluoride
	Stained teeth	↓Iron supplements
	Mottled, pitted enamel	↓Fluoride
	Hypoplastic enamel	↓Vitamins A, D
Tongue	Glossitis	↓Niacin, folate, riboflavin, vitamin B12
Skeletal	Costochondral beading	↓Vitamins C, D
	Craniotabes; frontal bossing; epiphyseal enlargement	↓Vitamin D
	Bone tenderness	↓Vitamin C
Muscles	Decreased muscle mass	↓Protein, calories
	Tender calves	↓Thiamin
Neurologic	Ophthalmoplegia	↓Thiamin, Vitamin E
	Hyporeflexia	↓Vitamin E
	Ataxia, sensory loss	↓Vitamins B12, E
Endocrine and other	Hypothyroidism	↓Iodine
	Glucose intolerance	↓Chromium
	Altered taste	↓Zinc
	Delayed wound healing	↓Vitamin C, zinc

Source: Compliments of AbbottNutritionHealthInstitute.org
With permission from Duggan C, et al. *Nutrition in Pediatrics* (2008)

of well-being is definitely improved in those children who are receiving adequate nutrition [2, 7, 9, 23]. Published studies in LIC have shown that malnutrition at cancer diagnosis could cause delays in cancer treatment, poor adherence to treatment and a negative impact on outcome [24].

Table 8.4 Short- and long-term consequences of malnutrition on the paediatric cancer survivor

Short-term consequences	Long-term consequences
Wasting of muscle- and fat mass	Growth impairment, reduced final height
Decreased tolerance of chemotherapy	Decreased long-term survival in several tumour types
Unfavourable response to chemotherapy	
Treatment delays	Impact on motor, cognitive and neurodevelopmental impairment
Fatigue	
Biochemical disturbances (*anaemia and hypoalbuminemia*)	Risk for metabolic syndrome
	Risk for secondary cancers
	Risk for ageing
Delayed recovery of normal marrow function	Increased mortality rate
Changes in body composition	Retardation of skeletal maturation
Drug dose alteration	Abnormal bone mineral density
Decreased quality and productivity of life	Decreased quality of life
Greater levels of psychological distress	
Higher susceptibility to infections	

Source: Bauer et al. [37]

Co-morbidities which are a result of malnutrition or result in malnutrition do need to be evaluated clinically [25]. These include the presence of infection, both chronic and acute, as well as organ dysfunction that may have resulted from infections and/or malnutrition. The lists of these co-morbidities relevant to poor nutrition are listed in Table 8.4.

Nutritional Assessment

There are many textbooks and review articles on nutritional assessment and nutritional requirements for paediatric patients which are relevant to children with cancer and are available for further background on the following guidelines in this chapter [10, 26–30].

Nutritional assessment of Paediatric Oncology patient's should commence at diagnosis, continue whilst on therapy as well as during survivorship. The A, B, C, D's of nutrition assessment consists of anthropometry-, biochemical-, clinical- and dietary assessment. Anthropometric measurements are tabulated in Table 8.5, biochemical indicators in Table 8.6 and current clinical examination as in Table 8.3. Nutritional assessment is required to identify nutrition-related health status and help in decision making for the appropriate nutritional interventions.

Table 8.5 Important anthropometric measurements and assessments in children

- Weight (*Wt*)
- Height/length (*Ht*)
- Head circumference (*<3 years*)
- Weight for height/length
- Ideal body weight (*IBW = patients actual Wt divided by the ideal Wt for Ht × 100*)
- Body mass index (*BMI = Wt in kg divided by Ht in metres squared*)
- Height and weight Z-score
- Triceps skin fold (*fat stores*)
- Arm circumference (*muscle stores*)
- Waist circumference
- Height velocity

Source: Sacks et al. [26]

Table 8.6 Parameters part of biochemical assessment in high income countries

- Complete blood count, hepatic biochemistry, renal and fluid biochemistry, sugar
  - Albumin (*half-life 14–21 days*)
  - Transferrin (*half-life 8–9 days*)
  - Pre-albumin (*half-life 2–3 days*)
  - Retinol binding protein (*half-life 12 h*)
- Fat status
  - Cholesterol
  - Lipoproteins
- Trace elements: Zn, Cu, Se, Mg
- Vitamins: A, C, E, Thiamine, Riboflavin
- Global biochemical assessment of antioxidants

Source: Sacks et al. [26]

Anthropometry Evaluation [26, 27]

The weight and height of the patient needs to be plotted on relevant WHO growth charts or

Table 8.7 Summary of categories for Z-scores to determine nutritional status according to WHO standards

Z-score	H/A	W/H	W/A	BMI/A
> +3 SD	Above normal	**Obese**	Possible growth problem	**Obese**
>+2 to +3	Normal height	**Overweight**	Possible growth problem	**Overweight**
−1 to ≤+2	Normal height	Possible risk of overweight	Possible growth problem	Possible risk of overweight
<−1 to ≥−2	Normal height	Normal weight	Normal weight	Normal weight
<−2 to ≥−3	**Stunted**	**Wasted**	**Underweight**	**Wasted**
<−3 SD	**Severely stunted**	**Severely wasted**	**Severely underweight**	**Severely wasted**

Source: WHO
Categories in bold indicate malnutrition and these patients need urgent nutritional intervention [28]

compared with WHO data tables for age and gender. The corresponding *Z*-scores must then be categorised according to Table 8.7 to determine nutritional status.

- *Stunting* (*low H/A*) reflects on a child's length or height and is associated with chronic malnutrition or long-term growth faltering, insufficient food intake and frequently associated with low socio-economic status.
- *Underweight* (*low W/A*) is when a child weighs less than the corresponding age- and gender group.
- *Wasting* (*low W/H*) is an indicator of acute or recent malnutrition. It is a measure of how skinny a child is when compared to the corresponding height.
- *Body mass index for age* (BMI/A) is determined by the following: *weight (kg)/length* (m^2). BMI growth charts are available from birth but are more appropriate for children older than 2 years of age. Low BMI is an indicator of wasting while BMI above the 85th percentile *(+2 Z-score)* indicates overweight and above the 95th percentile *(+3 Z-score)* indicates obesity.
- *Head circumference* should be plotted on growth charts and compared with previous readings. This should be done especially for children under the age of 2 years.
- *Triceps skin fold* (*TSF*) is measured by skin fold callipers.
- *Mid upper arm circumference* (*MUAC*) is measured by reference tape at the position of the mid upper arm.

The TSF and MUAC values must be evaluated according to age and gender reference values as on WHO charts or data tables and then categorised as seen in Table 8.8 to determine body stores. It is the preference that TSF and MUAC be undertaken by one consistent observer as these measurements will vary if they are taken by different observers.

Table 8.8 Categories of *Z*-scores and percentiles to determine fat and muscle stores according to WHO standards

Z-score	Percentile	TSF/AFA/MUAC
> +3 SD	≥97th	Excess
> +2 to +3	≥85 to <97th	Above average stores
<+2 to <−1	≥15 to <85th	Average stores
<−2 to ≥−3	≥3 to <15th	Below average stores
<− 3 SD	<3rd	Depleted stores

Source: WHO [28]

It is recommended that patient's anthropometric measurements be done on a regular basis and longitudinal. Guidelines for the time frames of these measurements are presented in Table 8.9.

Anthropometry of PEM [26, 27, 30]

- *Z*-score of <−2 SD below the reference median for all measurements is an indicator of severe malnutrition
- Decrease in percentile for weight/height or two major percentiles
- Height for age (H/A) <95 % of the median for gender and age
  - H/A <75 % an indicator of chronic malnutrition
  - H/A <5th percentile indicates chronic undernutrition

Table 8.9 Minimum guideline for assessing anthropometric data

Parameter	Diagnosis	Each subsequent in-patient admission	Out-patient clinic review	At least every 4 weeks
Weight	✓	✓	✓	
Height	✓			✓
Plot on centile chart/BMI chart	✓			✓
Body mass index/%weight:height	✓	✓	✓	
% Weight loss since diagnosis		✓	✓	
Mid upper arm circumference	✓			✓

Source: Selwood et al. [30]

- Weight for height (W/H) under 90 % of the median for gender and age
  - W/H <50th percentile
  - W/H <10th percentile indicates severe wasting
- Weight loss >5 % to pre-illness weight or in 1 month
- BMI <10th percentile for age and gender
- TSF <5th percentile for age and gender
- AFA <5th percentile for age and gender
- AMA <5th percentile for age and gender
- MUAC <5th percentile for age and gender
- PEM can also be seen by a single measurement, such as MUAC, where a low value in paediatric patients classify them as acute malnourished:
  - **<12.5 cm if <5 years**
  - **<13.5 cm if >5 years of age**
  - In Table 8.10 values are presented to determine differences in severe malnutrition in children with cancer

Biochemical Assessment for PEM [26, 27]

- Serum albumin under 3.2 mg/dL (*if no acute metabolic stress previous 2 weeks*) may be seen as an indicator of a patient's protein status. Careful interpretation of low serum albumin values are needed, because other non-dietary factors are often the cause for decreased values. Serum albumin half-life is approximately 2 weeks and and need to be used in conjunction with other parameters for nutritional status.

Table 8.10 Assessment of nutritional status—cut-offs

Age group	Acute malnutrition	Severe acute malnutrition
6 months to 5 years	MUAC <125 mm	MUAC <110 mm
>5 years without tumour mass[a]	Weight for height <−2 SD	Weight for height <−3 SD
>5 years with a tumour mass[b]	MUAC <135 mm[c]	MUAC <115 mm[c]

Source: Israels et al. [38]
[a]For example, ALL
[b]Clinical assessment is more important, MUAC is more variable than in younger group especially in pubertal children
[c]Empiric cut-off

- Pre-albumin, when available, can also be used which has a half-life of only 2 days and therefore a better indicator of acute change of protein status.

Clinical Assessment of PEM Is Seen as [26, 27]

- Loss of subcutaneous fat.
- Presence of muscle wasting.
- Resent weight change (*weight loss or-gain must not be related to fluid retention or loss of fluid*).
- Presence of oedema at ankles, sacrum or face.
- Hair changes.
- Conditions that may affect the nutritional status, e.g.: *inability to chew and swallow*; *loss of appetite*; *the presence of vomiting, diarrhoea, constipation, flatulence, belching or indigestion.*
- Signs or symptoms suggestive of vitamin and/or mineral deficiencies. *(As seen in Table 8.3).*

Table 8.11 Patients at high risk for malnutrition

- Patients with advanced disease, e.g. *metastatic*
- Malnutrition or evidence of cachexia present at diagnosis
- Patients expected to receive highly emetogenic regimens
- Patients treated with regimens associated with severe gastrointestinal complications such as *constipation, diarrhoea, loss of appetite, mucositis, enterocolitis*
- Patients with relapse disease
- Patients who are <2 months old
- Patients who are expected to receive radiation to oropharynx/oesophagus or abdomen
- Chemotherapy treatment protocol with high occurrence of gastrointestinal or appetite depressing side effects such *as Burkitt's Lymphoma, Osteogenic sarcoma and CNS tumours*
- Post-surgical gastrointestinal complications such as prolonged illness or short gut syndrome
- Patients receiving a stem cell transplant
- Inadequate availability of nutrients due to low socio-economic status
- Patients with behavioural or eating disorder

Source: Mauer et al. [7]

- Medications and their nutrient interactions.
- Gut dysfunction for longer than 5 days in well-nourished patients.

Dietary Assessment of PEM Is Seen as [26, 27]

- Food intake of *less than 70%* of a patient's requirements for 5 days.

Table 8.11 indicates cancer patients at high risk for PEM.

Nutritional Requirements of Children with Cancer [26, 30–34]

Energy Requirements

The resting energy expenditure (REE) and nutrient requirements should be defined for each cancer patient when possible. The recommended daily allowance (RDA) for energy requirements of healthy children is seen in Table 8.12. An appropriate activity factor (AF) as seen in Table 8.13 can be factored. This is required to compensate for the increased demands on the body due to the tumour and other co-morbidities. Factors such as fever, infection, stress, physical activity and catecholamine can elevate energy expenditure [30]. *For example*, a 4-year-old girl is admitted in the unit, she weighs 12 kg. RDA is 90 kcal, so 12 kg×90 kcal=1080 kcal×1.5 AF=1575 kcal/day.

Table 8.12 Recommended daily allowances for calories and protein for children

Category	Age (years)	Protein (g/kg/day)	Calories (kcal/kg/day)
Infant	0.0–0.5	2.2	108
	0.5–1.0	1.6	98
Child	1–3	1.2	102
	4–6	1.1	90
	7–10	1.0	70
Male	11–14	1.0	55
	15–18	0.9	45
Female	11–14	1.0	47
	15–18	0.8	40

Source: Data from World Health Organization (1985) and Nutrition Support Services (1995)

Table 8.13 Disease and physical activity factors for adjustment of resting energy expenditure

REE factor	Disease and activity factors
X 1.0–1.1	Well-nourished children, sedated on ventilator, extracorporeal membrane oxygenation; minimal stress
X 1.3	Well-nourished children with decreased activity, minor surgery, mild-to-moderate sedation; minimal stress
X 1.5	Ambulatory child with mild-to-moderate stress
	Inactive child with sepsis, cancer, trauma, extensive surgery
	Minimally active child with malnutrition and catch-up growth requirements
X 1.7	Active child with catch-up growth requirements
	Active child with severe stress

Source: Maqbool et al. [29]
Compliments of *AbbottNutritionHealthInstitute.org*

Protein Requirements

Protein requirements would be met by using the RDA as seen in Table 8.12. It can be multiplied by a factor of 1.2 to meet the increased needs due to increased catabolism caused by the tumour, infection and other co-morbidities. If the intake of the patient is sufficient, fat stores will be restored and muscle mass will increase during the initial phase of treatment, otherwise the body's fat and muscle stores will be depleted if oral intake does not meet the required intake.

Vitamin and Trace Elements

It is well documented that patients who have PEM may also have depleted stores of necessary vitamins, trace elements and sometime essential fatty acids [1, 33]. The health care providers (HCP) caring for these patients should clinically evaluate for this. Clinical manifestations are listed in Table 8.3 as discussed earlier (*see nutritional assessment*).

Nutritional Care During Cancer Treatment

Nutritional supportive care has been surveyed in both North America and the UK where both showed inconsistency of care [30, 35]. Nevertheless, there are excellent expert opinions on the need for appropriate nutritional support during cancer treatment on which the following recommendations are based. Textbook references and websites are available for additional information [10, 26, 32, 36, 37].

The aim of nutritional support in children with cancer is to reverse and/or prevent malnutrition, promote weight gain, growth and normal development, improve immune system, enhance tolerance to treatment and quality of life.

Table 8.14 Nutritional screening

The following criteria are used to identify children at risk [33, 34]
• Total weight loss of >5 % of the pre-illness body weight over the past month
• Weight <10th or >90th percentile for age
• Height <10th percentile for age
• Weight for height <10th or >90th percentile
• Weight <90 % of ideal body weight for height
• Triceps skinfold thickness <10th percentile and mid-arm circumference <5th percentile (*arm anthropometry appears to be more sensitive measure of malnutrition than weight for height in children with large solid tumours* [33])
• BMI <5th or >85th percentile for age
• Oral intake <80 % of estimated needs
Children receiving high-dose chemotherapy or combination therapy for aggressive cancers are at high risk of developing malnutrition and may need early nutrition intervention on the basis of their oral intake and the treatment protocol

Source: Kleinman. *Pediatric Nutrition Handbook* 6th Ed. (2009)

Benefits of Nutritional Care Include

- Minimising the catabolic effect of the tumour
- Minimising weight loss during treatment
- Maintaining of body weight and body tissue to prevent deteriorating of nutritional status to PEM [7]
- Prevent specific nutrient deficiencies
- Decrease treatment-related side effects.

Children have decreased energy reserves compared to adults. The body consists mainly of water and a low fat percentage, making paediatric patients more susceptible to malnutrition. Medical treatment can lead to deterioration of the nutritional status of the patient if nutritional intervention does not take place [6], therefore regular nutritional screening of patients' nutritional status is needed to prevent the deterioration as seen in Table 8.14.

It is important to remember that every child is unique and will tolerate cancer treatment differently. The challenge lies in maintaining or improving the child's nutritional status during cancer therapy. Nutritional assessment and intervention should commence at time of diagnosis and continue during treatment. Figure 8.1 is an algorithm for a process of nutritional care as developed by the Children's Oncology Group. Other algorithms are available [26].

Patients need to continue, as far as possible, with their normal life. One way is to ensure eating familiar food, to improve their morale and quality of life. Awareness of cultural difference from the HCP is important for appropriate local nutritional support [38].

The Side Effects of Treatment

Chemotherapy, radiotherapy and/or surgery can cause various nutritional side effects as seen in Table 8.15. The appropriate management thereof is important to prevent decreased oral intake, weight loss and eventually PEM.

As observed in Table 8.15, if patients have anorexia or loss of appetite, one of the best strategies is to increase nutrient density of the food they eat, as indicated in Table 8.16. Simple high protein food sources such as peanut butter and/or eggs are recommended as alternatives to commercial expensive supplements [38]. The use of high energy and protein diets, nutritional supplements, special diets, nasogastric enteral feeds (NG) or as a last resort parenteral nutrition (PN) is suggested.

Oral Intake

High Energy and Protein Diet

A high energy and protein diet can provide patients with sufficient energy, to meet their nutritional needs.

A study done on sick children in which feeding them a high energy, high protein diet led to a mean increase of 1.33 kg in weight and 0.98 cm in height, with a significant increase in muscle stores, but not in fat mass. It demonstrated that the body first restores the lean tissue or muscle stores and then the fat stores [39].

Nutritional Supplements

Nutritional supplements are nutrient dense beverages available in different flavours and packaging. Patients in a South African study received snacks (*muffins*, *cheese*, etc.) and nutritional drinks that lead to significant weight gain [30, 34].

It is important that patients are monitored to ensure compliance of intake of the supplements. A patient's favourite drink or food can be supplemented to improve compliance and tolerance [30] or freeze the supplements to taste like "*slush puppy*" or in the *form of ice cubes* that they can be eaten individually [30].

Neutropenic Diet

Neutropenic sepsis is mostly the result of bacteria in the patient's flora in his gastrointestinal track (GIT) and thus a neutropenic diet (*low bacterial diet*) has been developed. The diet contains no raw fruits or vegetables, no aged cheese, no cold meat, no take-away food, no undercooked meat products or unpasteurized milk or juice. There is no evidence that a completely sterile food preparation diminishes the risk of infection [40]. Food safety guidelines with focus on guidelines for shopping, storage of food, food preparation, cooking and serving of food [34] are shown in Table 8.17.

Nasogastric Enteral Feeds [10, 30, 36, 37]

Children experience periods during their treatment where they do not have an adequate oral intake. NG feeds are required to provide adequate nutrients and prevent malnutrition. A number of reports document the utility and safety of enteral tube feeding [41–43].

NG feeds should be considered in paediatric cancer patients in the following situations:

- Malnutrition not responding to oral intake.
- Severe oral mucositis, nausea and/or vomiting.

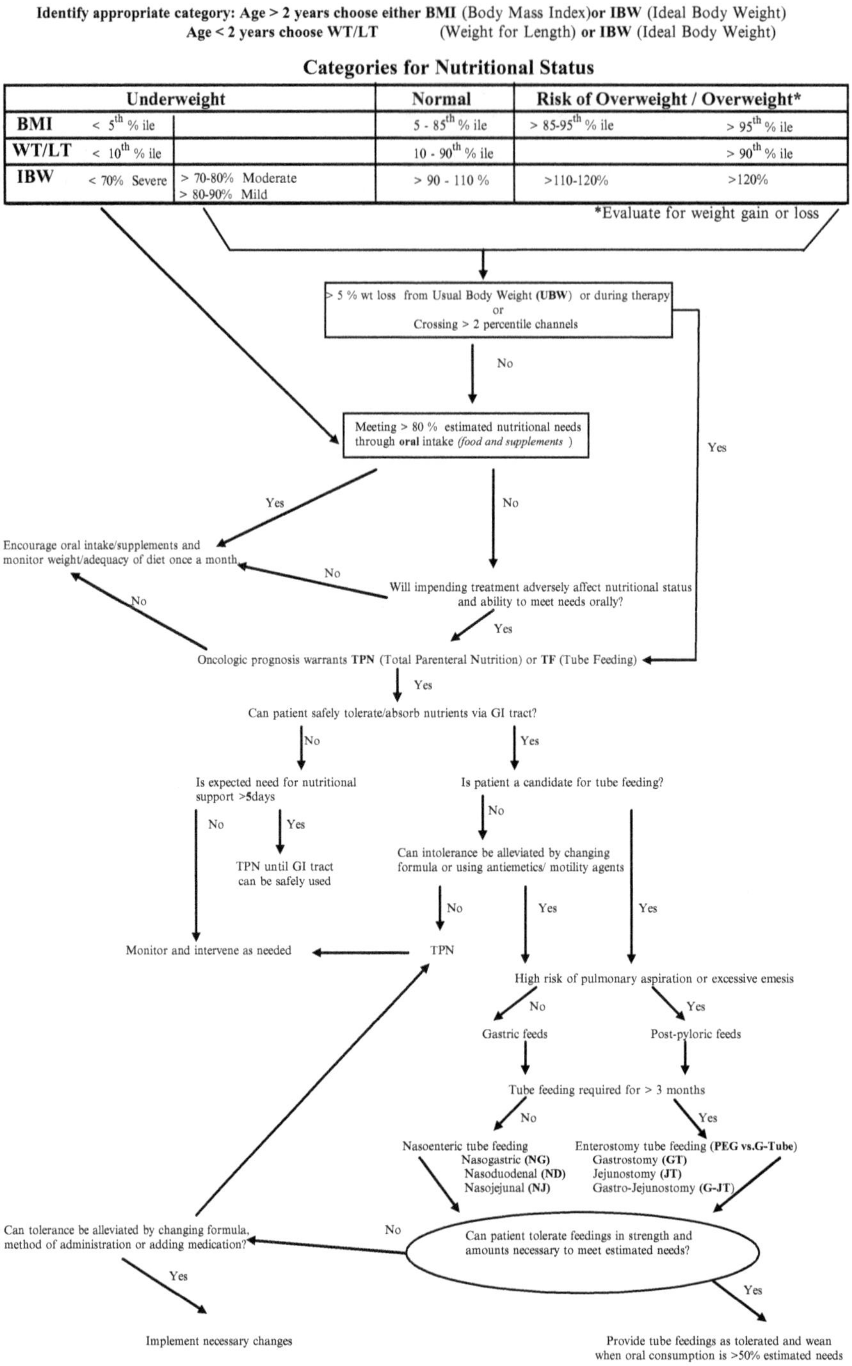

Fig. 8.1 Algorithm for nutritional intervention in the paediatric oncology

Table 8.15 Management of general nutrition-related side effects of treatment

Side effect	Description	Causative agents	What happen if not managed?	Strategies to cope
Nausea and vomiting	The vomiting centre is situated in the medulla oblongata near the respiratory centre and may be stimulated by • Chemoreceptor trigger zone • Vagal and visceral nerves • Cerebral cortex and limbic system	*Chemotherapeutic agents*: Cytarabine, Cytarabine with daunorubicin, Methotrexate, Methotrexate with mercaptopurine combination Methotrexate plus doxorubicin and Cisplatin Cyclophosphamide with doxorubicin, Dactinomycin Melphalan and Dacarbazine	Dehydration Metabolic abnormalities Children that vomited once lose their appetite and are one of the major reasons of anorexia because they are afraid to eat and drink, for the risk of vomiting again anxiety and stress Can lead to food aversion Can lead to refusal of treatment	Optimise antiemetic therapy Small amount of cold food Encourage slow eating Avoid strong odours Drink fluids between meals and not with meals Drink liquids with a straw and covered cup Children to develop strategies like "wishful thinking" to cope and activities like storytelling
Anorexia and low intake	*Anorexia is described as one of the following*: low appetite, early satiety, taste and smell alterations and meat aversions	The result of enlarged organs pressing on the stomach Shortness of breath Altered taste Constipation Nausea and vomiting Diarrhoea Pain and fatigue Metabolic disturbances Depression due to unfamiliar surroundings and continuous medical procedures	Decreased intake of food resulting in weight loss, muscle wasting and low albumins	Nutritional counselling can lead to increased oral caloric intake Provide small, frequent meals (*6–8 a day*) Serve food on a smaller plate Eat and make food more nutrient dense, e.g. *add margarine to porridge for breakfast or cheese to mash potatoes* Present food more attractively Mealtimes in a relaxed, pleasant environment or let children eat together at a table for social interaction Provide nutritional supplements or start with NG feed

(continued)

Table 8.15 (continued)

Side effect	Description	Causative agents	What happen if not managed?	Strategies to cope
Diarrhoea	Frequent loose stools, abdominal pains and flatus	*Chemotherapeutic agents*: Actinomycin, adriamycin, Methotrexate (*high dose*), Cytosine Result of mucositis, tumour infiltration in GIT, anxiety and malabsorption Infection, prolonged use of antibiotics = disturbance of the flora of the GIT Radiotherapy to GIT	Increased loss of nutrients Decreased oral intake due to fear of increasing diarrhoea Weight loss Breakdown of skin = infections	Adequate hydration Good hygiene Keep rectal area clean and dry Clear fluids Elemental or semi-elemental enteral diet NPO or TPN in worse case
Constipation	Decrease in frequency of stools or hard stools accompanied by pain and discomfort	*Chemotherapeutic agents*: Vincristine Intestinal obstruction Spinal cord compression Electrolyte imbalance Pain medication Lack of exercise Low fibre diet NOT sufficient time for defecation	Pain Low intake leads to weight loss	Prevention is best option Increase fluid and fibre intake Exercise Absolute privacy for child when going to toilet or use bedpan
Stomatitis/ mucositis	Chemotherapy damages the mucosa in the mouth by penetrating the epithelium cells and causing damage to the connective tissue Suppressing of bone marrow	*Chemotherapeutic agents*: Actinomycin Adriamycin Daunorubicin Epirubicin Bleomycin Melphalan Methotrexate	Leads to inadequate oral intake due to swelling, pain, ulcerations, dry, cracked lip and then causes nutritional depletion	BEST is to prevent oral mucositis with good oral hygiene and sucking ice cubes: *vasoconstriction takes place in the mouth, because of the cold ice cubes and prevents damaging by the chemotherapy* Optimal pain medication Give liquids or bland, pureed food Add butter, gravy, sauce or salsa dressing to moisten food Avoid highly seasoned food Avoid hard food Enteral nutrition

Altered taste	Chemotherapy damage the taste buds situated in the tongue and oropharynx due to fact that they have a high turnover	*Chemotherapeutic agents*: Vincristine, Carmustine, Dacarbazine, Cisplatin, Cyclophosphamide Antibiotics Nausea and vomiting Stomatitis Infection	Tendency to lower oral intake that leads to anorexia and then nutritional depletion Can lead to vomiting Learn aversion to some foods	Good oral hygiene Keep mouth moist at all times Use stronger seasoning on foods and serve food warm Avoid excessively sweet foods Offer salty or sour foods Try new flavours Use different cooking methods Use gravies and sauce to help with swallowing
Renal damage	Decreased output due to chemotherapy damage to nephrons	*Chemotherapeutic agents*: Cisplatin Cyclophosphamide Ifosfamide	Loss of protein through kidneys Loss of minerals (Mg, K, Ca, PO_4) through kidneys can lead to *Fanconi's renal syndrome* Can lead to chronic renal failure Adjustment to chemotherapy drugs and risk relapse	Protein and electrolyte controlled diet Supplementation of electrolytes

Sources: Ward [10], Selwood [36], Bechard et al. [47]

Table 8.16 Guidelines for increasing nutrient density

Butter, margarine and oils
• Add to soup, mashed and baked potatoes, hot cereal, grits, rice, noodles and cooked vegetables
• Stir into sauces and gravies
Cream
• Use on deserts, gelatin, pudding, fruit, pancakes, waffles and mashes potatoes
• Use in soups, sauces, egg dishes, batters, puddings and custards; put on cereals
• Mix with pasta, mash potatoes and rice
• Substitute for milk in recipes
• Makes cocoa with cream and add marshmallows
Sour cream
• Add to soups, bakes potatoes, vegetables, sauces, salad dressing, gelatin deserts, bread and muffin batter
• Use as dip for raw fruits and vegetables
Mayonnaise
• Add to salad dressing
• Spread on sandwiches and crackers
• Use in sauces and gelatin desserts
Honey (use in children over 1 year of age)
• Add to cereal, milk drinks, fruit desserts, smoothies or yogurt
• Use as a glaze for meats such as chicken
Granola
• Use in cookie, muffin and bread batters
• Sprinkle on vegetables, yogurt, ice cream, pudding, custard and fruit
• Mix with dried fruit and nuts for a snack
• Substitutes for bread or rice in pudding recipes
Dried fruits and nuts
• Cook and serve dried fruits for breakfast or as dessert
• Add to muffins, cookies, bread, cakes, rice and grain dishes, cereals, puddings and stuffing
• Bake in pies and turnovers
• Combine with cooked vegetables such as carrots, sweet potatoes or acorn and butternut squash
Milk and cheese
• Mix one cup dry milk powder in four cups of liquid milk; use this milk for cooking and baking
• Add milk powder directly to hot or cold cereals, scrambled eggs, soups, gravies, casserole dishes and dessert
• Add grated cheese or chunks of cheese to sauces, vegetables, soups, salads and casseroles
• Spread cream cheese on hot buttered bread

(continued)

Table 8.16 (continued)

Eggs
• Add eggs to soup or casseroles
• Slice boiled eggs in sauces and serve over rice, cooked noodles, buttered toast or hot biscuits
Peanut butter
• Add peanut butter to sauces; use on crackers, waffles or celery sticks
• Spread peanut butter on hot buttered bread

Source: Medical Nutrition Therapy Services Program, Seattle Cancer Care Alliance, Seattle, Washington

- Weight loss of 5 % since date of admission.
- Anticipate weight loss in patients on intensive treatment protocol.
- Decrease in MUAC of 10 %.
- Oral intake is less than 90 % of the nutritional requirements for 3–5 days.
- Bone marrow transplant (BMT) patients with intact guts unable to take adequate oral nutrition.

The step-by-step procedure with explanations to insert a NG tube is seen in Table 8.18.

Type of Enteral Feeds [10, 26, 34]

Different formulations of enteral feeds with unique characteristics are commercially available for children as seen in Table 8.19 and can be used for NG feeds. However, if not available or preferred some local foods can be pureed to a consistency that can be administered via NG tube.

Younger children tend to develop diarrhoea during the first few days of NG feeds which subsequently subsides. The GIT function decreases after every cycle of chemotherapy received due to damage to the intestinal mucosa. Flattening of the epithelial take place, atrophy of the villi can occur and down-regulation of enterocytes. Lactose intolerance may also occur. The digestion and absorption of oral intake is affected and then changes may have to be made to a different type of enteral feed used as indicated in Table 8.19 or change other local foods available.

Table 8.17 Food safety practices

Food shopping	1. Check expiry dates on food and do not buy or use if the food is out of date
	2. Do not purchase ready-to-eat food from bulk food bins (*Breads, nuts, dried fruits, candies*)
	3. Avoid produce that is bruised or damaged
	4. Bag fresh fruits and vegetables separately from meat, poultry and seafood
Food storage	1. Store perishable fresh fruits and vegetables (i.e. *cucumbers, tomatoes*) in a clean refrigerator at a temperature of 40 °F *(4.4° C)* or below
	2. Refrigerate all products that is purchased pre-cut or peeled
	3. Beef should be refrigerated at 40 °F *(4.4° C)* and use within 2 days. Beef can be frozen at 0 °F *(–18° C)* and use within 6 months of the purchase date
Food preparation	1. Wash hands with water and soap for 20 s before and after any food preparation
	2. Wash fruits or vegetables under running water even if you are going to peel them. Do not use soap, bleach or commercial produce washes to clean fruit
	3. Dry produce with a clean cloth or paper towel. This will reduce the spread of bacteria. Do not wash meat, poultry or eggs
	4. Defrost all meats in the refrigerator. Do not defrost at room temperature
	5. Food preparation surface must be cleaned first. Wash surface thoroughly with soap and water and thoroughly dry. As an extra precaution, you can *use a solution of one tablespoon of unscented, liquid chlorine bleach in one gallon of water to sanitise washed surfaces and utensils*
	6. Wash cutting boards, dishes, utensils and counter tops with hot, soapy water after preparing each food item and before you go to the next item
Cooking	1. Cook foods immediately after thawing
	2. All raw foods such as meats, poultry and entrees should be cooked until they are well done. Beef should be cooked to 160 °F *(71° C)*, depending on the cut. Chicken should be cooked to an internal temperature of 165 °F *(74° C)*. Cold food should be stored at <40° *(<4.4° C)*. Hot foods at >140° F *(>60° C)*. A home thermometer may help
Storage of cooked foods	• Store leftovers within 2 h. By dividing leftovers in several clean, shallow containers, you'll allow them to chill faster. Discard leftovers that were kept at room temperature for greater than 2 h
	• Perishable foods (*fruits, vegetables, meats, dairy*) should be put into the fridge or freezer within 2 h. In the summer months, cut this time to 1 h
	• Do not use leftovers prior to reheating to >165 °F *(> 74° C)* before serving
Baby food/ infant formula	• Never put baby food in the refrigerator if the baby doesn't finish it. Do not feed your baby directly from the jar of the baby food. Instead, put a small serving of food on a clean dish and refrigerate the remaining food in the jar. If the baby needs more food, use clean spoon to serve another portion. Throw away ant food in the dish that's not eaten. If you do feed the baby from the jar, always discard the remaining food
	• Prepare safe water for preparing formula. Bring tap water to a rolling boil and boil for 1 min. If you use bottled water, follow the same process. Cool the water to body temperature before mixing the formula
	• Sterilise bottles and nipples before first use. After that, wash them by hand or in a dish washer
	• Formula can become contaminated during preparation and bacteria can multiply quickly if formula is improperly stored. Prepare formula in smaller quantities on an as-needed basis to greatly reduce the possibility of contamination. Always follow the label instructions for mixing formula
Sanitary food practices for immunocompromised patients	
AVOID	
• Uncooked meats (*cook meat until well done*)	
• Avoid raw eggs	
• Avoid soft French style cheese, pates, uncooked hot dogs and sliced deli meats	
• Avoid alfalfa sprouts and unpasteurized juices	

Selected recommendations from the Federal Drug Administration's Clean, separate cook, chill are described above. Additional information may be found at *foodsafety.gov*

Source: Adapted from Bechard L. Oncology and bone marrow transplantation. In: Hendricks K, Duggan C, Walker W, eds. Manual of pediatric nutrition. 3rd ed. Hamilton, Ontario: B.C. Decker, 2000

Table 8.18 Nasogastric tube insertion

1.	IDENTIFY patient and EXPLAIN the procedure to child (*Engage child life therapist as needed*)
2.	OBTAIN help of second nurse as required
3.	WASH hands
4.	DETERMINE which nostril is most patent. A penlight may be used to check which nostril is more patent or occlude/ask child to occlude one nostril at a time and observe their breathing
5.	MEASURE the distance with the gastric tube from the nares to the earlobe, to a point midway between the bottom of the sternum and the umbilicus. Suggestions
	(i) #5 Fr for infants <2.5 kg
	(ii) #6–8 Fr for newborns—9-year-old
	(iii) #10 Fr for 9 years and up
	MARK tube with permanent ink. *NOTE*: *With weighted tubes, measure from the feeding port openings, not the end of the weight*
6.	PLACE incontinence pad or towel on patient's chest and have emesis basin available
7.	PLACE patient in high fowlers or sitting position or hold infant stabilising the head in the neutral or "sniffing" position
8.	GLOVE and coil the end of the tube around your index finger to produce a flexible curve
9.	LUBRICATE tip of tube 2–4 in.
10.	INSERT the tube
	(a) Instruct patient to hold head straight up with neck slightly hyperextended and facing forward or assist patient to hold this position
	(b) Hold the end of the tube above the lubricant and with the curve pointing downward, carefully insert the tube along the floor of the nostril, on the lateral side
	(c) Offer the patient sips of water to help move the tube past the oropharynx. Infants may suck on a pacifier during the procedure
	(d) Advance the tube each time the patient swallows until tube reaches marked length
	(e) Observe patient throughout procedure for signs of tube mal-positioning (*coughing*, *choking*, *inability to talk*). Withdraw tube immediately if changes occur in patient's respiratory status, if tube coils in mouth, or if the patient begins to cough, choke or changes colour
	(f) Gently remove guidewire (*when used*) and retain at bedside for future use. Never reinsert guidewire while tube is in situ
11.	CONFIRM tube placement
	(a) Flush tube with 1–5 mL of air using a 20–50 mL syringe
	(b) Aspirate 1–5 mL of fluid using a 3–5 mL syringe and note visual characteristics of aspirate
	(c) Place a few drops on ph test strip—gastric ph should be 5.5 or less
	(d) Refer to algorithm if unable to obtain aspirate or if pH is 6 or above
12.	Once placement in stomach is confirmed, SECURE tube
	(a) Curve and tape the tube with transparent tape, or securement device, taped to the child's cheek (*on same side as nostril with tube*) to prevent unnecessary tugging on the nostrils (*Do not tape to the patient's forehead as this will put pressure on the nares*)
	(b) Wrap a small piece of tape around the tube near the connection creating a tab and pin to the patient's gown/clothing
	(c) Measure the length of the tube from nose to hub
13.	CLAMP tube or CONNECT to suction or to feeds as ordered
14.	REMOVE equipment and DISPOSE appropriately. WASH hands
15.	DOCUMENT in appropriate record

Source: BC Children's Hospital Child & Youth Health Policy and Procedure Manual (2011)

Paediatric cancer patients tolerate elemental formula, lactose and gluten free, low residue, low fat and low osmolality feeds via NG tubes better than other feeds.

Schedule and Feeding Rates of Enteral Feeds [10, 26, 34, 37]

The feeding schedule and rate of enteral feeds is determined by the patient's oral intake, sleep patterns, medical procedures and lifestyle.

NG feeds should be started at 1–2 mL/kg/h and increased by approximately 1–2 mL/kg/day until the total volume the patient requires is reached. It should be increased slowly over a 3-day period to prevent the risk of gastric retention, nausea, vomiting, abdominal cramping and diarrhoea. Continuous, constant infusion of NG feeds with a feeding pump is better tolerated than bolus feeds and fewer complications occur. NG feeds can be administered at home depending on the social circumstances and parent level of competence. Nocturnal NG feeds are optimal for children, as they can then lead a more normal life and are not pressurised to eat at mealtimes.

Table 8.19 Type of enteral feeds to use

Type of feed	Characteristics	When to use	Studies done
Elemental enteral feeds	Consists of nutrients in simpler forms like glucose and amino acids	Mucositis After patient was on TPN Malabsorption Catabolic patients to increase absorption After patient had few cycles of chemotherapy or risk for malabsorption Protein losing enteropathy	Patients with mucositis had low absorption of nutrients and for them an elemental feed was chosen to increase absorption Mucositis did not alter the absorption of the amino acid leucine
Peptide-based enteral feed	Proteins are digested to amino acids and small peptides absorbed via the dual system on the membranes of the enterocytes	Suspected malabsorbtion After patient was on TPN Low albumin to improve absorption Protein losing enteropathy Suspect GIT toxicity after chemo	Patients with radiation enteritis received protein and had a N-balance of 4.4 g/day for the peptide diet and 1.5 g/day for the amino acid diet In critically ill patients the peptide-based diets increased their mucosal integrity and liver function After multiple traumas, no patients developed diarrhoea and an increase in pre-albumin, transferrin and albumin occurred and shorter hospital stay
Standard formula	Whole nutrients, contains 1 kcal/mL	Normal biochemistry Patient NOT malnourished, use as supplementary feeds due to low oral intake	Group received a standard formula showed significant improvement up to 4 weeks but not during the rest of the period
High energy feeds	Whole nutrients, contains 1.5 kal/mL	Patient who is volume sensitive To improve nutritional status of patient (*albumin normal*)	Group on high energy feeds had after 10 weeks significant weight gain, increased measurements in MUAC and TSF
Enteral feeds with fructo-oligosaccharides	Contains prebiotics that improve the defence mechanism of the GIT	Long-term enteral feeds On high-dose pain medication Constipation	Enteral feeds with 2 g/L FOS compared to a standard feed. After 30 days a significant increase in number of *Bifidiobacteria* and *Lactobacilli* in the FOS group, decreased infection markers and improved nutritional status by measuring Z-scores Further studies are needed to determine the dose of FOS children need to induce a bifidogenic effect

Sources: Ward [10] and Schoeman [34]

Enteral feeds have been shown to maintain an adequate nutritional status in patients and can reverse malnutrition. A correlation was found between the time periods that patients received NG feeds and the improvement in their nutritional status.

Advantages of Enteral Feeds

- Maintain normal digestive and absorption functions in the GIT.
- Safe in neutropenic patients and in patients with low platelet counts.
- Low risk for infections.
- Low risk for liver abnormalities.
- GIT-mucosa is maintained and growth promoted.
  - Low risk for bacterial translocation.
  - Prevents enterocyte atrophy.
  - Increases barrier function and immune function of the GIT.
  - Delivers nutrition beyond obstruction areas.
  - Delivery of nutrients is slow and GIT has time for absorption.
- Provided a route to give medication.

- Reduces the anxiety and pressure to eat.
- Low cost compared to PN.
- Improves the well-being of the child.
- The child can lead a "normal" hospital life and the dietician and HCP can relax, because nutritional needs are being met.

Complications of Enteral Nutrition

- Local irritation at nasal site.
- Poor compliance.
- Psychological distress due to body image.
- Difficult to maintain tube in site if persistent vomiting.
- Associated anxiety if frequent replacement required.
- Local infection at tube site area.
- Aspiration pneumonia.
- Tube dislodgement.

Percutaneous Endoscopic Gastrostomy Tube [10, 30, 36]

A percutaneous endoscopic gastrostomy (PEG) tube is a feeding tube inserted into the stomach with a gastroscope and is the preferred method for gastrostomy feeding. It is a useful alternative to a NG tube when prolonged tube feeding is anticipated or NG tubes are difficult to insert such as patients who have had head and neck surgery or radiation to oral or oesophageal regions.

The tube is inserted by the pull technique, usually under general anaesthesia. **Indications for the insertion of a PEG tube are:**

- On-going dysphagia due to cancer of the head and neck.
- Oesophageal stricture.
- A high risk for aspiration, intractable bleeding.
- The patient needs long-term enteral feeds, e.g. *Neuro-oncology patients.*
- Head and neck surgery and/or radiation.

PEG Tube Complications

- Local infections at tube site.
- Increased granulation at tube site.
- Localised bleeding.

Parenteral Nutrition [10, 26, 30, 36, 44, 45]

Some centres may have the capacity to deliver pre-prepared IV nutritional support or have it prepared in the local hospital pharmacy under sterile conditions. Parenteral nutrition (PN) should be considered as a last resort when all efforts to receive adequate oral or tube feeding have failed or are contraindicated. Total parenteral nutrition (TPN) refers only to those patients who have no enteral intake but is used interchangeably with PN.

Indications for PN

- Patients with GIT dysfunction due to tumour, chemotherapy or graft-versus-host disease (GVHD) of the GIT after BMT.
- Bowel obstruction.
- Neutropenic enterocolitis (*typhilitis*).
- Continuous vomiting or inability to access the GIT, chronic diarrhoea and impaired absorption of nutrients.
- Nutritional requirements that cannot be met by oral or NG feeding.

Patients with typhilitis, also called neutropenic enterocolitis, present with abdominal pain, sometimes ascites, diarrhoea and vomiting. Abdominal X-ray may be of use which may show thickened bowel wall, air in the bowel and sometimes free air if there has been perforation. The appendix is usually normal, but the caecum maybe thickened and the colon inflamed that can lead to perforation. Typhilitis originally referred to caecum involvement but enterocolitis can affect the small bowel as well. Perforation is a major complication of enterocolitis and can become a surgical emergency. Absolute bowel rest is needed for patients to heal while receiving appropriate antibiotics. TPN is prescribed until the patient's abdominal tenderness, fever or neutropenia has improved. The TPN can then be weaned by giving small amounts of enteral nutrition or oral clear fluids.

Table 8.20 TPN recommendations for children

Age	Energy (kcal/kg/day)	Protein (g/kg/day)	CHO	Fat (g/kg/day)
Baby—1st month	90–100	1.5–3	NPC 60–75 % (*See separate table*)	*NPC 25–40 %* 3–4 (*0.13-0.17 g/kg/h*)
2nd month–3 years	90–100, >1 year 75–90	1.5–2.5		3–4 (*0.13-0.17 g/kg/h*)
3–5 years	75–90	1–2 (*3 critically ill*)		2–3 (*0.08–0.13 g/kg/h*)
6–12 years	60–75	1–2 (*3 critically ill*)		2–3 (*0.08–0.13 g/kg/h*
12–18 years	30–60	1–2		2–3 (*0.08–0.13 g/kg/h*)
Parenteral recommendations for carbohydrates				
Weight (kg)	Day 1 (g/kg/day)	Day 2 (g/kg/day)	Day 3 (g/kg/day)	Day 4 (g/kg/day)
Up to 3	10	14	16	18
3–10	8	12	14	16–18
10–15	6	8	10	12–14
15–20	4	6	8	10–12
20–30	4	6	8	<12
>30	3	5	8	<10

Maximum infusion rate = 1.2 g/kg/h
Source: Koletzko et al. [44]

PN Requirements and Administration

Standard nutritional requirements for PN depend on the patient's weight and age as seen in Table 8.20. Nutrients are fed via the venous route and the energy from PN must be approximately the BMR of a patient. A level of 1.5–1.7 times the BMR is too high and leads to overfeeding. The parenteral protein requirements are lower than enteral, as the amino acids do not have to be digested. Overfeeding of glucose leads to lipogenesis and fat deposition and should be avoided.

Administration of PN

Careful planning, administration and monitoring of PN are required to prevent metabolic complications. Central venous catheters (CVCs) or peripheral venous access catheters (PVCs or PICC) are used to administer TPN. Peripheral CVCs are placed directly into the large central vein and may be used to give large volumes of intravenous fluid to patients, to administer medication directly into the vein and to measure central venous pressure.

Peripheral parenteral nutrition (PPN) is not used if a CVP is available and can only be given if the osmolarity of the PN is under 1,000 mOsmol/L or dextrose content less than 12.5 %. The problem with PVCs is that it can cause phlebitis, venous sclerosis and venous thrombosis.

It is important to prevent essential fatty acid deficiency in patients receiving only PN. A patient can experience a deficiency within only 20 days. Iron is not routinely supplemented in the PN bags because it can influence the stability of the nutrients inside the bags. Institutions that are capable of administering PN should establish their own specific guidelines for administration and monitoring for metabolic complications. Specific comprehensive guidelines for PN are available [44]. If possible a minimal amount of oral or NG feeding should be administered during PN to help maintain gut integrity.

The best way to wean a patient from PN is to start with elemental- or semi-elemental enteral feed at 1–5 mL/h. If NG feeds is not an option, the patient needs to be started on a clear fluid diet with supplements.

Complications of Parenteral Nutrition

- PN is expensive.
- May be harmful in children with PEM due to increased risk for infections.

- Complications of central lines.
  - Line access is not always possible, fluid overload, obstruction of catheters usually due to clots, arterial trauma and/or pneumothorax at the time of insertion.
- Metabolic complications:
- Refeeding syndrome can occur.
- Cholestasis/biliary cirrhosis and parenteral nutrition associated liver disease (PNALD).

PN serves a purpose in maintaining adequate nutrition but should only be used as a last resort when oral and enteral feeding is contraindicated or failed. A Cochrane review supported the use of PN in BMT patients but there was little evidence to support its routine use in other oncology patients [46, 47]. Patients receiving PN managed by a multi-disciplinary team have shown a decreased number of mechanical complications compared to other patients not managed by a team.

Cancer Survivors

Nutritional counselling and support should not end with the completion of the cancer therapy. Survivors may continue to be underweight and require supplementation to maintain growth or help in catch-up growth. Obesity can become a problem in survivors for a variety of reasons, such as reduced physical activity or endocrinological side effects of therapy [48–50]. Obesity is most frequently seen in patients who have has central nervous system or other head and neck radiation therapy [50]. Routine nutritional assessment should include a dietary history, basic anthropometrics and use of growth charts. Relevant dietary counselling should be part of a comprehensive long-term follow-up clinic.

Conclusion

Supportive care is an essential component of cancer therapy. In LIC the ability to deliver supportive care is dependent on resources, infrastructure and personnel available. It has to be adapted to the reality of the environment. Some guidelines have been published for LIC which include suggestions for nutritional support [38]. This chapter has expanded on those guidelines.

All paediatric patients with cancer have risk of malnutrition and it is recommended that they receive early and on-going nutritional assessment and intervention to maintain their nutritional status. The child's age, clinical condition and treatment received must be taken into consideration when the method of nutritional support is chosen. Institutions need to assess and intervene according to their capacity. Use of local foods that are well tolerated is encouraged. Parent education on appropriate foods and preparation is required. Enhanced oral or tube feeding is encouraged in the underweight patient. Nutritional assessment and support for children with cancer is an important part of his/her treatment regimen that can last for several months to years. Nutritional support aims to improve immune competence, tolerance and adherence to therapy, promote growth, development and improve quality of life.

References

1. Lochs H, Allison SP, Meier R, et al. Introductory to the ESPEN guidelines on enteral nutrition: terminology, definitions and general topics. Clin Nutr. 2006;25:180–6.
2. Van Eys J. Malnutrition in children with cancer: incidence and consequence. Cancer. 1979;4395(Suppl): 2030–5.
3. UICC International Workshop. Nutritional morbidity in children with cancer: mechanisms, measures and management. Int J Cancer. 1998;78 Suppl 11:66–8.
4. Sala A, Pencharz P, Barr RD. Children, cancer, and nutrition- a dynamic triangle in review. Cancer. 2004; 100:677–87.
5. Barr RD, Gibson B. Nutritional status and cancer in childhood. J Pediatr Hematol Oncol. 2000;22:491–4.
6. Zimmermann K, Ammann RA, Kuehni CE, De Geest S, Cignacco E. Malnutrition in pediatric patients with cancer at diagnosis and throughout therapy: a multicenter cohort study. Pediatr Blood Cancer. 2013;60: 642–9.
7. Mauer AM, Burgess JB, Donaldson SS, et al. Special nutritional needs of children with malignancies: a review. JPEN J Parenter Enteral Nutr. 1990;14(3): 315–24.
8. Barr RD, Ribeiro RC, Agarwal BR, Masera G, Hesseling PB, Magrath IT. Pediatric oncology in countries of limited resources. In: Pizzo PA, Poplack DG,

editors. Principles and practice of pediatric oncology. 4th ed. Philadelphia: Lipincott, Williams and Wilkins; 2002. p. 1541–52.
9. Donaldson SA, Wesley MN, Dewy WD, Suskind RM, Jaffe N, Van Eys J. A study of the nutritional status of pediatric-cancer patients. Am J Dis Child. 1981;135: 1107–12.
10. Ward E. Paediatric oncology. In: Shaw V, Lawson M, editors. Clinical paediatric dietetics. 3rd ed. Oxford: Blackwell Publishing; 2007.
11. Lange BJ, Gerbing RB, Feusner J, et al. Mortality in overweight and underweight children with acute myeloid leukemia. JAMA. 2005;293(2):203–11.
12. Lobato-Mendizabal E, Ruiz-Arguelles GJ, Marin-Lopez A. Leukaemia and nutrition. I: malnutrition is an adverse prognostic factor in the outcome of treatment of patients with standard-risk acute lymphoblastic leukaemia. Leuk Res. 1989;13(10):899–906.
13. Gomez-Almaguer D, Montemayor J, Gonzalez-Llano O, Ruiz-Arguelles GJ, Betz NL, Marfil-Rivera J. Leukemia and nutrition. IV: improvement in the nutritional status of children with standard-risk acute lymphoblastic leukemia is associated with better tolerance to continuation chemotherapy. Int J Pediatr Hematol Oncol. 1995;2:53–6.
14. Krishnaswamy K. Drug metabolism and pharmacokinetics in malnourished children. Clin Pharmacokinet. 1989;17 Suppl 1:68–88.
15. Murry DJ, Riva L, Poplack DG. Impact of nutrition on pharmacokinetics of anti-neoplastic agents. Int J Cancer Suppl. 1998;11:48–51.
16. Murphy AJ, White M, Davies PSW. Body composition of children with cancer. Am J Clin Nutr. 2010;92:55–60.
17. Mihranian MH, Wang YM, Daly JM. Effects of nutritional depletion and repletion on plasma methotrexate pharmacokinetics. Cancer. 1984;54(10):2268–71.
18. Kennedy D, Tucker K, Ladas EJ, Blumberg J, Rheingold S, Kelly K. Low antioxidant vitamin intakes are associated with increases in adverse effects of chemotherapy in children with acute lymphoblastic leukemia. Am J Clin Nutr. 2004;79:1029–36.
19. Sgarbieri UR, Fisberg M, Tone LG. Nutritional assessment and serum zinc and copper concentration in leukemic children. Sao Paulo Med J. 1999;117(1): 13–8.
20. Chandra RK. Nutrition as a critical determinant in susceptibility to infection. World Rev Nutr Diet. 1976;25:166.
21. Hughes WT, Price RA, Sisko F, et al. Protein-calorie malnutrition. A host determinant for pneumocystis carinii infection. Am J Dis Child. 1974;128:44–52.
22. Larson CP, Roy SK, Khan AI, Rahman AS, Qadri F. Zinc treatment to under-five children: applications to improve child survival and reduce burden of disease. J Health Popul Nutr. 2008;26(3):356–65.
23. Andrassy RJ, Chwals WJ. Nutritional support of the pediatric oncology patient. Nutrition. 1998;14:124–9.
24. Sala A, Rossi E, Antillon F, Molina AL, de Maselli T, Bonilla M, Hernandez A, Ortiz R, Pacheco C, Nieves R, Navarrete M, Barrantes M, Pencharz P, Valsecchi MG, Barr R. Nutritional status at diagnosis is related to clinical outcomes in children and adolescents with cancer: a perspective from Central America. Eur J Cancer. 2012;48:243–52.
25. Burke ME, Lyden ER, Meza JL, Elena J, Ladas EJ, Dasgupta R, Wiegner EA, Arndt CA. Does body mass index at diagnosis or weight change during therapy predict toxicity or survival in intermediate risk rhabdomyosarcoma? A report from the children's oncology group soft tissue sarcoma committee. Pediatr Blood Cancer. 2013;60:748–53.
26. Sacks N, Ringwald-Smith K, Hale G (2004). Nutritional Support. In: Altman A, Editor. Supportive Care of Children with Cancer (pp 243–261). Baltimore: The Johns Hopkins University Press.
27. Lee Rd, Nieman DC. Nutritional assessment. New York: McGraw Hill; 2010. p. 3, 176–7, 225–8, 315, 343, 348, 353–4.
28. WHO Antro 2005, Beta version 17 Feb 2006. Software for assessing growth and development of the world's children [Internet]. Geneva: WHO; 2006. http://www.who.int/childgrowth/software/en
29. Maqbool A, Olsen IE, Stallings VA. Clinical assessment of nutritional status. Compliments of AbbottNutritionHealthInstitute.org, with permission from Duggan C, et al. Nutrition in pediatrics. 4th ed. Hamilton, ON: BC Decker Inc.; 2008.
30. Selwood K, Ward E, Gibson F. Assessment and management of nutritional challenges in children's cancer care: a survey of current practice in the United Kingdom. Eur J Oncol Nurs. 2010;14:439–46. doi:10.1016/j.ejon.2010.04.004.
31. Rickard KA, Coates TD, Grosfeld JL, Weetman RM, Baehner RL. The value of nutrition support in children with cancer. Cancer. 1986;58(8 Suppl): 1904–10.
32. Ladas EJ, Sacks N, Meacham L, Henry D, Enriques L, Lowry G, Hawkes R, Dadd G, Rogers P. A multidisciplinary review of nutrition considerations in the pediatric oncology population: a perspective From children's oncology group. Nutr Clin Pract. 2005;20:377–93.
33. Otten JJ, Hellwig Pitzi J, Meyers LD. Dietary reference intakes: the essential guide to nutrient requirements. Washington, DC: National Academy Press; 2006.
34. Schoeman J. The effect of the nutritional status of paediatric patients with cancer at diagnosis on disease outcome. [MSc thesis—Dietetics]. Pretoria: Kitskopie; 2008.
35. Ladas E, Sacks N, Brophy P, et al. Standards of nutritional care in pediatric oncology: results from a nationwide survey on the standards of practice in pediatric oncology. A Children's Oncology Group study. Pediatr Blood Cancer. 2005;46(3):377–93.
36. Selwood K. Side effects of chemotherapy. In: Gibson F, Soanes L, editors. Cancer in children and young people. Chapter 4, side effects of chemotherapy. West Sussex: Wiley; 2008. p. 35–6, 43–55.

37. Bauer J, Jürgens H, Frühwald MC. Important aspects of nutrition in children with cancer. Adv Nutr. 2011; 2:67–77.
38. Israels T, Renner L, Hendricks M, Hesseling P, Howard S, Molyneux E. SIOP PODC: recommendations for supportive care of children with cancer in a low-income setting. Ped Blood Can. Published online in Wiley Online Library (wileyonlinelibrary.com). 2013; doi:10.1002/pbc.24501
39. Kabir I, Malek MA, Rahman MM, Khaled MA, Mahalanabis D. Changes in body composition of malnourished children after dietary supplementation as measured by bioelectrical impedance. Am J Clin Nutr. 1994;59:5–9.
40. Moody K, Charlson ME, Finlay J. The neutropenic diet: what's the evidence? J Pediatr Hematol Oncol. 2002;24:717–21.
41. Den Broeder E, Lippens RJ, van't Hof MA, Tolboom JJ, van Stavere WA, Hofman Z, Sengers RC. Effects of naso-gastric tube feeding on the nutritional status of children with cancer. Eur J Clin Nutr. 1998;52: 494–500.
42. Den BE, Lippens RJ, van't Hof MA, Tolboom JJ, Sengers RC, van Staveren WA. Association between the change in nutritional status in response to tube feeding and the occurrence of infections in children with a solid tumor. Pediatr Hematol Oncol. 2000;17: 567–75.
43. Deswarte-Wallace J, Firouzbakhsh S, Finklestein JZ. Using research to change practice: enteral feedings for pediatric oncology patients. J Pediatr Oncol Nurs. 2001;18:217–23.
44. Koletzko B, Goulet O, Hunt J, Krohn K, Shamir R. Guidelines on Paediatric Parenteral Nutrition of the European Society of Paediatric Gastroenterology, Hepatology and Nutrition (ESPGHAN) and the European Society for Clinical Nutrition and Metabolism (ESPEN), Supported by the European Society of Paediatric Research (ESPR). J Pediatr Gastroenterol Nutr. 2005;41:S1–69.
45. Christensen ML, Hancock ML, Gattuso J, Hurwitz CA, Smith C, McCormick J, Mirro Jr J. Parenteral nutrition associated with increased infection rate in children with cancer. Cancer. 1993;72:2732–8.
46. Jones L, Watling RM, Wilkins S, et al. Nutritional support in children and young people with cancer undergoing chemotherapy. Cochrane Database Syst Rev. 2010;7, CD003298.
47. Bechard L. Oncology and bone marrow transplantation. In: Hendricks K, Duggan C, Walker W, editors. Manual of pediatric nutrition. 3rd ed. Hamilton, ON: Decker; 2000. p. 492–502.
48. Demark-Wahnefried W, Werner C, Clipp EC, Guill AB, Bonner M, Jones LW, Rosoff PM. Survivors of childhood cancer and their guardians. Cancer. 2005;103:2171–80.
49. Hudson MM, Mertens AC, Yasui Y, Hobbie W, Chen H, Gurney JG, Yeazel M, Recklitis CJ, Marina N, Robison LR, Oeffinger KC. Health status of adult long-term survivors of childhood cancer: a report from the Childhood Cancer Survivor Study. JAMA. 2003;290:1583–92.
50. Rogers PC, Meacham LR, Oeffinger KC, Henry DW, Lange BJ. Obesity in pediatric oncology. Pediatr Blood Cancer. 2005;45(7):881–91.

Oncologic Emergencies

9

Inam Chitsike and Scott C. Howard

Introduction

Oncologic emergencies are defined as potentially life-threatening events that are directly or indirectly related to the underlying malignancy or its treatment or acute toxicities that require immediate management to minimize morbidity and mortality [1–3]. If oncologic emergencies are not anticipated, quickly recognized, and effectively treated, they may result in permanent morbidity or death. In this chapter, we classify emergencies into the following categories and describe the management of selected emergencies within each category:

1. Mass effects on vital organs and structures—superior vena cava (SVC) syndrome, central airway compression (CAC) syndrome, cardiac tamponade, pleural effusion, spinal cord compression, raised intracranial pressure
2. Metabolic emergencies—tumor lysis syndrome (TLS), hypercalcemia, hyponatremia, lactic acidosis, adrenal insufficiency
3. Gastrointestinal emergencies—typhlitis, intestinal obstruction, bowel perforation
4. Hematologic emergencies—hyperleukocytosis, febrile neutropenia, hemorrhage, and thrombocytopenia
5. Chemotherapy extravasation

Mass Effects

Superior Vena Cava Syndrome and Central Airway Compression Syndrome

SVC syndrome and CAC syndrome comprise signs and symptoms that result when a mediastinal mass compresses the right ventricular outflow tract, SVC, or the veins that drain into it leading to venous obstruction (SVC syndrome) or the trachea or main stem bronchi leading to airway compromise (CAC syndrome) [4–7]. Airway obstruction is divided into proximal or large airway obstruction (upper airway) or distal (lower) airway obstruction.

Etiology

SVC and CAC syndromes are most commonly caused by anterior mediastinal masses (Fig. 9.1), so in children, T-cell leukemias and lymphomas are the most common causes. However, other lymphomas, Kaposi sarcoma, Ewing sarcoma with bone tumor metastasis, teratomas, thyroid gland tumors, and rhabdomyosarcomas are also potential causes (Table 9.1). Kaposi sarcoma is

I. Chitsike, M.D., Ch.B., M.Med. Paeds
Department of Paediatrics and Child Health/Consultant Paediatric Oncology Unit, College of Health Sciences, University of Zimbabwe, Harare, Zimbabwe

S.C. Howard, M.D. (✉)
Department of Oncology, St. Jude Children's Research Hospital, University of Tennessee Health Sciences Center, Memphis, TN, USA
e-mail: Scott.Howard@stjude.org

D.C. Stefan and C. Rodriguez-Galindo (eds.), *Pediatric Hematology-Oncology in Countries with Limited Resources: A Practical Manual*, DOI 10.1007/978-1-4614-3891-5_9,

an increasingly common cause of lower airway obstruction where HIV infection is common. In areas endemic for tuberculosis, tuberculous adenitis should be considered, since it can also present with mediastinal mass and cause SVC syndrome and CAC with respiratory distress.

Signs and Symptoms

Symptoms and signs include cough, facial swelling, dyspnea, orthopnea, fatigue, and less frequently headache, dizziness, visual disturbances, hoarseness, and dysphagia [6, 7]. Symptoms can worsen abruptly when the patient is supine and improve when in the prone position. Physical examination findings can include edema of the head, neck, and upper extremities; venous distension; laryngeal edema; stridor; wheezing and anxiety.

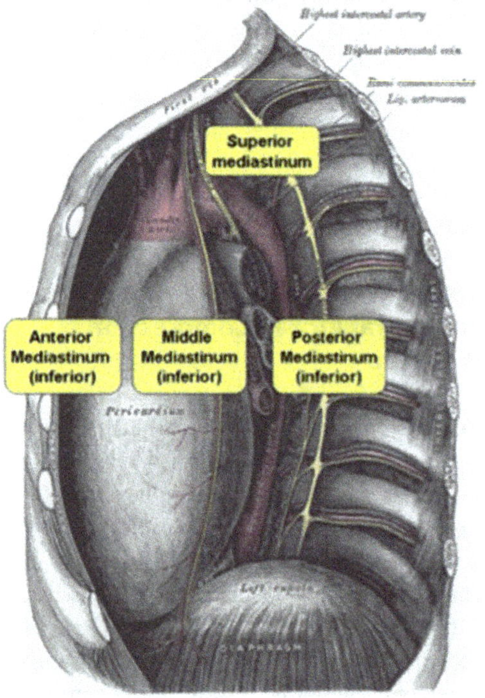

Fig. 9.1 Mediastinal anatomy. http://en.wikipedia.org/wiki/Mediastinum

Diagnosis

Symptoms and physical examination are sufficient to suspect the diagnosis of SVC or CAC syndrome, but patients with severe obstruction may be asymptomatic. Mediastinal masses compressing critical structures constitute an emergency even in patients with no symptoms or signs, and must be ruled out in any patient with suspected leukemia or lymphoma. A chest radiograph is sufficient to identify clinically important mediastinal masses, but rarely shows the degree of obstruction because most masses occur in the anterior mediastinum so that the tracheal width is normal. A lateral radiograph can sometimes show antero-posterior narrowing, but is neither sensitive nor specific. Chest radiography is useful for newly diagnosed patients because it can also identify pleural or pericardial effusions that may necessitate urgent intervention. Chest computed tomography (CT) allows adequate anatomical description of the mass and neighboring structures, and quantifies the degree of tracheal compression, and thus the risk of complete obstruction and sudden death. Such evaluation is critical to facilitate decisions regarding sedation or anesthesia.

Immediate Management

Great caution must be exercised during every phase of initial evaluation, since patients with CAC syndrome are at risk for worsened compression and sudden death. Painful procedures, or anything that increases patient anxiety, should be avoided, since rapid inspiration can decrease

Table 9.1 Some potential causes of mediastinal tumors in children

Etiology	Anterior mediastinal masses	Middle mediastinal masses	Posterior mediastinal masses
Malignant	Non-Hodgkin lymphomas Hodgkin lymphoma	Non-Hodgkin lymphomas	Neuroblastoma
	Teratoma Kaposi sarcoma	Kaposi sarcoma	
Benign	Tuberculosis	Tuberculosis	

pressure in the airways and precipitate collapse, which can be difficult to reverse. When transporting the patients to the radiology department, they should remain in upright position and the initial CT should be performed with the patient in the *prone* position to avoid worsening compression.

The main aim of management is to secure the airway of the patient and alleviate respiratory distress by maintaining an upright or prone position, or bed rest with elevation of the upper part of the body. These positions, and sometimes the left lateral decubitus position, help lift an anterior mediastinal mass off the airways and right ventricular outflow tract. Inability to tolerate the supine position is an ominous sign, and the supine position should be avoided. Patients with respiratory distress may feel better with oxygen via facemask, but if this increases anxiety it may be counterproductive.

If the patient experiences distress, he should be immediately placed in the prone position so that gravity will pull the mass away from the airways. If complete tracheal compression occurs, intubation is usually not possible without a rigid bronchoscope, so patients should be placed prone during any resuscitation attempt, since prone positioning itself may sometimes be sufficient to open the airway. Adequate IV access is important, but is not helpful in a resuscitation attempt, since opening the airway and relieving right ventricular outflow tract obstruction are the only measures that can reverse cardiac or respiratory arrest caused by a mediastinal mass.

Definitive Management

Making a correct diagnosis using the least invasive method possible and immediate initiation of appropriate therapy are the top priorities. A complete blood count and peripheral blood smear is noninvasive and can often diagnose acute leukemia. Pleural fluid aspiration using local anesthesia is also not very invasive, and cytology of pleural fluid is sufficient to diagnose T-cell lymphomas in many cases. Bone marrow aspiration or biopsy of a peripheral lymph node or testicular mass, if present, can also be performed under local anesthesia, but in some cases the only site of disease is the mediastinum, and the mass must be biopsied by an interventional radiologist or thoracic surgeon, with the attendant procedural and anesthetic risks. Empiric therapy (e.g., glucocorticoids) can lead to rapid improvement of symptoms in patients with lymphomas or acute leukemias, but the mass may shrink rapidly and make subsequent diagnosis and disease-specific therapy impossible, so every effort should be made to obtain a histological diagnosis prior to starting therapy.

If emergent antineoplastic therapy is needed to save the life of the child prior to making a diagnosis, radiotherapy to the central mediastinum (if available) using a daily dose of 2–4 Gy can lead to clinical improvement within 18 h. The radiation port can be limited so that peripheral disease is spared and thus available for biopsy when the patient's clinical condition has improved. If radiation-induced edema occurs, symptoms and signs may worsen and necessitate glucocorticoid therapy. In life-threatening cases for whom emergent radiation therapy is not possible, empiric treatment with intravenous methylprednisolone 50 mg/m^2/day in four divided doses may rapidly reduce the size of the mass and associated edema. Chemotherapy with cyclophosphamide, an anthracycline, vincristine, and prednisone (CHOP) can also be considered. Note that even when a residual mass is present and available for biopsy, prior glucocorticoids, chemotherapy or radiotherapy could change the histological findings and make it difficult to establish a definitive histological diagnosis.

Pericardial Effusion and Cardiac Tamponade

Although pericardial effusion is often asymptomatic, it represents an oncologic emergency when it causes cardiac tamponade [8, 9].

Pathophysiology

Pericardial effusion is seen with a variety of tumors including lymphomas and metastatic solid tumors and results from inflammation of the pericardium, obstruction of lymphatic drainage from the pericardium, or fluid overload. Malignant involvement of the pericardium rarely may be primary, but is usually secondary to spread from a nearby or distant focus of malignancy, which can involve the pericardium by contiguous extension from a mediastinal mass, nodular tumor deposits from hematogenous or lymphatic spread, and diffuse pericardial thickening from tumor infiltration (with or without effusion). In diffuse pericardial thickening the heart may be encased by an effusive-constricted pericarditis, but this is rare in children.

Symptoms, Signs, and Diagnosis

Pericardial effusion is usually asymptomatic, and most often diagnosed incidentally during evaluation of newly diagnosed cancer, and confirmed by echocardiogram. When the effusion is caused by pericarditis, patients often have chest pain and dyspnea, but otherwise usually effusions are asymptomatic unless they cause cardiac tamponade, defined as the inability of the ventricle to maintain cardiac output because of extrinsic pressure. Note that cardiac tamponade can also be caused by a mediastinal mass or an intrinsic mass. Fortunately, tamponade is rare in children with cancer. Findings in patients with tamponade resemble those of heart failure, including shortness of breath, cough, palpitations, chest pain improved by sitting, and nonspecific abdominal pain. Physical examination findings include tachycardia, low blood pressure, jugular venous distension, pulsus paradoxus, soft heart sounds, pericardial rub, and signs of low cardiac output, such as poor peripheral perfusion.

Investigations

In patients with significant pericardial effusions, the chest X-ray shows enlargement of cardiac silhouette, ECG demonstrates low voltage QRS complexes, and flattened or inverted T waves, and echocardiography shows the volume of pericardial effusion and whether there is atrial or ventricular collapse with hemodynamic compromise.

Treatment

Most patients can be treated by treating the underlying malignancy, but in those with refractory disease or life-threatening tamponade, a pericardial tap for one-time aspiration of fluid or percutaneous catheter drainage under echocardiographic guidance or fluoroscopic guidance may be considered. Fluid should be evaluated for malignant cells, which may affect treatment and prognosis of the underlying cancer.

Pleural Effusion

Pleural effusions can occur at diagnosis in children with lymphomas, and the effusion is usually malignant in patients with non-Hodgkin lymphomas and nonmalignant in those with Hodgkin lymphoma [10–12]. Effusions can also be caused by fluid overload with congestive cardiac failure, low albumin, infections (e.g., empyema, tuberculosis), and toxicity of chemotherapy (e.g., dasatinib, methotrexate, procarbazine, cyclophosphamide, bleomycin). Although pleural effusion is rarely life-threatening, sizeable and rapid accumulation of fluid can compress lung parenchyma and cause respiratory insufficiency.

Clinical Presentation and Evaluation

Symptoms are related more to the rate of pleural fluid accumulation rather than total volume of fluid, and can include dyspnea, orthopnea, cough, and pleuritic chest pain. The presence of fever suggests atelectasis or infection. Diagnosis can be suspected when basilar breath sounds are absent and the patient has shifting dullness to percussion [12]. Chest X-ray with lateral decubitus views can confirm the presence of a pleural effusion and estimate its extent. Ultrasonography and CT may be useful to differentiate fluid loculations from pleural masses, and should be performed if biopsy is planned to assure that the biopsy site is representative of the pathologic process.

Management

Small or asymptomatic effusions require no treatment and resolve once the underlying cause is addressed [10, 11]. Large, symptomatic effusions causing respiratory distress can be drained by thoracentesis. Initial drainage can be performed manually using a large bore needle, attached to a three-way stopcock and a large volume syringe. This may be followed by insertion of tube for more complete drainage if the patient is at risk for re-accumulation.

Spinal Cord Compression

Epidural spinal cord compression can occur in patients with a variety of solid tumors and in approximately 0.4 % of patients with newly diagnosed acute leukemia [13]. The spinal cord can be compromised at any site, but in children the thoracic vertebral segment is most often affected. Vertebral collapse resulting from tumor invasion of the vertebral bodies can also compromise the spinal cord. Symptoms and signs can include numbness, tingling, paresthesia, progressive pain at the level of the epidural lesion, radicular pain, weakness or paralysis of the upper and lower extremities, and neurogenic bladder. Deep tendon reflexes are hyperactive, and the Babinsky response is extensor.

Diagnosis and Treatment

Spinal cord compression is a medical emergency and should be evaluated promptly. Plain films and CT scans are not sensitive enough to identify spinal cord compression, so magnetic resonance imaging should be performed whenever possible. In patients with newly diagnosed cancers that are predicted to be chemosensitive, intensive systemic chemotherapy plus high-dose corticosteroids should be used. Intravenous dexamethasone reduces spinal cord edema. Radiotherapy and laminectomy are reserved for patients with resistant disease or when the diagnosis is unknown and biopsy is needed anyway.

Raised Intracranial Pressure

Raised intracranial pressure can cause cerebral herniation and rapidly lead to death or severe neurologic disability. Causes include intracranial masses, obstruction of outflow of cerebrospinal fluid, and obstruction of venous outflow, as can occur in SVC syndrome [14]. It can also complicate intrathecal chemotherapy administration or treatment with all-trans retinoic acid [15–17]. Management consists in urgently treating the underlying cause, though hyperosmolar therapy with hypertonic saline or mannitol, intubation, and hyperventilation can be temporizing measures [18, 19].

Metabolic Emergencies

Tumor Lysis Syndrome

Patients with TLS can present with nausea, vomiting, lethargy, agitation, somnolence, pain, and hypertension, but are usually asymptomatic and diagnosed after identification of hyperuricemia, azotemia, hyperkalemia, hyperphosphatemia, and hypocalcemia [20]. Hyperkalemia and hypocalcemia can cause cardiac dysrhythmia or cardiac arrest; hyperuricemia and hyperphosphatemia can cause acute kidney injury, which in turn leads to oliguria, fluid overload, pulmonary edema, respiratory failure, hypoxia, cerebral edema, and death. In addition, hyperphosphatemia exacerbates hypocalcemia and can cause ectopic calcification at many sites, including the kidneys [20]. It occurs most commonly in children with acute leukemia or lymphoma, but can occur in any bulky tumor that is sensitive to initial therapy and prone to rapid lysis.

Pathophysiology

Tumor breakdown causes release of potassium, phosphorus, and DNA, which is metabolized into uric acid. Hyperphosphatemia occurs frequently during the first few days of induction chemotherapy, and hypocalcemia in TLS results from precipitation of calcium phosphate in tissues [20–22]. In cases of severe hyperphosphatemia, despite a compensatory decrease in blood calcium levels, the calcium × phosphorus product can exceed 60 $(mg/dL)^2$, a level associated with calcium phosphate precipitation in soft tissues. Uric acid and calcium phosphate can cause acute kidney injury that in turn reduces renal excretion of uric acid, phosphate, and potassium, and puts the patient at risk for fatal hyperkalemia and hypocalcemia (secondary to hyperphosphatemia).

Management

The best treatment for TLS is prevention, and since precipitation of uric acid, phosphates, and xanthine causes acute kidney injury in TLS, rapid volume expansion to achieve normal blood pressure and adequate urine output remains the most effective strategy [20]. Hydration with normal saline boluses until the patient is euvolemic then slightly hypotonic IV fluids at 2,500–3,000 mL/m^2/day optimizes renal perfusion and urine output. Fluid input and output should be monitored closely, and a urethral catheter is helpful in patients at high risk. Maintaining adequate urine output may require administration of mannitol, furosemide, or both, but diuretics should not be used until the patient has adequate intravascular volume. Urine output should be kept above 100 mL/m^2/h.

Uric acid is much more soluble in alkaline conditions, but calcium phosphate is more soluble in acidic conditions; thus, calcium phosphate crystallizes more readily in alkaline urine and excessive alkalinization may do more harm than good in patients at risk for TLS [20]. Patients with hyperuricemia should be treated with rasburicase when it is available or with urinary alkalinization and allopurinol when it is not. If the phosphorus increases, alkalinization should be discontinued to reduce the risk of calcium phosphate precipitation.

Hyperkalemia can occur suddenly and cause cardiac dysrhythmia and sudden death, so all patients with TLS should be hospitalized, have continuous cardiac monitoring, and frequent electrolyte measurement [20]. Patients at risk for TLS should not receive potassium-containing intravenous fluids and their dietary potassium intake should be restricted. Symptomatic hyperkalemia or serum potassium levels near 6 mEq/L are indications for the use of potassium exchange resins such as sodium polystyrene sulfate (Kayexalate), at a dosage of 0.25–0.5 g/kg every 6 h (orally or as a retention enema in a 20 % sorbitol solution). If associated electrocardiographic abnormalities occur or if the serum potassium level exceeds 6.5 mEq/L, patients should immediately receive cardioprotective agents: $NaHCO_3$ at a dose of 0.5 mEq/kg over 10–15 min, followed by a 10 % calcium gluconate solution at a dose of 0.5 mL/kg over 5–10 min. These agents should be administered separately to avoid precipitation. These measures shift potassium into the intracellular compartment, but are temporary in effect and should be used until body potassium can be reduced by sodium polystyrene sulfate, forced diuresis with hyperhydration and furosemide, or dialysis.

Hyperphosphatemia and Hypocalcemia

Administering aluminum hydroxide, lanthanum, or sevelamer hydrochloride orally or through a nasogastric tube can control hyperphosphatemia. Asymptomatic patients with hypocalcemia are treated with oral calcium carbonate, but symptomatic patients should be treated with intravenous 10 % calcium gluconate at a dose of 0.5 mL/kg administered over 5–10 min. If intravenously administered calcium solutions extravasate, or if the local concentration of calcium × phosphate exceeds 60 $(mg/dL)^2$, soft-tissue calcification can occur. In cases of hypocalcemia unrelated to TLS, in addition to calcium supplementation, vitamin D should also be provided, especially in breast-fed infants or dark-skinned patients with a low-calcium diet.

Hypercalcemia

Mild hypercalcemia is defined as a total serum calcium <12 mg/dL, moderate hypercalcemia as 12.0–13.5 mg/dL, and severe hypercalcemia is >13.5 mg/dL. Hypercalcemia is a common life-threatening metabolic complication of malignancy in adults, but is rare in children [23]. It has been reported in leukemias, lymphomas, and solid tumors [24]. It can present at the initial diagnosis of the cancer as, for example, in ALL or it can occur during treatment or during relapse.

Mechanism

The mechanism is related to increased local release of skeletal calcium caused by direct erosion of bone plus the release of local and systemic endocrine factors that interfere with bone metabolism, renal calcium clearance, and intestinal absorption of calcium.

Symptoms and Signs

Symptoms of hypercalcemia depend on the serum level of serum calcium and its rate of rise.

Patients with mild hypercalcemia are usually asymptomatic. Those with moderate hypercalcemia may have weakness, anorexia, constipation, polyuria, and polydipsia. Severe hypercalcemia can manifest as a life-threatening metabolic emergency with cardiac and central nervous system effects including encephalopathy, seizure, and coma.

Treatment

Treatment of hypercalcemia includes vigorous hydration with normal saline (3,000 $mL/m^2/day$) until the patient is euvolemic with good urine flow, cardiac and electrolyte monitoring, and specific therapy to reduce calcium levels: furosemide 1–2 mg/kg IV TID or QID to increase urinary calcium secretion by blocking reabsorption of calcium in the ascending limb of Henle [24]. Calcitonin, bisphosphonates, or dialysis can be used in refractory cases, but are rarely necessary in children [25].

Lactic Acidosis

Lactic acidosis, a clinical condition with blood pH ≤7.35 and serum lactate level ≥5 mEq/L [26], is rare, occurs in patients with lymphoma and leukemia, and carries a poor prognosis. The pathogenesis of lactic acidosis is poorly understood but in one case series neoplastic involvement of the liver was observed in 24 of the 28 cases of lymphoma and 18 of 24 cases of leukemia, which suggests that hepatic underutilization of lactate may contribute [27].

Signs, Symptoms, and Treatment

Lactic acidosis may be associated with weakness, weight loss, low-grade fever, tachypnea, tachycardia, somnolence, and an altered mental state. Since it usually occurs in the setting of rapidly progressive, refractory hematologic cancer, many other symptoms may be present related to the underlying malignancy. Control of the underlying cancer is the only definitive treatment, but alkalinization with bicarbonate may reduce the severity of acidosis while awaiting response to therapy.

Hyponatremia and the Syndrome of Inappropriate Diuresis

Hyponatremia, defined as serum sodium below the lower limit of normal, can result from administration of excess hypotonic intravenous fluids or syndrome of inappropriate diuresis (SIAD), characterized by sustained release of excessive vasopressin, or antidiuretic hormone (ADH), from the posterior pituitary gland [28]. Vincristine is the most common cause of SIAD in cancer patients, but many other drugs can cause the syndrome. Azole antifungal drugs, such as itraconazole, fluconazole, ketoconazole, and voriconazole, inhibit the activity of the cytochrome p450 enzymes that metabolize vincristine and potentiate its toxicity.

Symptoms and Signs

Lethargy, weakness, headache, oliguria, and weight gain are early symptoms of SIAD, which can progress to confusion, seizures, coma, and death [29]. However, many patients with hyponatremia are asymptomatic, especially if it develops slowly.

Treatment of SIAD

SIAD is treated with fluid restriction, close monitoring (urine output, serum sodium concentration, neurologic status), and discontinuation of vincristine therapy until the episode has resolved [28]. Furosemide should be given if fluid overload is present. Hospitalization is indicated for patients with oliguria or neurologic symptoms. Hyponatremic seizures require emergent intervention, including anticonvulsants and, if necessary, 3 % sodium chloride solution intravenously (3–5 mL per kg of body weight given over 2–3 h) [30–32]. If such aggressive therapy is necessary, the patient should be monitored in the intensive care unit, and serum sodium measured every 1–2 h. Correction of sodium should be no faster than 0.5 mEq/dL/h to reduce the risk of central pontine myelinolysis [33].

Adrenal Insufficiency

Clinically important adrenocortical insufficiency, including the inability to mount a response to metabolic stress, is common after prolonged courses (4 weeks or more) of corticosteroid therapy and can last for weeks to months after they are discontinued [34]. Symptoms include malaise, fatigue, weakness, anorexia, nausea, vomiting, weight loss, abdominal pain, diarrhea, hypothermia or hyperthermia, hypotension, altered mental status, and coma. Hyponatremia, hypoglycemia, hyperkalemia, metabolic acidosis, and prerenal azotemia may occur [35–37].

Management

Whenever patients with prior glucocorticoid therapy develop a metabolic stress, such as infection, chemotherapy-induced toxicity, or surgery, clinicians should be vigilant for symptoms of adrenal insufficiency. Empiric treatment with IV hydrocortisone 30 mg/m^2/day (moderate stress) or 100 mg/m^2/day (severe stress) in three or four divided doses should be initiated whenever the degree of hemodynamic or neurologic compromise is out of proportion to the severity of the inciting illness, because untreated adrenal insufficiency in patients undergoing severe infection, surgery, or other physiologic stress can be fatal [38].

Gastrointestinal Emergencies

Typhlitis

Typhlitis, or neutropenic enterocolitis that affects the cecum, comes from the Greek word typhlon, or cecum. The triad of neutropenia, abdominal pain, and fever with compatible diagnostic imaging findings of a thickened bowel wall defines it clinically [39–41].

Pathogenesis

Typhlitis occurs most commonly in patients with prolonged and severe myelosuppression, especially when treatment includes anthracyclines or high-dose methotrexate, which can damage the gut mucosa. There is inflammation and sometimes necrosis of the bowel wall. Neutropenic colitis frequently involves the cecum (typhlitis) but often extends into the ascending colon and terminal ileum as well. The inflamed bowel wall can be infiltrated by pathogens including gram-negative and -positive bacteria, anaerobes (e.g., *Clostridium septicum*), and Candida, which can enter the bloodstream.

Signs and Symptoms

Typical symptoms include the following: watery or bloody diarrhea, fever, nausea, vomiting, and abdominal pain which may be localized to the right lower quadrant. There could be shock secondary to septicemia or colonic perforation. The symptoms often appear 10–14 days after cytotoxic drugs at a time when neutropenia is most profound.

Physical Examination

Abdominal distension, absence of bowel sounds, tympany, tenderness in the right lower quadrant, and occasionally a palpable mass can mark the presence of typhlitis. Diffuse direct and rebound tenderness suggest colonic perforation and peritonitis.

Differential Diagnosis and Evaluation

Typhlitis should be considered in the differential diagnosis of any profoundly neutropenic patient (absolute neutrophil count <500 cells/μL) with abdominal pain. Conditions that mimic typhlitis include appendicitis, pseudomembranous colitis, ischemic colitis, and amoebic typhlitis (in endemic areas). The method of choice for investigating typhlitis is by computed tomography (CT) or ultrasound [41, 42]. The hallmark of typhlitis is diffuse cecal wall thickening. Abdominal radiography is not generally useful, and barium enema and colonoscopy are relatively contraindicated due to risk of perforation. Other investigations include blood and stool cultures and assays for *Clostridium difficile* toxin.

Management

Patients with severe typhlitis uncomplicated by peritonitis, perforation, or severe bleeding are managed with broad-spectrum antibiotics that cover *Clostridium difficile*, bowel rest and nasogastric suction if vomiting, intravenous fluids, and nutritional support [43]. Empiric antifungal therapy should be considered if fever persists

>72 h despite broad-spectrum antibiotics and GCSF administered if neutrophil recovery is expected to be delayed. Anticholinergic, antidiarrheal, and opioid agents should be avoided, since they may aggravate ileus.

In patients with typhlitis complicated by perforation or life-threatening bleeding, a two-stage hemicolectomy may be considered with complete removal of all necrotic tissue. However, it should be noted that surgery is rarely needed to manage typhlitis, since the goal is to support the patient until neutrophil recovery and resolution of bowel inflammation. Typhlitis may recur with subsequent chemotherapy, so complete gut healing is necessary prior to resuming chemotherapy with agents that can cause toxicity to the gut, such as anthracyclines or methotrexate.

Bowel Perforation and Intestinal Obstruction

Solid tumors and Burkitt lymphoma can cause intestinal obstruction, intussusception, and bowel perforation, which are managed similarly to these conditions when they occur in patients without cancer.

Hematological Complications (Leukocytosis, Febrile Neutropenia, Thrombocytopenia, Severe Anemia)

Hyperleukocytosis

Patients with leukemia and hyperleukocytosis can develop leukostasis syndrome: progressive neurologic or respiratory symptoms or signs caused by small blood vessel infiltration and occlusion by leukemic blast cells that can cause intracranial bleeding or pulmonary insufficiency [44]. In acute leukemia in children with leukocyte counts that exceed 100×10^9/L, symptomatic pulmonary leukostasis occurred in 6 of 73 patients with myeloid leukemia and in none of 161 patients with lymphoid leukemia [45].

Pathophysiology

Leukostasis is a function of the number, deformability, size, surface markers, and tissue invasiveness of the leukemic cells, as well as the volume fraction of white blood cells (leukocrit), so it is much more common in AML than ALL or CML [46]. Adaptive mechanisms mitigate the effect of hyperleukocytosis on blood viscosity, such that patients with a high leukocrit usually have significant anemia (low erythrocrit), thus maintaining blood viscosity within normal limits [47]. Leukostasis most commonly damages the lungs and CNS.

Presenting Features and Evaluation

Symptoms and signs include shortness of breath, tachypnea, dyspnea on exertion, hypoxia, confusion, somnolence, delirium, and coma [46]. Interpretation of laboratory data from patients with hyperleukocytosis may produce spurious values for arterial oxygen tension (due to oxygen consumption in vitro by the white blood cells); serum potassium concentrations can be falsely elevated if excessive cytolysis occurs in vitro. Therefore, blood samples from such patients should be placed on ice and immediately hand-carried to the laboratory for expeditious analysis [48]. The differential diagnosis of pulmonary leukostasis includes pneumonia, pneumonitis, pulmonary edema, pulmonary hemorrhage, and pulmonary embolism, all of which occur with greater frequency among children with newly diagnosed leukemia who have elevated WBC counts, sometimes with fatal results [45, 49]. If pulmonary embolism is suspected, a spiral CT or angiogram should be performed, since immediate anticoagulation can be life-saving.

Management

Rapid treatment of the leukemia and implementation of supportive care measures reduce morbidity in hyperleukocytosis. Hydration by administration of intravenous fluids at a rate of 2,500–3,000 mL/m^2/day and careful monitoring of urine output to achieve and maintain a euvolemic state reduce blood viscosity to the extent possible prior to cytoreduction. Prophylactic transfusion of red blood cells should be avoided, because any elevation in hematocrit is accompanied by an increase in blood viscosity. Anesthesia complications are common among patients with hyperleukocytosis, so procedures that require anesthesia should be deferred when possible. The diagnostic lumbar puncture should be deferred until the patient is stable to reduce the risk of a traumatic LP with blasts, which can worsen the patient's prognosis.

Leukapheresis and exchange transfusion are not necessary in most patients, and have not been shown to reduce the risk of complications associated with hyperleukocytosis [49]. The WBC count can usually be reduced gradually without complications using glucocorticoids (in ALL) or by initiating remission induction therapy or hydroxyurea (in AML) [50].

Febrile Neutropenia

When fever occurs in patients with neutropenia (ANC <1,000 and falling or <500), it represents an emergency. In 10–20 % of patients it is caused by bacteremia, and fever may be the only warning sign before septic shock occurs [51, 52]. The definition of fever used for cancer patients differs across centers, but the hospital should have a written policy for cancer patients well known to doctors, nurses, and patients so that there is no question at the time of the emergency [53]. If there is any doubt, the patient should be treated for febrile neutropenia, especially if taking glucocorticoids, which can mask fever [53]. We favor a threshold of 38.3 °C (oral or tympanic membrane) as the definition of fever. Some gram-negative bacteria can double every 30 min in a neutropenic host, such that a delay of 2 h in delivery of the first dose of antibiotic permits a 16-fold increase in bacterial burden, and development of sepsis (Fig. 9.2). Another 2 h and the patient will develop septic shock, and 2 more hours will lead to inevitable death due to overwhelming endotoxin production.

Bacterial growth and clinical manifestations in neutropenic patients

Time (hours)	Organisms per mL	Clinical Manifestations
0	1	None
0.5	2	None
1.0	4	None
2.0	16	None
4.0	256	None
6.0	4096	Fever
8.0	65,536	Sepsis
10.0	1,048,576	Septic shock
12.0	16,777,216	Death

Fig. 9.2 Bacterial growth and clinical manifestations in neutropenic patients. Used with permission of St. Jude Children's Research Hospital (www.Cure4Kids.org)

Management

Immediate administration of broad-spectrum antibiotics is the cornerstone of febrile neutropenia management, and reduces morbidity and mortality. Written policies and procedures, a readily available supply of the preferred antibiotic on the inpatient wards and in the emergency department, and a rigorous quality control procedure can help achieve the standard of 30 min or less between onset of fever and the first dose of antibiotics. Ideally, blood cultures should be obtained prior to the first dose of antibiotic, but if this will delay the first dose of antibiotic, then culture may have to be delayed to protect the patient from an increased bacterial burden. Immediate administration of antibiotics is paramount. An important study in El Salvador documented delays for parents to decide to bring their child to the hospital when fever developed (median of 10 h), delays in transport to the hospital (1.8 h), and delays in administration of the first dose of antibiotic once the patient arrived (3.5 h, Fig. 9.3) [54]. Each of these components of the overall delay requires specific interventions, and every pediatric cancer center should identify these time intervals and develop strategies to minimize them.

Hemorrhage and Thrombocytopenia

Hematologic malignancies account for almost 40 % of all cancers in children, and hemorrhage is a common cause of early death in children with leukemia in low- and middle-income countries.

Causes of Hemorrhage

Causes of hemorrhage include thrombocytopenia and coagulopathy. Thrombocytopenia occurs at the time of diagnosis when the bone marrow is

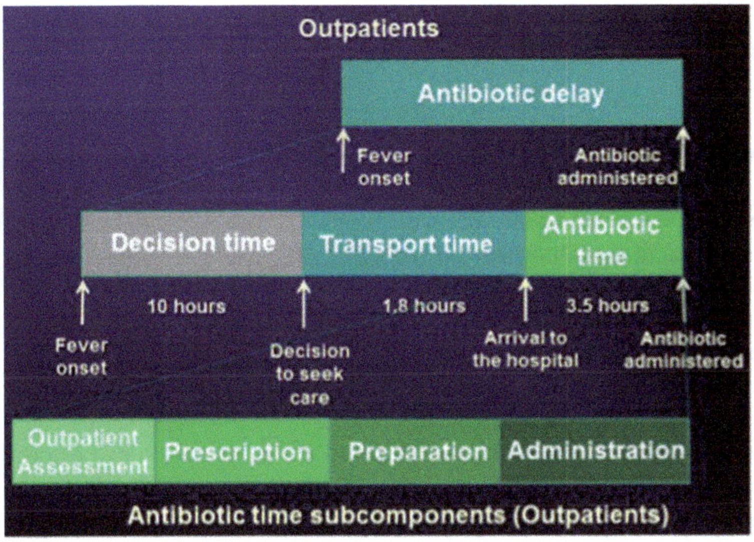

Fig. 9.3 Components of delay in administration of the first dose of antibiotic in children with cancer and febrile neutropenia in El Salvador. Information from Gavidia et al. [54]. Figure used with permission of St. Jude Children's Research Hospital (www.Cure4Kids.org)

infiltrated by leukemia or solid tumors (e.g., neuroblastoma, rhabdomyosarcoma), which displace normal hematopoietic precursor cells leading to cytopenias. Myelosuppression by chemotherapy is a common cause of thrombocytopenia during therapy. The nadir of platelets count is usually reached by 7–10 days except in carboplatin/cisplatin where there is prolonged thrombocytopenia. Radiotherapy when involves a large field (including craniospinal radiation in young children) can cause bone marrow suppression including thrombocytopenia.

Coagulopathies include disseminated intravascular coagulation (DIC), which occurs frequently in acute promyelocytic leukemia (AML M3) since promyelocytes contain a high number of granules whose release causes intravascular coagulation [55, 56]. Sepsis and hyperleukocytosis can also be associated with DIC. Other acute leukemias can cause coagulopathy at diagnosis by releasing cytokines and causing inflammation. During therapy, L-asparaginase can cause coagulopathy by decreasing synthesis of coagulation factors, including antithrombin, protein C, protein S, and fibrinogen. However, the net result of asparaginase therapy is almost always to produce a hypercoagulable state, rather than hemorrhage, and bleeding is rare in patients who are receiving asparaginase.

Management of Hemorrhage

Platelet transfusion is warranted for any thrombocytopenic patient who is actively bleeding, but indications for prophylactic platelet transfusions depend on the risk of major hemorrhage, the patient's distance to reach the hospital should bleeding occur, the availability of platelets and time needed to transfuse them at the particular center, and other logistical factors [57]. Guidelines developed in high-income countries must be adapted to each center based on these factors, and should be written and provided to clinicians and the family to assure appropriate locally adapted, personally applied management of thrombocytopenia. Bleeding due to thrombocytopenia that is refractory to random donor platelets may respond to cross-matched compatible platelets. In patients with coagulopathy caused by DIC, treatment of the underlying cause is key, but fresh frozen plasma can be administered in the meantime, and cryoprecipitate is preferred if the fibrinogen level is low.

Severe Anemia

Patients with severe, longstanding anemia can develop high-output cardiac failure that can be exacerbated by overly rapid red blood cell transfusion or hyperhydration, which both commonly occur soon after a cancer diagnosis. Patients who present with hemoglobin <6 g/dL (not due to bleeding) should be transfused slowly (5 mL/kg of packed red cells over 4 h) with careful monitoring of cardiorespiratory status. Hyperhydration is appropriate until the patient is euvolemic, but then fluid intake must be kept close to urine output to avoid decompensated heart failure [58, 59].

Chemotherapy Extravasation

Chemotherapy extravasation refers to the accidental leakage of the cancer drug from the vein into surrounding tissues with resulting injury that can range from a mild skin reaction to severe necrosis depending on the drug category and amount of extravasation [60]. Cancer drugs can be grouped into three categories based on their potential to cause tissue damage upon extravasation: nonirritants rarely produce an acute reaction if extravasated (all medications that can be given intramuscularly or subcutaneously); irritants cause pain, phlebitis, or local hypersensitivity reactions but not tissue necrosis; and vesicants cause pain, tissue damage, and extensive necrosis at the site of extravasation. Vesicants can be further sub-categorized into those with moderate potential to cause damage (dactinomycin, fluorouracil, mitoxantrone, and paclitaxel) and those with high potential to cause damage (anthracyclines, mitomycin C, vinca alkaloids [vincristine, vinblastine], etoposide if highly concentrated, and cisplatin). Vesicants with high potential to cause damage enter the cells at the site of extravasation, bind to nucleic acids, and initiate tissue necrosis and progressive ulceration that can persist for weeks or months. Significant levels of doxorubicin can be detected in surrounding tissues weeks and months after extravasation. The continuing release of drug from necrotic cells damages surrounding tissues (Fig. 9.4). Furthermore, extravasation in immunocompromised patients predisposes them to local infections and bacteremia.

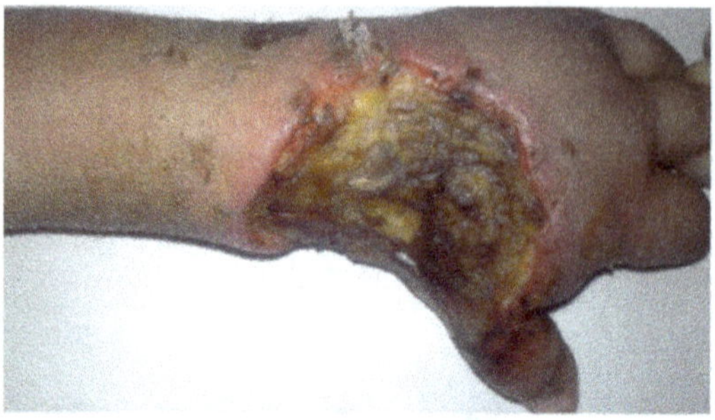

Fig. 9.4 Extravasation of vincristine in a child with acute lymphoblastic leukemia. Figure used with permission of St. Jude Children's Research Hospital (www.Cure4Kids.org)

Signs and Symptoms

The initial symptoms of extravasation occur immediately after the blood vessel has been breached. There may be discomfort or pain which ranges from mild to intense and permanent tissue damage and necrosis is common after vesicant extravasation.

Management

Vesicant extravasation must be recognized and managed promptly to minimize tissue damage, which can become so severe that surgical debridement and plastic surgery are required (Fig. 9.4) [60]. Treatment is summarized in Table 9.2. All incidents of extravasation should be documented and reported to senior staff.

Table 9.2 Treatment of extravasation of non-vesicant irritant drugs

Initial steps in the management of all types of extravasation:	
1. Stop the administration of the drug	
2. Disconnect the infusion, but do not remove the cannula/needle	
3. With the cannula/needle in place, aspirate as much of the drug as possible with a 10 mL syringe	
Drug category and selected examples	*Management of extravasation*
Vesicants, DNA binding	1–3. Initial steps for all types of extravasation
Alkylating agents (mechlorethamine, Bendamustine), anthracyclines (doxorubicin, daunorubicin, epirubicin, idarubicin); antibiotics (dactinomycin, mitomycin C, mitoxantrone)	4. Avoid corticosteroid injections, which may worsen tissue damage. Specific antidotes when available: • Anthracyclines—IV dexrazoxane within 6 h, if dexrazoxane not available apply topical dimethylsulphoxide (DMSO) to an area twice the size of the extravasation immediately then bid × 14 days • Mechlorethamine (sodium thiosulfate 10 %) SQ immediately 5. Remove the cannula/needle 6. Apply a cold pack to the affected area for 20 min 4 times daily for 1–2 days and elevate the limb
Vesicants, non-DNA binding	1–3. Initial steps for all types of extravasation
Vinca alkaloids (vincristine, vinblastine, vindesine, vinorelbine); taxanes (docetaxel, paclitaxel)	4. Immediately inject hyaluronidase SQ 150–1,500 IU diluted in 1 mL sterile water around the extravasated area to allow wider dispersion of the extravasated vinca 5. Remove cannula/needle 6. Apply a warm compress after hyaluronidase to the affected area for 20 min 4 times daily for 1–2 days and elevate the limb 7. Apply 1 % hydrocortisone cream and sterile dressing 3 times per day if skin is persistently red and inflamed 8. Avoid corticosteroid injections or cold compresses, since they may exacerbate tissue injury
Irritants	1–3. Initial steps for all types of extravasation
Alkylating agents (ifosfamide, melphalan, dacarbazine), fluorouracil, liposomal anthracyclines, platinum agents (carboplatin, cisplatin, oxaliplatin), topoisomerase I inhibitors (irinotecan, topotecan), topoisomerase II inhibitors (etoposide, teniposide)	4. Remove the cannula/needle 5. Apply a loose dry dressing 6. Apply cold compresses or elevate the limb to limit swelling
Non-vesicants	1–3. Initial steps for all types of extravasation
Any medication that can be administered IM or SQ plus bleomycin, bortezomib, cladribine, etoposide phosphate, gemcitabine, fludarabine, monoclonal antibodies, thiotepa, cyclophosphamide	4. Remove the cannula/needle 5. Apply a loose dry dressing 6. Apply cold compresses or elevate the limb to limit swelling

IM intramuscularly, *SQ* subcutaneously, *IV* intravenously

References

1. McCurdy MT, Shanholtz CB. Oncologic emergencies. Crit Care Med. 2012;40(7):2212–22.
2. Baldwin KJ, Zivkovic SA, Lieberman FS. Neurologic emergencies in patients who have cancer: diagnosis and management. Neurol Clin. 2012;30(1):101–28; viii.
3. Demshar R, Vanek R, Mazanec P. Oncologic emergencies: new decade, new perspectives. AACN Adv Crit Care. 2011;22(4):337–48.
4. Rachapalli V, Boucher LM. Superior Vena cava syndrome:role of the interventionalist. Can Assoc Radiol J . 2013 Feb 14. pii: S0846–5371(12)00108-8. doi: 10.1016/j.carj.2012.09.003.
5. Chaudhary K, Gupta A, Wadhawan S, Jain D, Bhadoria P. Anesthetic management of superior vena cava syndrome due to anterior mediastinal mass. J Anaesthesiol Clin Pharmacol. 2012;28(2):242–6.
6. Cheng S. Superior vena cava syndrome: a contemporary review of a historic disease. Cardiol Rev. 2009;17(1):16–23.
7. Wan JF, Bezjak A. Superior vena cava syndrome. Emerg Med Clin North Am. 2009;27(2):243–55.
8. Spottswood SE, Goble MM, Massey GV, Ben-Ezra JM. Acute monoblastic leukemia presenting with pericardial effusion and cardiac tamponade. Pediatr Radiol. 1994;24(7):494–5.
9. da Costa CM, de Camargo B, Lamelas R, et al. Cardiac tamponade complicating hyperleukocytosis in a child with leukemia. Med Pediatr Oncol. 1999;33(2):120–3.
10. Kaifi JT, Toth JW, Gusani NJ, et al. Multidisciplinary management of malignant pleural effusion. J Surg Oncol. 2012;105(7):731–8.
11. Muzumdar H. Pleural effusion. Pediatr Rev. 2012; 33(1):45–7.
12. McGrath EE, Anderson PB. Diagnosis of pleural effusion: a systematic approach. Am J Crit Care. 2011; 20(2):119–27.
13. Wide JM, Curtis J. Granulocytic sarcoma as a cause of cord compression. Clin Radiol. 1997;52(10):803.
14. Bartek Jr J, Abedi-Valugerdi G, Liska J, Nystrom H, Andresen M, Mathiesen T. Intracranial hemorrhage due to intracranial hypertension caused by the superior vena cava syndrome. J Clin Neurosci. 2013;20:1040–1.
15. Labrador J, Puig N, Ortin A, Gutierrez NC, Gonzalez-Diaz M. Multiple cranial neuropathy and intracranial hypertension associated with all-trans retinoic acid treatment in a young adult patient with acute promyelocytic leukemia. Int J Hematol. 2012;96(3):383–5.
16. Vartzelis G, Lancaster D, Fallon P. Intracranial hypertension in pediatric patients with acute lymphoblastic leukemia. Pediatr Blood Cancer. 2009;52(3):418–20.
17. Legrand F, Dorgeret S, Saizou C, Duval M, Vilmer E. Cerebellar herniation after intrathecal chemotherapy including cytosine arabinoside in a boy with T acute lymphoblastic leukemia. Leukemia. 2002;16(12):2454–5.
18. Fink ME. Osmotherapy for intracranial hypertension: mannitol versus hypertonic saline. Continuum (Minneap Minn). 2012;18(3):640–54.
19. Mercille G, Ospina LH. Pediatric idiopathic intracranial hypertension: a review. Pediatr Rev. 2007;28(11):e77–86.
20. Howard SC, Jones DP, Pui CH. The tumor lysis syndrome. N Engl J Med. 2011;364(19):1844–54.
21. Cairo MS, Coiffier B, Reiter A, Younes A. Recommendations for the evaluation of risk and prophylaxis of tumour lysis syndrome (TLS) in adults and children with malignant diseases: an expert TLS panel consensus. Br J Haematol. 2010;149(4):578–86.
22. Coiffier B, Altman A, Pui CH, Younes A, Cairo MS. Guidelines for the management of pediatric and adult tumor lysis syndrome: an evidence-based review. J Clin Oncol. 2008;26(16):2767–78.
23. McKay C, Furman WL. Hypercalcemia complicating childhood malignancies. Cancer. 1993;72(1):256–60.
24. Kerdudo C, Aerts I, Fattet S, et al. Hypercalcemia and childhood cancer: a 7-year experience. J Pediatr Hematol Oncol. 2005;27(1):23–7.
25. Andiran N, Alikasifoglu A, Kupeli S, Yetgin S. Use of bisphosphonates for resistant hypercalcemia in children with acute lymphoblastic leukemia: report of two cases and review of the literature. Turk J Pediatr. 2006;48(3):248–52.
26. Gokce M, Unal S, Gulsen H, et al. A rare metabolic complication of acute lymphoblastic leukemia in childhood: lactic acidosis. Turk J Pediatr. 2012; 54(1):61–3.
27. Sillos EM, Shenep JL, Burghen GA, Pui CH, Behm FG, Sandlund JT. Lactic acidosis: a metabolic complication of hematologic malignancies: case report and review of the literature. Cancer. 2001;92(9):2237–46.
28. Howard SC, Pui CH. Endocrine complications in pediatric patients with acute lymphoblastic leukemia. Blood Rev. 2002;16(4):225–43.
29. Krutisch G, Valentin A. Comatose state due to severe hyponatremia in a patient with the syndrome of inappropriate antidiuretic hormone secretion. Intensive Care Med. 2001;27(5):944.
30. Haycock GB. The syndrome of inappropriate secretion of antidiuretic hormone. Pediatr Nephrol. 1995; 9(3):375–81.
31. Moritz ML, Ayus JC. New aspects in the pathogenesis, prevention, and treatment of hyponatremic encephalopathy in children. Pediatr Nephrol. 2010;25(7):1225–38.
32. Moritz ML, Ayus JC. 100 cc 3% sodium chloride bolus: a novel treatment for hyponatremic encephalopathy. Metab Brain Dis. 2010;25(1):91–6.
33. Omari A, Kormas N, Field M. Delayed onset of central pontine myelinolysis despite appropriate correction of hyponatraemia. Intern Med J. 2002; 32(5–6):273–4.
34. Felner EI, Thompson MT, Ratliff AF, White PC, Dickson BA. Time course of recovery of adrenal function in children treated for leukemia. J Pediatr. 2000;137(1):21–4.
35. Krasner AS. Glucocorticoid-induced adrenal insufficiency. JAMA. 1999;282(7):671–6.
36. August GP. Treatment of adrenocortical insufficiency. Pediatr Rev. 1997;18(2):59–62.

37. Cooper MS, Stewart PM. Corticosteroid insufficiency in acutely ill patients. N Engl J Med. 2003;348(8):727–34.
38. Leman P. Addison's disease. Hydrocortisone should be started immediately adrenal insufficiency is considered. BMJ. 1996;313(7054):427.
39. Altinel E, Yarali N, Isik P, Bay A, Kara A, Tunc B. Typhlitis in acute childhood leukemia. Med Princ Pract. 2012;21(1):36–9.
40. Moran H, Yaniv I, Ashkenazi S, Schwartz M, Fisher S, Levy I. Risk factors for typhlitis in pediatric patients with cancer. J Pediatr Hematol Oncol. 2009;31(9):630–4.
41. Mullassery D, Bader A, Battersby AJ, et al. Diagnosis, incidence, and outcomes of suspected typhlitis in oncology patients–experience in a tertiary pediatric surgical center in the United Kingdom. J Pediatr Surg. 2009;44(2):381–5.
42. Alexander JE, Williamson SL, Seibert JJ, Golladay ES, Jimenez JF. The ultrasonographic diagnosis of typhlitis (neutropenic colitis). Pediatr Radiol. 1988;18(3):200–4.
43. Junpaparp P, Buppajarntham S, Madueno FV, Varadi G. Concomitant typhlitis and Clostridium difficile colitis developed after first R-CHOP chemotherapy in a non-Hodgkin lymphoma patient. BMJ Case Rep. 2013 Apr 17;2013. doi:pii: bcr2013008894. 10.1136/bcr-2013-008894.
44. Haase R, Merkel N, Diwan O, Elsner K, Kramm CM. Leukapheresis and exchange transfusion in children with acute leukemia and hyperleukocytosis. A single center experience. Klin Padiatr. 2009;221(6):374–8.
45. Krance RA, Hurwitz CA, Head DR, et al. Experience with 2-chlorodeoxyadenosine in previously untreated children with newly diagnosed acute myeloid leukemia and myelodysplastic diseases. J Clin Oncol. 2001;19(11):2804–11.
46. Porcu P, Cripe LD, Ng EW, et al. Hyperleukocytic leukemias and leukostasis: a review of pathophysiology, clinical presentation and management. Leuk Lymphoma. 2000;39(1–2):1–18.
47. Lichtman MA, Heal J, Rowe JM. Hyperleukocytic leukaemia: rheological and clinical features and management. Baillieres Clin Haematol. 1987;1(3):725–46.
48. Polak R, Huisman A, Sikma MA, Kersting S. Spurious hypokalaemia and hypophosphataemia due to extreme hyperleukocytosis in a patient with a haematological malignancy. Ann Clin Biochem. 2010;47(Pt. 2):179–81.
49. Lowe EJ, Pui CH, Hancock ML, Geiger TL, Khan RB, Sandlund JT. Early complications in children with acute lymphoblastic leukemia presenting with hyperleukocytosis. Pediatr Blood Cancer. 2005; 45(1):10–5.
50. Ozdemir MA, Karakukcu M, Patiroglu T, Torun YA, Kose M. Management of hyperleukocytosis and prevention of tumor lysis syndrome with low-dose prednisone continuous infusion in children with acute lymphoblastic leukemia. Acta Haematol. 2009; 121(1):56–62.
51. Cull LF, Nolan MB. Treating neutropenic fever in the emergency department: delays may be deadly! J Emerg Nurs. 2009;35(1):36–9.
52. Goldberg E, Gafter-Gvili A, Robenshtok E, Leibovici L, Paul M. Empirical antifungal therapy for patients with neutropenia and persistent fever: systematic review and meta-analysis. Eur J Cancer. 2008;44(15):2192–203.
53. Binz P, Bodmer N, Leibundgut K, Teuffel O, Niggli FK, Ammann RA. Different fever definitions and the rate of fever and neutropenia diagnosed in children with cancer: a retrospective two-center cohort study. Pediatr Blood Cancer. 2013;60(5):799–805.
54. Gavidia R, Fuentes SL, Vasquez R, et al. Low socioeconomic status is associated with prolonged times to assessment and treatment, sepsis and infectious death in pediatric fever in El Salvador. PLoS One. 2012;7(8):e43639.
55. Tallman M, Douer D, Gore S, et al. Treatment of patients with acute promyelocytic leukemia: a consensus statement on risk-adapted approaches to therapy. Clin Lymphoma Myeloma Leuk. 2010;10:S122–6.
56. Tallman MS. Updates on the treatment of acute promyelocytic leukemia. Clin Adv Hematol Oncol. 2010;8(2):89–90.
57. Green D. Management of bleeding complications of hematologic malignancies. Semin Thromb Hemost. 2007;33(4):427–34.
58. Agrawal AK, Hsu E, Quirolo K, Neumayr LD, Flori HR. Red blood cell transfusion in pediatric patients with severe chronic anemia: how slow is necessary? Pediatr Blood Cancer. 2012;58(3):466–8.
59. Weiskopf RB. Emergency transfusion for acute severe anemia: a calculated risk. Anesth Analg. 2010; 111(5):1088–92.
60. Perez Fidalgo JA, Garcia FL, Cervantes A, Margulies A, Vidall C, Roila F. Management of chemotherapy extravasation: ESMO–EONS clinical practice guidelines. Eur J Oncol Nurs. 2012;16(5):528–34.

Essential Medicines and Pharmacy Services

10

John T. Wiernikowski and Ronald D. Barr

Introduction

It is estimated that more than 80 % of children in the world live in low- and middle income countries (LMICs) where they carry a disproportionate burden of cancer-related morbidity and mortality [1, 2], and this is unlikely to change without significant interventions at national and regional levels. Indeed, deaths from cancer at all ages in LMICs now exceed deaths from malaria, tuberculosis, and HIV/AIDS (diseases prevalent in LMICs) combined [3] The last half century has witnessed remarkable progress in pediatric oncology, at least in resource-rich countries in which cure rates for children with cancer approximate 80 % [4]. The major goal now is to provide children living in LMICs a similar opportunity to be cured.

In 1999 the World Health Organization (WHO) declared "Some relatively rare but curable cancers require highly specialized facilities for optimal care, such as the acute leukemias and pediatric tumors" [5]; a laudable goal and one that is beginning to bear fruit through the efforts of numerous international outreach initiatives and the work of groups such as the Société Internationale d'Oncologie Pédiatrique (SIOP) which have established mechanisms specifically to address the challenges of Pediatric Oncology in Developing Countries (PODC). As a result, it is quite clear that diseases such as Burkitt lymphoma and acute lymphoblastic leukemia (ALL), and certain cancers more prevalent in adults (e.g., Breast Ca), can be treated effectively in resource-poor countries [6–9]. The opportunity to maximize pediatric cancer outcomes for a particular countries development index is being enhanced further through the efforts of the PODC Committee of SIOP and others through the establishment of "adapted" protocols/treatment guidelines for a number of malignancies prevalent in LMICs [10–14]. However, these successes are limited to a few centers of evolving expertise and not uniform across LMICs, and as such for ALL; cure rates in high income countries are on the order of 80–90 % but remain around 10 % in LMICs [15].

Financial and Other Barriers

While not the sole contributor, the lack of consistent, timely, and affordable access to antineoplastic and other drugs is a significant ongoing barrier to governments, non-governmental organizations (NGOs), and individual citizens who must pay for drugs out of pocket in providing health care,

J.T. Wiernikowski, B.Sc. Phm., PharmD (✉)
Department of Pediatrics, McMaster University,
1200 Main Street West, Hamilton, ON, Canada L8N 3Z5
e-mail: wierniko@hhsc.ca

R.D. Barr, M.B. Ch.B., M.D.
McMaster University, 1200 Main Street West,
Hamilton, ON, Canada L8N 3Z5
e-mail: rbarr@mcmaster.ca

D.C. Stefan and C. Rodriguez-Galindo (eds.), *Pediatric Hematology-Oncology in Countries with Limited Resources: A Practical Manual*, DOI 10.1007/978-1-4614-3891-5_10,

and this financial barrier contributes to the disparity in cancer (and other disease)-related outcomes in LMICs. Recent estimates indicate that drug expenditures in LMICs can range from 20 to 60 % of total health care expenditures [16] compared to less than 20 % in resource-rich countries [17], and that up to 90 % of those living in LMICs must pay for drugs out of pocket, making this the next biggest expense after food [18]. Indeed, in some low income countries; upwards of 60 % of children diagnosed with malignant disease will not even have treatment initiated due to the onerous costs to the family [19, 20]. While newer biologics and oral cytotoxics are prohibitively expensive, the majority of childhood cancers can be effectively treated with off-patent generic drugs; yet despite this, there remains significant price variance of 5–10-fold for arguably "staple" antineoplastics such as doxorubicin and cis-platinum [21]. Given that drugs are often curative (e.g., antimicrobials), or can lead to significant prolongation and quality of life (HIV/AIDS) or effect palliation when cure is not possible, they cannot be regarded as ordinary commodities.

In resource-rich countries drugs are now showing the most rapid increase in cost on a line item basis, yet the pharmaceutical industry remains one of the most profitable industries in the USA [18]. An exhaustive examination of factors affecting the pricing of pharmaceuticals is beyond the scope of this chapter. One important aspect of pricing that affects developing countries is the World Trade Organization (WTO). Trade-Related Aspects of Intellectual Property Rights (TRIPS) agreement, first ratified in 1994 then clarified in 2001 in the Doha Accord with respect to issues in public health. The agreement strengthened intellectual property law, procedures, and remedies. For resource-rich countries with established patent laws, the TRIPS agreement meant next to no change; however, in LMICs, especially those with well established and thriving generic drug industries such as India, it meant a significant curtailing in the activities of those companies. The TRIPS agreement has generated considerable debate with respect to its ultimate impact on the cost of drugs and access to medications by the poor in LMICs. A number of solutions have been proposed to mitigate the perceived or real negative impact of the TRIPS agreement. These include intensified loans/grants from organizations such as the World Bank to developing countries to purchase essential drugs that are still covered by patents; debt cancellation for poor nations to free up capital to purchase essential medicines; the purchasing of patents by a bank or an NGO; and providing licenses for patented drugs to generic manufacturers in LMICs. The favored solution currently is for the establishment of a global equity-based pricing system for high-, middle-, and low income countries [22–24] and should be relatively easy to implement given estimates for aggregate cost of drugs to treat ALL in LMICs to be around US$150 million per year; a tawdry amount given annual figures for international commerce [21].

Access to pharmaceuticals has been viewed as a fundamental human right and the focus of international policy development for several decades, starting with the WHO Model List of Essential Medicines that was first generated in 1977 [25]. Criticized initially by the pharmaceutical industry, it has been embraced since by governments, NGOs, and academia as a truly "workable" document upon which to base local/regional policy initiatives on access to drugs in LMICs. A number of newer initiatives have been put forward recently that are beginning to bear fruit also. The Millennium Declaration: "In co-operation with pharmaceutical companies, provide access to affordable essential drugs in developing countries" was one of several development goals established for LMICs. In conjunction with the World Health Assembly's resolution on "Better Medicines for Children" [26], which encourages the WHO and its member states to undertake activities to promote training and research in pediatric clinical pharmacology, improve drug regulation, access and rational use, such initiatives are bringing these issues to the forefront globally. Courtesy of a US$9.7 million grant from the Gates Foundation to the WHO and UNICEF, a Model List of Essential Medicines for children (EMLc) has been generated and has gone through several iterations already [27], and a follow-up document "The Model Formulary for Children" [28] has been produced.

Table 10.1 List of medications for the treatment of children with cancer in low and middle income countries

Antineoplastics	Section	Antimicrobials	Section	Supportive care agents	Section
Asparaginase	8.2	Acyclovir	6.4.1	Allopurinol	8.2
Bleomycin	8.2	Amikacin	6.2.4	Amitriptyline	24.2.1
Carboplatin	8.2	Amphotericin B	6.3	Codeine	2.2
Cisplatin	8.2	Cefotaxime	6.2.1	Diazepam	5
Cyclophosphamide	8.2	Ceftazidime	6.2.1	Docusate	8.4
Cytarabine	8.2	Ceftriaxone	6.2.1	Folinic acid	8.2
Dacarbazine	8.2	Clindamycin	6.2.2	Heparin	10.2
Dactinomycin	8.2	Fluconazole	6.3	Lactulose	8.4
Daunarubicin	8.2	Gentamycin	6.2.2	MESNA	8.2
Dexamethasone	8.3	Meropenem	6.2.1	Midazolam	8.4
Doxorubicin	8.2	Metronidazole	6.2.2	Morphine	8.4
Etoposide	8.2	Septra	6.2.2	Ondansetron	8.4
Hydrocortisone	8.3	Vancomycin	6.2.1	Senna	8.4
Hydroxyurea	8.2				
Ifosfamide	8.2				
Mercaptopurine	8.2				
Methotrexate	8.2				
Methylprednisolone	8.3				
Prednisolone	8.3				
Thioguanine	8.2				
Vinblastine	8.2				
Vincristine	8.2				

Section numbers refer to the WHO Model List of Essential Medicines

These were created to address the valid criticism that the original Essential Medicines List was too adult-focused. Drugs relevant to the care of children with cancer from the EMLc and their relevant sections are summarized in Table 10.1. The grant from the Gates Foundation is funding additional work that will impact children living in LMICs to develop methods for estimating body weight easily and accurately (when no scale is available) to dose drugs reliably; and the development of flexible, solid oral dosage forms as the formulation of choice [29].

In order to promote the development of drugs with pediatric indications and to provide more pediatric dosing, labeling, and safety data; regulators such as the United States Food and Drug administration (FDA) and the European Medicines Agency (EMA) have enacted legislation to mandate basic pediatric data for new drug submissions and financial incentives for drugs already licensed or "off-patent" [30–32]. The impact of this legislation is currently debatable, since all of the additional data provided by manufacturers have been for drugs that are still "on-patent"; and in Europe, of 29 new anticancer drugs licensed by 2009 only 6 had a pediatric indication. Furthermore, the new pediatric information (dosing, safety, labeling) generated by manufacturers as a result of these initiatives is not being filed in other jurisdictions because there is no financial gain to be had from doing so [33–35].

Infrastructure and Logistical Issues

Regulatory agencies in high income countries such as the FDA, the Health Protection Branch (Canada), and the EMA, undertake reviews of data submitted by drug manufacturers with respect to efficacy, safety, and quality, as well as performing cost-effectiveness analyses before

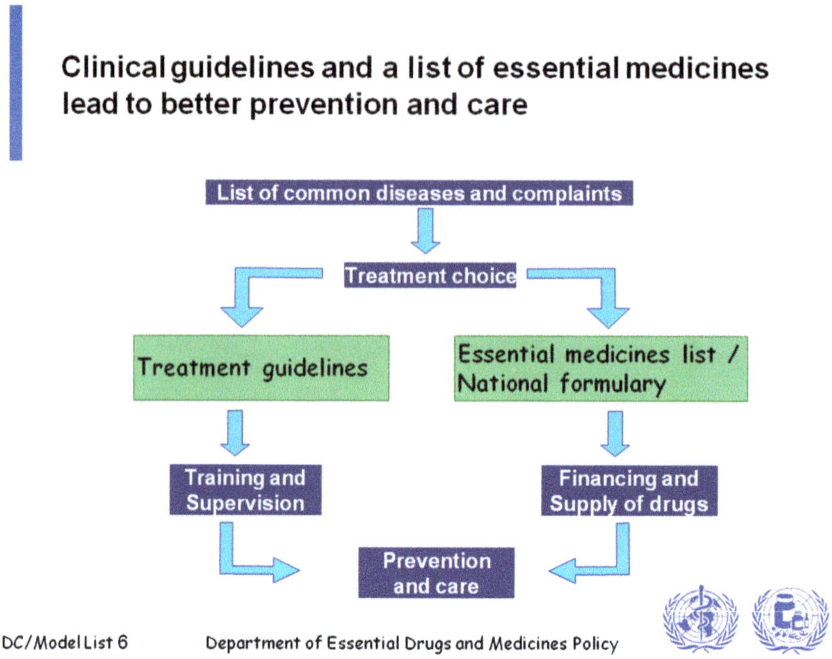

Fig. 10.1 Potential framework for policy development for medications in low and middle income countries

granting a notice of compliance (NOC) with their respective regulations and issuing a license to manufacture and/or sell the product within the respective country/jurisdiction. Developing countries may not have such agencies in place and, if they do, likely these will not have the capacity or expertise to adjudicate such submissions properly. These countries rely on international agencies such as the WHO for guidance and programs that can assist with drug evaluations. One of the fundamental guiding documents is the WHO Model List of Essential Medicines (adult and pediatric) [27, 28] which health ministries in LMICs can access and tailor to the needs of their populations. This is done best in conjunction with published evidence-based treatment guidelines that now exist for many medical conditions. A proposed framework is shown in Fig. 10.1 [36].

The quality of drugs available in developing countries is also of increasing concern [29, 37, 38]; since many chemotherapeutic agents are clear colorless solutions and, beyond emesis with certain agents (e.g., cis-platinum), have no immediate clinical/laboratory value correlates for "fraud," making them easy prey for counterfeiters, with estimates that up to 30 % of drugs in certain settings may be counterfeit or substandard [39]. Using the adage of "you get what you pay for" attempts have been made to use "low-price" together with "brand vs. generic" and "appearance" of the selling pharmacy as indicators of poor quality drug product in LMICs; with low price for a "brand" drug being somewhat useful, but none of these factors is highly helpful [40]. Due to the high cost of imported brand name drugs, some governments in LMICs have fostered the development of generic pharmaceutical industry capacity within their own borders (e.g., India), or import generic versions of drugs preferentially. This is sound policy and can result in significant cost savings [41]; however, no strategy is perfect and tragedies have occurred [42, 43]. To address the issue of access to high quality pharmaceutical products, the WHO developed a "Prequalification Program" in 2004 for manufacturers of drugs. The program encompasses all major aspects of drug manufacture and quality assurance and provides for inspections as well as employing quality control laboratories.

Drugs that pass quality control are published on the WHO prequalification website for reference by governments and NGOs purchasing drugs for LMICs [44].

Additional factors that impact on drug availability and access in developing countries are infrastructure issues. Due to lack of local production, many drugs in the developing world have to be imported. Once imported, distribution of such drugs to health care providers in hospitals, clinics, or other medical facilities may be problematic. Roads may be in poor states of repair; some drugs require storage under controlled temperature/humidity conditions or refrigeration, which may be problematic during transport; or, at the destination, if there is no refrigerator or provision of consistent electrical supply.

The social and economic conditions in developing countries often make them fertile breeding grounds for corruption. Life saving/prolonging drugs such as antineoplastics and antiretrovirals are often stolen and resold on the black market. Narcotic analgesics have high resale value and, coupled with concerns about addiction, many governments in LMICs have adopted overly restrictive drug control policies at the national level [45, 46]. This is particularly tragic as it results in pain being the most undertreated symptom in patients in the developing world; and, for the child (or adult) with cancer whose chances of cure are low, effective palliation is virtually impossible.

While the lack of child-friendly formulations is true for most drugs, it is particularly true for antineoplastics. Injectable drugs are available almost universally in sizes geared towards adult patients; this is problematic globally and not unique to LMICs. However, given the cost of these agents, and potential lack of proper storage facilities (e.g., refrigeration), enormous waste occurs if a second or third child cannot benefit from a dose of drug that has been reconstituted. In some cases, the provision of cancer care (adult and pediatric) is undertaken at a single center; this may be a preferable scenario in LMICs as it provides the opportunity to realize cost savings through minimization of waste. Indeed, in some settings, doses of chemotherapy for adults are rounded to the nearest vial size for this reason. Oral agents are equally problematic in the lack of appropriate dosage forms for children, necessitating the handling of antineoplastics to split tablets or open capsules by health care personnel or parents/caregivers without the availability of proper personal protective equipment.

The Role of Pharmacists in Cancer Care

Pharmacists are society's experts on medicines. They work at the interface between the vast global drug development and marketing apparatus, and the patients who are prescribed these drugs or consume "over the counter" preparations. Their primary role in today's health care environment is to promote and support the safe, effective, and rational use of medications. Globally however, there remains significant variability in how pharmacists actually practice. In many resource-rich countries, pharmacy practice has and continues to evolve with pharmacists now being more engaged in direct patient care, working together with physicians and nurses to ensure the best outcomes for patients in both hospitals and the community. Occurring in parallel with this evolution has been the development of credentialing bodies such as the Board of Pharmacy Specialties [47] in the United States which establishes criteria for specialty practice areas and standards for credentialing of pharmacy specialists; with oncology pharmacy practice being a specialty. Indeed, some of the fundamental dispensing functions performed by pharmacists are now being devolved to properly trained pharmacy technicians, freeing up pharmacists' time to devote to patients. Given the complexity of caring for patients with cancer, requiring multidisciplinary teams [48], the costs of antineoplastic drugs, the potential for severe drug toxicity in the event of a medication error, and requirements for the safe preparation, administration, and disposal of cytotoxics, pharmacists are critical members to include in the health care team. This is no less true in LMICs than it is in resource-rich countries; although it must be acknowledged that in some settings, access to a pharmacist is not possible, and the role of chemotherapy preparation and administration falls to a nurse. It can be argued that having pharmacists involved in the care of patients with cancer in LMICs is as (or more) vital than in a high income country. Given the risks for inadvertent exposure to antineoplastic drugs by health care personnel, establishing a dedicated oncology pharmacy and having a trained pharmacist (or pharmacy technician, depending on the setting) to prepare chemotherapy (ideally utilizing appropriate personal protective equipment and a biological safety cabinet or laminar flow hood) and properly dispose of used administration sets afterwards is of prime importance. Additional benefits of having a dedicated oncology pharmacist and pharmacy service relate to establishment of standard operating procedures and documentation of workload leading to better inventory control. By establishing and projecting drug needs, it may be possible to purchase drugs in bulk and realize additional cost savings. Additionally, having a secure central storage facility may prevent loss due to theft. The key elements in establishing an effective oncology pharmacy in an LMIC (Kenya) are listed in Table 10.2 and a core curriculum for pharmacists' training (Table 10.3) have been described recently by Strother et al. [49]. While there are no distinct standards of practice for oncology pharmacy in LMICs, the International Society of Oncology Pharmacy Practitioners (ISOPP) has developed and published Standards of Oncology Pharmacy Practice that take into account realities from both resource-rich and resource-poor settings. These standards address key issues for pharmacists and nursing personnel preparing and administering chemotherapy with respect to sterile preparation, personal protective equipment, waste and spill management as well as management of drugs and checking procedures to prevent medication errors [50]. A second edition of the standards is to be published in 2013. Beyond their primary functions described above, pharmacists in LMICs can participate in additional initiatives such as establishing pharmacovigilance programs [51] and contribute to patient care through the use of standardized assessment tools for toxicity and adherence, and in patient/parent education [52–55].

Table 10.2 Recommendations for development of an oncology pharmacy in a resource-limited setting

Procurement	• Bulk purchasing to reduce costs • Identification of reputable suppliers, particularly in areas at high risk of counterfeit • Placement of personnel on the procurement boards of hospital
Storage	• Physical security of storage location • Establish policy and procedures to buttress physical security measures
Preparation and dispensing	• Fixed dosing rounded to vial size to reduce waste and minimize potential for error • Pre-printed order sheets • Defined treatment protocols • Physical infrastructures to limit exposures (i.e., use of PPE and Class II laminar flow hood)
Disposal	• Defined disposal protocols for chemotherapy waste • A functional incinerator capable of safety destroying chemotherapeutics or a plan for long-term storage
Personnel training	• Safe handling of chemotherapeutics • Safe disposal of chemotherapeutics • Emergency procedures for events such as chemotherapy spills • Safe administration of chemotherapeutics (nursing) • Management of complications (e.g., extravasation)
Cost containment	• Bulk purchasing • Fixed dosing to minimize waste • Defined cost-effective treatment protocols • Disease guidelines and priorities

Table 10.3 Competency-based training elements for pharmacists in LMICs

Chemotherapy basics
• Mechanisms of cancer and chemotherapy
• Side effects of chemotherapy
• Risks of hazardous drug exposure
Appropriate and safe ordering of chemotherapy
• Body surface area and dose calculation
• Dose adjustment for organ function
• Laboratory value evaluation
Personal protective equipment
• Required personal protective equipment for preparation, administration and disposal of hazardous drugs
• Chemotherapy preparation area (glove box, laminar flow hood, etc.)
Preparation and administration of chemotherapy
• Sterile preparation techniques
• Negative pressure reconstitution(vs. venting vials)
• Use of chemotherapy compendium(diluent selection, fluid selection, infusion time/drip rate expiration dating)
• Vein assessment and selection
• Administration of vesicants
Disposal of chemotherapy
• Disposal of bulk hazardous waste, trace contaminated waste and sharps
• Chemotherapy spill clean up
Chemotherapy supportive care measures
• Chemotherapy requiring pre- and/or post-hydration
• Antiemetic selection
• Management of allergic and anaphylactic reactions
• Management of extravasation
Certification to handle hazardous drugs
• Completion of 2-day training course of the above topics
• Successful completion of chemotherapy competency exam

References

1. Barr R, Antillon F, Agarwal B, Mehta PS, Ribeiro R. Pediatric oncology in countries with limited resources. In: Pizzo PA, Poplack DG, editors. Principles and practice of pediatric oncology. 6th ed. Philadelphia: Lippincott Williams and Wilkins; 2011. p. 1463–73.
2. Kellie SJ, Howard SC. Global child health priorities; what role for paediatric oncologists? Eur J Cancer. 2008;44:2388–96.
3. Lingwood R, Boyle P, Milburn A, et al. The challenge of cancer control in Africa. Nat Rev Cancer. 2008;8: 398–403.
4. Gatta G, Zigon G, Capocaccia R, et al. Survival of European children and young adults with cancer diagnosed 1995–2002. Eur J Cancer. 2009;45:992–1005.
5. Sikora K, Advani S, Koroltchouk V, et al. Essential drugs for cancer therapy: a World Health Organization consultation. Ann Oncol. 1999;10:385–90.
6. Hesseling PB, Molyneux E, Tchintseme F, et al. Treating Burkitt's lymphoma in Malawi, Cameroon and Ghana. Lancet Oncol. 2008;9:512–3.
7. Dedicoat M, Newton R. Treatment of Kaposi's sarcoma in resource-poor settings. Trop Doct. 2005;35:60.
8. Howard SC, Pedrosa M, Lins M, et al. Establishment of a pediatric oncology program and outcomes of childhood acute lymphoblastic leukemia in a resource-poor area. JAMA. 2004;291:2471–5.
9. Omar S. The Fakous experience: meeting the challenge of cancer in a low resource setting. Breast J. 2007;13:318–9.
10. Molyneux E, Davidson A, Orem J, et al. The management of children with Kaposi sarcoma in resource limited settings. Pediatr Blood Cancer. 2013;60(4): 538–42.
11. Hesseling P, Israels T, Harif M, et al. Practical recommendations for the management of children with endemic Burkitt lymphoma (BL) in a resource limited setting. Pediatr Blood Cancer. 2013;60(3):357–62.
12. Israels T, Moreira C, Scanlan T, et al. SIOP PODC: clinical guidelines for the management of children with Wilms tumour in a low income setting. Pediatr Blood Cancer. 2013;60(1):5–11.
13. Chantada G, Luna-Fineman S, Sitorus RS, et al. SIOP-PODC recommendations for graduated-intensity treatment of retinoblastoma in developing countries. Pediatr Blood Cancer. 2013;60(5):719–27.
14. Hunger SP, Sung L, Howard SC. Treatment strategies and regimens of graduated intensity for childhood acute lymphoblastic leukemia in low-income countries: a proposal. Pediatr Blood Cancer. 2009;52(5):559–65.
15. Knaul F, Arreola-Ornelas H, Méndez O. Cancer survival need not be determined by income: lessons from developing countries and focusing on children. In: 42nd Congress of the International Society of Paediatric Oncology, Boston, MA; 22 Oct 2010. Data from Globocan 2010 and WHO Global Health Observatory. http://Apps.who.int/ghodata.
16. WHO. The world medicines situation. Geneva: World Health Organization; 2004.
17. Organization for Economic Co-operation and Development. Drug spending in OECD countries up by nearly a third since 1998, according to new OECD data. http://www.oecd.org/document/25/0,2340,en_2649_37407_34967193_1_1_1_37407,00.html. Accessed 30 Jan 2013.
18. WHO. Equitable access to essential medicines: a framework for collective action. Geneva: World Health Organization; 2004.
19. Mannan MA, Islam A, Gosh NK. Acute lymphoblastic leukemia—outcome of treatment with a "hybrid" protocol. Indian J Pediatr. 2002;69:51 (abstract).

20. Bonilla M, Rossell N, Salaveria C, et al. Prevalence and predictors of abandonment of therapy among children with cancer in El Salvador. Int J Cancer. 2009;125:2144–6.
21. Knaul FM, Gralow JR, Atun R, Bhadelia A, editors. Closing the cancer divide: an equity imperative. Cambridge: Harvard University Press; 2012.
22. Angell M. The pharmaceutical industry: to whom is it accountable? N Engl J Med. 2000;324:1902–4.
23. Ashcroft RE. Access to essential medicines: a Hobbesian social contract approach. Devel World Bioeth. 2005;5:121–41.
24. Cohen-Kohler JC. The morally uncomfortable global drug gap. Ethics. 2007;82:610–4.
25. Cohen-Kohler JC, Forman L, Lipkus N. Addressing legal and political barriers to global pharmaceutical access: options for remedying the impact of the Agreement on Trade-Related aspects of Intellectual Property Rights (TRIPS) and the imposition of TRIPS-plus standards. Health Econ Policy Law. 2008;3:229–56.
26. Laing R, Waning B, Gary A, et al. 25 years of the WHO essential medicines lists: progress and challenges. Lancet. 2003;361:1723–9.
27. Hoppu K. Pediatric clinical pharmacology: at the beginning of a new era. Eur J Clin Pharmacol. 2008; 64:201–5.
28. World Health Organization. The selection and use of essential medicines. Report of the WHO Expert committee, 2009 (including the 16th WHO Model list of Essential Medicines and the second WHO Model list of Essential Medicines for Children), Technical report series, Vol. 958. WHO, Geneva; 2009.
29. WHO. WHO Model formulary for children 2010. Geneva: WHO; 2010.
30. WHO. WHO report of the informal expert meeting on better medicines for children (Geneva, October 2010); 2008. http://www.who.int/childmedicines/progress/Dosage_form_reportDEC2008.pdf. Accessed 30 Jan 2013.
31. Ward RM, Kauffman R. Future of pediatric therapeutics: reauthorization of BPCA and PREA. Clin Pharmacol Ther. 2007;81:477–9.
32. US FDA. Pediatric Research Equity Act; 2003. http://www.fda.gov/downloads/Drugs/DevelopmentApprovalProcess/DevelopmentResources/UCM077853.pdf. Accessed 30 Jan 2013.
33. European Commission. Regulation (EC) no1901/2006 of the European parliament and of the Council on medicinal products for paediatric use and amending Regulation (EEC) no 1768/92, Directive 2001/20/EC, Directive 2001/83/EC and Regulation (EC) No 726/2004. 2006. http://ec.europa.eu/health/files/eudralex/vol-1/reg_2006_1901/reg_2006_1901_en.pdf. Accessed 30 Jan 2013.
34. Baker-Smith CM, Benjamin Jr DK, Grabowski HG, et al. The economic returns of pediatric clinical trials of anti-hypertensive drugs. Am Heart J. 2008;156: 682–8.
35. Olski TM, Lampus SF, Gherarducci G, et al. Three years of paediatric regulation in the European Union. Eur J Clin Pharmacol. 2011;67:245–52.
36. Vassal G. Will children with cancer benefit from the new European Paediatric Medicines Regulation. Eur J Cancer. 2009;45:1535–46.
37. Hoppu K, Hogerzeil HV. Global aspects of drug development. In: Seyberth HW et al., editors. Pediatric clinical pharmacology. Berlin: Springer; 2011.
38. Caudron JM, Ford N, Henkens M, et al. Substandard medicines in resource-poor settings: a problem that can no longer be ignored. Trop Med Int Health. 2008;13:162–72.
39. Gautem CS, Utreja A, Singal GL. Spurious and counterfeit drugs: a growing industry in the developing world. Postgrad Med J. 2009;85:251–6.
40. WHO. Counterfeit medicines. http://www.who.int/medicines/services/counterfeit/impact/ImpactF_S/en/index1.html. Accessed 30 Jan 2013.
41. Bate R, Zhe Jin G, Mathur A. Does price reveal poor quality drugs? Evidence from 17 countries. J Health Econ. 2011;30:1150–63.
42. Cameron A, Mantel-Teeuwisse AK, Leufkens HGM, et al. Switching from originator brand medicines to generic equivalents in selected developing countries: how much could be saved? Value Health. 2012;15: 664–73.
43. Sengaloundeth S, Green MD, Fernandez FM, et al. A stratified random survey of the proportion of poor quality oral artesunate sold at medicine outlets in the Lao PDR. Implications for therapeutic failure and drug resistance. Malar J. 2009;8:172.
44. Obaid A. Quality of ceftriaxone in Pakistan: reality and resonance. Pak J Pharm Sci. 2009;22:22–9.
45. WHO Prequalification program. http://apps.who.int/prequal/default.htm. Accessed 30 Jan 2013.
46. Board INC. Report of the International Narcotics Control Board on the availability of internationally controlled drugs: ensuring adequate access for medical and scientific purposes. New York: United Nations; 2011.
47. WHO. Access to Controlled Medications Programme. Quality assurance and safety: medicines. Department of Medicines Policy and Standards, WHO Briefing Note. Geneva: WHO; 2007.
48. American Board of Pharmacy Specialties. http://www.bpsweb.org/about/history.cfm. Accessed 30 Jan 2013.
49. American Society of Clinical Oncology, European Society for Medical Oncology. ASCO-ESMO consensus statement on quality cancer care. Ann Oncol 2006;17:1063–4.
50. Strother RM, Rao KV, Gregory KM, et al. The oncology pharmacy in cancer care delivery in a resource-constrained setting in western Kenya. J Oncol Pharm Pract. 2012;18:406–16.
51. International Society of Oncology Pharmacy Practicioners Standards Committee. ISOPP standards of practice for oncology pharmacy. J. Oncol Pharm Pract 2007;13(Suppl.):1–81.

52. Olsson S, Shanthi NP, Stergachis A, et al. Pharmacovigilance activities in 55 low and middle income countries. A questionnaire-based analysis. Drug Saf. 2010;33:689–703.
53. Mancini R. Implementing a standardized pharmacist assessment and evaluating the role of a pharmacist in a multidisciplinary supportive oncology clinic. J Support Oncol. 2012;10:99–106.
54. Pastakia SD, Schellhase EM, Jakait B. Collaborative partnership for clinical pharmacy services in Kenya. Am J Health Syst Pharm. 2009;66: 1386–90.
55. Tuffaha HW, Abdelhadi O, Al OS. Clinical pharmacy services in the outpatient pediatric oncology clinics at a comprehensive cancer center. Int J Clin Pharm. 2012;34:27–31.

Palliative and Supportive Care

11

Jan Du Plessis and David N. Korones

There is music everywhere—In a child's laugh or the wind in the trees—
And to survive, you must learn to dance to it.

—Hazel Mitchley (Nov 2004)

What Is Paediatric Palliative Care

Paediatric palliative care is a holistic and active approach to care, with the aim to improve quality of life [1–3]. The World Health Organization (WHO) defines it as the active and total care of the child's body, mind and spirit, which also involves the family [2, 4]. Paediatric palliative care considers the child and family as a unique entity whose members require care throughout the course of an illness, and if the child dies, at and beyond the time of death [1]. It is child- and family-centred care that is based on shared decision making and sensitivity to the family's cultural and spiritual beliefs, values and practises. It complements curative and life-prolonging interventions from the time of diagnosis onwards and can be provided in the home or hospital [5–8].

In paediatric oncology palliative care addresses the needs of children who suffer from their disease and the toxicity of therapy as well as the needs of children for whom cure is no longer possible [5]. Good palliative care affirms life and regards dying as a profoundly personal experience for each child and family [5, 6]. Paediatric palliative care is multidisciplinary. It is delivered collaboratively with other professionals (e.g. nurses, nurse practitioners, child life specialists, social workers, chaplains, teachers, ethicists), because no one person has the expertise to address all the care needs of the child and family. It can be delivered together with measures aimed to cure or reduce illness or it may be the only focus of care. The actual mix will vary for each child/family, based on their expectations and needs, goals of care and treatment priorities. Figure 11.1 demonstrates the relative focus of care over time; however, the balance of palliative versus curative care may change over time (not necessarily in a linear fashion). Both palliative and cancer-directed care play important roles throughout a child's illness, although the child's care may focus more on palliation as the disease progresses [5]. Regardless

J. Du Plessis, M.D.
Department of Paediatrics and Child Health, Universitas Hospital, University of the Free State, Bloemfontein, Free State, South Africa

D.N. Korones, M.D. (✉)
Department of Pediatrics, Golisano Children's Hospital, University of Rochester Medical Center, Rochester, NY, USA
e-mail: david_korones@urmc.rochester.edu

D.C. Stefan and C. Rodriguez-Galindo (eds.), *Pediatric Hematology-Oncology in Countries with Limited Resources: A Practical Manual*, DOI 10.1007/978-1-4614-3891-5_11,

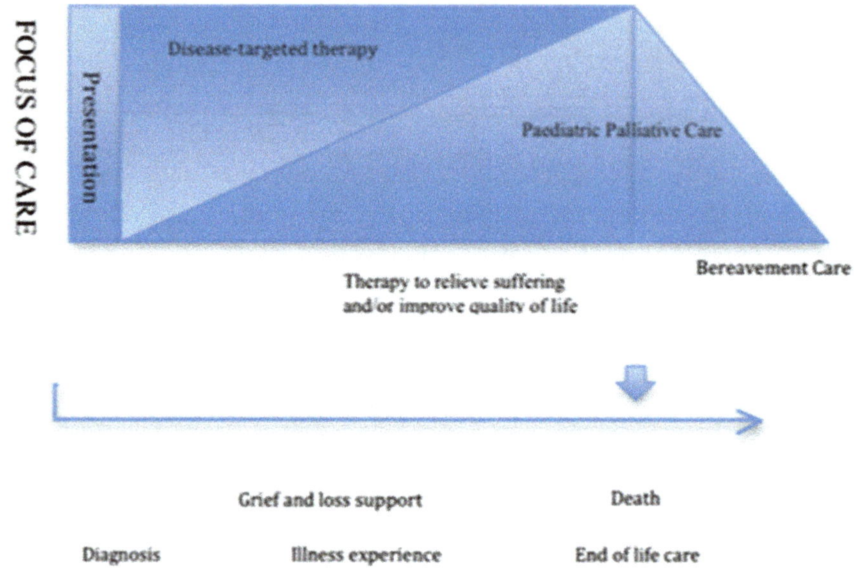

Fig. 11.1 The integration of disease-targeted and paediatric palliative care [2]

of the clinical situation, palliative care recognizes that there is always care to provide, such as relieving physical or emotional distress [6].

There is a tremendous need for the integration of palliative care into paediatric oncology services in developing countries. This is in large part due to the relatively high mortality of children with cancer in these countries, and the frequent association of cancer and its treatment with pain and other symptoms [9]. While palliative care teams have expertise in symptom management, communication and end-of-life care, such services often are not available in developing countries, and it therefore falls to the paediatric oncology team to provide these services.

Communication and Palliative Care

Communication with seriously ill children and their families is a central part of providing good palliative care. While palliative care physicians have expertise in this realm, it is incumbent upon paediatric oncologists to develop some level of comfort and expertise as well, because they are usually the physicians directing care of the child with cancer, and families look to them for information and guidance. Communication can be a daunting challenge, because paediatric oncologists must often communicate difficult news (new diagnosis of cancer, recurrence, limits of treatment options), and must discuss goals and limits of care. It is important to reach out to the parents and child, and explore their hopes, concerns and goals of ongoing care. Information should be shared adjusting the style of communication to the family's level of knowledge and prior understanding/misunderstandings. Families rarely hear or understand all that is said to them, even after much repetition. They often find it difficult to formulate questions in context of an emotional interview carried out in a hospital [10]. Perhaps the two most common and challenging areas of communication are delivering bad news and discussing goals and limits of care (e.g. resuscitation), each of which are discussed below.

Sharing bad news. Paediatric oncologists are frequently required to share difficult news with children and families, whether it be the initial diagnosis of cancer, recurrence of disease or that the child's disease is no longer curable.

Regardless, communication at this point needs to be handled sensitively [4]. The news must be given clearly and should respect the family's coping strategies. Many physicians follow a six-step protocol, described by Buckman et al. [11]: (1) *Prepare*. Find a quiet place, turn beepers off or on silent, making sure that one has the time needed to devote to a family, and that the family has the people they want/need present at the meeting. (2) *Find out what the patient/family knows*. Ask them what they already know, understand and perceive. This gives insight into their factual knowledge as well as their understanding of what is happening. (3) *Find out what the patient/family wants to know*. Allowing families to assist in "setting the agenda" can transform the "bad news" discussion into an opportunity to reassure and support. (4) *Share the information*. Information should be given to families at a level, pace and amount they can assimilate easily and accurately. The message they receive is not always the message that is given. For example, families may know that multiple metastases have developed, but may not know that means cure is impossible [12]. Check in with them along the way, saying things such as "Does this make sense so far?" or "Do you want to ask me anything about what I have just said?" It is not uncommon for families to misinterpret or not remember what is said. It is not because the oncologist failed to speak clearly, but because they find it hard to take everything in. (5) *Respond to emotions*. Perhaps the most important aspect of a "bad news" conversation, this is a time to listen, support and allow periods of silence for parents who are too emotionally overwhelmed to process what they have just been told. (6) *Provide a follow-up plan*. Families may leave a difficult conversation like this stunned and lost. It is vital to have a specific follow-up plan so they know they are not being abandoned and so they can ask questions they might not have had the presence of mind to ask at the initial meeting. Table 11.1 outlines a few key points in "How to deliver bad news", similar to the approach taken by Buckman et al. [11]. Regardless of the precise protocol followed, the key to effective communication is to be sensitive, listen, have empathy for the child and family's concerns, respect their cultural and spiritual beliefs and do not be judgemental [2].

Table 11.1 The "how to" of sharing bad news [12]

Set the scene	• Find a private and quiet place
	• Invite relevant others—child, social worker, ward staff, etc.
	• Ensure eye-contact on the same level (ideally all sit)
	• Speak in an unhurried way
	• Never look at clock or watch
	• No interruptions (give bleep to someone else)
Alignment (let the family talk)	• What does the family already know?
	• What does the family understand?
	• What are they expecting from you in this interview?
Exchanging information	• Acknowledge what is already known and understood
	• Use it as basis for giving new information—use the family's vocabulary
	• Prioritize: what are most important and/or immediate concerns?
	• Repeat and summarize as often as necessary
Checking back	• What has the family understood?
	• Did they receive the message you intended to give?
	• Have you answered what they needed to hear?
	• Go back to step 3 as often as necessary
Closing	• Reassure the family that they are not expected to remember everything
	• Invite further questions (go back to step 3 if necessary)
	• "Permit" further questions in the future—of you, ward staff, etc.
	• Make arrangements to meet again
	• Summarize once again

Talking to children. Many parents and professionals find it difficult to involve children in discussions about a diagnosis of cancer, particularly if their prognosis is poor. It is the instinct of parents and professionals alike to protect children from "badness". However, there is a wealth of evidence that suggests most children know when they are dying, feel isolated when such information is withheld and fare better when they are told what is happening [13]. Much of this evidence comes from the United States and western Europe and may not hold true for other parts of the world where cultural norms regarding sharing information may differ. As for who and how to talk to children, it need not be the physician, and in fact, for older children it is best to explore their hopes and fears with whomever they feel comfortable and have a connection. That might be their parents, a chaplain, a nurse, psychologist or social worker [10]. For younger children, child life therapists are particularly skilful in helping children express themselves through play therapy.

Siblings. Just as it is difficult to involve children with cancer in discussions of poor prognosis, so, too, is it difficult to have these discussions with their siblings. There are data which suggest that siblings, too, fare better when they are fully informed about their brother's or sister's illness. SIOP has issued suggested guidelines for helping siblings cope with their siblings' illness and/or impending death [14].

Challenges regarding communication in developing countries. The approach to sharing bad news directly with patients, be they adults, parents or children, is highly variable from country to country and culture to culture (even within the same country) [15]. In the United States and western Europe only a minority of physicians disclosed a diagnosis of cancer or a poor prognosis as recently as the 1950s and 1960s. But since that time, there has been a trend toward full disclosure to the point that now full and open communication with patients (even children) is standard practice. However, this approach does not hold true in many parts of the world where full disclosure of diagnosis and prognosis is often withheld from the patient (although shared with the family) [15, 16]. With such cultural variability in how difficult news is approached, it is essential for the paediatric oncologist to ask parents how much detail they want about their child's illness, and how to approach these issues with their ill child and his/her siblings.

Goals of care. When a child with cancer is not doing well, when treatment options are limited or when it appears that the child's disease is not curable, it is important for the physician to communicate this to the parents and the child (if appropriate). At this point the paediatric oncologist must work with the family to decide what sort of medical interventions make sense to do and which ones do not. For example, will it really help the child with refractory leukaemia to receive one more round of chemotherapy, or will this most likely have significant toxicity and little efficacy. Or does it make sense to give a child artificial nutrition or hydration if it does not enable the child to live longer and does not provide comfort. In a developing country where resources may not be available for curative treatment, these conversations may need to take place early in children's course, even at presentation.

Do not resuscitate orders. Perhaps one of the most emotionally charged aspects of goals-of-care discussions is cardiopulmonary resuscitation (CPR). For children who have relapsed and who have incurable disease, the benefits of CPR are questionable, and the potential toxicity considerable. Whenever possible, discussion of CPR should be done in advance to allow parents and children to make decisions that would fit with their values and goals of care.

When having such a discussion, it is important to honestly assess the likelihood of benefit versus harm performing CPR. It should be handled as any other medical recommendation: the physician should take responsibility for the process and not put undue responsibility for any decision on the parents. It should be a process of shared decision making with the medical team taking the lead, guiding the family, but also listening to and including them. It should be pointed out to the parents that it would be the uncontrolled cancer causing the death and not their decision not to resuscitate. In addition they should be reminded that "Do not resuscitate" (DNR) status does not mean "do nothing". It simply means that one does not proceed with this intervention because it is unlikely to work and is likely to cause harm. Even if parents are unable to make a decision, it is helpful for them to have heard that they may have to face such a decision in the future [2, 6].

The appropriateness of DNR discussion may also depend on the resources available in a given country. For example, in some resource-poor countries a child with ALL might have a very poor prognosis. In such a case, DNR might be discussed early in the child's course. In other countries resources for conducting advanced CPR might not be available so such a discussion is not relevant. In addition, laws may vary from country to country regarding the legal requirement to discuss resuscitation status with families [17].

Location of Care for the Dying Child

Whether a child dies at home or the hospital, early discussion and planning of location of death is highly recommended. When such early discussion takes place, families and children fare better at end of life and children are more likely to die in their preferred location [18].

If families opt for home care, the paediatric oncology team is obligated to ensure that good palliative care is provided in the child's home and/or community. For many families the paediatric oncologist will still remain their key medical professional. Most of the time the key team members in the community will be the community nurse, general practitioner (GP), paediatrician, etc., with the paediatric oncologist simply providing occasional guidance and support. Some children and families require input from psychologists, chaplains and, if available, pain specialists and child life specialists. Where available an outreach nurse and/or children's hospice are valuable resources to provide effective palliative care [12].

Although the inpatient paediatric oncology unit may not seem to be the ideal place for end-of-life care, for some families that may be where they are most comfortable. In addition, sometimes hospital admission is unavoidable (due to pain control, the need for transfusions, etc.). In this instance, the goal should be to create a home-like environment. If available a single room should be set aside and allow the family to decorate it with toys and home furnishings, etc. as they see fit. It is important for team members to take time to talk to the family members each day, even though there is no active treatment of the cancer. Generally, this does not take as long as one might expect and a great deal can be said in a 5- or 10-min encounter [12].

Symptom Management

Management of symptoms is a very big part of paediatric palliative care. Children with cancer experience a myriad of symptoms (physical and psychologic) from the tumour and the therapy from the time of diagnosis until the time of cure or death. A good working knowledge of the most common symptoms experienced by children with cancer, how to assess these symptoms and how to treat them is a cornerstone of good paediatric palliative care.

Pain

Pain is one of the most common and most debilitating of symptoms. While there are many definitions of pain, perhaps the most compelling one was written by a nurse over 40 years ago: "Pain is whatever the experiencing person says it is, existing whenever the experiencing person says it does" [19]. In the United States, pain is now considered "the 5th vital sign", and is assessed regularly in US hospitals and clinics along with pulse, blood pressure, respiratory rate and temperature. Optimal pain management begins with a good assessment including biological, psychological, social, cultural and spiritual factors that influence the way a child perceives pain. Such assessment is simple, takes little time and is feasible in resource-limited settings [12].

Pain assessment

The purpose of pain assessment is to determine the severity and nature of pain. The assessment

Table 11.2 The following aspects of pain should be recorded and is summarized by the useful mnemonic "PQRST" [4]

Precipitating or relieving factors	• Abdominal pain relieved by defecation suggests that constipation is the cause
	• A pathological fracture can be suggested by pain on movement of the affected limb
	• Also pay attention to medications that have been effective in the past
Quality	• Children can be surprisingly clear in their descriptions of what the pain feels like
	• An intense, well-localized pain can suggest bone pain
	• Neuropathic pain can be described as numbness, burning, paraesthesia or hyperaesthesia (change of sensation)
Radiation	• Neuropathic pain is typically distributed in a recognizably dermatome pattern
Severity	• Use age-appropriate pain measurement tools
	• Record the measurements in the child's clinical charts or journal (kept by the child or his/her parents)
Timing	• Neuropathic and bone pain are usually constant in nature
	• Causes of intermittent pain:
	– Cause is episodic in nature, e.g. intestinal colic due to constipation, stimulant laxatives, or pathological fracture that is only painful when it is moved
	• Management of these differ and it is important to distinguish between them

should include a detailed pain history (see Table 11.2 which highlights the PQRST mnemonic) and a physical examination. Further investigation of the underlying cause of the pain depends on where a child is in the course of his/her illness. For example, evaluation of abdominal pain in a child who has just started chemotherapy for a newly diagnosed malignancy might be extensive, whereas exhaustive evaluation of the cause of bone pain in a child with end-stage leukaemia is not necessary [12].

A challenge in assessing pain in children is that many children are non-verbal and therefore cannot directly report their pain. Even young children, who are verbal, might not understand the standard 0–10 numeric scale used in adults. A number of pain assessment scales have been developed for young children and non-verbal children. These include the CRIES scale for infants (Crying, Requires oxygen, Increased vital signs, Expression, Sleeplessness), the FLACC scale for very young and non-verbal children (Face, Legs, Activity, Cry Consolability), the Faces Pain Scale-Revised for children 3–8 years old and the standard numeric scale for older children and adolescents [20]. Figure 11.2 illustrates the Faces Pain Scale-Revised (Bieri Faces scale), one of the most frequently used measures of pain in young children.

Pain management. Like all aspects of medical care pain management requires a systematic and analytical approach. The approach must be sensible and realistic, with careful attention to the principles and evidence that support our understanding of the pathophysiology of pain [12]. Optimal pain management requires a comprehensive approach comprising judicious use of non-opioid, opioid analgesics, adjuvants and non-pharmacological strategies. Such an approach is possible in resource-limited settings [8].

The World Health Organization (WHO) guidelines on the pharmacological treatment of persistent pain in children with medical illnesses have become the gold standard in the pharmacological treatment of persistent pain, including cancer pain. In the new guidelines (2012) the WHO recommends using analgesic treatments in two steps (see Table 11.3) [4].

This simple guideline is straightforward. For mild pain (1–3 on a scale of 10) non-opioids such as paracetamol (acetaminophen) and/or ibuprofen should be used. For moderate pain (4–6), a low dose of an opioid should be considered, and for more severe pain (7–10) opioids are definitively indicated. For children with persistent or frequent moderate to severe pain, opioid dosing should be scheduled at regular intervals (e.g. morphine every 4 h) to insure continuous control

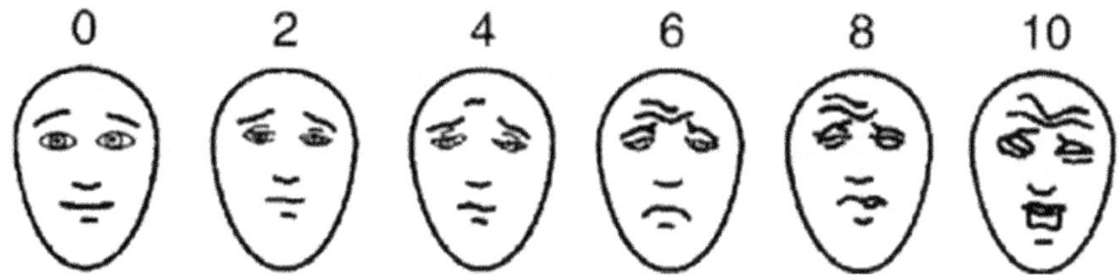

Fig. 11.2 The Faces Pain Scale-Revised [21]

Table 11.3 WHO guidelines [4]

Step	Pain severity	Medications	
1	Mild	Non-opioid analgesics, e.g. paracetamol (acetaminophen) and ibuprofen	Provide only limited analgesia Fixed maximum dosage
2	Moderate to severe	Opioid, e.g. morphine	Use a weight appropriate starting dose Lower doses for moderate pain than severe pain. Increase by increments of not more than 50 % per 24 h if pain is not controlled

of the pain. In addition, provision should be made for additional doses to be given on an as-needed basis for breakthrough pain.

Adjuvants should always be considered for a child in pain. An adjuvant is a medication that targets a specific type of pain. Hence an accurate diagnosis of the likely nature of pain should be made in order to select the appropriate adjuvant. For example, non-steroidal anti-inflammatory drugs (NSAIDs) are effective adjuvants against bone pain; gabapentin is an effective adjuvant for neuropathic pain. Adjuvants may be used *in addition* to opioids or as an alternative to them.

Specific Analgesics

A detailed description of all the available analgesics and appropriate doses is beyond the scope of this book. Frequently used analgesics are described below.

Simple analgesics/non-opioids. Paracetamol (acetaminophen) and NSAIDs are the analgesics of choice as initial therapy for mild pain. Paracetamol (acetaminophen) is a safe and effective analgesic in children and is also antipyretic. NSAIDs (e.g. ibuprofen and diclofenac) are useful for mild pain, and as adjuvants in the management of cancer-related bone pain, joint and inflammatory pains. NSAIDs should be avoided if the platelet count is less than 20,000/μL and used with caution in patients with impaired renal function. Both ibuprofen and paracetamol (acetaminophen) are inexpensive and widely available [9, 12].

Opioids. There are many available opioids. Although they differ in formulation, mode of delivery, half-life and range of toxicities, they are fairly similar and there is seldom a compelling reason to start one specific type of opioid over another.

Morphine. Morphine is generally acknowledged as the gold standard of opioid management, and therefore it is the opioid of choice in the management of moderate to severe pain in children with cancer [3, 4, 10, 12]. It comes in many formulations: an immediate release (short acting) form in liquid (inexpensive) and tablets (expensive) and a sustained release form. In addition it can be infused intravenously and subcutaneously. Morphine is very safe and usually well tolerated in children [9]. It can cause drowsiness

Table 11.4 A practical guideline for the use of morphine for children with moderate–severe pain [9]

1. Start with 0.2–0.5 mg/kg/dose orally immediate release morphine given scheduled every 4 h (start with lower doses, e.g. 0.1–0.2 mg/kg/dose in opioid naïve children. For infants use 0.1–0.2 mg/kg/dose and give every 6 h)
2. Provide dosing for breakthrough pain (same dose as above) every 2 h as needed
3. The dose can be increased 30–50 % every 24–48 h based on the child's previous daily morphine dose (scheduled + breakthrough doses) and level of pain
4. Start a laxative when starting the morphine
5. If sustained release morphine is available, start it 24–48 h after starting the above immediate release morphine. Sustained release morphine is given twice daily, and the total dose should be equivalent to the child's 24-h requirement of immediate release morphine
6. If sustained release morphine is available, the child should also continue to receive immediate release morphine for breakthrough pain. Typically this dose is about 10 % of the 24-h morphine dose and is given as often as every 2 h

and nausea, but tolerance to these side effects usually develops within 48 h, without requiring dose-adjustment [10]. The immediate release formulation should be used initially and given every 4 h (or every 6–8 h in infants) with breakthrough doses given as necessary in between scheduled doses [9, 12]. Even in low-income countries, with morphine alone, effective control of pain can be achieved in the majority of children. See Table 11.4 for a practical guideline for starting morphine in a child in moderate to severe pain.

Other opioids used for children with pain include fentanyl, diamorphine, buprenorphen, oxycodone, hydromorphone and methadone. The WHO recommends that codeine and tramadol should no longer be used for children.

Methadone. Methadone deserves special mention. It is unique among opioids in that it also blocks NMDA receptors, resulting in an adjuvant effect against neuropathic pain and potentially in bone pain [12]. It is also less sedating than morphine, has a long (but variable) half-life and in contrast to most other opioids is not renally cleared. It is available as tablets and liquid and can be given intravenously [4]. Many case series have been published in children [10]. The pharmacokinetics of methadone is variable from child to child. Consultation by a pain specialist or palliative care specialist is recommended if one is contemplating using methadone.

Adverse effects of morphine (and other opioids). Like any drug morphine (and other opioids) does have side effects. Constipation is the most common toxicity. Tolerance to constipation does not develop. Laxatives should always be prescribed when a child is started on an opioid. This should be a combination of a stimulant and a softener such as co-danthrusate. Other possible side effects include nausea, vomiting, pruritus, urinary retention, lethargy, myoclonus and delirium [10]. Morphine is not recommended for children with renal insufficiency because it is cleared through the kidney. Some of the most feared toxicities such as respiratory depression and addiction do occur but are uncommon.

Opioid equivalence and conversions. Sometimes it is necessary to convert from one opioid to another (e.g. due to toxicity), or from one route of administration to another (e.g. oral to intravenous for a child who has emesis). In these instances opioid conversion charts serve as a useful reference [21, 22].

Unique challenges of pain control in lower-income countries. Unfortunately access to opioids, even inexpensive ones, remains a challenge in low-income countries. For example, the worldwide consumption of morphine is 5.98 mg per capita compared to only 0.33 mg per capita in Africa [23]. Some of the obstacles include over-inflated fears of addiction, lack of healthcare practitioner experience prescribing opioids, crushing government regulation for manufacture and distribution as well as requirements for prescribing and concerns about theft. Paediatric oncologists can be advocates in their institutions and countries for the safety and effectiveness of opioids for children with cancer.

Adjuvant Drug Therapies

Adjuvants are medications that target specific types of pain. For example, somatic pain (pain due to bone and soft tissue injury) can be effectively treated with NSAIDs or glucocorticoids [13, 14]. Neuropathic pain is pain due to nerve injury, and is often described as shooting, burning, tingling, prickly or like pins and needles. The most commonly used medications for neuropathic pain include gabapentin and amitriptyline. Methadone is unique among opioids in its ability to control neuropathic pain. Visceral pain is due to distension of viscera. While visceral pain is effectively treated with opioids, glucocorticoids can also be effective (e.g. a child with malignant bowel obstruction). Glucocorticoids are also effective for headaches due to brain tumours or metastases. It is important to note that adjuvant drug therapies need not be given alone. More often than not, they are given in addition to opioids for moderate to severe pain.

Cancer-Directed Therapy

Although one does not typically consider cancer-directed therapy as a means of pain relief or other symptom management, it very definitely can have such a role. Many chemotherapy agents are relatively non-toxic and can cause significant symptom relief when used properly. For example, for the child with relapsed leukaemia and bone pain, vincristine and prednisone might provide significant pain relief. Radiation therapy plays a similar role. Radiation can provide significant relief of pain due to bone metastases. Larger fractions can be given over a short period of time since late-arising complications are not a concern in the terminally ill child [2]. In these contexts, radiation or chemotherapy is an example of "palliative therapy" the primary purpose of which is to relieve pain, not prolong life. However, this is a distinction that a family might find difficult to grasp, and might hope for as life-prolonging therapy as well. It is imperative to explain that while such therapies might prolong life, that is not their primary purpose and that is not what typically happens [12].

Psychological and Other Non-pharmacologic Interventions for Pain

Depression is an understandable response to terminal cancer and intractable pain. Whenever possible the child's understanding of pain and its causes should be explored, because fear, anger, guilt, grieving, sadness and lack of understanding are all part of the pain experience. Child psychologists and play therapists are particularly skilled in eliciting the source of a child's worry. In some children depression, anxiety, issues of guilt or anger may coexist and may be under-diagnosed in children. Uncontrolled pain can cause depression and if the depression is untreated it may make the pain experience worse. Doctors should be prepared to offer counselling and, if indicated, medications in managing depression in children [12]. Other non-pharmacologic interventions for pain include acupuncture, reiki therapy, massage, guided imagery and biofeedback. While there is not a strong evidence base for the effectiveness of many of these therapies, they are safe and inexpensive.

Gastrointestinal Problems

Nausea and Vomiting. Nausea and vomiting are significant symptoms in children with cancer throughout their course of illness. The pathophysiology of vomiting is complex and can be triggered by the stimulation of receptors in the gastrointestinal tract, chemotherapy trigger zone (located at the floor of the fourth ventricle), and the vestibular apparatus. Emesis is triggered by impulses from these areas, which in turn travel to the emesis centre and induce vomiting. Each of these areas has receptors, which can be blockaded by medications that bind to and block these receptors and decrease the likelihood of emesis. For example, 5-hydroxytryptamine receptors (5-HT3) are located in the chemotherapy trigger zone and can be blocked by a 5HT3 receptor blocker such as ondansetron [24]. In order to treat nausea and vomiting effectively, it is necessary to have a systematic approach to diagnosis of the cause. This is the basis for rational prescribing of antiemetic therapy [3, 10, 12].

Table 11.5 Drugs (and receptor targets) commonly used in management of nausea and vomiting

Drug	Receptor blocker	Dosage	Frequency	Route
Metoclopramide	D_2 dopamine	0.1–0.2 mg/kg/dose	Every 6 h	PO/SC/IV
Haloperidol	D_2 dopamine	0.05–0.15 mg/kg/day	BD/TDS	PO/SC/IV
Ranitidine (if gastritis)		2–4 mg/kg (max 8 mg/dose)	BD	PO
Ondansetron	5HT3 serotonin	0.15 mg/kg/dose	Every 8 h	IV
Dexamethasone		Wide range 0.25 mg/kg/dose	BD	PO/SC/IV

The most commonly used anti-emetics include ondansetron, metoclopromide, promethazine and hydroxyzine (Table 11.5). A typical starting regimen might be metoclopramide or ondansetron given on a scheduled basis. Glucocorticoids are also helpful adjuvants in the management of nausea and vomiting. Although not blocking receptors directly, they are synergistic with ondansetron and other 5HT3 receptor blockers and can reduce emesis with their anti-inflammatory effect. Lorazepam can also be effective when anxiety contributes to the nausea.

Constipation. Constipation is common among children with cancer and is defined as the infrequent and difficult passage of hard stools [12]. Causes include medication (opioids, vincristine), poor oral intake, dehydration, electrolyte imbalances, immobility and emotional distress. Prevention is the most important part of treatment and where appropriate increased fluid intake and exercise should be encouraged [9].

As with any symptom, a history and physical exam to determine the aetiology of the constipation is an essential first step. Constipation, in addition to infrequent stooling, may manifest as irritability, abdominal pain or generalized discomfort. Health care practitioners use many different regimens. It is important to have a stepwise plan of interventions that is coordinated with the parents and the healthcare team. The initial choice of medication for constipation is largely empiric. Many recommend starting with a laxative such as senna because it stimulates bowel motility, along with bisacodyl that softens stool. If these are not available as liquid formulations, another effective option is polyethylene glycol, an osmotic laxative powder that can be dissolved in most liquids. Suppositories can provide more immediate relief. Mobility and hydration are important when feasible. It is also important to remember that any child on an opioid should also be receiving a laxative.

Dyspnoea

Dyspnoea is a very common symptom, frightening to the child and not easy to treat. It is defined as the unpleasant subjective sensation of the inability to breathe adequately. The pathophysiology of dyspnoea is complex and not completely understood. There is a strong cerebral component to dyspnoea, and the higher cortical centres which process anxiety and fear and the respiratory centre are mutually influential. Because of this a vicious cycle could be established when anxiety exacerbates dyspnoea and vice versa [3, 10].

Management of dyspnoea should start with simple investigation of underlying correctible causes. For example, reactive airways might respond to albuterol inhalers, or congestive heart failure might respond to furosemide. Other possible causes include anaemia, effusion and infection. When there is no known underlying correctable cause, it is best to start with non-pharmacologic approaches such as repositioning, reassuring the child and ensuring some airflow across the child's face by using a fan or placing the child near an open window. Oxygen may or may not be helpful [3]. Regarding pharmacologic therapies, opioids are the treatment of choice.

The dose required is about half of that required for pain relief. While morphine is the standard opioid used, dyspnoea can be relieved by other opioids. Benzodiazepines are also helpful in relieving the anxiety associated with dyspnoea.

Fatigue

Fatigue is a very common and distressing symptom for children with cancer [2, 6]. Unfortunately, it is also the symptom that is the least likely to be addressed by health care teams. The cause is usually multifactorial including anaemia, infection, pain, poor nutrition, deconditioning, depression and medications. Treatment should be focused on treating the underlying cause/s (e.g. depression, anaemia). Non-pharmacological approaches include modifying the child's social/play activities, and encouraging the child to rest and take naps as appropriate [6]. Pharmacologic approaches are few. Methylphenidate has been shown to be effective in small clinical trials in adults and older children [2].

Other Symptoms

Delirium. Delirium is an altered state of consciousness characterized by sudden onset, waxing and waning, periods of inattention and periods of confusion. The most common cause is medications (e.g. opioids, benzodiazepines), electrolyte abnormalities and lack of change of environment. Haloperidol is the treatment of choice for delirium. Also adequate hydration (when appropriate) will ensure renal excretion of toxic metabolites [3, 12].

Convulsions. Convulsions are relatively common in children with brain tumours and brain metastases, and can also occur in children with other malignancies during therapy and at the end of life. They can be extremely frightening to the family. When convulsions are likely (for example, a child with multiple brain metastases or leptomeningeal disease), prophylactic anticonvulsant therapy should be considered. Frequently used agents include leviteracetam, benzodiazepines, phenytoin, valproate, carbamazepine and phenobarbital. It is important to inform the parents about the possibility of convulsions, and to guide them on what a convulsion might look like. They will also need a practical management plan. Strategies include positioning of the child in a safe place and not to place objects in the child's mouth. Parents should be trained on how to administer benzodiazepine rectally, or buccal application of lorazepam or injectable midazolam [3].

Anaemia and bleeding. In the advanced stages of many cancers suppression of red cell and platelet production is common, specifically in lymphoproliferative disorders such as leukaemia [12]. A red blood cell transfusion may relieve symptoms such as weakness, fatigue, breathlessness and drowsiness when the child is anaemic. As the cancer progresses, the symptomatic benefit from a transfusion may decrease [6]. Deciding whether to transfuse or not can be very challenging. Although there may be benefits, transfusions can also be burdensome (trips to the hospital, insertion of a needle and taking of blood for cross-matching, need or the presence of an indwelling central venous catheter, transfusion reactions). The pros and cons must be carefully weighed with the family.

Platelet transfusions should be considered to prevent bleeding, or if spontaneous bleeding is occurring. For less severe bleeding the antifibrinolytic drug tranexamic acid can be used [9]. When the bleeding is localized to the oral mucosa, use a 5 % solution mouthwash by dissolving a 500 mg tablet of the tranexamic acid in 5 mL of water. To prevent clot breakdown in more widespread bleeding use tranexamic acid 20 mg/kg every 8 h, enterally or intravenously (it can be given as often as hourly if needed) [9]. Epistaxis can be managed with nasal plugs or ribbon gauze. Topical applications of 1:1,000 epinephrine [12] can be used for bleeding cutaneous ulcers. A wet tea bag can be pressed onto bleeding gums at home; the tannins in black tea can also help to stop the bleeding [6].

Massive bleeding. Families should be counselled and adequately prepared if sudden massive bleeding is a possibility. Massive bleeding can be extremely frightening for a child and family. In order to relieve a child's anxiety associated with massive bleeding, the use of benzodiazepines may be indicated. To mask the colour and quantity of blood, practical measures include using dark-coloured sheets and towels [3, 12].

End-of-Life Care

For some children, cure is not possible and the goals of care shift from disease-targeted treatment to primarily comfort measures. Care at the end of life is focused on comfort and minimizing suffering for both the child and family. Common symptoms include pain, fatigue, nausea, constipation, anxiety and depression (management of these symptoms is detailed above). But care of the dying child goes far beyond symptom management; it requires understanding and anticipating the needs of the child and family and supporting any social, spiritual and emotional needs of the child and family [6]. When a child dies the psychological and physical wellbeing of the family members (particularly parents, siblings and grandparents) are affected for the rest of their lives. Positive and negative events that occur around the time of death are highly important to the family members. There are some basic needs regarding the end-of-life care which are important to attend to: honest communication and complete information are needed; basic symptom control; good access to staff; emotional expression and support by the staff; coordination of services; the integrity of the parent–child relationship, faith and meaningfulness should be preserved [25].

Final Days

The final days can be particularly physically and emotionally demanding for a child and family. Symptoms particularly prominent in the last few days of a child's life include fatigue, weakness, loss of appetite and pain. A few simple medications can provide a lot of comfort for a child as death nears: morphine for pain and shortness of breath, a benzodiazepine (e.g. lorazepam) for anxiety and haloperidol for delirium. Of these medications, morphine is most important because it can effectively relieve pain and dyspnoea. Some children develop rattling respirations as death nears. Although this is not thought to be uncomfortable, it can be very difficult for a family to listen to. Such rattling can be relieved with glycopyrrolate or a scopolamine patch. Although there may be little in the way of medical management for the paediatric oncology team, the presence of the oncologist and his/her team can be a tremendous source of comfort to the child and family.

Bereavement

The death of a child is an unimaginably stressful event, producing a crisis of meaning in which parents search for cognitive mastery and renewed purpose. Grief is a lifelong process; parents typically never get over the loss of a child but rather learn to adjust and to integrate the loss into their lives [1]. During this period of mourning and reorganization, parents and siblings can be supported in many ways [12]. Resumption of everyday function, derivation of pleasure from life and establishment of new relationships are all signs of healing from grief [1]. In most cases families are able to mourn and find meaning and purpose in life again.

Siblings are similarly bereaved. They may experience social isolation and withdrawal since much of the sadness is focused on their ill or deceased sibling. Families should be encouraged to involve siblings throughout the illness trajectory, allowing them to have safe outlets for their feelings and creating opportunities for their needs to be identified and met [6]. As they grow up they will probably find it helpful to reprocess the death in light of their newfound knowledge and emotional capabilities.

It is a challenge for paediatric oncologists to maintain contact with bereaved families, since their training and focus is traditionally on the treatment of children with cancer, and not bereavement. However, even brief periodic contact can

Table 11.6 Resources to help grieving families [3, 6, 12]

Resources to help grieving families include:
• Continued contact with the care team. Many families value the chance to meet with the paediatric oncologist. For some it may simply be an opportunity to say thank-yous and goodbyes to members of the team. Other families continue to have medical questions or misconceptions following the death, which a trusted team member can address
• Support groups. Invite parents and siblings to receive support from others. It is well known that parents who have access to psychosocial support prior to the child's death are better able to work through their grief
• Offer educational materials about the process of grief and mourning. There are resources that are written for both adults and children
• Grief counselling with therapists and/or clergy
• Establish memorial services and organized opportunities for families of deceased children. They provide both a power reaffirmation of the importance of the deceased child and a time when parents and siblings can reunite with those who cared for their child

have real meaning for families. In addition, it is the responsibility of the paediatric oncologist and his/her team to ensure that bereaved families receive ongoing support, whether it is informal or professional [3]. Table 11.6 lists some specific ways to support bereaved families.

Support for Staff

Paediatric oncology remains a field with high emotional casualties, despite improvements in cure rates [12]. There is little doubt that repeated losses become a significant source of personal stress for staff. They may find it difficult to talk to parents or distance themselves from difficult emotional situations in an effort to cope with the many losses they experience. Some physicians and staff may question the meaning of their work or even their own skills, when treatment fails and death is imminent. Relatively high rates of burnout (emotional exhaustion, depersonalization and diminished feelings of personal accomplishment) have been reported among paediatric oncologists [26].

Yet despite the sadness involved, dying children seem to find a way to live in the "precious moment" and through them and their families' caregivers have the rare opportunity to find meaning and fulfilment in their work. So much can be learned from the family and the child by simply acknowledging the burdens they face, communicating honestly and sensitively and by simply listening [6].

Providing support for the team can minimize compassion fatigue and burnout. This can be done through regular input from "skilled" supervisors and also by encouraging the team through helping them feel confident in their own skills. Adequate education in aspects such as listening, communication and symptom control can lead to such confidence [12]. Mindfulness-based stress reduction (a technique which teaches people to be in the present) is simple and inexpensive, and has been shown to reduce physician burnout [27].

> We need to take care not only of ourselves, but also of one another.
>
> When we strengthen ourselves, we nurture the strength to help others—Numfundo Wasala

Summary

The paediatric oncology team has a unique role in supporting a child and family throughout the course of his/her illness, whether it ends in cure or death. Part of that support is providing palliative care, relief of physical, emotional, social and spiritual suffering. Communication and symptom management are cornerstones of good palliative care. To provide such care, the team may often need to call upon the expertise of others, including psychologists, bereavement counsellors, chaplains, child life specialists and social workers, as well as paediatric palliative care specialists (if available), GPs, children's hospices and adult palliative medicine teams [12].

References

1. Himelstein BP, Hilden JM, Boldt AM, Weissman D. Pediatric palliative care. NEJM. 2004 [cited 2012 May 11];350(17):1752–62. Available from: http://www.nejm.org/doi/full/10.1056/NEJMra030334.
2. Wolfe J, Sourkes B. Palliative care for the child with cancer. In: Principles and practice of pediatric oncology. 6th ed. Philadelphia: Lippincott Williams & Wilkins; 2011; Chapter 49. p. 1404–27.

3. Goldman A, Hain R, Liben S, editors. Palliative care for children. 2nd ed. New York: Oxford University Press; 2012.
4. World Health Organization. Persisting pain in children. Geneva: World Health Organization; [cited on 2012 Sept 30]. Available from: http://whqlibdoc.who.int/publications/2012/9789241548120_Guidelines.pdf.
5. Pediatric Oncology Palliative Care Guidelines. BC Children's Hospital; April 2005 [cited 2012 Sept 30]. Available from: www.bcchildrens.ca/NR/rdonlyres/749DC4F5-6CAF-4E20-9109-89AE7E529D3A/11879/PaliativeCareNormsofPractice3.pdf.
6. Wolfe J, Grier HE, Klar N, Levin SB, Ellenbogen JM, Salem-Schatz S, Emanuel EG, Weeks JC. Symptoms and suffering at the end of life in children with cancer. NEJM. 2000[cited 2012 Sept 30];342(5):326–33. Available from: http://www.nejm.org/doi/full/10.1056/NEJM200002033420506.
7. Mellor C, Heckford E, Frost J. Developments in paediatric palliative care. Paediatr Child Health. 2011[cited 2012 Sept 30]; 22(3);115–20. Available from: http://journals.ohiolink.edu/ejc/search.cgi?q=authorExact:%22Mellor%2C%20Charlotte%22.
8. Temel JS, Grier JA, Muzikansky A, Gallegar ER, Admane S, Jackson PA, Dahlin CM, Blinderman CD, Jacobson J, Pirl WF, Billings JA, Lynch TJ. Early palliative care for patients with metastatic non-small-cell lung cancer. NEJM. 2010 Aug 19[cited 2012 September 30];363(8):733–42. Available from: http://www.nejm.org/doi/full/10.1056/NEJMoa1000678.
9. Amery J, editor. Children's palliative care in Africa. New York: Oxford University Press; 2009.
10. Hain RDW, Jassal SS. Paediatric palliative medicine. New York: Oxford University Press; 2010.
11. Baile WF, Buckman R, Lenzi R, Glober G, Beale EA, Kudelka AP. SPIKES—a six-step protocol for delivering bad news: application to the patient with cancer. Oncologist. 2000;5:302–11.
12. Hain RDW, Hardy J. Palliative care in paediatric oncology. In: Pinkerton R, Plowman PN, Pieters R, editors. Paediatric oncology. 3rd ed. London: Arnold; 2004.
13. Waechter EH. Children's awareness of fatal illness. Am J Nurs. 1971;71:1168–72.
14. Spinetta JJ, Jankovic M, Eden T, et al. Guidelines for assistance to siblings of children with cancer: SIOP working committee on psychosocial issues in pediatric oncology. Med Pediatr Oncol. 1999;33:395–8.
15. Mystakidou K, Parpa E, Tsilika E, Katsouda E, Vlahos L. Cancer information disclosure in different cultural contexts. Support Care Cancer. 2004;12:147–54.
16. Aljubrain AH. The attitude towards disclosure of bad news to cancer patients in Saudi Arabia. Ann Saudi Med. 2010;30:141–4.
17. Adhikar SD, Raviraj R. Do not resuscitate orders. Indian J Med Ethics. 2006;3:100–1.
18. Dussel V, Kreicbergs U, Hilden JM, et al. Looking beyond where children die: determinants and effects of planning a child's location of death. J Pain Symptom Manage. 2009;37:33–43.
19. Carson MG, Mitchell GJ. The experience of living with persistent pain. J Adv Nurs. 1998;21:695–701.
20. Friebert S, Bower KA, Lookabaugh B. Caring for pediatric patients. In UNIPAC 8, a resource for hospice and palliative care professionals. AAHPM, Chicago; 2012.
21. Hicks CL, von Baeyer CL, Spafford PA, van Korlaar I, Goodenough B. The Faces Pain Scale-Revised: toward a common metric in pediatric pain measurement. Pain. 2001;93:173–83.
22. http://www.compassionandsupport.org/pdfs/professionals/pain/PedsEquiTable.pdf.
23. DDungu H. Palliative care: what approaches are suitable in developing countries? Br J Haematol. 2011; 154:728–33.
24. Management of nausea and vomiting in patients at the end of life: "I was feeling nauseous all the time . . . nothing was working." JAMA 2007;298:1196–207.
25. Liben S, Papadatou D, Wolfe J. Paediatric palliative care: challenges and emerging ideas. Lancet. 2008 [cited 2012 Sept 30];371:852–64. Available from: http://www.northeastintegrativemedicine.org/resources/ResearchReferences/Pediatrics/PediatricPalliativeIdeas.pdf.
26. Roth M, Morrone K, Moody K, et al. Career burnout among pediatric oncologists. Pediatr Blood Cancer. 2011;57:1168–73.
27. Krasner MS, Epstein RM, Beckman H, et al. Association of an educational program in mindful communication with burnout, empathy, and attitudes among primary care physicians. JAMA. 2009;302: 1284–93.

12 Psycho-Social Aspects/Parent Support Groups

Kenneth Dollman, Wondu Bekele, and Kazuyo Watanabe

Why should I belong to and how can a parent group help me?

Cancer Facts: Realities

The vast majority of children, and 80 % of those who get cancer, live in developing countries [1] where the survival rate is much lower than those in developed countries. Childhood cancer is highly curable when diagnosed early and adequate access to treatment and care is available, yet most children living in countries with limited resources will not be saved as these conditions do not exist in their countries. As a starting point, in order to be able to tackle this challenge successfully, the realities and needs based on the resources currently available in these resource-limited countries needs to be carefully researched and accurately recorded. Cancer impacts on all aspects of the life of a child with cancer and his or her family. In this chapter, psycho-socio-economic and cultural aspects are addressed so that both medical and nonmedical support can be provided as part of a holistic approach to cancer care for the child and family.

Circumstances: Information, Materials, Finances, and Human Resources

Even among countries with limited resources, the situation at local and national level differs from country to country; therefore, what needs to be considered is what factors are common among all resource-poor countries. Some of these are highlighted under the categories: "Human," "Material," "Financial," and "Information" resources.

Information Resources

The management of childhood cancer care is often impeded by prevailing myths regarding childhood cancers. Such myths would include: (1) cancer is just a healthy life-style issue; (2) cancer is a disease of the wealthy, elderly, and is more common in developed countries; (3) cancer is a

K. Dollman (✉)
The International Confederation of Childhood Cancer Parent Organizations, CHOC Childhood Cancer Foundation South Africa, P.O. Box 2417, Durbanville 7550, Cape Town, South Africa
e-mail: aps02@iafrica.com

W. Bekele
Mathiwos Wondu-YeEthiopia Cancer Society, Getu Commercial Center 10th Floor, Room Number 1004, P.O. Box 80571, Addis Ababa, Ethiopia
e-mail: wondu@mathycancersoc.org; mathycancersoc@ethionet.et

K. Watanabe
Asian Children's Care League-Japan (ACCL), 1-36-9-601 Nihonbashi kakigaracho, Chuo-ku, Tokyo 103-0014, Japan
e-mail: accl@accl.jp; KazuyoW@aol.com

D.C. Stefan and C. Rodriguez-Galindo (eds.), *Pediatric Hematology-Oncology in Countries with Limited Resources: A Practical Manual*, DOI 10.1007/978-1-4614-3891-5_12,

death sentence; and (4) cancer is one's fate [2]. The mistaken belief that childhood cancer is a deadly illness or too difficult to cure can result in parents abandoning treatment or not seeking treatment at all. Stigma and misconceptions abound among cancer patients and their families which makes the provision of accurate information to parents and patients by medical staff so vitally important. Sadly, such misbeliefs are still accepted as fact, even in the medical profession [3].

Materials Resources

Material resources are crucial to and play a significant role in the provision of adequate treatment. Often medical centers that offer diagnosis and treatment cannot provide adequate access to care. Due to the lack of beds in these hospitals, parents of in-patient children face a particularly difficult challenge in that when in between treatments, the lack of beds does not allow them to keep their children in hospital for long periods of time and they have to find accommodation outside of the hospital environment. Some of the parents are not able to return to rural areas due to lack of transport and they are forced to endure hardship and some are often homeless during these times. Often the over utilization of available space leads to issues with infection control. It is here that the provision of a "family house" becomes an important consideration as a place where such families can stay during these relatively short periods between treatments.

Critical shortages of basic diagnostic and treatment equipment is common at treatment centers in resource-limited countries despite the fact that such equipment has proven instrumental in dramatically changing treatment outcomes. Although such basic equipment can be sourced from resource-rich countries, the logistics and paperwork involved often discourages overworked medical staff from exploring these options. It is here that support groups from resource-rich countries can play an important role.

Across low- and middle-income countries, access to essential medicines is often limited [4]. Treatment may fail due to the shortage and/or the unavailability of drugs. To this must be added: insufficient dosages given, counterfeit branded drugs, and the timing of the medications during treatment which may lead to the ultimate termination of treatment and the death of the child. Expanding sustainable access to safe, affordable, and effective essential medicines is one of the keys to increased survival and improved outcomes in childhood cancer [4].

Financial Resources

Financial issues often form a major part of families' problems and anxieties and can cause much distress at the time of diagnosis and throughout the treatment process. The question arises whether or not medical costs, which include among others, hospital fees, costs for examinations, medicines, blood products, and medical materials, can be afforded by families from resource-poor countries and where families have no or minimal social health insurance and often live a subsistence lifestyle. During hospitalization, families are faced with loss of income as often either the mother or father or both lose their jobs because they wish to be with their ill child. In addition, there are many "hidden costs" of treatment [5], for example, traveling, accommodation away from home, meals, additional nutritional requirements of the ill child, and so on. Abandonment of treatment is one of the significant issues that countries with limited resources are facing and often one of the reasons cited is the financial burden on the family, especially in cases of lengthy treatment.

Human Resources

Without quality medical care by specifically trained professionals, many children cannot benefit from advances in the field of pediatric oncology in terms of diagnostic techniques, treatment methods, and comprehensive support such as supportive and palliative care. The number of permanent medical specialists, including doctors, nurses, and laboratory staff who have undergone specialized training in the field of pediatric oncology, is very small when compared to the number of pediatric cancer patients in the world. A lack of sufficiently qualified staff negatively impacts on the quality of treatment and care currently given in low- to middle-income countries—this is mentioned not to distract from the invaluable interventions that those hospitals and the staff qualified in other fields have had in the lives of many children with cancer. The lack of physicians, nurses, and social workers is a factor which is one of the top five challenges, as reported by sites in countries with limited resources [6]. The many examples of twinning that exists between resource-rich treatment centers and resource-poor treatment centers in developing countries is a very positive step in the right direction [7]. However, in order to avoid late detection, incorrect diagnosis, and inappropriate treatment and care, well-trained medical staff is essential in the long term.

Creating Partnership and Communication

The effective management of resources is vital to achieving one's objectives and goals successfully. Specifically, "people" are the most importance resource. In the pediatric oncology field too, creating a good partnership with patients and families may bring about a cooperative atmosphere that contributes positively to the overall outcome of the disease.

The diagnosis of cancer in a child is a shocking and terrifying experience for families. Many of the parents in countries with limited resources think that childhood cancer is a deadly disease and that there is no hope whatsoever. Therefore, ensuring adequate knowledge of both the disease and its treatment at the time of diagnosis is crucial to ensuring mutual understanding of the process that needs to be followed. In addition, further education, which would include hygiene, infection control, nutrition, and highlighting certain behaviors that should be avoided, would need to be shared with families so that any additional factors that could impact on a successful outcome can be kept to a minimum. Assessment of families, including the level of education, lifestyle, strengths, and weaknesses, is necessary so that the appropriate psycho-social care and interventions can be provided according to the needs of the family. Decisions involving treatment and care often are not made alone and members of the extended family, especially grandparents, are often included in conversations prior to critical decisions being made by the parents of the ill child. Therefore, detailed information, such as procedures to be followed, diagnosis, prognosis, and treatment protocols, should be shared with the extended family wherever possible.

Understanding each other and close cooperation reduces numerous emotional burdens such as stress, disruptions, anxiety, depression, and bewilderment. Hope is heightened, and abandonment and/or nonadherence to the treatment process can be avoided.

The cornerstone of good care is good communication. Effective, open communication among health-care providers, patients, and families, is essential and should form a part of any treatment regime, no matter from where the patient and family comes. Sharing information about the child's condition makes it possible for the family to weather the hardships and plan effectively for all future outcomes.

Unfortunately, pain in children with cancer is often treated inadequately, and unrelieved pain during treatment places enormous emotional stress on children and their families [4]. In 1998, the World Health Organization (WHO) issued a comprehensive guide to the relief of pain and other symptoms in children suffering from cancer [8]. Frank communication among physicians and families is a nonnegotiable must where pain care management is involved.

Coping: Connection to Parents/Family Groups

What is an organization for parents/family support?

These are groups that are formed by like-minded individuals who wish to improve conditions in their countries as regards the total care of children with cancer and their families. The type of groups that can be formed will differ according to the objectives, skills available, laws, and conditions in the countries where they are formed.

The composition of such groups differ as well, and whereas some are run and have as members only parents of children with cancer, others have no parent involvement at all, but share the same drive to help families of children with cancer.

Support beyond medical interventions plays an important role in alleviating the distress experienced by patients and their families. Such support can be made available through parent/family support groups and peer support [9].

The experience of a child undergoing cancer treatment is traumatic, distressing, and can also isolate parents, siblings, and patients from friends and society. The impact of treatment on the whole family has been well understood by health professionals for many years, as have the medical needs of the child. Lately, the necessity to provide services which look after the emotional and social needs of the family of the child has now also become generally accepted as part of the therapeutic process. Parent support groups have been formed over the past 30 years that now provide a wide range of support to enable patients and families to cope with the difficulties associated with lengthy treatment, such services include, among others but not limited to, information; practical, emotional, and financial support for families; homes away from home; sourcing and supply of drugs where these are not supplied by the treatment center; advocacy on behalf of patients and their families; on-going support for bereaved families; and long-term support of survivors [ICCCPO Web] [10].

The step-by-step guide, *Your Group is Not Alone* [3] which ICCCPO (The International Confederation of Childhood Cancer Parent Organizations) compiled is a very practical tool intended to be of value to all those involved in the establishment and development of support groups involved with childhood cancer, especially in developing countries [3]. As the title states, patients and families are not alone. By joining parent/family support groups, families can not only share their feelings and gain hope, courage, and resilience but also learn how to cope with the disease and resulting stress, and obtain the information and knowledge necessary for the journey ahead.

Parent/family groups organize activities that provide opportunities for recreation, learning new skills, a respite from the rigors of ward life and contribute to a welcoming, warm atmosphere that contributes significantly towards a more positive experience. Families who have already gone through the cancer journey become mentors to newly diagnosed families to help them cope better and make their cancer journey a little easier.

Parents, siblings, and other close family members should always be encouraged to play an active role in the discussion of future plans and in the design and implementation of psycho-social interventions. In addition, survivors and parents have an important role to play by sharing information and life skills, helping to empower other survivors and parents, and in the design and implementation of future services. Parents and advocacy groups should be included as active members in the multidisciplinary health-care team [11].

Parent/family groups also play a role in opening a path for health-care professionals wishing to embark on short- to long-term education and training as they progress towards becoming dedicated and skilled specialists in the treatment of childhood cancers and blood disorders.

Parent/family groups will need to rise to the challenges of often not having the manpower to deliver the services they wish to offer, the scarcity of required volunteers, and insufficient funds. However, it is encouraging that despite the many challenges, parent support groups and similar organizations in countries with limited resources still manage to provide support services to patients and their families. Networking and collaboration with other similar and related organizations does and must always form part of any parent support group's activities that wish to source support and resources elsewhere in order to provide a better quality of life for their patients and families.

Community Involvement: Society and Global Initiatives

Childhood cancers in developing countries do not receive sufficient attention and are almost always low down on the health priority list where the burden of childhood cancer is not recognized. However, this should not be a reason for silence and inaction; there is much that can be done to improve the situation of children and their families, even in such constrained circumstances it is still possible to make a real difference [3].

By bringing people, i.e., medical professionals, patients, survivors, and families, and volunteers together locally and internationally, and through all working together, such groups can become powerful advocates to help improve the care and cure of childhood cancer patients globally, and specifically in countries with limited resources. In addition, in order to make childhood cancer medicine available and accessible, mobilization and collaboration with multi-sectoral stakeholders to ensure the presence of policies, programs, and resources for improved availability and accessibility to safe, affordable, effective, essential medicines, and easy access to information as well as the availability and prices of childhood cancer drugs across countries [4], must form part of global advocacy.

Even from a purely economic standpoint, investment in childhood cancer treatment makes sense as the number of life years saved by survivors of childhood cancers is very high as these children will go on to become productive members of society contributing to the well-being of their communities and their own families. Having community and government involvement in promoting positive changes will increase the chances of optimal care and cure rates for children with cancer.

Raising awareness and providing education about childhood cancer in the community and among health professionals helps towards removing the stigma and discrimination, such as parents' guilt reactions [12] associated with childhood cancer, especially in rural areas. Furthermore, it will not only increase early detection, referral and diagnosis, the prevention of discontinuance of treatment, fund-raising activities, favorable legislative and policy making, but many other positive outcomes as well.

International activities, such as World Cancer Day (WWC) [13] and especially International Childhood Cancer Day (ICCD) [14], aim to raise awareness of childhood cancer and to help create a commitment to improving access to the best possible treatment and care of all children with cancer no matter where they may live. Attempts to place children with cancer on the global Non-Communicable Diseases (NCD) agenda has alerted the world to childhood cancer and is a step forward in drawing the attention of health ministers globally to the plight of childhood cancer and to the resultant implementation of practical steps to improve conditions for childhood cancer patients in their countries.

Challenges: Combined Efforts and Care

Every child with cancer, no matter where, deserves adequate treatment and care and a chance to survive. Continued psycho-socio-economic and cultural support interventions with comprehensive medical and palliative care, from diagnosis and continuing throughout treatment and recovery, makes a significant difference to the lives of children with cancer and their families. Appropriate care from when further treatment is no longer a viable option to the grief stage must not be neglected or forgotten.

Care and support services based on psycho-socio-economic and cultural aspects needs to be integrated with medical care at all stages of the disease and the treatment thereof. Such services should be effective, accessible, cost-efficient, high-quality, and be managed within a multidisciplinary approach [15].

Concluding Remarks

Combining the wisdom, experience, and resources of all stake-holders involved with childhood cancer and working together as a team is the only way that this devastating disease will be beaten. What will result is a renewed spirit of hope and determination to bring to each child in the world affected by the disease, the effective care they so richly deserve.

References

1. American Cancer Society. Global cancer facts and figures 2007. Atlanta, GA: American Cancer Society; 2007.
2. Union for International Cancer Control (UICC). World Cancer Day [Internet]. 2013. Available from: http://www.worldcancerday.org/
3. The Executive Committee of ICCCPO (The International Confederation of Childhood Cancer Parent Organizations). Your Group is Not Alone [Internet]. 2008. Available from: http://cms.onlinebase.nl/userfiles/c1icccpo/file/Handbook_FINAL.pdf
4. ICCCPO (The International Confederation of Childhood Cancer Parent Organizations). Every child with cancer deserves a chance [pamphlet]. The Netherlands; 2012. Available from: http://cms.onlinebase.nl/userfiles/c1icccpo/file/WHO_leaflet.pdf
5. Childhood Cancer Foundation of South Africa ("CHOC"). CHOC's guide for parents [Internet]. 2006. Available from: http://www.choc.org.za/pdf/parent_handbook.pdf
6. St. Jude Children's Research Hospital International Outreach Program. Annual report; 2006.
7. Ribeiro RC, Pui C-H. Saving the children—improving childhood cancer treatment in developing countries. N Engl J Med. 2005;352:2158–60.
8. World Health Organization (WHO). Cancer pain relief and palliative care in children. Geneva: WHO; 1998.
9. A global challenge: treating children with cancer in developing countries. HemOnc today, 25 April 2012.
10. ICCCPO (The International Confederation of Childhood Cancer Parent Organizations). http://icccpo.org, ICCCPO, was set up in 1994 as a worldwide umbrella organization currently representing 158 members from 85 countries (30/10/2012). ICCCPO's mission is to share information and experiences in order to improve access to the best possible treatment & care for children with cancer everywhere in the world. It also offers practical assistance and guidance in the establishment of new support groups. ICCCPO representatives sit on committees that determine cancer policy globally, as well as at local and regional government level.
11. Haupt R, et al. Long term survivors of childhood cancer: cure and care. The Erice statement. Eur J Cancer. 2007;43:1778–80.
12. Pisani P, Hery C. The burden of childhood cancer. Childhood cancer: rising to the challenge. Geneva: International Union Against Cancer (UICC); 2006. p. 9–14.
13. World Cancer Day (WCC). 4 Feb. http://www.worldcancerday.org. World Cancer Day was initiated by the Union for International Cancer Control (UICC). http://www.uicc.org aiming to raise awareness and education about cancer and to encourage its prevention, detection and treatment.
14. International Childhood Cancer Day (ICCD). 15 Feb. A campaign to raise public awareness throughout the world of childhood cancer. ICCD was initiated by the International Confederation of Childhood Cancer Parent Organizations (ICCCPO) in 2002 and has been held on 15th February ever since. In 2010 the idea of a Global Fundraising event linked to this day was initiated to not only promote global awareness of childhood cancer, but also to create an opportunity for individual member childhood cancer organizations to raise funds.
15. SIOP Working Committee on Psychosocial Issues in Pediatric Oncology. Aims and recommendations for psychosocial care; 1993.

Suggested Reading

Childhood Cancer Foundation of South Africa ("CHOC"). CHOC's guide for parents [Internet]. 2006. Available from: http://www.choc.org.za/pdf/parent_handbook.pdf

The Executive Committee of ICCCPO (The International Confederation of Childhood Cancer Parent Organizations). Your Group is Not Alone [Internet]. 2008. Available from: http://cms.onlinebase.nl/userfiles/c1icccpo/file/Handbook_FINAL.pdf

World Health Organization (WHO). Cancer pain relief and palliative care in children. Geneva: WHO; 1998.

13 Nursing Care of Children with Cancer

Lisa Morrissey, Julia M. Challinor, Eleanor De Beer, and Colleen Nixon

Pediatric Oncology Nursing in Resource-Limited Settings

Overview

Childhood cancer care requires a multidisciplinary team of highly trained professionals to ensure safe and effective care along the treatment continuum. Nurses represent the largest workforce in health care, and are uniquely positioned to evaluate patient and family response to disease and treatment in the context of the social and cultural environment [1].

In low-and mid-income countries (LMIC), high nurse–patient ratios and the absence of specialized oncology nurse training programs are factors that contribute to suboptimal outcomes [2, 3]. Multiple robust studies have shown that low nurse staffing is associated with increased mortality and adverse patient outcomes, highlighting the need to match staffing with patient needs for nursing care [4]. Increasing the numbers of specialized nurses has also been shown to contribute to increased survival rates [5]. However, local schools of nursing or hospitals in LMIC often do not recognize the need for pediatric oncology specialization [6]. Nurses in LMIC must rely on short-term visiting teaching programs, or establish partnerships with expert nurses through twinning programs, to compensate for the lack of formalized training.

Collaborative relationships, or twinning, between nurses in resource-rich centers and those in resource poor settings is a successful model for providing education and mentoring to pediatric oncology nurses. St. Jude Children's Research Hospital developed a twinning approach which has been successful in many resource poor countries; this model has been replicated by cancer institutes and foundations throughout the world [7, 8]. Twinning for nursing involves the selection of a nurse educator in the resource-limited setting who collaborates with a nurse leader from the partnering site. Nurses in partnerships must prioritize the retention of specialized nurses and the development of pediatric oncology nursing specialty programs in local nursing schools or hospitals,

L. Morrissey, M.S.N., M.P.H., R.N., CPON® (✉)
Department of Hematology/Oncology, Boston Children's Hospital, 300 Longwood Avenue, Boston, MA 02115, USA
e-mail: lisa.morissey@childrens.harvard.edu; colleen.nixon@childrens.harvard.edu

J.M. Challinor, Ph.D., R.N., M.A. in Ed, M.Sc. Medical Anthropology
School of Nursing, University of California, San Francisco, 2 Koret Way #N-611Y, San Francisco, CA 94143, USA
e-mail: jmchallinor@gmail.com

E. De Beer, R.N. • C. Nixon, M.S.N., R.N., CPON®
Tygerberg Hospital, P.O. Box X3, Francie van Zyl Avenue, Tygerberg 7507, Cape Town, South Africa

C. Nixon, M.S.N., R.N., CPON®
Department of Hematology/Oncology, Boston Children's Hospital, Boston, MA

D.C. Stefan and C. Rodriguez-Galindo (eds.), *Pediatric Hematology-Oncology in Countries with Limited Resources: A Practical Manual*, DOI 10.1007/978-1-4614-3891-5_13,

where the culture and priorities of the country are embedded into the program [3, 9, 10]. Cost-effective, local innovations built into educational programs have been found to be effective in LMIC [11].

Along with shortages of technology and sufficient supplies to carry out nursing responsibilities [12, 13], lack of respect and low prestige for nurses within health care teams are also substantial obstacles to optimal nursing care in LMIC [14–16]. Opportunities for nursing leadership and networking on an international level are few for nurses in LMIC. However, Steward and Usher noted, "Empowerment of nursing leaders and managers, increased focus on the patient…. exploring conditions for frontline nurses and the direct relationship between improved nursing conditions and increased patient safety [in developing countries] mirrors literature from developed countries" [17].

Pediatric oncology nurses are involved in all aspects of cancer care, including early detection, physical and psychosocial care throughout treatment, management of disease and treatment-related side effects, long-term survival, and palliative therapy. Although cancer care settings vary in the availability of resources and technology, pediatric oncology-specific education and training for nurses is necessary to ensure the provision of quality patient care. This chapter will outline the essential elements of pediatric oncology nursing which are applicable in low-, middle-, and high-income settings.

Standards of Care

To ensure the delivery of safe, effective, and family-centered nursing care, standards for nursing practice are essential. The Association of Pediatric Hematology/Oncology Nurses (APHON) published the updated "Pediatric Oncology Nursing: Scope & Standards of Nursing Practice" in 2007 [18]. APHON defines the highest standards for care, education, and professional practice. Joint Commission International standards have also been successfully adapted to guide pediatric oncology nursing standards in resource-limited settings [19]. Nursing leadership must be involved in decision-making around the appropriate standards for pediatric oncology nursing in a given setting, taking into account the availability of resources and the nature of the care environment.

Effective pediatric oncology care incorporates guidelines for nursing assessment, diagnosis, outcomes identification, planning, and implementation. Principles for communication and coordination of care, along with guidelines for patient and family teaching and health promotion, are essential. Nurses are expected to evaluate the child and family's progress toward optimal health outcomes (Table 13.1).

Standards for Professional Performance

Professional performance standards address competency, promotion of quality practice, and collaboration with patients, families, and the medical team. Inherent in professional performance is recognition of the rights of children and families to participate in decision-making in accordance with ethical principles, the integration of research into clinical practice, and management of a safe, effective care environment that it is mindful of resource utilization. Nurses also serve as leaders, mentors, and educators through modeling professional performance in nursing practice (Table 13.2).

Standards for Nursing Education

Ideally, nurses new to pediatric oncology will receive formal training to develop a sufficient knowledge base and clinical skills, and ongoing education will be provided. Although the needs will vary depending on the availability of resources and technology, basic content should include an overview of growth and development, review of common pediatric cancers, safe handling and administration of chemotherapy, assessment and management of pain and distressing symptoms, venous access management, nutritional assessment and management, and infection control and prevention. Nurses should

Table 13.1 Pediatric oncology nursing standards of practice

Nursing process	Standards of practice
Assessment	The pediatric oncology nurse collects and documents data regarding the child and family to guide the development of an appropriate plan of care
Diagnosis	The pediatric oncology nurse uses assessment data from nursing and other disciplines to identify problems and determine diagnoses and appropriate interventions
Outcomes identification	The pediatric oncology nurse identifies expected and desired outcomes specific to the patient and family. These include adequate education, optimal growth and development, physical and emotional health, minimal suffering and distress due to symptoms of disease and treatment, and optimal quality of life for dying children
Planning	The pediatric oncology nurse develops an individualized plan that prescribes interventions to attain expected outcomes
Implementation	The pediatric oncology nurse implements the plan of care to achieve the expected outcomes for the child and family, with the goal of improving the child's health, promoting quality of life, and facilitating optimal family functioning
Coordination of care	The pediatric oncology nurse coordinates the delivery of care to support transition across the continuum of care and promotes optimal communication among caregivers
Health teaching and health promotion	The pediatric oncology nurse employs strategies to educate families about maintaining health and providing a safe environment of care
Evaluation	The pediatric oncology nurse evaluates the child and family's progress toward attainment of expected outcomes

From Association of Pediatric Oncology Nurses, American Nurses Association. Scope and Standards of Pediatric Oncology Nursing Practice. Glenview, IL, 2007

Table 13.2 Pediatric oncology nursing: standards of professional performance

Standard of practice	Description
Quality of practice	The nurse participates in activities that improve the quality, safety, and effectiveness of nursing care in all settings
Education	The pediatric oncology nurse demonstrates competency in pediatric oncology nursing practice and maintains current knowledge gained from publications, research findings, and professional activities
Professional practice evaluation	The pediatric oncology nurse evaluates own nursing practice in relation to professional practice standards, relevant statutes, and regulations
Collegiality	The pediatric oncology nurse interacts with and contributes to professional development of peers, colleagues, and others
Collaboration	The pediatric oncology nurse collaborates with children, families, and multidisciplinary team members in providing care
Ethics	The pediatric oncology nurse respects the rights of all children and families and makes decisions and designs interventions that are in agreement with ethical principles
Research	The pediatric oncology nurse contributes to nursing through participation, review, and integration of research

From Association of Pediatric Oncology Nurses, American Nurses Association. Scope and Standards of Pediatric Oncology Nursing Practice. Glenview, IL, 2007

also learn to recognize the early signs of sepsis and other oncologic emergencies. Instruction in assessing and managing the psychosocial, emotional, and spiritual aspects of cancer care, including supporting patients and families at end of life, helps to provide nurses with skills to manage the myriad of emotions that families experience during the cancer journey. If the creation of a nurse education program is not possible, the presence of standard policies and procedures that are available to nurses on the ward should be prioritized to promote safe, consistent patient care.

Pediatric oncology nursing involves caring for children with cancer across a continuum, from diagnosis to cure or a peaceful death. Nurses orchestrate multiple aspects of care and advocate for effective patient and family education, communication, and quality care. Nurses may also act to increase early diagnosis of cancer through public awareness, by promoting local cancer treatment options and partnering with parent groups and other nonprofit organizations in their countries to spread the message that childhood cancer is treatable and often curable [20].

Symptom Management and Supportive Care

Bone Marrow Suppression

Bone marrow suppression, or myelosuppression, is a common and potentially life-threatening complication of cancer and cancer treatment in children and adolescents. Bone marrow function may be impaired both by the disease process and chemotherapy, interfering with healthy production of white blood cells (WBCs), red blood cells (RBCs), and platelets. Complications include the increased risk of infection due to a reduction in the circulating number of neutrophils, anemia from decreased RBCs necessary for tissue and organ oxygenation, and an increased risk of bleeding due to diminished platelets that are required for blood clotting. Recognition and prompt response to the complications of myelosuppression is essential [21].

Anemia and Thrombocytopenia

Packed RBC transfusions at 10–15 mL/kg of body weight may be given if symptoms of anemia are present, such as pallor, tachycardia, fatigue, or shortness of breath. Platelet transfusions may be needed for patients who are severely thrombocytopenic or who are at high risk for bleeding due to infection, surgical procedures, or the presence of intracranial tumors.

Assurance that the donor blood supply has been appropriately screened for pathogens such as hepatitis, HIV, cytomegalovirus, and bacteria is essential to minimize transfusion risks. Nurses are responsible for monitoring complications of blood product support such as transfusion reaction or hypersensitivity and to monitor symptoms such as fever, chills, rigors, urticaria, hemolytic reactions, and volume overload [21]. A transfusion policy which provides guidelines for safe verification and administration of blood products, including vital sign parameters and standard procedures for transfusion reactions, is essential in patient care settings where transfusions are administered.

Fever and Neutropenia (F&N)

There are numerous causes of fever in neutropenic patients, yet the risk of severe bacterial infection makes rapid detection and urgent intervention essential [22]. The Infectious Diseases Society of America defines fever as a single oral temperature of ≥38.3 °C (101 °F) or a temperature of ≥38.0 °C (100 °F) over a 1-h period [23]. Axillary temperatures are not considered as an accurate measure of core temperature and rectal temperatures are discouraged to prevent colonizing gut organisms from entering the surrounding mucosa and soft tissues. Neutropenia is defined as a neutrophil count of less than 500 cells/mm^3 or a count of 1,000 cells/mm^3 with a predicted decrease to 500 cells/mm^3 in the next 48 h. The risk of serious bacterial infection increases when the ANC is ≤500 cells/mm^3 [24]. Management includes prompt, thorough evaluation for evidence of infection, initiation of broad-spectrum intravenous antibiotics, and hospitalization until the neutrophil count has sufficiently recovered. The risk for infection and infection-related mortality increases with the duration and severity of neutropenia. Other risk factors include the presence of central venous access devices, impaired skin or mucosal integrity, active disease with bone marrow involvement, use of corticosteroids, and asplenia [25].

Nursing management: A thorough nursing history is completed upon admission and a complete assessment is conducted daily throughout the course of hospitalization. A nursing physical exam should include assessment of the skin, oral mucosa, lungs, and perineum. Signs of infection include fever, oral lesions, redness at the site of tubes and lines (i.e., central venous access devices, gastrostomy tubes, and chest tubes), skin lesions, perirectal irritation or abscess, cough, rhinorrhea, ear or throat pain, and diarrhea [26]. Timely communication to the medical team of new or persistent fever or other infectious symptoms is essential.

Patient and family education: Caregivers must demonstrate understanding that fever in the setting of neutropenia is an emergency and can signal a life-threatening infection. Upon discharge from the hospital, they must provide reliable contact information and confirm that transportation to an emergency room is available. Written information with instructions on when and how to contact the doctor is recommended. Caregivers should be instructed to call the doctor before administering any fever-reducing medicine at home, and to be aware of the signs and symptoms of infection, including fever, fatigue, body aches, shaking chills, cough or shortness of breath, redness or swelling at the site of an injury or tube site, belly pain, mouth sores, diarrhea or rectal pain, and dizziness [27]. Special consideration must be given to children who live in rural areas or who do not have access to transportation to a local hospital or emergency room. Alternate arrangements should be considered during predicted episodes of neutropenia to ensure that access to medical care is available in the event of a fever.

Infection Control

The nurse is responsible for promotion of good hand washing and serves as a role model for infection control by thorough demonstration of hand sanitation techniques for the patients, families, visitors, and other health care personnel on the unit. If water, soap, and a disposable towel are not available, the use of alcohol-based hand sanitizer is recommended [28]. It is essential that nurses demonstrate and observe good hand washing with newly diagnosed patients and families so the crucial role of hand washing in preventing the spread of infection is understood [29]. The nurse must also be vigilant about the presence of an adequate supply of hand washing/sanitizing materials in the patient care area to promote proper hand hygiene by clinicians, family members, and visitors [27]. Children and adolescents may arrive on the unit with contagious infections. Adequate measures must be taken to isolate patients who potentially contagious, particularly in crowded settings where bathrooms are shared or plumbing are suboptimal. In addition, visitors should be screened for symptoms of infections conditions, such as fever, cough, runny nose, sore throat, diarrhea, skin rashes, or open wounds. Other preventative strategies include prohibiting the use of rectal thermometers or suppositories, educating the patient and family to avoid contact with people who are ill, and encouraging good mouth care and daily hygiene.

Gastrointestinal Complications

Gastrointestinal (GI) disruption is a common complication of cancer therapy. Mucosal cells divide rapidly, so are particularly sensitive to chemotherapy and radiation. Compromise of the mucosal barriers increases the risk of infection, dehydration, pain, bleeding, and malnutrition.

Mucositis is the inflammation of the mucous membranes and is a common side effect of chemotherapy. It can be mild to severe, and may be dose-limiting, particularly in children receiving high dose, intensive chemotherapy, radiation of the head and neck, or undergoing bone marrow transplant. Stomatitis refers specifically to an inflammation of the oral mucosa. Clinical manifestations include redness, edema, and ulceration of the mucus membranes, gums, and tongue. Symptoms include pain, changes in taste, cracked lips, and sore throat.

Nursing interventions include assessment of the oral cavity at least daily, pain assessment, promotion of good oral hygiene (including use of a soft toothbrush and toothpaste), and evaluation of oral intake and hydration status [29]. Topical agents or systemic analgesics ranging from acetaminophen to continuous intravenous narcotics are often prescribed to minimize pain until mucositis resolves. In some studies, the use of topically applied vitamin E has been found to be helpful to reduce or prevent mucositis [30]. Coconut water, applied topically, has also been reported to relieve mucositis as it promotes wound healing [31].

Constipation is noted as a decrease in the frequency of bowel movements, or hard, dry stools, often accompanied by abdominal discomfort, straining, rectal pain, or cramping. Constipation is often related to decreased gastric motility due to medications (especially vinca alkaloids and narcotics) or may also be caused by tumor compression, electrolyte imbalance, decreased physical activity, changes in appetite, and disruption of normal routine due to hospitalization. Laxatives and stool softeners are often used as prophylaxis against constipation. Drinking warm tea or prune juice and increasing dietary fiber (beans, cereals, and whole-grain crackers) can also help address constipation [32]. It is also important to stay well hydrated by drinking fluids and water throughout the day.

Nursing assessment includes close monitoring of frequency, volume, and consistency of stool output. Report any abnormal signs, such as bleeding or perirectal pain or fissure to the medical team. Interventions include promotion of adequate hydration and a rigorous bowel regime, such as a diet high in fiber and administration of preventative stool softeners or laxatives if constipation is expected before chemotherapy, such as with repeated doses of vincristine [33].

Nausea and vomiting are common and highly distressing side effects of chemotherapy. Acute nausea and vomiting typically begins within several hours of chemotherapy administration and resolves within 24–48 h. However, delayed symptoms can last up to 2 weeks. Poorly controlled nausea may result in complications such as dehydration, poor nutritional intake, electrolyte imbalance, and severe discomfort. Once the cycle of nausea and vomiting has begun, it is difficult to manage. Therefore, prevention before symptoms begin is the most effective approach. Premedication for children who either have a history of nausea or vomiting or who will receive known highly emetic chemotherapy is highly recommended.

Several drug classes of antiemetics are effective. Serotonin receptor antagonists, such as ondansetron and granisetron are highly effective, yet may be limited in availability due to cost. Dopamine antagonists, such as prochlorperazine (Compazine), and glucocorticoids such as dexamethasone, may also be useful in preventing symptoms before chemotherapy is administered. Metaclopramide with diphenhydramine is an effective combination that is often readily available, yet requires monitoring for the risk of dystonic reaction. Nurses are responsible to know the action and side effects of antiemetics and to monitor patients for hyperemesis and dehydration, reporting symptoms to the medical team [33].

Diarrhea is an increase in the quantity, frequency, or fluid content of stool that differs from the usual bowel pattern. Chemotherapy, bowel surgery, radiation therapy, and infection may all be causes of diarrhea [33]. Complications include dehydration, malnutrition, intestinal infection, electrolyte imbalance, and social withdrawal due to disrupted daily routines. Children with severe diarrhea must be closely monitored for signs and symptoms of dehydration and electrolyte imbalance. Nurses must track intake and output carefully and report imbalances to the medical team. Daily weights and careful monitoring of abdominal symptoms and perirectal breakdown are usually indicated. Patients with diarrhea should be isolated until infectious causes can be ruled out. Dietary measures to control diarrhea include eating small frequent low fat snacks, limiting milk products, and eating food at room temperature [32].

Nutritional Support

Providing children with food and nourishment is a fundamental parental task. In the hospital setting, nourishment may become a difficult issue. Children and adolescents may refuse to eat unfamiliar foods; in addition, chemotherapy and other treatments may change a child's taste sensations turning formerly favorite foods to unpleasant or unusual tasting. Many treatment-related factors may impact the child/adolescent's nutritional status, such as type of tumor, nausea/vomiting, constipation, and oral and gastrointestinal toxicities of medications [34].

Children in countries with limited resources may already be malnourished when diagnosed with cancer, although obesity is on the rise and may also impact nutritional status [35]. Poor oral intake increases the risk of dehydration, infection, and gastrointestinal symptoms such as constipation. In settings where food is scarce, the nurse must be particularly observant about what the patient is eating since parents and visitors may also have limited food supplies. Careful evaluation, monitoring, and documentation of the patient's nutritional status are important upon admission and throughout treatment. It may be necessary to consider supplementing the child's diet, particularly during induction therapy or in malnourished children with insufficient protein intake. Options may include oral intake of a high-calorie diet with additional protein (such as adding one egg a day or supplements such as Plumpy Nut), nasogastric enteral feeds, or total parenteral nutrition [36, 37].

Parents must be educated about safe storage and handling of foods during cancer treatment, such as washing fruits and vegetables before eating. They should be advised to avoid bringing food prepared under potentially unhygienic conditions into the hospital. Food preparation areas on the pediatric oncology unit stocked with snacks, juice, and bottled water are helpful to parents who want to supplement the child's hospital diet. Parents are the experts on their child's food preferences; partnering with parents to address nutritional issues in the hospital will enhance the child's dietary health [38].

Pain Management

Pain is one of the most frightening and debilitating consequences of childhood cancer. Uncontrolled pain can result in decreased physical activity, poor appetite, fear, loneliness, depression, isolation, and mistrust of the medical team [38]. Pediatric oncology nurses are critical in the assessment, treatment, and evaluation of pain in children with cancer.

Clinical Presentation

Pain can be acute or chronic, or both, and may be the result of tissue damage or nerve injury. Pain originating in the bones, joints, muscles, skin, tissue, or viscera is usually receptive to pain medication, such as non-opioids and opioids. Neuropathic pain is the result of nerve injury and is often described as burning or shooting pain. Neuropathic pain is usually more difficult to manage, as it is less responsive to opioids and non-opioids [39].

Nursing Assessment and Intervention

Pain assessment must take into consideration the patient's developmental level and ability to express pain (Table 13.3). Pain evaluation ideally is completed routinely by nursing as the "fifth vital sign," using a validated pain scale such as the Wong-Baker faces scale for younger children (Fig. 13.1), the numeric scale for older children, or the FLACC scale for nonverbal children.

Pain location, quality, and intensity, along with medications or non-pharmacological interventions and subsequent response must be communicated to the medical team and documented appropriately by the nurse. Ongoing evaluation of pain and symptom relief is essential to quality patient care.

Chemotherapy Administration

Chemotherapy Safety

Safe administration of chemotherapy is an essential aspect of caring for children, adolescents, and young adults with cancer. The health care team shares responsibility in assuring patient safety by adhering to error prevention practices throughout the chemotherapy process. Pediatric oncology nurses have an important and active role in the patient's pretreatment evaluation, the administration of chemotherapy and supportive care, as well as post-chemotherapy monitoring. The complexity of chemotherapy and the risk of adverse effects make a process for safe and effective administration of chemotherapeutic agents essential [40]. Ideally, a pharmacist should prepare all chemotherapy under a chemical hood with ventilation systems designed to reduce exposure and protect against toxic fumes. Awareness of the need for trained pharmacists is growing and should be strongly advocated for by pediatric oncology care teams [41].

Table 13.3 Pain assessment by developmental level

Developmental level	Expression of pain
Infant	Intense crying, inconsolable, draws his or her knees to the chest, hypersensitivity or irritability, unable to eat or sleep
Toddler	Verbally aggressive, regressive behavior or withdrawal, guarding of painful areas
Preschooler	May verbalize the intensity of the pain, view the pain as a punishment, and understand that there can be a secondary gain associated with the pain
School-age child	Verbalizes pain, can use an objective measurement of pain, resists movement. Can be influenced by cultural beliefs and can experience nightmares associated with pain
Adolescent	Can verbalize pain but may not request pain medications or may deny pain in the presence of peers. May experience changes in sleep patterns and in appetite or may display regressive behavior in the presence of family members

Reprinted with permission from "Essentials of Pediatric Hematology/Oncology Nurses: A Core Curriculum" (3rd edition), p. 151. Association of Pediatric Hematology/Oncology Nurses, Glenview, IL, 2008

When a nurse is responsible for preparing chemotherapy, training in chemotherapy preparation and personal safety is necessary. Along with a properly installed, ventilated biosafety hood, adequate personal protection equipment (PPE), which includes chemo safe gowns, disposable gloves, and protective eye gear are critical to minimize personal risk [42]. Adequate staffing of nurses per shift when chemotherapy is being prepared and administered is also essential for patient and nurse safety [43]. The allocation of a designated chemotherapy preparation nurse has been found to improve efficiency, reduce costs, minimize the risk of medication errors, and promote safety for both patients and nurses. The nurse preparing the chemotherapy can serve as the double check to the nurse administering the chemotherapy by verifying the patient name, route, dose, date, and time of chemotherapy medications [44].

Chemotherapeutic agents are administered in a variety of settings, including inpatient units, ambulatory clinics, and in the home. All nurses who administer chemotherapy must be educated about chemotherapeutic agents, the route of administration, side effects, and safe handling practices. A process for assessing the nurses' knowledge and competency of chemotherapy administration is imperative before they are allowed to administer chemotherapy to a patient.

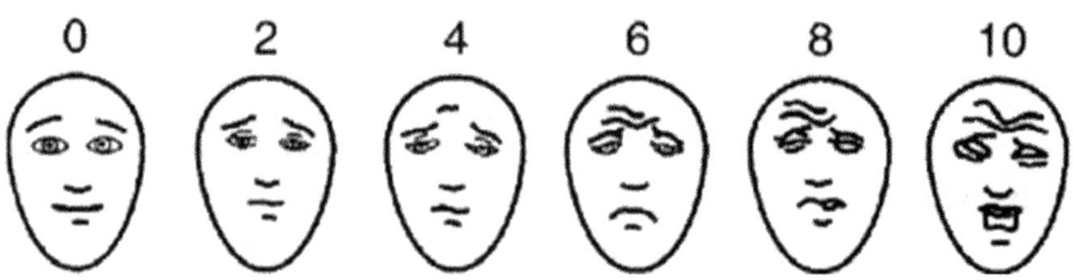

Fig. 13.1 Wong-Baker Faces Pain Rating Scale

Table 13.4 Components of the pre-chemotherapy treatment assessment

Components	Comments
Obtain and document baseline vital signs and pain assessment	Use validated pain tool for assessment
Evaluate past medical history (PMH)	
Evaluate current health history	• Recent illnesses
	• Current medications
	• Use of complementary and alternative therapies
	• Allergies (drugs, foods, products [i.e., latex])
	• Immunization status
	• Nutritional status
Obtain height and weight	For initial chemotherapy treatment, obtain two unique heights and weights
	Remeasure height and weight before each chemotherapy cycle
	Notify physician if >5–10 % difference since previous measurement
Assess need for rehydration	Dependent on chemo agents to be administered, yet twice maintenance is the standard used [51]
	Review orders, consult with prescribing MD
Calculate maintenance fluid using body weight method	• 4 mL/kg for the first 10 kg of a patient's weight
	• 2 mL/kg for the next 10 kg of a patient's weight
	• 1 mL/kg for the rest of the patient's weight
	Example: Maintenance for 32 kg patient:
	$4mL\ \ for\ \ first\ \ 10kg = 40mL$ $+2mL\ \ for\ \ second\ \ 10kg = 20mL$ $+1mL\ \ for\ \ remainder = 12mL$ $= 72mL/\text{h}$
Review patient's previous chemotherapy experience (if any)	Focus on side effects and effectiveness of the supportive care regime.
Ensure adequate fluid status by evaluating patient's ability to tolerate oral fluids or receive IV hydration.	Monitor fluid status by assessing:
	• Skin turgor
	• Fluid intake and urine output
	Families must be instructed to save urine in urinals or bottles to ensure that urine output is at 1–2 mL/kg/h

Chemotherapy Administration Process

Pretreatment assessment of the chemotherapy administration process starts with a patient assessment (Table 13.4) including past medical history, allergies, hospitalizations, and current medications. If the patient has received chemotherapy or radiation therapy in the past, it is important to assess for previous use and effectiveness of antiemetics, presence of side effects, and overall tolerability of treatment. This allows the nurse to determine if adjustments should be made for the current chemotherapy administration.

Chemotherapy Orders and Treatment Plan Review

Chemotherapeutic agents have a narrow therapeutic index and are considered high-risk medications, meaning there is a small difference between the desired treatment dose and a dose that can cause severe or fatal complications. For high-risk medications, an independent dose calculation by each chemotherapy competent clinician who prescribes, dispenses, and administers chemotherapy has been shown to reduce and prevent errors [45].

The administration of chemotherapy requires two clinicians to independently verify the correct patient and medication. When checking the medication, confirm the dose, route, scheduled administration time, correct fluid/volume, and compatibility. Ensure informed consent for treatment has been obtained and is available for review. The essential elements of chemotherapy orders include the following [5]:

- Patient name and unique patient identifiers (such as birth date and medical record number)
- Date and time order is written with the intended start date
- Patient diagnosis
- Protocol name and number (if applicable), treatment regimen, cycle, week, and day
- Criteria based on treatment and specific patient information
- Height (documented in centimeters), weight (documented in kilograms), body surface area (BSA), or other variables (age) necessary to determine dosage
- The generic name of the drug (abbreviations are not acceptable)
- Dosage of all agents in the regimen are clearly written (i.e., milligrams or grams, or units) as well as dosing parameters (i.e., ___ mg/m^2 = ___mg)
  - Leading zeros are acceptable (i.e., 0.4 rather than 0.4)
- Chemotherapy diluent, volume, and rate
- Number of doses to be administered, treatment duration, including start and stop date, total amount of drug administered per course and if applicable, cumulative doses
- Supportive care medications necessary for treatment
- Monitoring parameters (i.e., vital signs, intake and output requirement, when to notify the physician)

Other safety measures to incorporate into chemotherapy orders include prohibiting verbal chemotherapy orders, avoiding hand written orders, and requiring written documentation for any adjustment(s) to the order.

Chemotherapy Dosing Considerations

Pediatric chemotherapy drug doses are determined based on BSA in milligrams per meter square (mg/m^2) or milligrams per kilogram (mg/kg). The formula to calculate BSA is:

$$BSA\left(\mathrm{m}^2\right) = \sqrt{\frac{Weight\ (kg) \times Height\ (cm)}{3{,}600}}$$

Children under 12 months or less than 6 kg are often dosed using mg/kg formula [46]. Dose per m^2/30 is typically used, unless otherwise specified in the protocol or treatment plan. The dosing for intrathecal and intra-Ommaya chemotherapy is determined by the patient's age [47].

Dose reductions may be made based on organ toxicity or toxicity from prior therapy. Agents, such as doxorubicin, (Adriamycin), dactinomycin (Actinomycin-D), the taxanes, docetaxel and paclitaxel, and gemcitabine (an antimetabolite), are dose-reduced or stopped during radiation therapy to prevent radiation recall. Symptoms of radiation recall may range from a mild rash or desquamation to painful, edematous vesicles or papules. Delaying the time between completion of radiotherapy and the start of chemotherapy can decrease the risk of radiation recall [48]. Lack of evidence exists supporting the need for adjusted dosing in obese patients compared with non-obese patients [49]. *Dose escalation* maybe protocol-specific or made if the absolute neutrophil count or platelet count does not decrease as expected.

Chemotherapy Administration

To safely administer chemotherapy, a designated chemotherapy preparation area away from any food or beverages must be identified. The chemotherapy drugs are brought to this area in a sealed plastic bag with a sticker labeled as "cytotoxic" in order to ensure proper handling by others [45]. This area must be equipped with PPE, chemotherapy hazardous waste container, and a chemotherapy spill kit. Ideally, all chemotherapy infusions are administered via an infusion pump with Luer Lock tubing connections [50]. Before administering chemotherapy and/or supportive care medications, review the medication label for the name of the drug, dose, and expiration date. Inspect the medications for discoloration and particulate matter. The last step is for two chemotherapy-competent clinicians to compare the chemotherapy product to the chemotherapy order, checking patient identification, name of the drug, route, dose, and correct infusion rate [51].

Routes of Administration

Chemotherapy may be given by mouth or by injection (i.e., intramuscularly, intravenously, intrathecally, or subcutaneously). Special considerations apply for each route.

Oral chemotherapy can be given as a liquid, tablet, or capsule. It is essential to evaluate the patient's ability to swallow pills before oral medication are prescribed, as pediatric patients often are unable to swallow pills or tablets. Guidelines with instructions for how and when to repeat a dose of oral chemotherapy if the patient vomits are helpful. For patients who cannot tolerate oral medications, a nasogastric tube or gastrostomy tube may be necessary. Successful oral chemotherapy administration contributes to a sense of control for the patient and family.

Health care providers must wear PPE when administering oral chemotherapy. Pills and/or tablets are to be crushed and/or dissolved under a biological safety hood. Prescriptions need a double-check process to verify accuracy [50].

Subcutaneous (SC) chemotherapy is an injection that is given into any area with sufficient subcutaneous tissue, inserting the smallest gauge needle for the child's size (typically a 26–30-gauge needle) at a 45° or 90° angle. Sites that are frequently used are the center third of the lateral aspect of the upper arm, the center third of the anterior thigh and the abdomen.

Intramuscular (IM) chemotherapy is an injection that is given into the muscle. The age of the child is often what determines the site chosen [52, 53].

Recommended sites based on age include the following:

- Vastus lateralis (anterior, lateral aspect, middle third of thigh); desired site for children less than 2 years of age, as well as small or sick children
- Deltoid (lateral aspect of upper arm, begins about two finger breaths below the lower edge of the acromion process); desired site for children greater than 2 years of age, who have sufficient muscle mass
- Ventrogluteal: place palm of hand over greater trochanter [thumb facing toward patient's groin], index finger over anterior superior iliac spine and the middle finger stretched toward but below the iliac crest. The "V" formed by the second and third finger is the injection site, desired site of adult administration. The length and gauge of the needle is dependent on viscosity of the medication to be administered and age and size of the child
- Volume for a single intramuscular (IM) injection is dependent on the site of injection and the amount of muscle tissue. The pharmacist should prepare drugs in the minimum allowed volume of diluent. If two injections are needed, administer the injections simultaneously. Maximum volumes are:
  - Deltoid: 0.5–1 mL (children/adolescents)
  - Vastus lateralis: 0.5 mL (infants), 2 mL (children/adolescents)
  - Ventrogluteal: 0.5 mL (infants), 2 mL (children/adolescents)
  - Dorsogluteal: 2 mL (children/adolescents)

Always rotate sites and avoid giving an injection into an area of preexisting tenderness and/or an ecchymotic area. When administering an IM injection, be cognizant of the patient's platelet count. Patients who are thrombocytopenic should have pressure directly applied to the injection site to prevent the hematoma formation. Document the injection site, needle size, medication, and patient response. Provide patient education as needed.

Use of PPE, safety needles, and chemotherapy waste disposal in accordance with regulatory and institutional policies are essential when administering SC or IM chemotherapy. Vesicant and irritant chemotherapy agents are not administered subcutaneously or intramuscularly [52].

Intrathecal (IT) chemotherapy is administered into the cerebrospinal fluid (CSF) via a lumbar puncture (LP) or a ventricular reservoir (i.e., Ommaya reservoir). The sterile procedure should be limited to the operating or treatment room. Other parenteral chemotherapy must not be brought into the area until the IT procedure is complete [45]. Most notably, it is imperative that vincristine is never brought to the location where an IT procedure is being performed. **Vincristine administered intrathecally is 100 % fatal**. Safety measures must be built into chemotherapy practices to ensure that this event never occurs.

The optional site for IT injections is at the point of intersection on the spinal column between the tops of bilateral iliac crests at lumbar vertebrae L3–L5. The length and gauge of the spinal needle depends on the size of the child and amount of tissue the needle needs to get through to reach the spinal space. Patient positioning is very important when LPs are performed. The side lying position has the patients on their side with their spine flexed and hips aligned one on top of the other to maximize access to spinal space. Support the patients in a curled position by helping them to bring their knees up into the abdomen and while flexing their neck toward their chest. For older or larger patients, a sitting position is an alternate option. The patients sit upright, leaning forward to open the spinal space [52].

Be aware of the patient's platelet count before administration of an IT injection, typically the platelet count should be at 50,000. To help minimize injection pain, apply ice or a topical anesthetic to the injection site before administration. Sedation and/or pain medications are administered as prescribed. Monitor patient as specified per institutional policies and guidelines. There is little evidence that supports lying flat after lumbar puncture prevents post-lumbar puncture headache (PLPH), but for some patients this may help minimize PLPH [54].

Wear appropriate PPE and dispose of chemotherapy waste in accordance with regulatory and institutional guidelines for IT medication handling and administration.

Intravenous (*IV*) access must be established via a peripheral IV (PIV) or a central venous catheter (CVC) prior to administration of parenteral chemotherapy. Before administering any chemotherapy, the vein and catheter patency is assessed by flushing and checking for blood return [55].

Management of Venous Access Devices

Central Venous Catheter

Vascular access devices are vital to the delivery of cancer treatment to children. There are three types of CVC's typically used during pediatric cancer treatment; they are external tunneled catheters (e.g., Groshong, Broviac, and Hickman), implanted ports (e.g., Port-a-Cath and Mediport), and peripherally inserted central catheters (PICCs). PICCs are considered a temporary line although they can be used throughout treatment [50].

While CVCs have greatly improved the quality of pediatric oncology care, the potential for serious complications exist, including infection, occlusion, pneumothorax, and air embolism. Catheter-associated bloodstream infections (CLABSI) are a serious and potentially life-threatening complication of CVCs. Nurses play an important role in the care and maintenance of CVCs, including prevention of infections. O'Grady et al. [56] describe that the following indicators are effective in reducing the incidence of CLABSI:

- Implementation of educational programs for those who insert and care for CVCs
- Use of maximal sterile barrier precautions during catheter placement
- Use of chlorhexidine for skin antisepsis at the time of insertion and during maintenance care
- Removal of the catheter when it is no longer required for treatment

Nursing policies and procedures for care of central lines, including flushing, dressing changes, and cap changes, promote consistent and safe practice. If a child is discharged from the hospital with a CVC, teaching for the caregiver at home will be necessary. Standardization of line care between hospital and home will reduce confusion and minimize the risk of complications. Many resources for the care and maintenance of central lines are available via the Internet, such as on the Center for Disease Control website (www.cdc.gov) the St. Jude's Cure4kids website (www.cure4kids.org).

PIV access for chemotherapy administration is dependent on expert venipuncture technique [57]. When choosing the IV site, the following considerations are important:

- The optimal site for a PIV is the lower forearm sites.
- Avoid sites distal to any recent venipuncture, as integrity of the vein may be compromised and lead to leakage of medications and fluids into the surrounding tissue.
- Avoid areas of joint flexion. If there are no other PIV placement options, secure the site with an arm board to reduce the risk of thrombosis and infiltration [55, 58].
- A new IV should be restarted if any site(s) that has signs of redness, pain, or inflammation or if there is concern about the integrity of the IV [50].
- Warming the child's arm may make the veins easier to view. A transilluminator or an ultrasound when available can be useful to help visualize the veins of children.
- To minimize needle pain, apply ice or a topical anesthetic to the IV site.
- Site is covered with a transparent dressing, if available, to allow visualization and to promptly identify signs of infiltration [57].
- An institutional policy with criteria for new IV placement is highly recommended.

IV infusions of chemotherapy may be administered as IV push, intermittent infusion, or continuous infusion. Irrespective of the infusion method, the following safeguards must be in place:

- Use safety needles when available to minimize accidental needle exposure.
- Don appropriate PPE in accordance with regulatory and institutional guidelines during medication administration and disposal of contaminated materials.
- Secure all IV tubing with Luer Lock connections.
- To minimize exposure to the patient's skin, use gauze and/or a plastic-backed drape beneath the CVC and tubing/syringe connections during access or de-access procedures.
- Flush CVC per institutional standards.
  - 10 mL syringes must be used to flush a CVC to decrease pressure on the catheter [50].
- Chemotherapy waste is disposed in accordance with regulatory and institutional guidelines.
- Document the injection site, needle size, medication, patient response, and other pertinent information, including blood return before, during, and after medication administration.
- Document the appearance of the catheter or IV site.
- Ensure discharge teaching is completed with patient and family.

Extravasation refers to the infiltration of fluid or drug, which can cause tissue damage if it leaks outside of the vein. The class, concentration, and the amount of drug determine the extent of tissue damage when extravasation occurs. Symptoms such as tingling, burning, pain, swelling around the catheter site, redness at the catheter site and/or lack of blood return are signs that require immediate evaluation [45]. If extravasation occurs or is suspected, follow the acronym-**SLAPP**:

- S = stop the infusion
- L = leave the needle
- A = aspirate
- P = pull the needle
- P = notify the provider

The management of an extravasation includes hot or cold packs as indicated. Some chemotherapeutic agents have specific antidotes. An extravasation kit should be available if needed. If a blister develops, this should remain intact and covered if possible. Evaluate the site at regular intervals, i.e., 24, 48, 72 h, as some agents can cause more damage as tissue invasion progresses [51]. Document the event noting the agent, size of needle, site, amount of drug that infiltrated, who was notified of the event, nursing, and medical interventions. The complications that can develop from extravasation include infection, tissue necrosis, and a loss of function.

The importance of educating the patient and family about extravasation cannot be underestimated. It is important for patients to understand that any pain, redness, swelling, or abnormal sensation at the infusion site should be reported immediately.

Psychosocial Care of the Child and Family

Overview

A diagnosis of childhood cancer is a life-changing event for the entire family. The patient, parents, caregivers, siblings, extended family, and friends are all affected and may react quite differently. Disrupted school, home and work routines, financial stress, and delegation of responsibilities such as care of siblings and other family members are just a few of the concerns that families face. An evaluation of the family's support system and coping strategies by the health care team is essential. Partnering with families along the treatment continuum is the most effective means to promote adaptation to "the new normal."

Family-centered care is defined as "An approach to… health care that is grounded in mutually beneficial partnerships among health care providers, patients, and families" [59]. Patient and family involvement in decision-making is critical to the delivery of effective cancer care.

Communication with Patients and Families

Diagnosis

Childhood cancer is rare and symptoms often look similar to common childhood diseases, such as fever, pain, or swelling [60]. The parents are usually the first to recognize that something is wrong. The anticipation with which they wait for a diagnosis is a very stressful period. When families are receiving news of a new diagnosis or recurrence of cancer, it is important to show empathy, respect, and compassion for the family. The age and developmental level of the child are important considerations. For example, adolescents are often treated on adult oncology units, yet they have unique developmental needs that should be acknowledged by nurses who care for them [61, 62]. A nurse should be present when the family first learns about the child/adolescent's diagnosis to ensure a clear understanding of what the patient and the family has been told. This avoids the dilemma of the family misinterpreting the information and the nurse being unaware of what the physician actually said [63]. Nurses can facilitate a meeting that promotes effective communication [64]. The meeting should be at a time that is convenient for the family, and held in a quiet, private, comfortable setting, with a minimum or no interruptions [65]. Language, cultural and religious beliefs, as well as the family's previous experience with cancer and knowledge about their child's illness are important factors to consider. Ideally, information will be shared in clear, understandable terms at a pace that is determined by the family. Reassurance that nothing they did or failed to do has led to the diagnosis of cancer is very important [66]. The goals of treatment and plan of care will often need to be repeated several times after the initial meeting to ensure clear understanding among family members.

Stigma and Isolation

In many countries, significant stigma is associated with a cancer diagnosis [67, 68]. Families can be ostracized or feel isolated from their community during their child's treatment. Patients, particularly adolescents, may experience diminished social contact with friends and their community during long hospitalizations or periods of recovery at home [69]. Communicating and working with families and communities to decrease stigma through education and role modeling is an important nursing task.

Relapse

Children and adolescents who relapse need extra support when facing a second round of treatment and may react differently than during their first treatment [70]. The patient and family members may be angry that they are back in the hospital or feel hopeless since the first treatment failed and a cure is less likely [71]. In a study in Australia, De Graves et al. found that "The most significant finding…was the profound impact of uncertainty. The families fluctuated between two states of reality—hoping for a cure and contemplating death—as they faced the uncertainty that surrounded their child's prognosis" [72]. Sensitive exploration of these issues with the families can help to identify issues that may require attention from a social worker or psychologist. If professional experts are not an option, the health care team can work to develop specific strategies to help these patients and families. After a relapse, families may have increased interest in exploring the use of alternative therapies [73].

Patient and Family Education

Clear and consistent communication with children, adolescents, parents, and siblings is essential. Families in low- and middle-income countries may not have experience with tertiary health care centers and formal medical treatments. The use of medical jargon and unfamiliar regimens can be quite difficult for families with a newly diagnosed child or adolescent [69]. Strict hospital policies for visitation, infection control, meal times, and medication administration can be threatening to the family's normal routine of caring for an ill member [74]. It is critical that nurses diligently explain and re-explain treatment and medical information. When giving instructions, the nurse evaluates the patient and family's understanding, especially when giving the families discharge instructions for care at home. Techniques to ensure that the information has been well understood include asking the family to repeat the instructions or information in their own words. Re-demonstration of a procedure (e.g., dressing change) by the parent or caregiver to the nurse is also an effective strategy. Home visits by nurses can ensure continuity in care and will confirm whether educational information has been clearly communicated and is being carried out appropriately. This is an effective strategy to minimize complications and unplanned hospital admissions [75].

Extended family members, such as grandparents, aunts, and uncles (whether blood relations or connected through social ties), can offer critical support to the child/adolescent with cancer and their parents [76]. Acknowledging the extended family's role and including them in teaching sessions can help reinforce learning.

Low level of education or language issues: A language barrier may interfere with effective patient and family education. Migrants, indigenous populations, or ethnic minorities who do not speak the local language may experience significant stress when trying to negotiate their child's treatment and side effects [77]. The use of professional interpreters or health care professionals within the hospital to translate can significantly reduce the sense of powerlessness and dependence that families may have and improve trusting relationships in the care of the patient [78]. Families who do not have formal education can also experience stress trying to learn about their child's cancer and treatment [79]. Simple and clear language should be used; metaphors may be helpful. For example, describing chemotherapy as a medicine that kills cancer cells just as weed-killer removes the unwanted plants from a crop, or describing the position of the sun for timing medication administration when the child is at home may make explanations more meaningful. The health care team is responsible for ensuring that the family has a good understanding of their child's cancer so they are able to make informed care decisions [80]. Nurses who commit to working with the patient and family over time, providing clear and consistent educational support and ensuring active family inclusion and collaboration in the child/adolescent's care will maximize the caregiver's ability to succeed [81].

Traditional medicine: Families who have consulted traditional healers and practice traditional cures during their child/adolescent's cancer treatment may need nursing support to share their practices with the medical team, in order to prevent conflicting treatments [82]. Open and ongoing communication that includes active listening about cultural issues combined with education for the patient, parents, siblings, and extended family members is key to a successful treatment experience [83].

Multidisciplinary Communication

Nurses must communicate clearly among themselves, particularly during clinical hand-offs between shifts. Nurses review and document clinical information in the patient's medical record, including nursing assessments, observation of abnormalities, disease or treatment symptoms or side effects, and changes to the plan of care [84]. Consistent documentation of teaching and issues that have been raised by the family promotes continuity of education and communication.

Effective communication among the multidisciplinary team is essential to quality care and patient safety. Nursing presence at daily rounds promotes team cohesiveness in carrying out the plan of care. For complex or private information that cannot be discussed in rounds, multidisciplinary team meetings are a valuable mechanism to ensure consistency and team consensus in the communication of information to families [65].

Psychosocial Support

The cancer journey evokes powerful feelings and emotions for families that are important to recognize and acknowledge. Age¸ gender, cultural and socioeconomic factors will influence how people express, define, describe, or recognize their emotions [85]. The news of a cancer diagnosis is overwhelming, and the initial reaction will differ from person to person. Some react with disbelief or the possibility of a wrong diagnosis, while others will initially revert to "How long do I have to live?" The nurse encourages the patient to ventilate his or her feelings, and may guide the patient toward positive thinking, such as things to be thankful for [84, 86].

The first treatment is often anticipated with doubt and trepidation, due to fear of the unknown. Numerous people involved in the patient's treatment, along with other cancer patients and families, may tell various stories of their own experiences, often leaving families bewildered and unable to remember much of what was said. Advise the patient and the family to ask for explanations to be repeated until they are satisfied [84, 87]. Guilt feelings may often be foremost; the parent's natural reaction is to protect and nurture the child who is facing the reality of cancer [88]. Although the child has a life-threatening disease, he or she is still growing and developing and has needs similar to those of healthy siblings and peers. Each family member will develop methods of coping; adjustments will be made that in turn affect the others. Even the well-adjusted families will experience significant emotional stress.

Although each age group expresses emotions in distinct ways, secrecy tends to isolate children of all ages, increasing their fears. The young child may not be able to express his or her concerns verbally, but is still in need of reassurance and support. Caregivers of children must create an atmosphere where the child can express his or her worries and emotions [88].

Hospitalization and treatment can be very difficult for the parents and the siblings of the patient. When parents spend a great deal of time in the hospital with the sick child, siblings may develop feelings of jealousy, guilt, and fear toward the ill child. Encourage siblings to attend the hospital for visits if possible, so that they may have an idea of what is happening. Parent and sibling support groups can play a significant role to help family members cope. Reassurance that "you are not alone" on the cancer journey often provides comfort. Likewise, it is helpful to alert parents that behavior problems in siblings often arise at home or at school when the family routine is disrupted by a hospitalization [86].

Pediatric Palliative Care

Palliative care practices are now common around the world. The concept of palliative care "includes physical, psychological, educational, social, and spiritual goals and is provided concurrently with disease-modifying therapies or as the main goal of care. This care aims to enhance life, decrease suffering, optimize function, and provide opportunities for personal and spiritual growth" [71]. The age and developmental stage of the dying child are important considerations when developing palliative care strategies.

Infants work to develop a sense of trust, established when their needs for food, comfort, and caring are met. Allow the caregiver to stay with the baby, and provide support as he or she attends to the basic needs of the infant. Nursing staff can take over the infant's care for periods of time to allow parents to visit with relatives and family, or to go home and rest. Suggest this option to the caregiver, but refrain from forcing a caregiver to leave the hospital.

Toddlers work to develop a sense of independence and self-mastery. Explain procedures in very simple terms to the toddler. When possible, allow the toddler to handle any apparatus that will be used in his or her care. It can be helpful to provide consistent nurses with whom the toddler has established a trusting relationship to tend to his or her needs [19].

Preschoolers develop mastery over physical skills and tasks. They experience guilt if they overstep the limits of their behavior. Encourage children to voice their fears about illness and death, so they can be reassured. Young children may demonstrate regressive behavior and find comfort in resuming old habits that they have outgrown, such as sleeping with a teddy bear or a night lamp. Ensure that all procedures are fully explained to the child. Preschoolers have a strong ego and may regard the procedures (or even the illness) as punishment for previous behavior. Ease guilt feelings by allowing the child to participate in his or her treatment. Encourage parents to spend as much time as possible with the child as they are capable of the most reassurance and comfort [89].

School-age children are becoming increasingly independent of their parents. They may feel inadequate if they are unable to perform social, physical, and academic tasks. Encourage the children to set short-term goals for as long as possible, providing the opportunity to maintain interest in their personal lives, such as friends, families, and activities, even at the end of life. School is an essential part of a child's life, representing normal routines and continued relationships with peers, which is essential for appropriate behavioral, social, and emotional growth and development. Staying in contact with friends and peers helps the school-age child to strengthen his or her self-image and have faith in the future.

Allow school-age children to do things for themselves to gain skills and maintain self-respect. Answer their questions about their disease and treatment honestly to reinforce their confidence throughout this period. Signs of anxiety should be stilled with the assurance that the nurse or the parent will stay with the child at all times [89, 90].

Adolescents are often treated on adult oncology units, yet they have specific needs that should be acknowledged by nurses who care for them [61, 62]. Self-image is very important to the adolescent, so body changes such as hair loss, weight gain due to steroids, or scars from surgical procedures should be addressed. Encourage contact with friends, since adolescents identify strongly with friends and peers and rely on their acceptance. If appropriate, offer adolescents the service of a religious worker, since their understanding of death approaches that of an adult. However, do not force religious counseling. Allow adolescents to indicate when they are ready to address the issues at hand [86, 90, 91].

Healthy adolescents are experiencing issues of independence from their parents or caregivers. This can be problematic during cancer therapy since adolescents have limited choices and significantly restricted activities and social experiences. Nurses should be sensitive to the specific challenges that adolescents face when they are receiving cancer treatment [61, 62].

Spirituality

Often when families are faced with a difficult situation or health problems, they draw strength from their religious beliefs and practices [92]. Religious beliefs and practices can help families manage emotions of helplessness and restore meaning and order to their lives while also promoting a sense of control. For some families, spirituality can be a powerful source of strength for facing life's challenges [93]. It is important to differentiate between religion and spirituality. A religion is a set of strongly held beliefs, values, and attitudes that one lives by. Spirituality refers to the inner experience and is not bound to religious tradition [90].

During the tumultuous cancer journey, the patient's emotions can be labile. It is normal to ask "Why is this happening to me?" or "Why does God allow this to happen to me?" [87] When coming to terms with bad news, it is not uncommon to have thoughts that challenge beliefs and faith. Suffering brings certain spiritual needs to the fore. Spiritual care is part of the nurse's core role in holistic nursing care. Preparing nurses to provide spiritual care in a palliative care setting allows them to support patients and families while acting as a resource to other clinicians [94].

Prayer is considered one of the most common forms of intervention to promote healing and well-being [87, 95]. The patient's spiritual needs during hospitalization may include a desire to be visited by a minister or religious worker, eating a special diet, receiving a sacrament, or listening to or participating in religious ceremonies. The patient's religious preferences should be obtained on admission. When appropriate, allow time for devotion during which the patient should not be disturbed [94].

When offering spiritual care to their patients, nurses must base their actions on sensitivity, compassion, and respect, acknowledging that cultural beliefs of others may differ from one's own standards. For example, when a patient or family chooses not to proceed with chemotherapy, it may be difficult for the health care team to accept. However, it is important to honor and respect the beliefs of the patient and family [94]. Abandonment of care is a complex issue and currently being studied in many low- and middle-income countries [96].

Death, Dying, and Bereavement

Although death and dying are natural components of the life process, the thought of dying is an uncomfortable concept to many people. According to Kübler-Ross, the emotional responses of a person facing death can be traced through five stages: denial and isolation, anger, bargaining, depression, and acceptance [97]. A patient's response to death and dying has been learned from his or her family or the culture from which he or she has come. It can also reflect the family's response to their pending loss [97]. Nurses are better able to provide care and support to dying patients and their families when equipped with specialized training in palliative care [98]. This training is an essential component of a pediatric oncology nursing curriculum.

The nurse strives to build a trusting relationship with the patient and family. When trust has been established, the patient and his or her family will be more comfortable sharing their beliefs and disclosing feelings to the nurse. Feelings the family may experience include sadness, anger, fear, relief, and acceptance of death [98]. Nurses provide comfort by acknowledging that people experience their feelings differently. There are no right or wrong feelings or patterns that a person must follow in respect to the end of life [99].

Nurses may also help families to maintain bonds through "legacy-making" activities before a child dies, such as creating handprints or memory boxes. Completing unfinished business may be important for the child or teen for whom a cure is not possible. As in treatment, hope remains for most children and adolescents throughout the end of life period [100]. With adolescents, awareness that cure is not the only hope may facilitate the efforts of the clinical to help the teen share his or her wishes. A well-tested clinical prompt to facilitate a discussion about hopefulness and the hoped-for object is, "please share with me what you are hoping for now" [71].

Bereavement: The goal of nursing is not "cure" but "care." For families whose children do not survive bereavement rituals can be comforting and meaningful. Nurses are important to this process since they are commonly acutely aware of cultural norms for the patients in their care. Nurses who attend bereavement services can be quite powerful in their support of the family at this time. The family recognizes that their child is not forgotten. In addition, nurses also need a time and space for remembrance since they are also affected by the loss of the child [101].

Survivorship: The number of children surviving cancer in countries with rich resources approaches

81 % [102], which contrasts dramatically with rates in resource-poor countries where survival rates may be as low as 10 % [103]. Nevertheless, children who have survived cancer bring happiness and satisfaction to all who participated in their treatment. Having a survivors' day celebration at the hospital can bring hope to families whose children are still receiving treatment and reinforces all hospital personnel's commitment to curing children with cancer. It is also essential to remain cognizant that a child or adolescent who has survived cancer will require long-term surveillance by a health care professional who is familiar with pediatric cancer treatment and long-term effects such as neurologic squeal [104], infertility [105], secondary neoplasms [106], and abnormal cardiac function [107] to maximize his or her health throughout adulthood.

Summary

The role of nursing in the care of children and adolescents with cancer cannot be underestimated. Specialized education and training for nurses is essential to ensure optimal care for this vulnerable patient population. Nurses who are well integrated in the health care team and have clear lines of communication with their professional colleagues are able to provide consistent and coordinated nursing care. This level of care supports patients, their families, and extended families through the complicated and stressful experience of cancer therapy. Thus, the expert pediatric oncology nurse "has confidence in his or her knowledge, provides high-quality care, and is given opportunities for professional growth" [108].

References

1. Day SW, Segovia L, Viveros P, Banfi A, Rivera GK, Ribeiro RC. Development of the Latin American Center for pediatric oncology nursing education. Pediatr Blood Cancer. 2011;56(1):5–6.
2. Wilimas JA, Donahue N, Chammas G, Fouladi M, Bowers LJ, Ribeiro RC. Training subspecialty nurses in developing countries: methods, outcome, and cost. Med Pediatr Oncol. 2003;41(2):136.
3. Rodriguez-Galindo C, Friedrich P, Morrissey L, Frazier L. Global challenges in pediatric oncology. Curr Opin Pediatr. 2013;25(1):3–15.
4. Needleman J, Buerhaus P, Pankratz VS, Leibson CL, Stevens SR, Harris M. Nurse staffing and inpatient hospital mortality. N Engl J Med. 2011;364(11): 1037–45.
5. Kendall-Gallagher D, Aiken LH, Sloane DM, Cimiotti JP. Nurse specialty certification, inpatient mortality, and failure to rescue. J Nurs Scholarsh. 2011;43(2):188–94.
6. Day SW, Garcia J, Antillon F, Wilimas JA, McKeon LM, Carty RM, et al. A sustainable model for pediatric oncology nursing education in low-income countries. Pediatr Blood Cancer. 2012;58(2):163–6.
7. St. Jude Children's Research Hospital. International partner sites. 2013. Available at: http://www.stjude.org/stjude/v/index.jsp?vgnextoid=9e566f9523e70110VgnVCM1000001e0215acRCRD&vgnextchannel=48a9f8f281901110VgnVCM1000001e0215acRCRD. Accessed 10 May 2013.
8. Stefan D, Shalongo S, Ribeiro R. Twinning in paediatric oncology—an African experience. S Afr Med J. 2012;102(1):28–9.
9. Ribeiro R, Wilimas J, Razzouk B, Rodriguez C, Rivera G, Pui C, et al. Pediatric oncology as a model for cancer care: cooperation between low-resource and high-resource countries. 2006. Available at: http://2006.confex.com/uicc/uicc/techprogram/P10439.HTM. Accessed 16 Feb 2013.
10. Colquhoun S, Ogaoga D, Tamou M, Nasi T, Subhi R, Duke T. Child health nurses in the Solomon Islands: lessons for the Pacific and other developing countries. Hum Resour Health. 2012;10(1):45.
11. Tran TQ, Scherpbier A, Van Dalen J, Wright PE. Teacher-made models: the answer for medical skills training in developing countries? BMC Med Educ. 2012;12(1):98.
12. Ider B, Adams J, Morton A, Whitby M, Clements A. Perceptions of healthcare professionals regarding the main challenges and barriers to effective hospital infection control in Mongolia: a qualitative study. BMC Infect Dis. 2012;12(1):170.
13. Kevany S, Murima O, Singh B, Hlubinka D, Kulich M, Morin SF, et al. Socio-economic status and health care utilization in rural Zimbabwe: findings from Project Accept (HPTN 043). J Public Health Africa. 2012;3(1):46.
14. Walton-Roberts M. Contextualizing the global nursing care chain: international migration and the status of nursing in Kerala, India. Glob Netw. 2012;12(2): 175–94.
15. Ng'ang'a N, Byrne MW. Prioritizing professional practice models for nurses in low-income countries. Bull World Health Organ. 2012;90(1):3–3A.
16. Kronfol N. Historical development of health professions' education in the Arab world. East Mediterr Health J. 2012;18(11):1157–65.
17. Stewart L, Usher K. The impact of nursing leadership on patient safety in a developing country. J Clin Nurs. 2010;19(21–22):3152–60.

18. Nelson MB, Forte K, Freiburg D, Hooke MC, Kelly KP, Brace O'Neill JB. Pediatric oncology nursing: scope and standards of practice. Glenview, IL: Association of Pediatric Hematology Oncology Nurses; 2007.
19. Day SW, McKeon LM, Garcia J, Wilimas JA, Carty RM, de Alarcon P, et al. Use of joint commission international standards to evaluate and improve pediatric oncology nursing care in Guatemala. Pediatr Blood Cancer. 2012;60(5):810–5.
20. Kulkarni KP, Arora RS, Marwaha RK. Survival outcome of childhood acute lymphoblastic leukemia in India: a resource-limited perspective of more than 40 years. J Pediatr Hematol Oncol. 2011;33(6):475–9.
21. Kline N, Hobbie W, Hooke M, Rodgers C, Shea J. Essentials of pediatric hematology/oncology nursing: a core curriculum. 3rd ed. Glenview, IL: Association of Pediatric Hematology Oncology Nurses; 2008.
22. Pizzo P, Robichaud K, Wesley R, Commers J. Fever in the pediatric and young adult patient with cancer: a prospective study of 1001 episodes. Medicine. 1982;61(3):153–65.
23. Freifeld AG, Bow EJ, Sepkowitz KA, Boeckh MJ, Ito JI, Mullen CA, et al. Clinical practice guideline for the use of antimicrobial agents in neutropenic patients with cancer: 2010 update by the Infectious Diseases Society of America. Clin Infect Dis. 2011;52(4):e56–93.
24. Hughes W, Armstrong D, Bodey G, Bow E, Brown A, Calandra T, et al. 2002 guidelines for the use of antimicrobial agents in neutropenic patients with cancer. Clin Infect Dis. 2002;34:730–51.
25. Koh A, Pizzo P. Infectious complications in pediatric cancer patients. In: Pizzo PA, Poplack DG, editors. Principles and practice of pediatric oncology. 6th ed. Philadelphia: Lippincott Williams & Wilkins; 2011. p. 1190.
26. Kline NE, editor. The pediatric chemotherapy and biotherapy curriculum. 2nd ed. Glenview, IL: Association of Pediatric Hematology Oncology Nurses; 2007.
27. Simon C. Neutropenia. In: Tomlinson D, Klein NE, editors. Pediatric oncology nursing: advanced clinical handbook. 1st ed. Heidelberg: Springer; 2005. p. 133–7.
28. Allegranzi B, Pittet D. Role of hand hygiene in healthcare-associated infection prevention. J Hosp Infect. 2009;73(4):305–15.
29. Bloomfield SF, Aiello AE, Cookson B, O'Boyle C, Larson EL, Bloomfield SF, et al. The effectiveness of hand hygiene procedures in reducing the risks of infections in home and community settings including handwashing and alcohol-based hand sanitizers. Am J Infect Control. 2007;35(10):S27–64.
30. El-Housseiny AA, Saleh SM, El-Masry AA, Allam AA. The effectiveness of vitamin "E" in the treatment of oral mucositis in children receiving chemotherapy. J Clin Pediatr Dent. 2007;31(3):167–70.
31. Esquenazi D, Wigg MD, Miranda MM, Rodrigues HM, Tostes JB, Rozental S, et al. Antimicrobial and antiviral activities of polyphenolics from *Cocos nucifera* Linn. (Palmae) husk fiber extract. Res Microbiol. 2002;153(10):647–52.
32. Dana Farber Cancer Institute. Planning meals and managing cancer side effects. 2013. Available at: http://www.dana-farber.org/Adult-Care/Treatment-and-Support/Patient-and-Family-Support/Nutrition-Services.aspx#bowel. Accessed 1 April 2013.
33. Landers R, O'Hanlon-Curry J. Gastrointestinal complications. In: Kline N, Hobbie W, Hooke M, Rodgers C, Shea J, editors. Essentials of pediatric hematology/oncology nursing: a core curriculum. 3rd ed. Glenview, IL: Association of Pediatric Hematology Oncology Nurses; 2008. p. 98–108.
34. Tazi I, Hidane Z, Zafad S, Harif M, Benchekroun S, Ribeiro R, et al. Nutritional status at diagnosis of children with malignancies in Casablanca. Pediatr Blood Cancer. 2008;51(4):495.
35. Hossain P, Kawar B, El Nahas M. Obesity and diabetes in the developing world—a growing challenge. N Engl J Med. 2007;356(3):213–5.
36. Sala A, Rossi E, Antillon F, Molina AL, de Maselli T, Bonilla M, et al. Nutritional status at diagnosis is related to clinical outcomes in children and adolescents with cancer: a perspective from Central América. Eur J Cancer. 2012;48(2):243–52.
37. Schoeman J, Dannhauser A, Kruger M. Malnutrition in paediatric oncology patients: malnutrition at the diagnosis of cancer is not an uncommon finding in childhood cancer in the developing world. SA J Contin Med Educ. 2011;28(8):385–8.
38. Rembert D. Pain in children with cancer. In: Tomlinson D, Kline NE, editors. Pediatric oncology nursing: advanced clinical handbook. 1st ed. Heidelberg: Springer; 2005. p. 397–405.
39. Jacob E. Pain. In: Kline N, Hobbie W, Hooke M, Rodgers C, Shea J, editors. Essentials of pediatric hematology/oncology nursing: a core curriculum. 3rd ed. Glenview, IL: Association of Pediatric Hematology Oncology Nurses; 2008. p. 148–52.
40. Jacobson JO, Polovich M, McNiff KK, LeFebvre KB, Cummings C, Galioto M, et al. American Society of Clinical Oncology/Oncology Nursing Society chemotherapy administration safety standards. Oncol Nurs Forum. 2009;36(6):651–8.
41. Strother RM, Rao KV, Gregory KM, Jakait B, Busakhala N, Schellhase E, et al. The oncology pharmacy in cancer care delivery in a resource-constrained setting in western Kenya. J Oncol Pharm Pract. 2012;18(4):406–16.
42. Kline NE. Promoting patient safety through the development of a pediatric chemotherapy and biotherapy provider program. J Pediatr Oncol Nurs. 2004;21(2):65–6.
43. Friese CR, Himes-Ferris L, Frasier MN, McCullagh MC, Griggs JJ. Structures and processes of care in ambulatory oncology settings and nurse-reported exposure to chemotherapy. BMJ Qual Saf. 2012; 21(9):753–9.
44. Leape LL, Kabcenell AI, Gandhi TK, Carver P, Nolan TW, Berwick DM. Reducing adverse drug events:

lessons from a breakthrough series collaborative. Jt Comm J Qual Patient Saf. 2000;26(6):321–31.
45. Ettinger AG, Echtenkamp D, Harley J, Wills MS, McNeil SB. Chemotherapy. In: Baggott C, Fochtman D, Foley G, Patterson K, editors. Nursing care of children and adolescents with cancer and blood disorders. 4th ed. Glenview, IL: Association of Pediatric Hematology Oncology Nurses; 2011. p. 326–80.
46. Smart M. Verification and maintenance of treatment as planned. In: Plovich M, Whitford JM, Olson M, editors. Chemotherapy and biotherapy guidelines and recommendations for practice. 3rd ed. Pittsburg: Oncology Nursing Society; 2009. p. 84–93.
47. Dreyer Z, Indelicato DJ, Reaman GH, Bleyer WA. Infants and adolescents with cancer: special considerations. In: Pizzo PA, Polackand DG, editors. Principles and practice of pediatric oncology. 6th ed. Riverwoods, IL: Lippincott Williams & Wilkins; 2011.
48. Burris HA, Hurtig J. Radiation recall with anticancer agents. Oncologist. 2010;15(11):1227–37.
49. Griggs JJ, Mangu PB, Anderson H, Balaban EP, Dignam JJ, Hryniuk WM, et al. Appropriate chemotherapy dosing for obese adult patients with cancer: American Society of Clinical Oncology clinical practice guideline. J Clin Oncol. 2012;30(13):1553–61.
50. Stiver W. Pretreatment and treatment. In: Plovich M, Whitford JM, Olson M, editors. Chemotherapy and biotherapy guidelines and recommendations for practice. 3rd ed. Pittsburg: Oncology Nursing Society; 2009. p. 93–103.
51. Nixon C, Rae ML. Administration considerations. In: Kline NE, editor. The pediatric chemotherapy and biotherapy curriculum. 3rd ed. Glenview, IL: Association of Pediatric Hematology Oncology Nurses; 2011. p. 73–103.
52. Brown TL. Pediatric variations of nursing interventions. In: Hockenberry MJ, Wilson D, editors. Wong's essentials of pediatric nursing. 8th ed. St. Louis: Mosby; 2009. p. 686–751.
53. Barron C, Cocoman A. Administering intramuscular injections to children: what does the evidence say? J Child Young People Nurs. 2008;2(3):138–44.
54. Sudlow CLM, Warlow CP. Posture and fluids for preventing post-dural puncture headache. 2010. Available at: http://onlinelibrary.wiley.com/doi/10.1002/14651858.CD001790.pub4.pdf. Accessed 9 April 2013.
55. Hadaway L. Infiltration and extravasation. Am J Nurs. 2007;107(8):64–72.
56. O'Grady NP, Alexander M, Patchen Dellinger E, et al. Guidelines for the prevention of intravascular catheter-related infections. Pediatrics. 2002;110:1–24.
57. Froiland K. Extravasation injuries: implications for WOC nursing. J Wound Ostomy Continence Nurs. 2007;34(3):299–302.
58. Gorski L. Standard 37: site selection. J Infus Nurs. 2009;32(3):125–6.
59. Institute for Patient- and Family-Centered Care. What is patient- and family-centered care? 2010. Available at: http://www.ipfcc.org/faq.html. Accessed 29 April 2013.
60. Feltbower R, Lewis I, Picton S, Richards M, Glaser A, Kinsey S, et al. Diagnosing childhood cancer in primary care—a realistic expectation? Br J Cancer. 2004;90(10):1882–4.
61. Sanchez AM. Cancer in adolescents. 2011. Available at: http://www.cure4kids.org/ums/oncopedia/case_detail/chapter/?id=33. Accessed 7 Jan 2013.
62. Goodall S, King M, Ewing J, Smith N, Kenny P. Preferences for support services among adolescents and young adults with cancer or a blood disorder: a discrete choice experiment. Health Policy. 2012;107(2–3):304–11.
63. Davis AJ. The clinical nurse's role in informed consent. J Prof Nurs. 1988;4(2):88–91.
64. Kodish E, Eder M, Noll RB, Ruccione K, Lange B, Angiolillo A, et al. Communication of randomization in childhood leukemia trials. JAMA. 2004;291(4):470–5.
65. Booyens S. Communication. In: Booyens SW, editor. Dimensions of nursing management. 2nd ed. Cape Town: Juta and Company Ltd.; 1998. p. 267–9.
66. Mack JW, Grier HE. The day one talk. J Clin Oncol. 2004;22(3):563–6.
67. Knaul F, Anderson B, Bradley C, Kerr D. Access to cancer treatment in low-and middle-income countries—an essential part of global cancer control; 2010. Available at: http://papers.ssrn.com/s013/papers.cfm?abstract_id=2055441.
68. Bekibele CO, Ayede AI, Asaolu OO, Brown BJ. Retinoblastoma: the challenges of management in Ibadan, Nigeria. J Pediatr Hematol Oncol. 2009;31(8):552.
69. Gannoni AF, Shute RH, Gannoni AF, Shute RH. Parental and child perspectives on adaptation to childhood chronic illness: a qualitative study. Clin Child Psychol Psychiatry. 2010;15(1):39–53.
70. Haddy TB, Mosher RB, Dinndorf PA, Reaman GH. Second neoplasms in survivors of childhood and adolescent cancer are often treatable. J Adolesc Health. 2004;34(4):324–9.
71. Foster TL, Lafond DA, Reggio C, Hinds PS. Pediatric palliative care in childhood cancer nursing: from diagnosis to cure or end of life. Semin Oncol Nurs. 2010;26(4):205.
72. De Graves S, Aranda S, De Graves S, Aranda S. Living with hope and fear—the uncertainty of childhood cancer after relapse. Cancer Nurs. 2008;31(4):292–301.
73. Paisley MA, Kang TI, Insogna IG, Rheingold SR. Complementary and alternative therapy use in pediatric oncology patients with failure of frontline chemotherapy. Pediatr Blood Cancer. 2011;56(7):1088–91.
74. Williams AM. Therapeutic landscapes as health promoting places. Soc Sci Med. 2009;43(9):1193–203.
75. Yilmaz MC, Ozsoy S. Effectiveness of a discharge-planning program and home visits for meeting the physical care needs of children with cancer. Support Care Cancer. 2010;18(2):243–53.
76. Moules NJ, Laing CM, McCaffrey G, Tapp DM, Strother D. Grandparents' experiences of childhood cancer, Part 1 doubled and silenced. J Pediatr Oncol Nurs. 2012;29(3):119–32.

77. Senior K. Health migration and childhood cancer. Lancet Oncol. 2006;7(11):889.
78. Pergert P, Ekblad S, Björk O, Enskär K, Andrews T, Pergert P, et al. Protecting Family Interests: an interview study with foreign-born parents struggling on in childhood cancer care. Int J Pediatr. 2012;2012:681301. doi:10.1155/2012/68/301. Available at: http://www.ncbi.nlm.nih.gov/pubmed/22518180.
79. Panganiban-Corales A, Medina MFJ. Family resources study: part 1: family resources, family function and caregiver strain in childhood cancer. Asia Pac Fam Med. 2011;10:14.
80. Pyke-Grimm KA, Stewart JL, Kelly KP, Degner LF. Parents of children with cancer: factors influencing their treatment decision making roles. J Pediatr Nurs. 2006;21(5):350–61.
81. Kelly P, Kelly D. Childhood cancer-parenting work for British Bangladeshi families during treatment: an ethnographic study. Int J Nurs Stud. 2012;50(7):933–44.
82. Genc RE, Senol S, Turgay AS, Kantar M, Genc RE, Senol S, et al. Complementary and alternative medicine used by pediatric patients with cancer in western Turkey (online exclusive article) (report). Oncol Nurs Forum. 2009;36(3):E159–64.
83. Landier W, Tse A. Use of complementary and alternative medical interventions for the management of procedure-related pain, anxiety, and distress in pediatric oncology: an integrative review. J Pediatr Nurs. 2010;25:566–79.
84. Dolamo BL. Unit records, reports and statistics in health services. In: Booyens SW, editor. Introduction to health care service management. 3rd ed. Cape Town: Juta and Company Ltd.; 2008. p. 138–42.
85. Grieve K, Van Deventer V. A student's A–Z of psychology. 1st ed. Bhisho: Juta Academic; 2005.
86. Hynson JL. The child's journey: transition from health to ill-health. In: Goldman A, Hain R, Liben S, editors. Oxford textbook of palliative care for children. 1st ed. New York: Oxford University Press; 2006. p. 18–20.
87. Stringfield M. Cancer and me. 1st ed. Bloomington, IN: Xlibris Corporation; 2011.
88. Buckman R. How to break bad news: a guide for health care professionals. 1st ed. Baltimore: The John Hopkins University Press; 1992.
89. Kelly KP, Hooke MC. Pediatric symptoms and responses. In: Varricchio CG, editor. A cancer source book for nurses. 8th ed. Sudbury, MA: Jones and Bartlett Publishers Inc.; 2004. p. 491–4.
90. Lanctot D, Morrison W, Koch KD, Feudtner S. Spiritual dimensions. In: Carter BS, Levetown M, Friebert SE, editors. Palliative care for infants, children, and adolescents: a practical handbook. 2nd ed. Baltimore: The John Hopkins University Press; 2011. p. 227.
91. Barraclough J. Cancer and emotion: a practical guide to psycho-oncology. 3rd ed. West Sussex: Wiley; 1999.
92. Van Schalkwyk D. Counselling and support of patients and family. In: Pervan V, Cohen LH, Jaftha T, editors. Oncology for health care professionals. 1st ed. Cape Town: Juta and Company Ltd.; 1995. p. 643–53.
93. Foyle L, Hostad J, editors. Innovations in cancer and palliative care education. 1st ed. Milton Keynes, UK: Radcliffe Publishing Ltd.; 2007.
94. O'Brien ME. Spirituality in nursing: standing on holy ground. 4th ed. Sudbury, MA: Jones & Bartlett Learning; 2011.
95. Eden O, Black I, MacKinlay G, Emery A. Communication with parents of children with cancer. Palliat Med. 1994;8(2):105–14.
96. Arora RS, Pizer B, Eden T. Understanding refusal and abandonment in the treatment of childhood cancer. Indian Pediatr. 2010;47(12):1005–10.
97. Kübler-Ross EK. Death: the final stage of growth. 1st ed. Englewood Cliffs, NJ: Prentice-Hall; 1975.
98. Brayne S. The D-word: talking about dying—a guide for relatives, friends and carers. 1st ed. London: Continuum International Publishing Group; 2010.
99. O'Neill B, Fallon F. ABC of palliative care. London: BMJ Books; 1998.
100. Hinds PS. The hopes and wishes of adolescents with cancer and the nursing care that helps. Oncol Nurs Forum. 2004;31(5):927–34.
101. Wenzel J, Shaha M, Klimmek R, Krumm S, Wenzel J, Shaha M, et al. Working through grief and loss: oncology nurses' perspectives on professional bereavement (online exclusive) (report). Oncol Nurs Forum. 2011;38(4):E272–82.
102. Kaatsch P. Epidemiology of childhood cancer. Cancer Treat Rev. 2010;36(4):277–85.
103. Knaul FM, Frenk J, Shulman L for the Global Task Force on Expanded Access to Cancer Care and Control in Developing Countries. Closing the cancer divide: a blueprint to expand access in low and middle income countries. Boston, MA: Harvard Global Equity Initiative; 2011.
104. Goldsby RE, Liu Q, Nathan PC, Bowers DC, Yeaton-Massey A, Raber SH, et al. Late-occurring neurologic sequelae in adult survivors of childhood acute lymphoblastic leukemia: a report from the Childhood Cancer Survivor Study. J Clin Oncol. 2010;28(2):324–31.
105. Oeffinger KC, Nathan PC, Kremer LC. Challenges after curative treatment for childhood cancer and long-term follow up of survivors. Hematol Oncol Clin North Am. 2010;24(1):129.
106. Friedman DL, Whitton J, Leisenring W, Mertens AC, Hammond S, Stovall M, et al. Subsequent neoplasms in 5-year survivors of childhood cancer: the Childhood Cancer Survivor Study. J Natl Cancer Inst. 2010;102(14):1083–95.
107. van der Pal HJ, van Dalen EC, Hauptmann M, Kok WE, Caron HN, van den Bos C, et al. Cardiac function in 5-year survivors of childhood cancer: a long-term follow-up study. Arch Intern Med. 2010;170(14):1247.
108. Enskär K. Being an expert nurse in pediatric oncology care nurses' descriptions in narratives. J Pediatr Oncol Nurs. 2012;29(3):151–60.

Paediatric Radiotherapy

14

Jeannette Parkes and Julie Wetter

Introduction

General

Availability of Radiotherapy (RT) Services in Africa

Radiotherapy is an essential part of oncology treatment. It is frequently used together with surgery and/or chemotherapy as curative treatment for cancer, and its use in the palliative setting is vital for relieving symptoms. In the paediatric setting, its use is vital to many treatment protocols [1].

RT may be delivered via external beam, such as Cobalt units and linear accelerators (Linacs), or via brachytherapy (internal use of radioactive sources). Providing safe, reliable, and effective RT is complex and extremely expensive. It requires specialised building structures for radiation protection, investment in expensive machinery, trained staff capable of using and maintaining such equipment, and a budget for doing so. It also requires ongoing quality assurance and training programs for such staff.

For all of these reasons, RT infrastructure in general, is very poor in low- and middle-income countries (LICs and MICs), with many such countries not having any services at all. Africa is the continent with the poorest radiotherapy services of all, with about 28 out of 48 countries having no services at all, and several countries having non-operational units due to lack of funds for maintenance of machines or lack of skilled staff to run them [2].

Currently, Africa is home to approximately one seventh of the world's seven billion population, and 40 % of Sub-Saharan Africans are under 15 years of age. However, only four countries in Africa treat more than 100 children per year with RT, due to lack of infrastructure and services [3].

Challenges Facing Paediatric RT Services in Developing Countries

Allied Services

Imaging is one of the greatest challenges in managing oncology patients in poorly resourced countries. Many intra-abdominal and head and neck tumours may be diagnosed by clinical examination and confirmed using the relatively inexpensive modality of ultrasound. Chest tumours are often visible on plain X-ray. However accurately diagnosing brain tumours requires CT scan availability and this requires infrastructure. Furthermore, once a diagnosis has been made, CT is needed for RT localisation of tumours unless only simple parallel opposed/2D planning is done.

Pathology services are also frequently problematic. Increasingly, LICs and MICs are sending clinicians for training in better-resourced

J. Parkes, M.D. (✉) • J. Wetter, M.D.
Department of Radiation Oncology, Groote Schuur and Red Cross Children's Hospitals and University of Cape Town, Cape Town, South Africa
e-mail: jeanette.parkes@uct.ac.za

D.C. Stefan and C. Rodriguez-Galindo (eds.), *Pediatric Hematology-Oncology in Countries with Limited Resources: A Practical Manual*, DOI 10.1007/978-1-4614-3891-5_14,

countries, but on returning home, they find that they are unable to confidently diagnose tumours because of lack of trained pathologists, and/or lack of funding for complicated immunohistochemical staining to aid diagnosis. In some instances, twinning programs with well-resourced countries can partly overcome this problem, by providing expert opinions, or by reviewing slides.

Medical physicists and technical engineers are in short supply internationally. All RT programs require these trained staff to maintain their machines and to provide quality assurance of the treatment machines and planning programs. *Radiation therapy technicians* (*RTTs*) are also highly trained staff, responsible for planning RT treatment and for operating the machines which administer it. Unfortunately skilled staff is frequently attracted away to better-resourced countries that are able to provide superior individual payment packages for these sought-after individuals.

Basic Health Care Availability

In LICs and MICs it is not only the oncology programs which are poorly resourced. In general, access to all aspects of tertiary health care in these countries is challenging, with patients having to travel vast distances, at great personal expense, to seek medical opinion. As a result, many cancers are diagnosed late and only palliative treatment is appropriate. The cost of such treatment may have to be borne, at least partly, by the patient and his or her family. Thus, many families may choose not to investigate or to treat obvious tumours.

For patients who do access oncology services, treatment may be hampered by poor general health; with coexisting malnutrition and infections such as HIV and tuberculosis prevalent. Side effects of oncology treatment may be extreme in these cases and supportive supplements and drugs are frequently not available. Oncology treatment protocols have to take these factors into account when offering treatment. Protocols available in a first world setting may be inappropriate and dangerous in under-resourced countries.

Practical Problems

For RT treatments in particular, radical courses of radiotherapy usually involve daily treatments for 5 or more weeks. Accommodation for the patient and accompanying adult is frequently problematic. In some countries, different charity organisations have been able to help with accommodation and transport for these patients. But in many countries, where RT services are many miles away, and families are large, it may not be practical for one parent to stay with the child for the duration of the treatment. Abandonment is a problem as parents are not readily contactable [2].

Where travelling distances are large, follow-up is also a problem. Personnel at local clinics are usually excellent at primary health care, but may be ignorant about the potential for post-radiotherapy (and post-chemotherapy) problems. Detailed referral letters back to local clinics, outlining potential side-effects as well as the types of follow-up tests and the appropriate interval between such tests does much to help this.

Technical Challenges in Treating Children with RT in Poorly Resourced Settings

The Time Challenge!

The biggest challenge that staff face when doing paediatric RT in any department is the length of time that is required. Children (and their parents) are far more likely to be co-operative when they are not being rushed, and when the team takes the time to explain everything in detail, and is patient and accommodating of their fears and anxieties.

For younger children, susceptibility to oral sedation is individual and quite variable, so that the team has to be ready to proceed as soon as the child is asleep!

In general it is essential to:

1. Allocate sufficient time and experienced staff on mark-up day.
2. Have all the required clinical information at hand, so that the process is not held up.
3. Get the patient's sedation history from other departments (e.g. Paediatric Oncology, Radiology, Surgery), so that it is known before-

hand whether the child is likely to co-operate, and how easily they can be sedated. A half-sedated child is harder to deal with than an unsedated child.

4. It is always helpful to get the child in for a "play" appointment prior to mark-up day, so that they familiarise themselves with staff and the machines. However, this is not always practical.
5. Children of 6 years and older, will generally co-operate without sedation, especially if the parents help to prepare them. They should always be told the precise steps of what will happen to them during the process; especially if any discomfort or pain is anticipated (e.g. tattoos/drip needles etc.).
6. Children under 5 years of age almost always need sedation. Between 5 and 6 years is variable.
7. Obtaining an anaesthetist on a daily basis for radiotherapy treatments is very difficult in many institutions. We resort to this only after several attempts at sedation have been tried.

Sedation for RT [4]

This may be oral or intravenous. The American Society of Anesthesiologists has proposed a grading system for sedation use by non-anaesthesiologists. The following categories are used:

1. *Minimal sedation/anxiolysis*: A drug-induced state during which patients respond normally to verbal commands. Cognitive and co-ordination function may be impaired but ventilator and cardiovascular functions are unaffected.
2. *Moderate sedation/analgesia*: A drug-induced depression of consciousness during which patients respond purposefully to verbal commands, either alone or accompanied by light tactile stimulation. No interventions are required to maintain a patent airway, and spontaneous ventilation is adequate. Cardiovascular function is usually maintained.
3. *Deep sedation/analgesia*: A drug-induced depression of consciousness during which patients cannot easily be aroused but respond purposefully following repeated or painful stimulation. Ability to independently maintain ventilator function may be impaired. Patients may require assistance in maintaining a patent airway and spontaneous ventilation may be inadequate. Cardiovascular function is usually maintained.
4. *General anaesthesia*: A drug-induced loss of consciousness during which patients are not rousable, even by painful stimulation. Ability to maintain adequate ventilatory function is often impaired. Patients often require assistance in maintaining a patent airway, and positive pressure ventilation may be required because of depressed spontaneous ventilation or drug-induced depression of neuromuscular function. Cardiovascular function may be impaired.

For RT planning, the mark-up, cast, and planning scan appointment can take up to an hour, and immobilisation and correct positioning is essential. Proper sedation is therefore essential.

Treatment visits are far shorter, and sedation is typically required only for about 10–15 minutes. Lighter sedation may be possible for these visits. Agents used for RT sedation:

(a) Clonidine is used as an anxiolytic and mild sedative. This is given orally about an hour (h) prior to the procedure. In older children, this may be all that is required (Category 1 sedation).
(b) Oral agents such as a combination of Droperidol (0.2 mg/kg) and Trimeprazine (2–4 mg/kg) are convenient and work well for mild to moderate sedation, but cause a long acting sedation which can be a problem if given for a protracted period, as children are not awake long enough during the day to take in adequate food. However, no monitoring equipment is required. The drugs must be administered 2 h prior to the procedure. Top up sedation at 2 h, with Chloral hydrate (50 mg/kg) can be given if sedation is inadequate. Caution must be taken when sedating children with brainstem dysfunction, as maintaining an adequate airway, and normal ventilation may already be impaired. For these children, electronic monitoring is recommended.

(c) Chloral hydrate is a cheap oral medication that works well as a top-up sedation after Droperidol/Trimeprazine or on its own at higher doses and has a shorter period of action than (b) above. It should be given approximately half an hour prior to the procedure. Doses from 50 mg/kg can be used for simple simulation with a supine child. However, when a face cast is required, doses of 100 mg/kg are needed. Use of this agent also does not require electronic monitoring. However it tastes terrible and may need to be delivered via nasogastric tube as many small children will spit it out!

(d) Shorter-acting agents such as IV Midazolam have become popular. At sedation dose (0.05 mg/kg) an anaesthetist is not required. However IV access is required, and electronic monitoring by an anaesthetic nurse or junior doctor is recommended, which makes it more labour-intensive. A repeat dose may be given if required, up to a maximum of 0.2 mg/kg.

(e) Ketamine may also be used intravenously. A single initial dose of 0.5–0.75 mg/kg is usually enough for short daily treatments. For longer procedures, an infusion may be used or an additional bolus of 0.25 mg/kg given. This has been safely and effectively used at many institutions without an anaesthetist, but with either an anaesthetic nurse or a junior doctor present. Electronic monitoring (e.g. pulse oximeter) is recommended. In older children Ketamine should be combined with a benzodiazepine to prevent post-procedure delirium. Tolerance may develop requiring higher doses for adequate sedation as the weeks go by. Intramuscular Ketamine is also effective, but when required daily, can cause severe anticipatory distress and therefore is seldom used.

(f) If anaesthesia is required, it must be remembered that anaesthetists are extremely infrequent visitors to the radiotherapy suite and frequently feel extremely vulnerable without the usual access to monitors, etc. The entire procedure needs to be discussed in advance and planned on site so that they are aware of the procedure, length of anaesthesia required, and possible cast covering the face. A decision regarding the type of anaesthetic will need to be made. Usually IV drugs, e.g. Propofol, Dexmedetomidine, or Ketamine are used. Inhalation anaesthesia may also be appropriate for some children. It is preferable to have the same anaesthetist available daily, so that the process becomes expedited, preventing delays on a busy RT machine unit [5].

Radiotherapy for Wilms Tumour

The development of protocols for the treatment of Wilms tumour has been extremely successful in the developed world. This has occurred mainly through research initiatives and clinical trials run by the SIOP (Societe Internationale d'Oncologie Paediatrique) in Europe and COG (Children's Oncology Group) and its precursors in the USA. Most centres treating Wilms tumours should attempt to follow the guidelines and treatment principles of one of these groups [6].

RT is an integral part of the management of Wilms tumour for selected individuals. However, only about 15–20 % of non-metastatic Wilms tumour patients will require RT. In general, the doses required for radiotherapy the in treatment of Wilms tumour are quite low, and the volumes are large. This means that sophisticated RT equipment is not a prerequisite and adequate therapy can be planned using fluoroscopy or a simulator, and delivered by Cobalt-60 machines.

Indications for RT for Wilms Tumour

Although direct outcome comparison of SIOP and COG protocols is not possible due to differing staging principles and timing of treatment, it is generally considered that in terms of outcome, they are equivalent. In LICs/MICs the decision of which protocol to follow usually lies with logistical considerations: In SIOP protocols, chemotherapy is administered first, and this is followed by surgery and staging. The decision for RT is based on findings at surgery. In COG protocols, surgery is done first, unless the tumour is deemed irresectable. Surgical staging then provides the basis for staging and further management. Either way, RT is done post-operatively. In some centres, it is

Table 14.1 COG radiation therapy guidelines—Wilms tumour

Tumour stage/histology	Radiotherapy (RT) dose and fields
1/FH and/2 FH	No RT
3/FH, 1–3/FA 1–2/DA 1–3/CCSK	10.8 Gy flank RT
Ascites (cytology +ve)	10.50 Gy whole abdomen RT (WART)
Pre-op tumour rupture	If residual tumour, boost with further 10.50 Gy
Diffuse surgical spillage	
Peritoneal seeding	
3/DA 1–3/RTK	19.8 Gy (infant 10.8 Gy)
4 (Lung, FH)	12 Gy whole lung irradiation (WLI) if no complete remission (CR) at week of 6 triple chemo
4 (Lung, UH)	12 Gy WLI regardless of (CR) or not
4 (Brain)	21.6 Gy whole brain + 10.8 Gy boost <16-year-old
4 (Bone)	25.2 Gy (tumour + 3 cm)
4 (Liver)	19.8 Gy to focal metastases if unresectable
Unresected LN	19.8 Gy
Resected LN	10.8 Gy
Abdominal relapse	12–18 Gy (>12 m)

RT radiotherapy, *FH* favourable histology, *FA* focal anaplasia, *DA* diffuse anaplasia, *CCSK* clear cell sarcoma of the kidney, *RTK* rhabdoid tumour of the kidney, *WLI* whole lung irradiation, *UH* unfavourable histology, *CR* complete remission, *LN* lymph node

convenient to biopsy, stage, and do the administration of chemotherapy first at a satellite centre and refer patients to large centres for planned surgery and possible RT. In other centres, children are referred to a large centre for diagnosis and immediate surgery and any necessary RT is performed immediately, and they are then sent closer to home for ongoing chemotherapy [7].

The radiotherapy method used for either protocol is the same, although doses differ slightly.

Indications for RT

1. COG Radiation therapy guidelines [8]

In COG protocols, the decision for RT is based on post-surgical histological sub-type and staging (Table 14.1).

Table 14.2 Radiotherapy guidelines SIOP and risk assessment [8, 9]

Tumour stage/histology	Radiotherapy dose and fields
2 HR except blastemal	Flank 14.1 Gy
3, IR	Flank 14.4 Gy ± boost 10.8 Gy
2, 3, HR	Flank 25.2 Gy/14#
3 with diffuse spillage	WART 14.1 Gy ± boost for gross disease up to 21 Gy
	Max 12 Gy for <1 year
Peritoneal metastases	WART 14.4 Gy ± boost
4 (Lung) persistent at 9 weeks, any histology	WLI 15 Gy/10#
4, Any HR tumour regardless of whether lung metastases present	WLI 15 Gy/10#
New lung metastases	WLI 15 Gy/10#
4, Brain	25.5 Gy ± boost of 4.5 Gy
4, Liver	20.05 Gy

HR high risk, *IR* intermediate risk, *WART* whole abdomen radiotherapy, *WLI* whole lung irradiation, # fractions

2. SIOP radiotherapy guidelines [8]

For SIOP, the decision for RT is also based on post-operative risk assessment, but this is *post-chemotherapy*:

- Risk assessment
- *Low risk* (*LR*): Mesoblastic nephroma, cystic partially differentiated nephroblastoma and completely necrotic nephroblastoma.
- *Intermediate risk* (*IR*): Epithelial, stromal, mixed, regressive, or focal anaplasia type nephroblastoma.
- *High risk* (*HR*): Blastemal, diffuse anaplasia (DA), clear cell sarcoma of the kidney (CCSK), rhabdoid tumour (Table 14.2).

Timing and Technique of Radiotherapy

For non-metastatic Wilms tumour, tumour bed RT, when required, should be commenced within 10 days of surgery.

Flank RT

Volumes

These are the same for COG and SIOP. They may be defined using simulator or image intensifier;

however, CT-based planning allows superior definition of volumetric doses to organs at risk.

- *Tumour bed* (*TB*) = outline of kidney + tumour as defined from *pre-operative* imaging
- *Clinical target volume* (*CTV*) = TB + 1–2 cm margin taking into account:
  - Pretreatment tumour size
  - Surgical findings and clips
  - Pathology report
- *Planning target volume* (*PTV*) = CTV + margin for movement and set-up error (about 1 cm) as well as:
  - Must include full width and length of vertebral bodies included in the radiation field (in order to prevent growth asymmetry later in life).
  - Must include the lateral abdominal wall.
- AP/PA parallel opposed fields are used and prescription is to a central dose (Fig. 14.1).

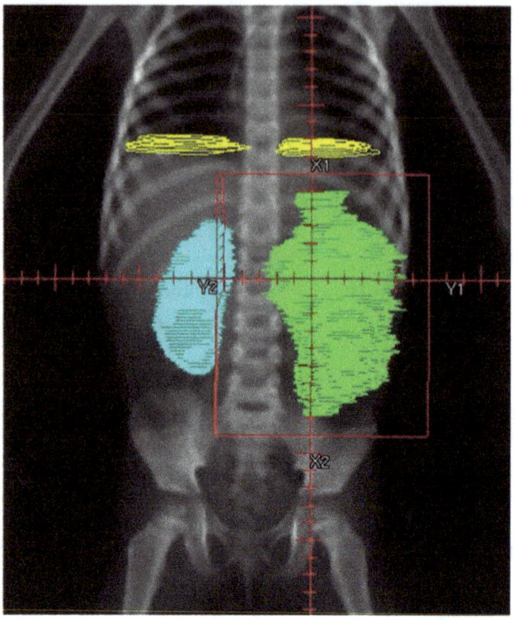

Fig. 14.1 Left flank radiotherapy for left-sided Wilms tumour. Gross tumour volume (GTV) shown in *green*. Opposite kidney shown in *blue*. From Halperin et al. [8]

Whole Abdomen Radiotherapy (WART)

Volumes

The entire abdominal contents with all peritoneal surfaces are included. Care must be taken to include the entire dome of the diaphragm, and extend down to the peritoneal reflection at the obturator foramina. The heads of femur are blocked. Anterior and posterior fields are used. Note that a margin of 2 cm is required if Cobalt-60 is used (Fig. 14.2).

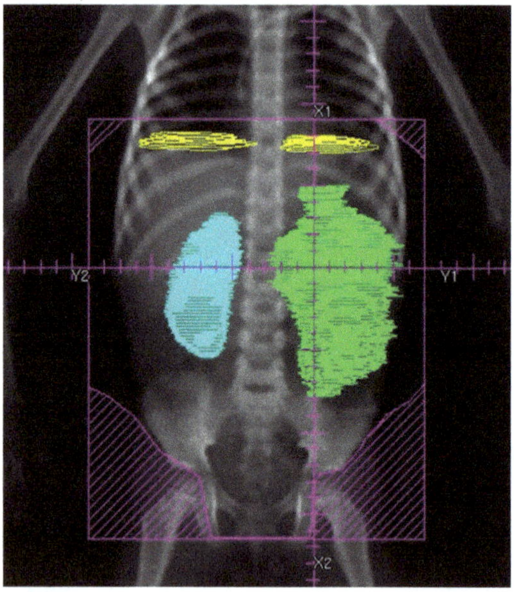

Fig. 14.2 Whole abdomen radiotherapy (WART) for diffuse spillage of a left-sided Wilms tumour. From Halperin et al. [8]

Whole Lung Irradiation (WLI)

This includes both entire lung fields and is treated with anterior and posterior fields. Care must be taken to extend fields to adequately cover both lung apices and inferior recesses. Posterior lung recesses are best seen on a lateral simulation view. If Cobalt-60 radiation is used, a margin of 2 cm on the target is required (Fig. 14.3).

If both lung and flank RT are required, these should be simulated and treated simultaneously as a single field. If whole lung and whole abdomen RT are required, these can be treated simultaneously, but in a child with any co-existing problem such as TB or malnutrition, it is advisable to plan the fields simultaneously but treat them sequentially with a 2 week gap between courses. Ideally, the lower half of the field is blocked for lung RT

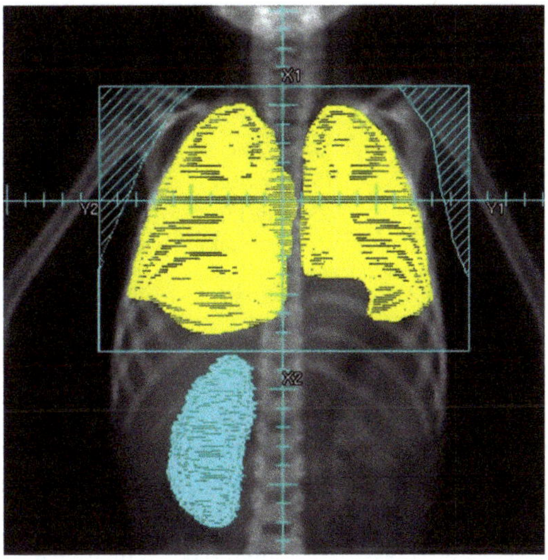

Fig. 14.3 Field for whole lung irradiation (WLI). Lung volumes indicated in *yellow*. Note that inferior recesses are best seen on a lateral view. From Halperin et al. [8]

and the upper for the abdomen RT. However, on Cobalt machines, this means very large and heavy lead blocks which are difficult for radiographers to lift. It may therefore be necessary to use two separate fields which require matching. Care must be taken not to overlap fields over the liver.

Boost Volumes

For boost volumes, or treatment volumes requiring higher doses, it is always preferable to use 3-D CT-based planning in order to adequately protect surrounding organs at risk, e.g. single residual kidney or lung. This allows the use of oblique treatment fields, if necessary.

If CT-planning is not available, then simulation or intensifier-based planning is used. This means parallel-opposed fields. Careful plotting of organs at risk is necessary using CT pictures and/or IVP.

Organs at Risk

There is very little literature available on tolerance doses of RT in children. Table 14.3 incorporates information from COG protocols.

Table 14.3 Paediatric radiotherapy tolerance doses (based on COG protocols)

Organ	Dose (cGy)
Single organs	
Bladder	4,500
Heart	3,000
Liver-whole	2,340
Liver-partial (50 %)	3,060
Spinal cord	4,500
Rectum	4,500
Peritoneum (whole abdomen pelvis)	2,400
Small bowel	4,500
Paired organs	
Kidney-whole	1,440
Kidney-partial (50 %)	1,980
Lung—whole	1,200
Lung (when PTV >1/2 bilateral lung volume)	1,500
Lung (when PTV <1/2 bilateral lung volume)	1,800

- When the whole abdomen or liver dose exceeds 1,440 cGy, the renal dose should be limited to 1,440 cGy by using appropriate renal shielding.
- Several techniques may be used for renal shielding when the whole abdomen irradiation (WAI) dose is >1,440 cGy. The use of posterior partial transmission kidney blocks for the entire course of treatment is recommended.
- The thickness of the block will be determined by the treatment plan. The dimensions of the block should be 0.5 cm wider than the projection of the kidney on a PA digitally reconstructed radiograph.

RT for Medulloblastoma

A prerequisite for radical treatment of medulloblastoma is the availability of a fairly sophisticated health system, including all of the items listed below:

- Adequate imaging (at least a CT scan) for diagnosis and planning, as well as portal field verification for quality assurance.
- Adequate surgery (trained surgeons, anaesthetist, and ICU services).
- Pathology services.
- Ability to plan craniospinal RT and to treat at least four fractions per week.

Table 14.4 Staging post-surgery in medulloblastoma—Tait and Evans stratification [8]

High risk	<3 years
	Leptomeningeal disease
	Residual tumour >1.5 cc
Average risk	≥3 years
	M0 on staging investigations
	Gross total resection

Table 14.5 Dose of craniospinal irradiation (CSI) in medulloblastoma

	Craniospinal axis	Posterior fossa boost
Full dose CSI (high risk)	36 Gy/20# (5× per week)	19.8 Gy/11# (5× per week)
Reduced dose CSI (average risk)—given with chemotherapy	23.4 Gy/13# (5× per week)	30.6 Gy/17# (5× per week)

- Availability of mould room services to manufacture blocks and/or compensators, as well as immobilisation devices adequate for reproducible and accurate field matching.

Craniospinal irradiation (CSI) is one of the most difficult techniques for any radiotherapy planning department or treatment floor. It requires advanced planning techniques in order to limit toxicity and these have evolved considerably over the past 15 years. It also requires reproducibility, and accurate set-up, in order to match fields [10].

Although CSI can be planned using an image intensifier or simulator together with a 2D planning system alone, this is extremely challenging and is associated with increased side effects. CT-based three-dimensional (3D) planning is easier and less time-consuming; however, it requires specialised equipment and software which is expensive and therefore is not available in many LICs. Similarly, although it is possible to administer CSI from a Cobalt-60 machine as opposed to a linear accelerator (Linac), it is much more difficult to achieve an acceptable plan and toxicity is greater.

General principles of treatment:

- Patients usually present acutely to neurosurgery with hydrocephalus. Initial diagnosis is made on imaging and then confirmed by histology after resection. Ideally spinal staging using MRI is done preoperatively, but in LICs and MICs this is frequently not feasible. Staging CSF sampling is done by lumbar CSF tap at least 2 weeks post-surgery. Immediate cytospin and microscopy of CSF may show tumour cells.
- Staging is done post-surgery (Table 14.4) [11]
- All children with medulloblastoma require CSI if cure is the aim.
- It is arguable that radical surgery should not be attempted in situations where CSI is not available, as no cure is possible. In this event, hydrocephalus should be shunted to relieve symptoms, and the child palliated.
- Children under 3 years of age require chemotherapy and surveillance until they are over 3 years of age, when they should receive CSI. They are classified as high risk. In many LICs and MICs, this may not be feasible. In such cases, these children should be palliated.

Dose of CSI

1. The dose used for CSI depends on several factors:
   (a) Ability to accurately stratify patients into average risk and high risk groups. (This requires MRI spinal imaging and/or CSF cytology.)
   (b) Availability of chemotherapy.
   (c) The ability of the family to bring the child for 6 cycles of adjuvant chemotherapy after CSI.

If the answer to any of the above is "no", then full dose CSI is given regardless of risk assessment. For patients who receive full dose CSI for logistical/practical reasons, no concurrent chemotherapy is administered (Table 14.5).

- For patients assessed as "average risk", and who are able to get chemotherapy, reduced dose CSI is given, together with weekly Vincristine during CSI and 6 cycles of adjuvant chemotherapy thereafter [12].
- For patients who are assessed as "high risk", they should receive full-dose craniospinal RT as well as 6 cycles of adjuvant chemotherapy.

Timing of RT

- RT treatment should be commenced within 40 days of surgery, and preferably within 28 days of surgery. Delays may lead to a worse prognosis.

- If delays are expected due to the patient's condition or planning delays, 1–2 cycles of chemotherapy can be given prior to starting radiotherapy.

During RT

- All patients require weekly full blood count (FBC) testing as a significant amount of bone marrow is in the field and pancytopenia may result. Delays are reserved for the unusual cases of extreme cytopenias and are avoided if at all possible.
- Many patients require anti-emetics during the CSI as a significant amount of small bowel and stomach is in the field and nausea/anorexia is a common side-effect. Treatment checks are done weekly and should include weekly FBC to look for bone marrow suppression due to treatment.
- Skin reaction around the pinna and neck is treated with 1 % hydrocortisone cream.
- Food and fluid intake and a weekly weight should be monitored in children, as many don't eat due to anorexia, nausea, or prolonged sedation.
- All patients require long-term follow-up for late toxicity of treatment including:
  - Neuro-cognitive problems
  - Psychosocial problems
  - Pituitary and thyroid hypofunction
  - Osteoporosis
  - Cardiovascular problems
  - Second malignancy

Technique for CSI

- Patients may be treated prone or supine for CSI. Supine treatment has many advantages [13], but requires that the beams are treated through the treatment couch and head rest. The treatment planning system must therefore have the ability to account for transmission through the couch or immobilisation devices that are in the posterior fields. This is not possible for older couches which have metal inserts. In this instance, prone treatment is mandatory and a custom-made body foam/shell and prone head cast are required for patient positioning and immobilisation. For supine treatment, an orfit cast can be used and is extended to below the shoulders.
- CT-planning is preferable, although several techniques for simulation and 2D planning have been widely used [10].
- The patient MUST be positioned straight with the help of lasers.
- The head should be placed in a slightly extended position and such that the cervical spine is as flattened as possible.

Beam Arrangement

- CSI is composed of two lateral head fields and a contiguous spinal posterior spinal field (Figs. 14.4 and 14.5).
  - The lateral head fields have a collimator rotation to match the superior beam edge of the spinal field. The head fields must be positioned to clear the shoulders.
  - Face shielding is accomplished by custom-made lead blocks if MLC (multi-leaf collimator) is not available.
    - The superior edge of the block should be situated 0.5 cm below the cribriform plate. It is important not to underdose the cribriform plate as this is bathed in CSF and is a site for recurrence in medulloblastoma.
    - The block should be placed 1 cm anteriorly to the middle cranial fossa, 1 cm inferiorly to the base of skull and extend posteriorly down the posterior pharyngeal wall. These bony structures should be identified when placing the block (Fig. 14.6).
  - The spinal fields, if not 3D planned, are simulated with a daily small couch rotation, alternately clockwise and anticlockwise, to match the beam divergence of the lateral head fields.
  - The junction between head and spine fields should be "feathered" by moving the junction by 1 cm at least twice during the course of CSI in order to minimise cold or hot spots caused by the junction/set-up error, etc.

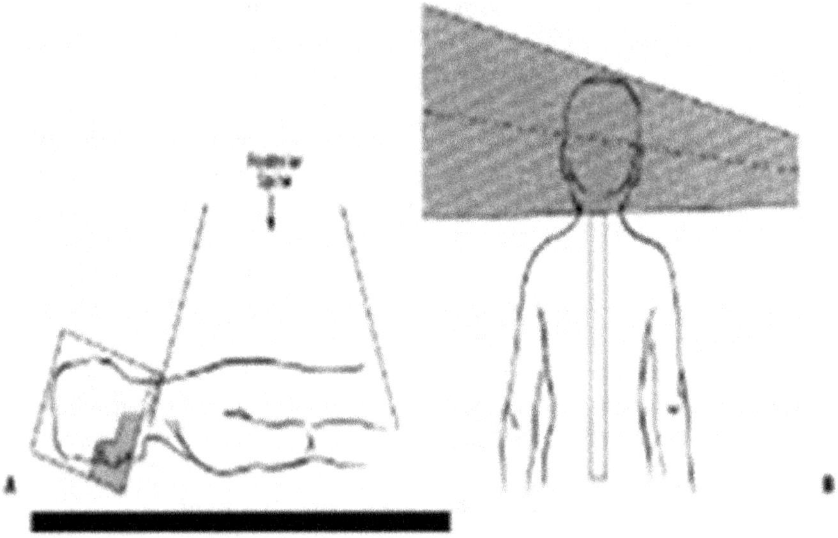

Fig. 14.4 Beams for prone craniospinal irradiation. From Halperin, 5th ed. [8]

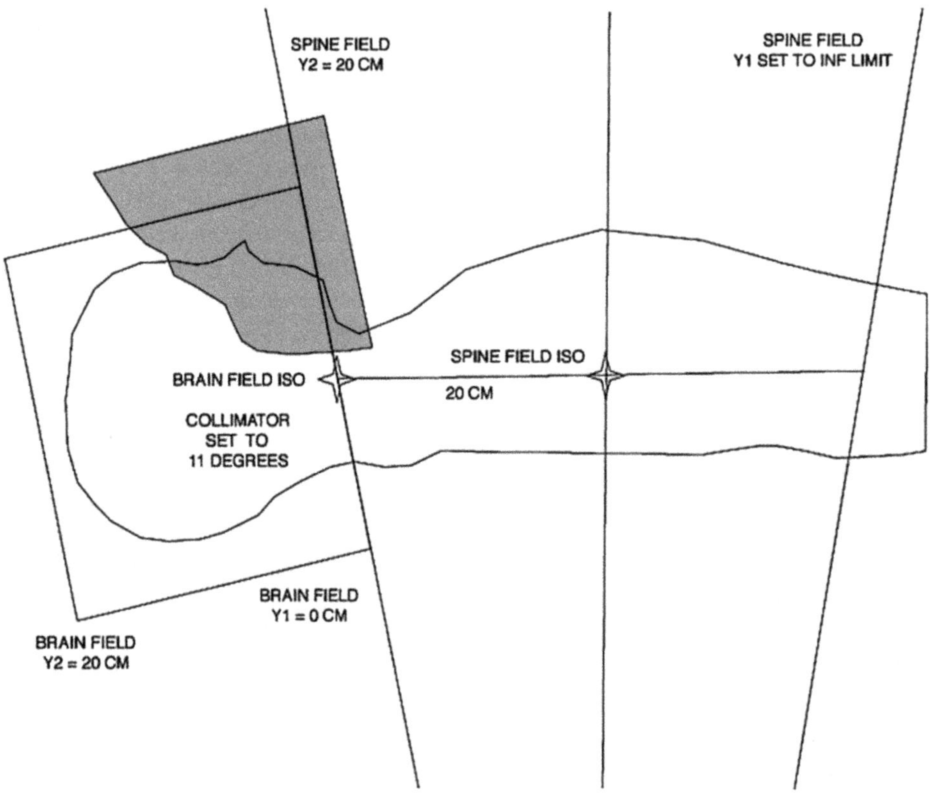

Fig. 14.5 A simple technique for supine craniospinal irradiation. From Parker et al. [13]

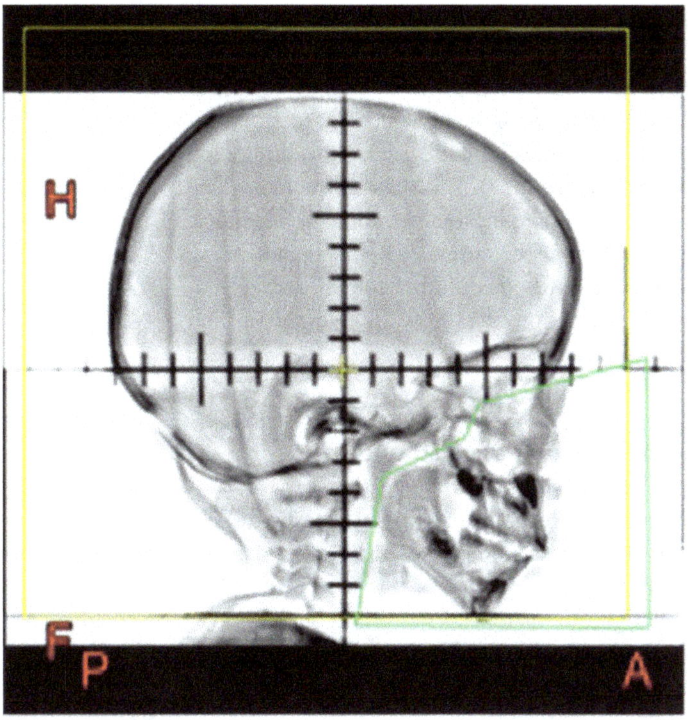

Fig. 14.6 Customised face block for lateral head fields

- The boost field can be treated as two parallel opposed lateral fields, with the posterior fossa field defined on a lateral skull X-ray, OR by a more conformal 3D planned volume (tumour bed + margin of 2 cm), defined on CT and planned with 3–5 fields [14].
- Ideally all fields should be summed and a total Gy plan produced.

Treatment

- It is critical to check the position of the fields prior to treatment. This is done on the simulator prior to starting treatment, or by portal imaging on the machine.
- The position of the axes as well as the position of the block relative to bony structures is checked. This is accomplished in the head fields, by a double exposure with and without the block, in order to visualise the bony anatomy behind the block.
- It is often helpful to see the projected light beams on the face at set-up.
- Lens doses may be measured using TLDs (thermo luminescence dosimetry) placed on the lateral canthus of the eye at the first or second treatment. This is not done in many first world centres where access to surgery for cataracts is easy. However in LICs and MICs, this may be less available and so keeping lens dose below 10 Gy is desirable.

The difficulty of treating medulloblastoma in LICs and MICs is that many countries do not have CT for RT planning even though it is available for diagnosis. Some do not have a working simulator although they may have competent surgeons and working cobalt machines. It could be argued that CSI should not be attempted in such a situation, as late effects of CSI are increased with 2D planning due to wider volumes and poorer dose homogeneity. It is preferable to refer these patients to centres where 3D planning and Linac-based RT is available.

Hair loss, growth and hormonal problems, coupled with poor learning ability make many of these children dependent on their families and the health care system for the rest of their lives.

RT for Rhabdomyosarcoma

Rhabdomyosarcoma (RMS) comprises about 3.5 % of cases of malignant disease in childhood. In a questionnaire sent to radiotherapy units in Africa in 2011, RMS was quoted as one of the four commonest indications for paediatric RT in African countries [2]; the others being Wilms tumour, medulloblastoma, and retinoblastoma, followed closely by lymphoma and palliation.

Principles of Management

Current COG studies stratify children with RMS into three risk groups according to prognostic factors [8].

Prognostic factors taken into account:

- *Histology*: Favourable (embryonal, botryoid, spindle cell) vs. unfavourable (alveolar, undifferentiated).
- *Stage*: Using site, invasiveness, tumour size, lymph node status, and presence/absence of metastases.
  - *Stage 1*: Localised or regional lymphatic spread in patients with orbit, head and neck (excluding parameningeal), genito-urinary (excluding bladder and prostate), biliary tract tumours.
  - *Stage 2*: Localised bladder or prostate, extremity, parameningeal head and neck, other.
  - *Stage 3*: As for Stage 2 but with lymphatic spread.
  - *Stage 4*: Any patient with distant metastases.
- *Clinical group*: IRS grouping system based on resectability.
  - *Group 1*: Localised disease, completely resected.
  - *Group 2*: Gross total resection with microscopic residual and/or resected regional lymphatic spread.
  - *Group 3*: Biopsy only or incomplete resection with gross residual disease.
  - *Group 4*: Distant metastases present at onset (Table 14.6).

Table 14.6 Risk groups in rhabdomyosarcoma [15]

Low risk	Localised AND embryonal AND favourable site OR Group 1 or Group 2 occurring at an unfavourable site
Intermediate risk	Embryonal at unfavourable site AND Group 3 OR Non-metastatic alveolar histology at any site
High risk	Metastatic disease, i.e. Group 4 or Stage 4

Treatment

Curative treatment almost always requires multidisciplinary therapy with combinations of chemotherapy, surgery and/or radiotherapy. Only RT treatment is discussed here, but comprehensive management is essential for these cases.

Radiotherapy

- Radiotherapy, together with surgery, is used in RMS to provide local and regional control.
- Chemotherapy is always used as part of the treatment protocol. Multi-modality treatment has the capacity to cause profound normal tissue damage, and ongoing COG study protocols have therefore been designed to try to minimise treatment for patients with low risk disease, while adequately treating patients with high risk disease.
- Current COG treatment protocols omit radiotherapy only for patients with Group 1, favourable histology disease [8].

Technique of RT

Because RMS can occur at any site in the body, and because it is critical that damage to normal tissue is minimised, it is highly recommended that RT is volume based (i.e. CT planning is preferable).

Minimum requirements:

- Immobilisation device
- CT scan for planning purposes

Table 14.7 Volumes and doses used in COG protocols ARST 0331 and ARST 0531 (rhabdomyosarcoma) [8]

GTV (gross tumour volume)	Pre-chemotherapy visible tumour
CTV (clinical target volume)	GTV + 1 cm. Include all proven nodal disease
PTV (planning target volume)	CTV + ITV (margin for organ motion) + institutional margin for set-up error

Table 14.8 Doses for planning in rhabdomyosarcoma

FH with microscopic residual (Group 1)	36 Gy/20#
FH with nodal disease	41.4 Gy/23#
Group 3 orbital tumours	45 Gy/25#
All other Group 3 tumours	50.4 Gy/28#

FH favourable histology

- 3D planning system
- Linac treatment preferable but Cobalt-60 adequate

Volumes used in Planning

The volumes and doses used as specified in current COG protocols ARST 0331 and ARST 0531 are summarised in Table 14.7.

A volume reduction after 36 Gy may be used for patients receiving 50.4 Gy who have had a substantial reduction in tumour size after surgery/chemotherapy (Table 14.8).

RT at Specific Sites

Bladder and Prostate

This represents about half of genito-urinary RMS and the exact origin of the tumour may be difficult to determine. Many of these children are also very young (<5 years of age). Therapeutic approaches have changed over time with these children. Aggressive surgery often led to good survival but terrible morbidity. More recent treatment protocols have been aimed at cure with preservation of bladder function. This is achieved with up-front chemotherapy and often preoperative RT, followed by conservative surgery.

Special considerations for RT technique:

- 3D planning is preferred for better target and normal structure delineation.
- Gross tumour volume (GTV) is defined as pretreatment tumour extent, but accounts for shifting structures, e.g. no need to cover area where previously displaced bowel has shifted to occupy area after chemotherapy or surgery.
- Depending on tumour position, better normal sparing may be obtained with either empty or full bladder, but this should be constant through treatment and is best managed with an in-situ catheter which may be clamped for treatment.
- Critical structures for delineation include bladder, rectum, bowel, pelvic and femoral growth plates, penile bulb, and testes.
- AP/PA or parallel opposed slightly oblique fields often give best shielding of femoral growth plates (tolerance is 10–20 Gy in young children).

Paratesticular RMS

This type of RMS is almost always of embryonal sub-type but has a relatively high rate of lymphatic spread to para-aortic nodes. CT of the abdomen is therefore an essential staging tool. This may however fail to demonstrate small involved nodes. The risk is higher for children over 10 years of age and therefore current practice is for any child with suspicious lymph nodes on CT AND all children >10 years to undergo ipsilateral retroperitoneal lymph node dissection. Any child who has had a scrotal biopsy is deemed to have group 2 disease and should be considered for hemi-scrotectomy or radiotherapy to the scrotum.

The commonest indication for RT is nodal disease and all patients with nodal disease should receive RT irrespective of response to chemotherapy.

Special considerations for RT technique:

- CT-planning is advised.
- Lymph nodes usually follow vessels and are found within 2 cm of vessels. Vessels and any involved lymph nodes should be contoured.
- AP/PA opposed fields are usually used.
- Critical structures include bowel, kidneys, bladder, femoral growth plates.

Vaginal/Vulval RMS

This is a rare tumour of very young girls (usually <2 years). Nodal involvement is uncommon. They are almost always embryonal and often botryoid. Current COG protocols aim to preserve organ function and therefore surgery in the primary setting is very conservative. Treatment is usually chemotherapy followed by non-mutilating surgery or RT.

Special considerations for RT technique:

- These tumours may be suitable for intracavitary brachytherapy if available.
- For external beam radiotherapy, CT-planning should be used.
- Doses are low (see guideline above).
- Critical structures include uterus, ovaries, rectum, bladder, bowel, bones.
- Consider ovary transposition prior to radiotherapy as doses >2–4 Gy may cause sterility.

Extremity RMS

This comprises 20 % of paediatric RMS and tends to have a poorer prognosis than other RMS because most of these tumours are of alveolar subtype, and there is a high incidence or lymphatic and distant metastases at presentation.

Special considerations for RT technique:

- Amputation should be considered in patients where limited excision and radiotherapy would have unacceptable functional results.
- Current COG studies require regional lymph node sampling as part of staging.
- CTV includes tumour or tumour bed with a 1.5 cm margin and includes involved regional lymph nodes only.
- A strip of soft tissue along the extremity should be spared from any dose to avoid future lymphoedema.
- CT planning with 3D conformal radiotherapy should be used. Fields are usually AP/PA or oblique parallel opposed fields.

Parameningeal RMS

These account for about half of the head and neck RMS tumours in children. They arise in areas where intracranial spread is a risk. The main areas are middle ear, nasal cavity, nasopharynx, infratemporal fossa, pterygopalatine fossa, and the parapharyngeal area. Many of these tumours invade through the base of skull, and these patients should be assessed for leptomeningeal seeding. Resection of these tumours is not usually feasible.

Special considerations for RT technique:

- CTV is defined as the pre-chemotherapy tumour volume + 1 cm margin.
- There is a cone-down to the post-chemotherapy volume + 1 cm after 36 Gy.
- Planning is complex and CT-planning is required.
- There is some evidence that earlier initiation of RT may improve results in patients with clear evidence of intracranial extension; however, if there is likely to be any delay in the start of radiotherapy due to planning constraints/waiting lists, then chemotherapy should be initiated. Furthermore, where tumours cause profound contour irregularities that may change with chemotherapy due to tumour shrinkage, it is not practical to replan, and RT is best delayed until after 1–2 courses of chemotherapy.
- Craniospinal radiotherapy is not indicated.
- Critical structures include eyes, lenses, chiasm, optic nerve and tracts, brain, temporal lobes, pituitary gland, cochleas, brainstem, parotid glands, and spinal cord.

Orbital RMS

This tumour comprises about 10 % of RMS and is often diagnosed early. It may be of embryonal or alveolar histology. Many of these patients are Group 3 at diagnosis and treatment consists of biopsy, chemotherapy, and RT [8].

Special considerations for RT technique:

- CT-planning should always be utilised because of the close proximity of normal structures. Advanced techniques may vastly improve late effects.
- Dose is 45 Gy in 28 fractions to both histological sub-types, although chemotherapy may differ.
- Critical structures include lens, lacrimal gland, cornea, retina, optic nerve, optic chiasm and brain.
- Treatment with the eyelids open may be preferred to limit the bolus effect.
- Brachytherapy should be considered for small localised tumours, or proton therapy if available.

Radiotherapy for Retinoblastoma

Introduction

Retinoblastoma is the commonest intra-ocular malignancy in childhood and is one of the commonest malignancies diagnosed in the first year of life. The incidence of retinoblastoma is quoted as approximately 1 in 18,000 live births. However, recent population-based studies have shown an apparently higher incidence of retinoblastoma in some developing countries compared to Western Europe. Decreased intake of fruit and vegetables during pregnancy and exposure to HPV have been suggested but not proven to play a role.

In developed countries retinoblastoma is usually diagnosed at an early stage and the disease-free survival is >80–90 %. In these countries a range of technologically advanced treatments are often used to conserve affected eyes with useful vision—but these techniques are not the reason for the high disease-free survival figures—simple enucleation of the diseased eye is curative. Whatever treatment is applied, the key to survival is early detection.

In developing countries the diagnosis of retinoblastoma is often made when the disease is already advanced and there is extra ocular extension. When retinoblastoma has spread outside the globe, it is difficult to cure. As a consequence the survival rates are correspondingly lower. In developing countries families are also more likely to withdraw from treatment. In some African or Asian countries the survival is almost zero because patients do not complete treatment or are lost to follow-up [16, 17].

Treatment Options for Retinoblastoma

Radiotherapy for retinoblastoma may take the form of external beam RT or brachytherapy. Brachytherapy is complex to plan and requires specialised expertise and equipment to execute accurately. It is therefore only performed in a few centres in the world and patients may require referral to other countries for treatment.

The advantages of brachytherapy are the relative sparing of normal tissue and the consequent reduction in the cosmetic side-effects of external beam radiotherapy as well as the risk of developing second malignancies in later life.

The retinoblastoma gene predisposes the carrier to the development of sarcomas—especially osteosarcomas—and this risk is significantly increased by exposure to radiation: 35 % of patients with retinoblastoma who undergo external beam RT will die of second malignancies within 40 years. For this reason, these children should be followed up for life [16, 18].

External beam RT is more readily available in LICs and MICs. Relatively simple planning techniques—using either Linacs or Cobalt machines—can be useful in both the radical and palliative settings. In LICs and MICs, retinoblastoma most commonly presents as advanced disease and consequently the non-availability of brachytherapy is less important the therapy is a value in this situation.

It must be mentioned that new localised treatment options for retinoblastoma have come into use recently. These include intra-arterial Melphalan (administered directly into the ophthalmic artery) and intra-vitreal Methotrexate. In several specialised centres these are being used—sometimes in combination with cryotherapy and/or laser therapy—in the place of brachytherapy. These two therapies are used for different presentations of the disease and are not interchangeable as treatment options [19].

Systemic chemotherapy also plays a vital role in the treatment of this disease and is incorporated into the management of almost all stages of retinoblastoma. The most commonly used chemotherapy drugs are Vincristine, Etoposide and Carboplatin (VEC). Detailed discussion of the used of chemotherapy in retinoblastoma is beyond the scope of this chapter [19].

Indications for RT for Retinoblastoma

The treatment protocols for retinoblastoma—including the application of radiotherapy—are dependent on the staging (and grouping) of the

Table 14.9 Retinoblastoma staging system according to the New Group Classification and the International Retinoblastoma Classification

Stage 0 (disease localised to the eye)	Group A	Tumour ≤3 mm; at least 3 mm from fovea; > 1.5 mm from disc
	Group B	Tumour >3 mm at any site, no vitreous seeds ± <5 mm sub-retinal fluid
	Group C	Focal vitreous seeds and/or <1 quadrant sub-retinal fluid
	Group D	Extensive vitreous/sub-retinal seeds and/or massive non-discrete tumour
	Group E	Destruction of the eye—requires enucleation—therefore Stage I
Stage I (eye enucleated, completely removed histologically)	C0	No choroidal infiltration
	C1	Minimal choroidal infiltration (<3 mm in any diameter)
	C2	Extensive choroidal infiltration (>3 mm in any diameter)
	S0	No scleral infiltration
	S1	Microscopic scleral infiltration
	N0	No involvement of optic nerve
	N1	Invasion of nerve up to/into the lamina cribros
	N2	Invasion of nerve beyond lamina cribros
Stage II (eye enucleated, microscopic residual tumour)	S2	Microscopic extra-scleral extension
	N3	Involvement of the cut end of optic nerve and/or subarachnoid invasion
	NX	Unknown
Stage III (laco regional extension)	(a) Overt orbital disease	
	(b) Pre-auricular/cervical node metastases	
Stage IV (metastatic disease)	(a) Haematogenous metastases (no CNS involvement)	1. Single lesion 2. Multiple lesions—includes bone marrow involvement
	(b) CNS extension (±other metastatic disease)	1. Pre-chiasmatic lesion 2. CNS mass 3. Leptomeningeal and CSF disease

disease. Many staging systems have been developed and used over the years. The current staging systems used world wide, the New Group Classification [20] and the International Retinoblastoma Classification [21] are summarised in Table 14.9. Note that in bilateral retinoblastoma each eye is grouped separately but staged according to the worse eye.

Stage 0

In Stage 0 disease the affected eye(s) often has useful vision and in specialised centres a combination of focal therapies are used in an attempt to salvage the eye(s). Focal therapies include brachytherapy, cryotherapy and trans-pupillary thermotherapy (laser)—with/without systemic chemotherapy.

In LICs and MICs this type of treatment is usually not available. If possible, patients should be referred to a specialised centre, but if this is not feasible then the options are: (a) simple enucleation if unilateral disease or, in the case of bilateral disease, (b) external beam radiation to both eyes, or (c) enucleation of worst affected eye with external beam radiation to the other eye.

Brachytherapy for Stage 0

(a) A custom-built plaque (gold loaded with I-125 seeds) is used to deliver 35–40 Gy to the apex of the tumour over 4 days. (Note: ready-made plaques in various sizes/shapes, e.g. Ruthenium plaques are also available.) The plaque must be inserted and removed under general anaesthetic by a specially trained opthalmologist. The radiotherapy planning requires specialised medical physics input. Eye plaques are used:

- As focal therapy for tumours too large to be treated with cryo-/laser therapy only.
- For treatment failures after cryotherapy or laser therapy [19, 22, 23].

(b) Whole-eye irradiation uses an I-125 applicator ("claws") to deliver 35–40 Gy to the whole eye over 4 days. The "claws" applicator was developed at Goore Schuur Hospital [24]. It is made of gold and consists of a pericorneal ring and four arms (claws) loaded with I-125 seeds. The ring is sutured to the 4 extraocular muscles and the 4 claws are inserted arived the eye between each of the extraocular muscles and sutured to the ring. The procedure is done under anaesthetic by an opthalmologist. Whole-eye radiation is indicated for:

- Consolidation of Group D eyes after chemotherapy
- Multiple tumours too large to treat with an I-125 plaque
- Posterior pole tumours—Groups B, C (these are difficult to cover with an adequate margin using a plaque); proton therapy would also be an option for these tumours [4].

External Beam RT for Stage 0

In LICs and MICs, retinoblastoma most commonly presents as advanced disease and consequently the unavailability of brachytherapy is less important. The availability of external beam RT (and chemotherapy) is of value in this setting.

The Schipper technique has long been associated with external beam RT treatment for retinoblastoma in an intact eye [26]. But the specialised equipment and need for general anaesthesia for each treatment makes it impractical for use in LICs and MICs. Alternative external beam techniques are more practical although the dose coverage of the eye is not as food.

For all external beam RT techniques, immobilisation in a thermoplastic/Perspex cast is essential to protect adjacent vital structures. The child is positioned supine—with the neck in a neutral or slightly flexed position.

Unilateral Disease

In some cases enucleation may be recommended– the aim being to cure the disease with one procedure. In instances where this is not deemed appropriate, and brachytherapy is not an option, or if the family refuse enucleation, external beam RT may be useful.

(a) Single lateral field with half-beam blocking: In unilateral disease a single lateral field may be used to treat tumours in the posterior part of the eye [25, 27, 28]. There are some limitations to this technique—these are discussed below.

If a Cobalt machine is to be used for treatment, then the smallest field size available is usually 5×5 cm. Half-beam blocking is used to shield the anterior half of the field to create a sharp beam edge—thus treating as much of the involved eye as possible—while simultaneously protecting the lenses of both eyes. However, because the smallest field size is 5×5 cm, even the half-beam blocked field will extend further posteriorly than is necessary to treat intra ocular retinoblastoma. The only way to prevent this is for the machine to be calibrated for smaller fields—which may not be possible in most centres. A fixed SSD technique is used. In order to get coverage of as much of the eye as possible—while minimising dose to the lens—the field is positioned so that the 10 % isodose passes through the lens and the 20 % isodose passes just behind the lens. The prescription is 40–45 Gy in 1.8–2 Gy per fractor as a given dose. However, because of the lower energy of Cobalt-60, only the 70 % isodose will cover most of the posterior part of the eye. The 50 % isodose will extend into the contralateral eye and orbit. If the dose is then prescribed to a depth or a specific isodose (to obtain better coverage), correspondingly, the dose to the lens as well as to the contralateral eye will also increase. Dose to the contralateral eye may compromise treatment to that

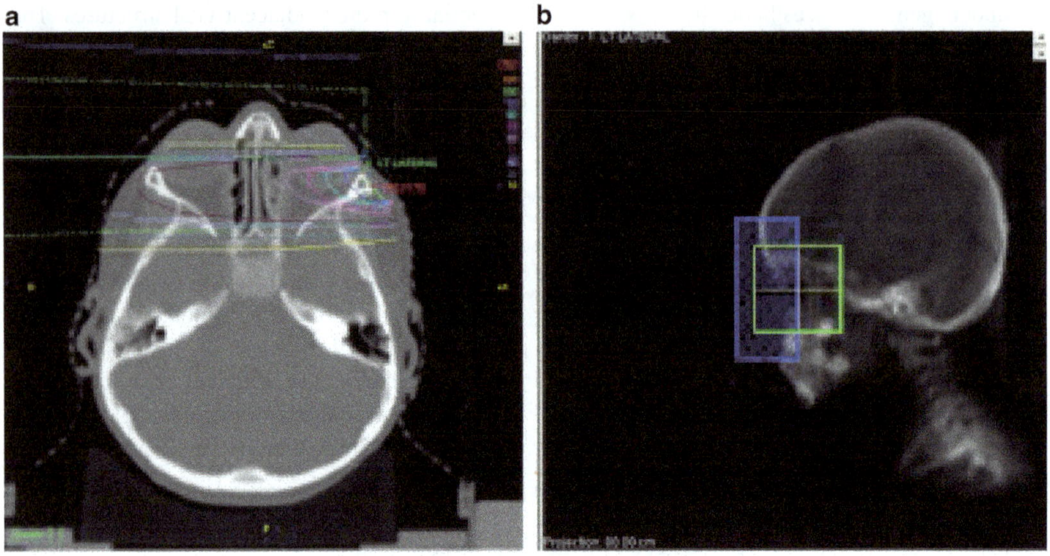

File Edit View	
Beam	1. LT LATERAL
Unit	Theratron III, Co-60
Rad Type / Algorithm	Isotope / PB
Nom. Acc. Pot.(MV)	2.600
FSDD (cm)	80.00
Weight	1.000
Width (cm)	5.00
-x Jaw (cm)	-2.50
+x Jaw (cm)	2.50
Length (cm)	5.00
+y Jaw (cm)	2.50
-y Jaw (cm)	-2.50
X (cm)	4.27
Y (cm)	-124.00
Z (cm)	5.60
SSD (cm)	80.00
Depth (cm)	0.00
Gantry (degrees)	90.0
Collimator (degrees)	0.0
Couch (degrees)	0.0

Fig. 14.7 Cobalt-60 single lateral beam with half-beam blocking

eye/orbit in the future which must be taken into consideration if the patient has known bilateral retinoblastoma—or a high risk for developing contralateral disease in the future (Fig. 14.7).

If 3D conformal RT planning is available, the beam dimensions and positions are determined using the measurements from the planning CT scan.

If 3D conformal RT is not available, it is possible to mark up the patient at the simulator. A clinical mark-up potentially does not have the same accuracy as can be achieved with CT-guided planning but is sufficiently accurate to be a safe and useful technique. When marking up a patient at the simulator, the middle of the field should be positioned approximately 3 mm behind the limbus (the posterior edge of the half-beam block will lie along this middle line). This will result in an isodose distribution as close as possible to that described above for CT-guided planning.

The two advantages of using a 6 MV beam in place of Cobalt-60 in this situation

a

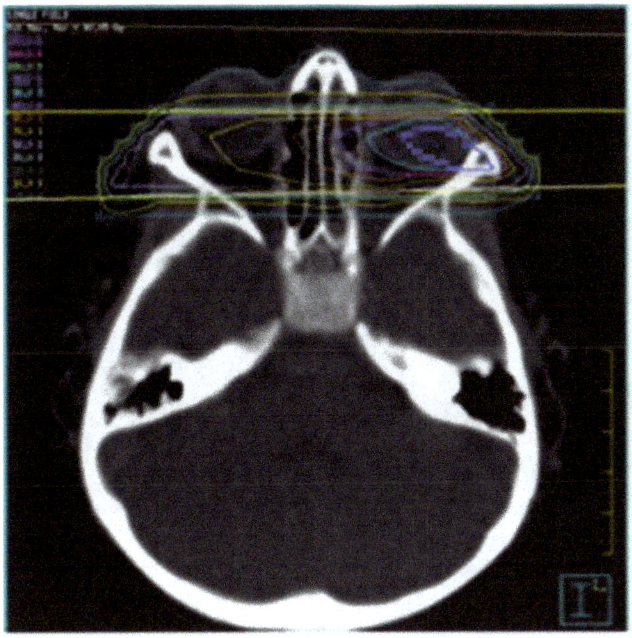

b

Field Order/Type	1 / Treat
Field ID	1 LT LATERAL
Field Name	
Technique	STATIC
Scale	IEC61217
Energy	6X
Dose Rate [MU/min]	600
MU	
Time [min]	
Tol. Table	
Calculated SSD [cm]	96.0
Planned SSD [cm]	96.1
Gantry Rtn [deg]	90.0
Coll Rtn [deg]	0.0
Field X [cm]	4.0
X1 [cm]	
X2 [cm]	
Field Y [cm]	4.0
Y1 [cm]	
Y2 [cm]	
MLC	NONE

Fig. 14.8 Single lateral 6 MV beam with half-beam blocking

are (i) the higher energy beam gives much better dose coverage of the eye (although at the expense of a higher dose to the contralateral eye) and (ii) the availability of a smaller field size (4×4 cm) means that less tissue behind the eye is unnecessarily included in the treatment field. The field set-up is the same as that described above for Cobalt-60 (Fig. 14.8) except that the SSD is not fixed.

(b) Single lateral field angled 5° posteriorly:
If half-beam blocking is not available, then this technique can be used to treat tumours in the posterior part of the eye. By angling the lateral field 5° posteriorly the dose to the contralateral lens is reduced [27, 28]. A fixed SSD technique is used with no wedge in the field. Similar to the half-beam blocked field described above, the beam is positioned so that the 10 % isodose passes through the lens and the 20 % isodose is just behind the lens. In a small child the 90 % isodose will cover the back of the eye. The smaller available field size of the 6 MV beam makes this the only beam option for this technique—but more normal tissue is treated than with the half-beam blocked technique described above. Cobalt-60 should *not* be used as the smallest available field (5×5 cm) when angled 5° covers too large an area of normal tissue posteriorly see Figure (X).
Note: tumours in the anterior part of the eye will not be adequately treated using a single lateral field—anterior tumours should be treated with cryotherapy and/or laser therapy (if small enough) with/without chemotherapy, or alternatively, by means of enucleation if too large for these treatment modalities.

Bilateral Disease

(a) Parallel-opposed lateral fields with half-beam blocking:

In bilateral disease two parallel-opposed lateral fields may be used to treat tumours in the posterior part of the eye [25, 28].

If a Cobalt machine is to be used for treatment, then the smallest field size available is usually 5×5 cm. Half-beam blocking is used to shield the anterior half of the field to create a sharp beam edge—thus treating as much of the involved eyes as possible—while

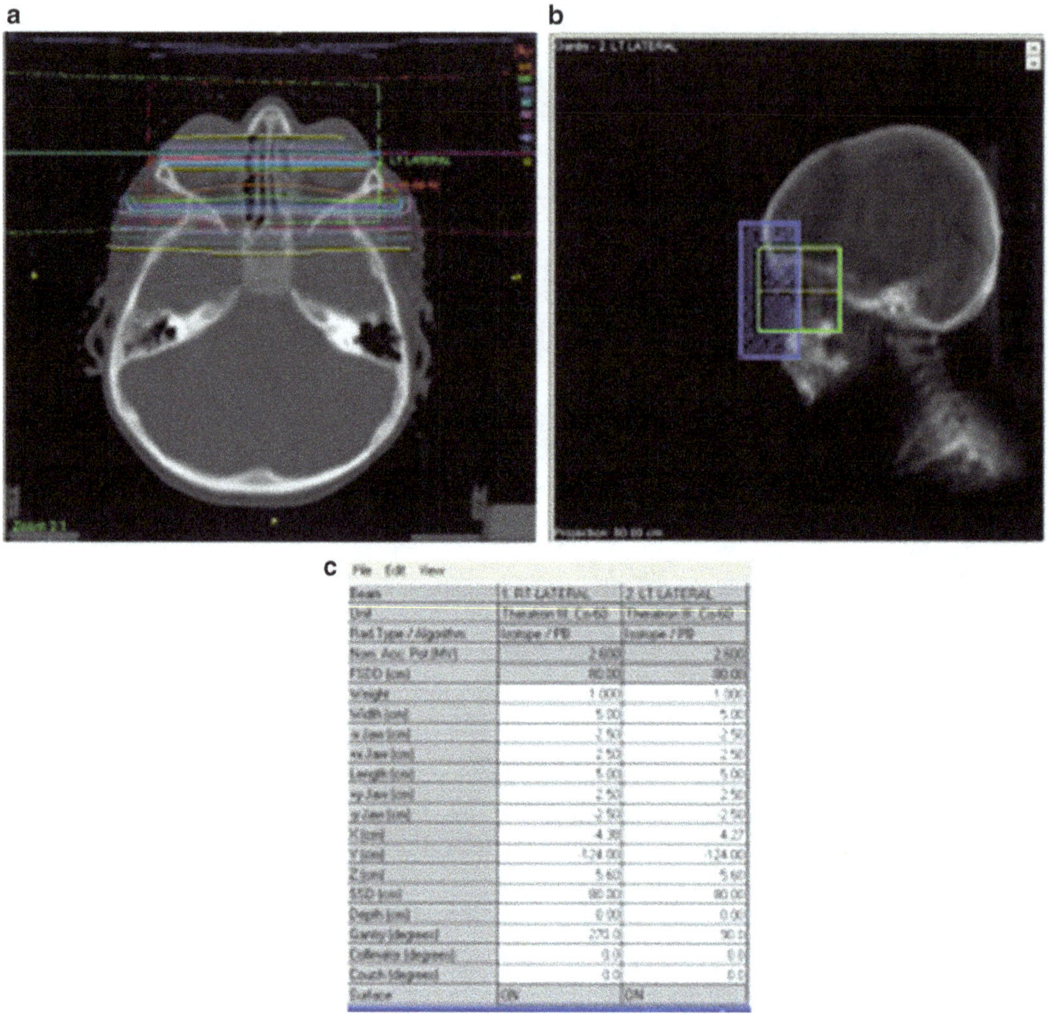

Fig. 14.9 Cobalt-60 parallel-opposed lateral beams with half-beam blocking

simultaneously protecting the lenses. However, because the smallest field size is 5×5 cm, even the half-beam blocked field will extend further posteriorly than is necessary to treat intra ocular retinoblastoma. A fixed SSD technique is used. A central dose of 40–45 Gy in 1.8–2 Gy fractions is prescribed. The dose is normalised at the centre of the volume. In order to get coverage of as much of the eye as possible, the field is positioned so that the 10 % isodose passes through the lenses and the 20 % isodose passes just behind the lenses of both eyes. The 90 % isodose will cover most of the posterior part of both eyes (as well as the superior nasal cavity/ethmoid sinus between the eyes) (Fig. 14.9).

The main advantage of using 6 MV beams in place of Cobalt-60 in this situation is the availability of a smaller field size (4×4 cm) which means that less tissue behind the eyes is unnecessarily included in the treatment field. The dose distribution is also more homogenous. The field set-up is the same as that described above for Cobalt-60 except that an isocentric technique is used (if available) and the dose (40–45 Gy in 1.8–2 Gy fractions) is prescribed to the ICRU point (Fig. 14.10).

a

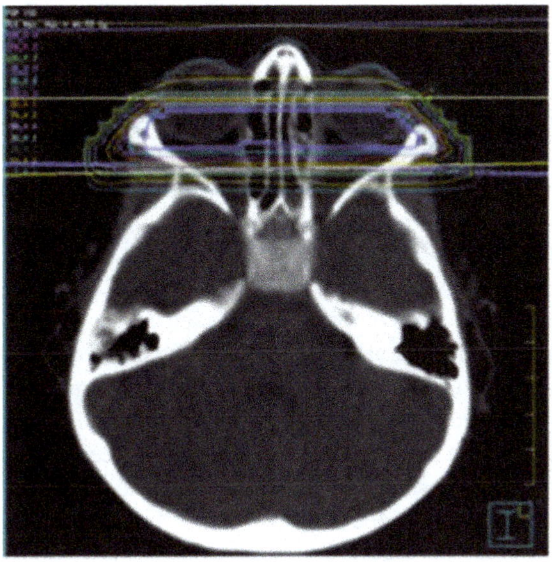

b

Field Order/Type	1 / Treat	2 / Treat
Field ID	1 RT LATERAL	2 LT LATERAL
Field Name		
Technique	STATIC	STATIC
Scale	IEC61217	IEC61217
Energy	6X	6X
Dose Rate [MU/min]	600	600
MU		
Time [min]		
Tol. Table		
Calculated SSD [cm]	95.9	96.0
Planned SSD [cm]	96.0	96.1
Gantry Rtn [deg]	270.0	90.0
Coll Rtn [deg]	0.0	0.0
Field X [cm]	4.0	4.0
X1 [cm]		
X2 [cm]		
Field Y [cm]	4.0	4.0
Y1 [cm]		
Y2 [cm]		
MLC	NONE	NONE

Fig. 14.10 6 MV parallel-opposed lateral beams with half-beam blocking

If 3D conformal RT planning is available, the beam dimensions and positions are determined using the measurements from the planning CT scan.

If 3D conformal RT is not available, it is possible to mark up the patient at the simulator. A clinical mark-up potentially does not have the same accuracy as can be achieved with CT-guided planning but is sufficiently accurate to be a safe and useful technique. When marking up a patient at the simulator, the middle of the field should be positioned approximately 3 mm behind the limbus (the posterior edge of the half-beam block will lie along this middle line). This will result in an isodose distribution as close as possible to that described above for CT-guided planning.

(b) Parallel-opposed lateral fields angled 5° posteriorly:

If half-beam blocking is not available, then this technique can be used to treat tumours in the posterior part of both eyes. By angling the lateral fields 5° posteriorly the dose to the lenses is reduced [28]. A fixed SSD or an isocentric technique with 30° wedges is used. Similar to the half-beam blocked fields described above, the beams are positioned so that the 10 % isodose passes through the lenses and the 20 % isodose is just behind the lenses. In a small child the 90 % isodose will cover the back of the eyes. The smaller available field size of the 6 MV beam makes this the only beam option for this technique—but more normal tissue is treated than with the half-beam blocked technique described above. Cobalt-60 should *not* be used as the smallest available field (5 × 5 cm) when angled 5° covers too large an area of normal tissue posteriorly see Figure (Y).

Stage I

The enucleated eye is examined histologically and if N0, N1, C0 or C1 disease then no further treatment is needed. If there is C2 or S1 disease then systemic chemotherapy is warranted. In addition to chemotherapy, orbital RT is necessary for S1. Orbital radiotherapy is also indicated for N2 disease if there is tumour <4 mm from the resection line [4]. It is preferable to administer orbital RT by means of brachytherapy but if this is not available, then external beam RT is suitable. These two radiotherapy techniques are described below under "Stage II".

Stage II

Systemic chemotherapy and orbital radiation is indicated in all patients. Intrathecal chemotherapy may be necessary for N3 disease. Orbital RT is preferably given by means of brachytherapy but external beam RT is a suitable alternative [4].

Orbital Brachytherapy for Stage I and II

The availability of brachytherapy for Stage I and II disease although ideal, is not essential. The technique used at Goore Schuur Hospital (Cape Town) is described briefly here for completeness only. Six plastic tubes loaded with 1–125 seeds, each opproximately 3 cm long, are inserted anteriorly through the eyelid towards the apex of the orbit posterionty under general anaesthetic. They are positioned at equal intervals around the rim of the orbited cavity. If there is no prosthetic implant attached to the extra ocular muscles, then a slightly shorter train is also inserted into the centre of the orbit. A 1.5 cm lead disc loaded with I-125 seeds on its posterior surface is sutured behind the eyelids to complete the implant [29]. The positioning of the tubes is checked in theatre using radiographic screening. A dose of 35–40 Gy is given over approximately 4 days whereafter the implant is removed (again under general anaesthetic). The technique requires the specialised expertise of a Madical Physicist and rould Room technician for preparation and planning.

External Beam RT to the Orbit for Stage I and II

Once the orbit has healed after enucleation—approximately 3 weeks—orbital radiotherapy can commence [27, 28]. Two wedged fields give adequate coverage of the orbit in a small child whether using a Cobalt-60 or a 6 MV beam. The medial edge of the field is parallel to the medial wall of the orbit. Dose to the optic chiasm and the pituitary area is kept as low as possible. With the beam arrangement as shown below, the 10 % isodose passes behind the contralateral eye. This means that the opposite eye/orbit could still be treated with radiation in the future—should it ever become necessary. A fixed SSD technique is used when treating with Cobalt-60 and an isocentric technique when treating with a 6 MV beam (Linac) (Figs. 14.11 and 14.12). A dose of 35–40 Gy in 1.8–2 Gy fractions is given.

Stage III

In the case of Stage IIIa (overt extra ocular disease), the treatment of choice is enucleation. One/two cycles of chemotherapy may be necessary first to make surgery easier (the course of 6 cycles chemotherapy is completed post-enucleation). External beam RT to the orbital contents (±10 Gy) can be used in addition to or instead of chemotherapy to facilitate enucleation. CT planning is the easier way to determine the ideal beam arrangement but it is also possible to mark the patient up at the simulator. The technique is similar to that used for orbital external beam RT post-enucleation about the dose increased to 45 Gy.

If it is confirmed after enucleation that no tumour extended into/beyond the orbital apex or into bone, then orbital radiotherapy in the form of either brachytherapy or external beam RT is given. If there is bony involvement or extension of tumour into/beyond the orbital apex, then only external beam RT is appropriate.

Extenteration is rarely indicated. Orbital radiotherapy can also be used to palliate inoperable disease.

The techniques for orbital RT (brachytherapy and external beam RT) for Stage IIIa are as described above for Stage I and II.

Stage IIIb disease requires loco regional treatment of pre-auricular and/or cervical lymph nodes—in addition to treatment of the orbit. Enucleation is indicated (as for Stage IIIa) but a neck dissection is contraindicated. Systemic chemotherapy is given and the orbit and involved nodal areas are treated with external beam radiotherapy. The technique for irradiating the preauricular and cervical nodes is similar to that for tumours/nodes in the parotid gland with associated nodes in the neck and is not described here. Radiation to the orbit is described above (for Stage I and II retinoblastoma). Palliative radiation to the orbit is described below under Stage IV.

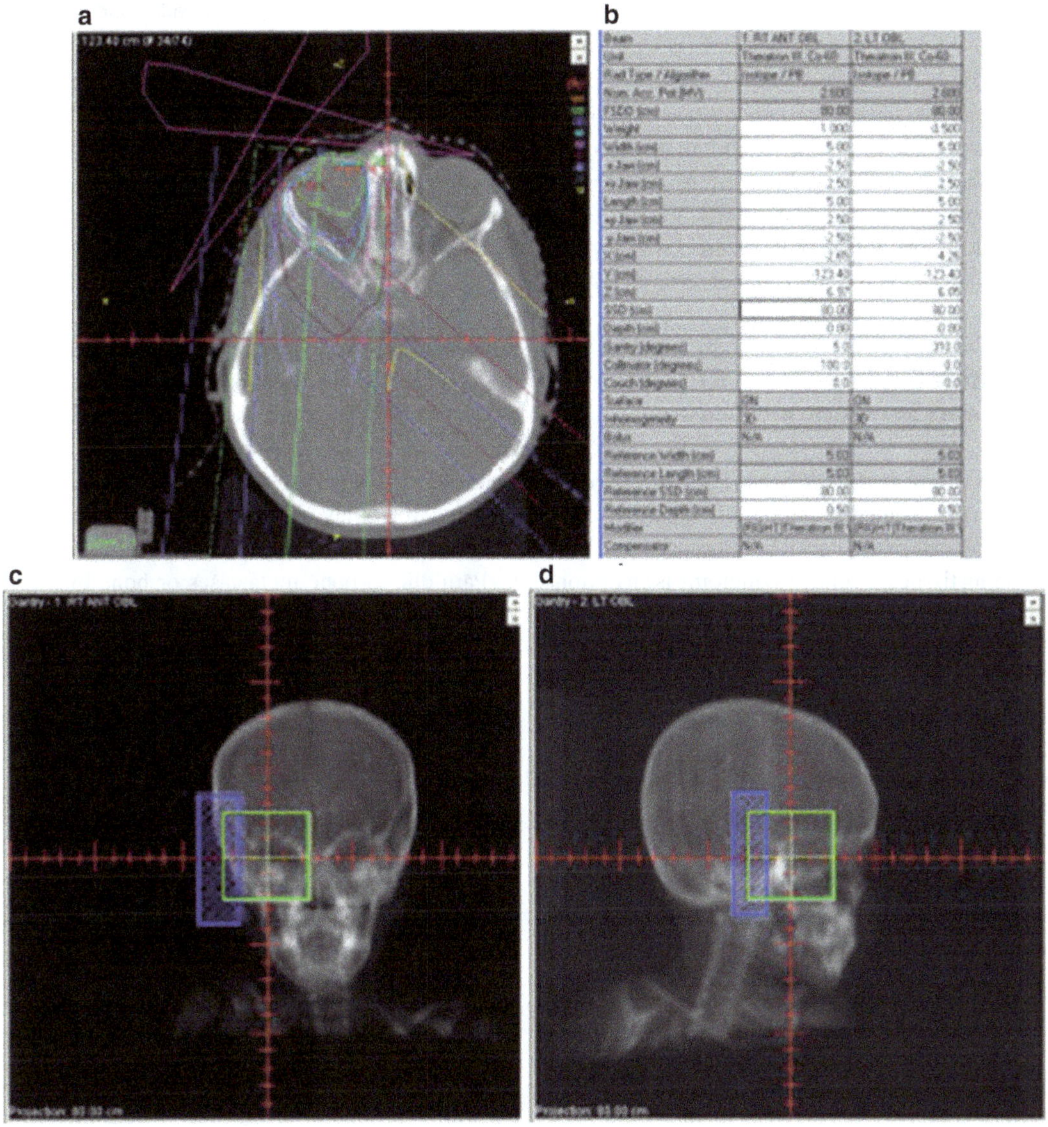

Fig. 14.11 Orbital radiotherapy: Cobalt-60

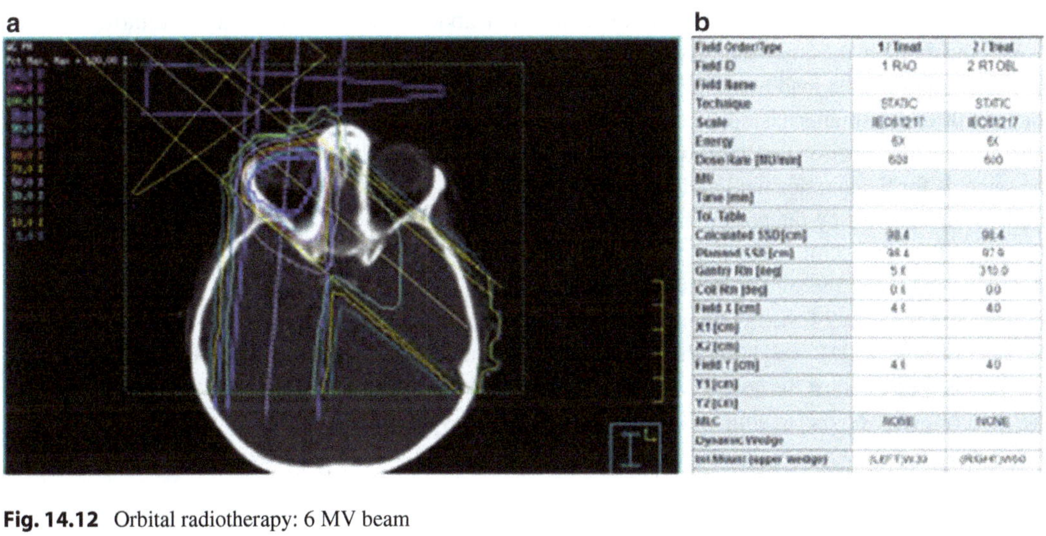

Fig. 14.12 Orbital radiotherapy: 6 MV beam

Stage IV

These patients have metastatic disease. The treatment approach is palliative and in addition to chemotherapy, RT can be used to relieve the symptoms associated with bone and/or CNS metastases. The RT techniques used will depend on the site(s) involved and are not described here.

Palliative External Beam RT to the Orbit and Surrounding Tissues

If there is gross orbital disease but surgery (enucleation) is deemed inappropriate or impossible, palliative external beam RT to the orbit and surrounding tissues to relieve symptoms is an option.

CT-guided planning is the easier way of planning radiotherapy to the orbit but it is possible to mark the patient up clinically at the simulator. The technique described below was originally developed to deliver palliative RT to patients with advanced tumours of the maxillary antrum but it can be adapted to treat the orbit. This particular technique is only applicable if one orbit is to be treated. A fixed SSD technique is used and either Cobalt-60 or 6 MV beams are appropriate for administering treatment. An anterior field is marked up to encompass all gross disease (preferably determined from a diagnostic CT scan if available—but otherwise from clinical examination) with a 1–2 cm margin. If necessary, the ipsilateral intra-parotid nodes and cervical nodes can be treated at the same time as the orbit using this technique (by extending the treatment volume laterally and inferiorly to cover these areas). If the medial border of the field crosses the midline, the contralateral eye should be shielded (using simple lead blocks). The gantry is rotated 90° and a smaller lateral ("boost") field is marked out: the superior and inferior borders are the same as for the anterior field and the posterior border is determined by the posterior extent of the disease within the skull. The anterior border is placed 4 cm behind the most anterior part of the tumour. The majority of the treatment is given by the anterior field 100 % weighting the smaller lateral field is used to boost the dose as it tapers off in the posterior part of the treatment volume 30 % weighting. A given dose is prescribed to the 85 % isodose and a manual dose calculation is done. The usual prescription is 4 Gy × 5 fractions or 3 Gy × 10 fractions at 85 % [30].

Palliative RT in Paediatric Oncology

In MICs and LICs, palliative RT is extremely important as many more children present late in the course of their disease and will not be amenable to cure. The cure rates seen in paediatric cancers in the developed world do not apply. Because of this, paediatric palliative RT is required relatively frequently. The commonest indications for this are:

- Pain due to bone metastases or bone marrow infiltration
- Large masses restricting function
- Nodal masses causing pain and/or oedema
- Control of neurological symptoms

Palliation is frequently achieved with a single fraction of 8 Gy or a course of 4–5 fractions (total = 20 Gy) [13]. Single fractions work well for pain, and relief can be almost immediate. This can be repeated later if necessary, if pain recurs at the same site. For masses restricting function, it is preferable to use several fractions so that a longer lasting effect is obtained. In these cases, maximum response is usually seen 1–2 weeks following treatment.

Side effects, although temporary, may be distressing and should be avoided if possible. For example, if the field covers the chest, the patient and parents must be warned about oesophagitis. For abdominal fields, nausea or vomiting should be prevented with anti-emetics. Head or neck radiotherapy can cause mucositis, dry mouth and loss of taste. Field shaping using simple lead blocks may help prevent some side effects.

Special Situations

- *Spinal cord compression*: If prompt, treatment can cause reversal of symptoms. This is especially true if RT is started within 48 h of onset of symptoms. This indication constitutes a radiotherapy emergency.

- *Whole lung RT*: Usually used in osteosarcoma/Ewing sarcoma when chemo has failed. 12–15 Gy in 1.5 Gy per fraction, given to the whole lung fields can give excellent palliation.
- *Parallel opposed radiotherapy for brainstem glioma*: It gives good temporary symptom relief. The diagnosis is usually a radiological one made on CT scan. There is a dose response for treatment, but outcome is almost always fatal within 2 years. A cast should be used for this and lateral fields encompassing the brainstem and extending down to the C2 vertebra are used. Doses may vary from 30 Gy/10# to full fractionation of 54 Gy as a dose response is observed for this disease. For full fractionation, CT-planning is preferred. Sedation should be used cautiously in these children.

Conclusion

- The availability of RT services in developing countries is extremely varied.
- Accessibility of specialised paediatric RT services is virtually non-existent and most paediatric patients are treated in large general radiotherapy referral centres.
- The setting up of multidisciplinary paediatric oncology meetings is essential in order to create centre-specific protocols for patients.
- For certain diseases requiring high levels of sophistication with respect to planning and delivery of RT (e.g. medulloblastoma, RMS), it may be appropriate to allocate regional centres of excellence to treat these paediatric patients.
- Twinning with regular meetings with international centres of excellence can help to overcome some of the problems with access to expertise; however, it MUST be remembered that not all first world protocols are necessarily applicable to patients in MICs and LICs where resources are limited, and back-up services are frequently non-existent.

Acknowledgments

1. Dr. Dafaalla Omer Abuidris, Associate Professor of clinical oncology and Dean National Cancer Institute, University of Gezira, Wad Medani, Sudan.
2. Prof. Clare Stannard, Department Radiation Oncology, Groote Schuur Hospital, Cape Town, South Africa.
3. Ms. W. Begg Groote Schuur Hospital, Cape Town, South Africa.

References

1. Sullivan R, et al. Improving cancer care for children and young people 4. New policies to address the global burden of childhood cancers. www.thelancet.com/oncology. Published online 20 Feb 2013. http://dx.doi.org/10.1016/S1470-2045(13)70007-X
2. Parkes J. Developing radiotherapy in Africa. In: Presented SIOP Africa 2012, Cape Town.
3. Magrath I, et al. Improving cancer care for children and young people 2. Paediatric cancer in low-income and middle-income countries. www.thelancet.com/oncology. Published online 20 Feb 2013. http://dx.doi.org/10.1016/S1470-2045(13)70008-1
4. Gross J et al. Practice guidelines for sedation and analgesia by non-anesthesiologists. An updated report by the American Society of Anesthesiologists Task Force on sedation and analgesia by non-anesthesiologists. Anesthesiology. 2002;96:1004–17.
5. Harris EA. Sedation and anesthesia options for pediatric patients in the radiation oncology suite. Int J Pediatr. 2010;2010:1–9.
6. Pritchard-Jones K, et al. Improving cancer care for children and young people. 1. Sustaining innovation and improvement in the treatment of childhood cancer: lessons from high-income countries. www.thelancet.com/oncology. Published online 20 Feb 2013. http://dx.doi.org/10.1016/S1470-2045(13)70010-X
7. Israels T, et al. SIOP PODC: clinical guidelines for the management of children with Wilms tumour in a low income setting. Pediatr Blood Cancer. 2013; 60:5–11.
8. Halperin EC, et al. Pediatric radiation oncology. 5th ed. Philadelphia: Wolters Kluwer/Lippincott Williams and Wilkins; 2011. p. 209–29.
9. SIOP. Nephroblastoma clinical protocol. Zurich: SIOP; 2001.
10. Dobbs J, et al. Practical radiotherapy planning (Chapters 21 and 36). 3rd ed. Arnold Pub 1999.
11. Packer RJ, et al. Medulloblastoma: present concepts of stratification into risk groups. Pediatr Neurosurg. 2003;39:60–7.
12. Packer RJ, et al. Treatment of children with medulloblastomas with reduced-dose craniospinal radiation therapy and adjuvant chemotherapy: a Children's Cancer Group study. J Clin Oncol. 1999;17:2127–36.
13. Parker W, et al. A simple technique for craniospinal radiation in the supine position. Radiother Oncol. 2006;78:217–22.
14. Merchant TE, et al. Multi-institution prospective trial of reduced-dose craniospinal irradiation (23.4 Gy) followed by conformal posterior fossa (36 Gy) and

primary site irradiation (55.8 Gy) and dose-intensive chemotherapy for average-risk medulloblastoma. Int J Radiat Oncol Biol Phys. 2008;70(3):782–7. Epub 2007 Sep 24.

15. Neville HL, et al. Preoperative staging, prognostic factors, and outcome for extremity rhabdomyosarcoma: a preliminary report from the Intergroup Rhabdomyosarcoma Study IV (1991–1997). J Pediatr Surg. 2000;35(2):317–21.
16. Strategies to manage retinoblastoma in developing countries. Chantada G et al. Pediatr blood cancer 2011;56:341–348.
17. Chantada G, et al. SIOP-PODC recommendations for graduated-intensity treatment of retinoblastoma in developing countries. Pediatr Blood Cancer. 2013; 60(5):719–27.

Procedures in Pediatric Oncology: Practical Guidelines

15

Furqan Shaikh, Kalid Asrat, and Chifumbe Chintu

Introduction

The procedures used in the diagnosis and management of children with cancer are:

1. Lumbar puncture
2. Bone marrow aspiration and trephine biopsy
3. Pleural tap thoracentesis
4. Abdominal paracentesis
5. Intravenous lines

The Lumbar Puncture

Indications

Lumbar punctures (LPs) are used to diagnose the presence of central nervous system (CNS) infiltration in acute lymphoblastic leukemia (ALL), acute myeloid leukemia (AML), brain tumors, non-Hodgkin lymphomas, and some solid tumors [1]. In addition, LPs are utilized to deliver intrathecal (IT) chemotherapy directly into the subarachnoid space as either treatment or prophylaxis of CNS disease [2]. In a child with cancer, an LP may also be performed for general indications, e.g., to diagnose meningitis, subarachnoid hemorrhage, or idiopathic intracranial hypertension [3].

Precautions

Increased Intracranial Pressure

In cases of increased intracranial pressure (ICP), an LP can cause a sudden drop in intraspinal pressure due to the rapid release of CSF and lead to fatal cerebral herniation [4]. However, routine neuroimaging to rule out increased ICP is not indicated. Rather, the clinical examination can guide the clinician as to whether increased ICP should be suspected. In the absence of headache, vomiting, any focal neurological findings, altered mental status, papilledema, or recent seizures, increased ICP is unlikely and the LP can be performed without first performing neuroimaging [5–7]. In the presence of these findings, an LP should not be performed.

Local Infection

Infection at the intended puncture site is a contraindication. To avoid infectious complications, a sterile technique should be used and gloves, a gown, and facemask should be worn [8, 9].

F. Shaikh, M.D., M.Sc. (✉)
Division of Haematology/Oncology, The Hospital for Sick Children and the University of Toronto, 555 University Avenue, Toronto, ON, Canada M5G 1X8
e-mail: furqan.shaikh@sickkids.ca

K. Asrat, M.D.
University of Botswana School of Medicine, Department of Paediatrics, Gabarone, Botswana

C. Chintu, M.D.
Division of Haematology and Oncology, Department of Paediatrics and Child Health, School of Medicine, University of Zambia, Lusaka, Zambia

D.C. Stefan and C. Rodriguez-Galindo (eds.), *Pediatric Hematology-Oncology in Countries with Limited Resources: A Practical Manual*, DOI 10.1007/978-1-4614-3891-5_15,

Coagulopathy

Although spinal hematomas are rare, their significant morbidity warrants proper attention to minimize the risk of hemorrhagic complication. Hematomas are associated with the presence of an underlying coagulopathy or the use of anticoagulation [10–13]. A coagulation profile, i.e., international normalized ratio (INR) and activated partial thromboplastin time (aPTT), should always be performed prior to an LP in children with a cancer diagnosis. If a coagulopathy is detected, an LP should not be performed until the coagulopathy has been reversed with appropriate therapy such as fresh frozen plasma transfusion or factor replacement [14, 15]. After the initial presentation, however, for a child in whom a normal coagulation profile has been documented and there is no new suspicion of a bleeding diathesis, coagulation testing prior to each LP is not warranted.

Anticoagulation

Approximately 5 % of children with ALL will experience a thrombotic complication and will require the use of anticoagulation at either therapeutic or prophylactic doses [16]. An LP is contraindicated for patients on anticoagulation. Therefore, a practice of suspending anticoagulation for a certain time period prior to an LP should be adopted. The American Society of Regional Anesthesia and Pain Medicine (ASRA) guidelines, though written for anesthesiologists performing neuro-axial procedures, may be a reasonable guide for this context as well. These guidelines state that a spinal procedure should be performed more than 24 h after the last treatment dose, or 12 h after the last prophylactic dose of low-molecular weight heparin (LMWH). Post-procedure, the first LMWH dose should be administered 6–8 h after the procedure and the second dose 24 h following that [13].

Thrombocytopenia

Severe thrombocytopenia is also associated with an increased risk of hemorrhagic complications. However, the exact platelet count below which an LP is contraindicated is controversial. A study by Howard et al. examined 5,223 LPs, including 941 with a platelet count less than 50×10^9/L, and found no serious hemorrhagic complications. The authors concluded that a prophylactic platelet transfusion was not necessary in children with platelet counts higher than 10×10^9/L (except for first LPs in newly diagnosed ALL; see below) [17]. The C17 Guideline for platelet transfusion thresholds for pediatric hematology/oncology patients [18] recommends that, for stable patients requiring an LP, the threshold to receive prophylactic platelet transfusions is 20×10^9/L. Transfusions at higher levels may be required for patients with concomitant bleeding disorders.

First LPs in ALL

The performance of a first LP in a child with newly diagnosed ALL is a special situation with unique considerations. In this setting, a traumatic lumbar puncture with blasts (TLP+, defined as ≥10 red blood cells (RBCs) per microliter of CSF together with visible leukemic blasts in the cytospin) is an undesirable event. The presence of RBCs and blasts in the CSF can obscure the diagnostic information sought from the procedure and make it difficult to accurately classify the child's true CNS status. Secondly, multiple studies have shown that the presence of a TLP+ is a risk factor for leukemia relapse [19–22]. These studies observed a 7–17 % decrease in event-free survival (EFS) in children who had a TLP+ compared to those who had CNS1 status. Lastly, according to many current treatment protocols, children with TLP+ receive additional therapy [2]. For all these reasons, the first LP in a child with newly diagnosed ALL should be performed only with strict optimization of all procedural conditions.

A study by Howard et al. [23] investigated risk factors for traumatic lumbar punctures in children with ALL and found that the risk was increased for LPs performed in an earlier era when sedation was not used, if the platelet count was less than 100×10^9/L and if the operator was inexperienced. The authors of the study described their institutional practice for first LPs as using sedation or general anesthesia, transfusing patients for platelet counts less than 100×10^9/L, administering IT treatment immediately after CSF collection, and having the most experienced clinicians perform the procedure [1].

Methods

Before the Procedure

Patient Assessment

The procedure and its risks should be explained to the patient and/or family. The patient's identity must be verified, known allergies reviewed, and the presence of contraindications should be considered. In particular, any allergies to antiseptic solutions or local anesthetics such as lidocaine should be noted. The protocol should be checked to ensure the indication for the procedure, and the chemotherapy agent and dose should be double-checked against the order with a second health care provider.

Sedation

Where resources are available, the use of sedation or general anesthesia should be strongly considered for all procedures on pediatric oncology patients. Sedation reduces discomfort, anxiety, and movement during the procedure [24–29]. Because children with cancer will undergo multiple LPs, sedation may also reduce anticipatory anxiety. If sedation is not used, local anesthesia such as EMLA® or intradermal lidocaine should be utilized. See Table 15.1 for a list of common sedatives and anesthetics and their doses.

Chemotherapy Safety

The inadvertent administration of vincristine as IT chemotherapy is a catastrophic event. From 1968 to 2007, this error was reported 55 times in several international settings, resulting in death in nearly all cases. Therefore, every pediatric oncology institution must ensure that maximal structural and procedural safeguards are in place to prevent this error. In 2007, the World Health Organization (WHO) issued an alert on this topic and recommended that syringes should not be used for vincristine administration, that where possible this drug should be prepared by dilution in small volume intravenous bags ("minibags"), and that labeling should include a clear warning [30].

Table 15.1 Guide to procedural analgesia and sedation

Sedatives	
Benzodiazepams	
Diazepam	0.2–0.3 mg/kg (maximum 10 mg) orally 45–60 min before the procedure
Midazolam	0.2–0.4 mg/kg (maximum 15 mg) orally 30–45 min or 0.05 mg/kg IV 3 min before the procedure
Ketamine	1–2 mg/kg given 3 min before procedure
Opioids	
Morphine sulfate	0.05–0.1 mg/kg IV over 1–2 min given 5 min before the procedure
Fentanyl	1–2 μg/kg IV 3 min before the procedure
Meperidine	0.5–1 mg/kg IV over 1–2 min given 2–5 min before the procedure
Local anesthetics	
Lidocaine 1 % (without epinephrine)	1–3 mg/kg infiltrate skin and periosteum; wait 4–5 min

Equipment

The equipment to be collected for procedures are shown in Table 15.2. The operator should ensure that the required equipment is available and properly set up prior to the procedure. For LPs, a large body of literature has focused on determining the ideal needle to be used, mainly from the perspective of reducing the risk of post-dural puncture headache (PDPH), which is the most common complication.

Needle Length

The following needle lengths are widely available: 1.5, 2.5, or 3.5 in. A longer needle is more challenging to use, as it is more likely to bend upon insertion. Therefore, the shortest needle that is likely to reach the target space should be selected. Generally, a 1.5 in. needle can be used for most patients weighing less than 35 kg, a 2.5 in. needle can be used for patients 35–70 kg, and a 3.5 in. needle is usually required for patients weighing more than 70 kg.

Table 15.2 Equipment required for procedures in pediatric oncology

For all procedures	Sterile tray
	Skin prep (chlorhexidine or iodine)
	Requisitions, consent forms, procedure notes
	Labels
	Specimen bags or containers
	Mask, gown, sterile gloves, sterile towels or drapes
	Sharps bin or container
For lumbar punctures	LP tray and extra needles
	Chemotherapy, orders, protocol
	20 mL syringe for chemotherapy
	Sterile gauze
For bone marrow aspirations	Two 18-gauge drawing needles and one 25-gauge injecting needle
	Local anesthetic and heparin vials
	Many 5 or 10 mL syringes (to draw samples)
	BMA needle(s)
	Slides, slide tray, pencil
	EDTA tubes, heparinized tubes, research tubes if indicated
For bone marrow trephine biopsies	Bone marrow biopsy needle(s)
	Formalin specimen jar
For thoracentesis and paracentesis	21-Gauge needle and 50 mL syringe
	Cannula
	3-Way tap
	Tubes and containers

Needle Type

Most practitioners are familiar with the traditional cutting tip LP needles (Quincke or bevel-tip) which are commonly available. Nevertheless, the atraumatic needle (Whitacre, Sprotte, or pencil point) has been shown in multiple randomized control trials to reduce the rates of PDPH. Using an atraumatic needle requires some learning for practitioners who are more used to cutting needles. An introducer may be required to pass the atraumatic needle through the skin, and the tactile feedback from subcutaneous tissues is different.

Needle Size

LP needles can be found in 20, 22, and 26 gauge (smallest size). As expected, a smaller sized needle is associated with lower rates of PDPH, likely because the smaller dural hole causes less CSF leakage. Switching to atraumatic needles or smaller gauge needles (or both) for patients who have experienced a moderate to severe PDPH after a prior LP is strongly advised. However, smaller gauge needles can bend upon insertion, decrease the rate of CSF flow, and increase the resistance felt when injecting chemotherapy. Therefore, a 22-gauge needle may be the optimal needle size for most LPs.

During the Procedure

Like most procedures, the LP is a practical skill that is best learned by observation and practice. Institutions should develop best practices to impart education and training on new staff members.

Positioning the Patient

While LPs can be performed in the sitting position, the lateral decubitus position is used when the patient is to be sedated. Furthermore, this position allows better distribution of injected chemotherapy through the CSF. The patient's legs are flexed toward the chest, and the shoulders and pelvis are square and perpendicular to the bed, as shown in Fig. 15.1 [31]. In this position, an imaginary vertical line drawn between the posterior superior iliac crest would approximately cross the L4 spinous process. LPs can be done in the L3-L4, L4-L5, or L5-S1 interspace. LPs should be avoided at higher interspaces, as this risk injuring the conus medullaris. Conversely, LPs performed at lower interspaces increase the difficulty of palpating the spinous processes.

Performing the LP

Wearing sterile gloves and a mask, the operator should cleanse the puncture site with an antiseptic solution. Sterile drapes should be applied, leaving the intended puncture site exposed.

The stylet should be in place within the needle. The needle should only be advanced with the

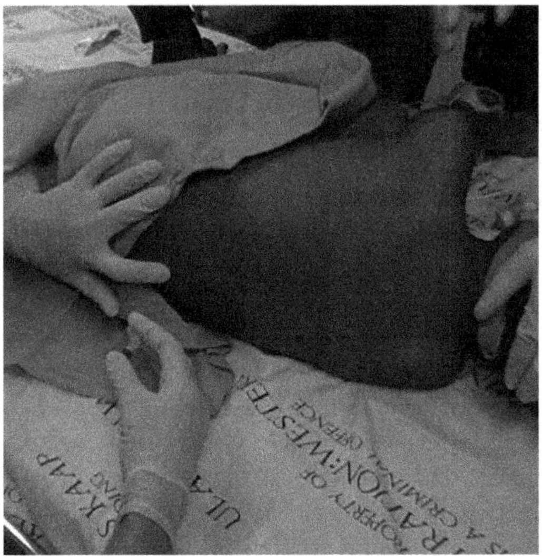

Fig. 15.1 A lumbar puncture needle being inserted

stylet in place, or else the needle bore can become obstructed with a core of tissue and increase the risk of developing an epidermoid cyst.

The tip of the spinous process superior to the chosen interspace should be palpated. The needle should be inserted inferior to this tip, midway between two spinous processes.

If a traditional Quincke or bevel-tip needle is used, the bevel face should be oriented parallel to the long axis of the spine, so as to separate the longitudinal fibers of the dura rather than transect them. Thus, in a child lying in a left lateral decubitus position, the bevel should face up toward the ceiling. Several studies have shown that this bevel orientation helps reduce the rate of PDPH [32, 33].

The needle should be advanced slowly at a slight cephalic angle so as to move parallel to the angle of the spinous processes and avoid bony contact [34]. In most patients, this angle can be approximately achieved by advancing the needle as though aiming for the umbilicus. If bony contact occurs or resistance is felt, the needle should be withdrawn to the subcutaneous position and reinserted at a slightly different angle.

Usually, a pop is felt when the needle penetrates the ligamentum flavum. However, in young children or in patients who have had repeated LPs, the pop may not be a reliable sign. Therefore, once the needle has reached close to the estimated depth of insertion, the stylet should be removed to check for CSF flow. If there is no fluid, reinsert the stylet and advance the needle slightly, withdrawing the stylet and checking for fluid after each movement.

If a bloody tap occurs, it is advisable to remove the needle, obtain a new needle, and reattempt the LP at a different interspace. If the LP fails a second time, a different person should attempt it, especially if a more experienced operator is available. After a bloody tap, however, the presence of a small hematoma may make a successful procedure more difficult in spite of the operator's proficiency. In such cases, the LP should be attempted again after a few days, allowing time for the hematoma to resolve.

Pressure Measurements

ICP can be measured by connecting a manometer to the needle or via a stopcock, and allowing CSF to flow into the manometer until the fluid level ceases to rise. This procedure is not often used in practice, but may be performed in cases of suspected ICP. There will be normal variation in the fluid level with respiration. After the measurement is obtained, the CSF in the manometer should be released into a collection tube using the stopcock rather than be wasted.

ICP should be measured with the patient in the lateral decubitus position. It can be falsely elevated if the patient is in the sitting position [35] or if the head is elevated above the level of the needle. The range of normal opening pressure is 11.5–28 cm of water [36].

Collecting Samples

CSF should be allowed to drip into the collecting tubes. It should never be aspirated into a syringe as this could result in significant negative pressure. For most LPs performed for delivery of intrathecal chemotherapy, a tube is collected for cytospin and another for biochemistry (protein and glucose). With LPs done for patients with brain tumors or solid tumors, a tube for cytology should also be obtained. In the case of suspected meningitis, additional tubes for bacterial studies (gram stain, culture, and sensitivity) and/or viral studies should be obtained.

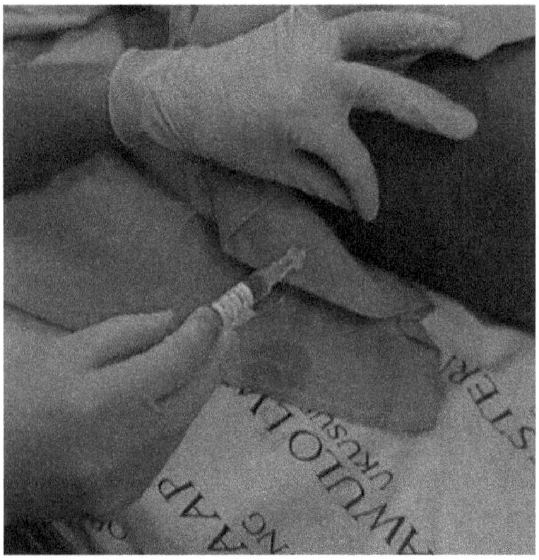

Fig. 15.2 Intrathecal chemotherapy being injected through a lumbar puncture needle

Volume of CSF

For a diagnostic LP, only the minimal required CSF volume should be collected. Excess CSF removal will increase the risk of a PDPH. Conversely, where intrathecal chemotherapy is to be administered, it is advisable to remove a CSF volume equal to the volume of drug that will be administered. Theoretically, a large net positive infusion volume may increase the risk of intracranial hypertension. Recognizing the limitations of time in the procedure room, some leukemia protocols recommend that clinicians should aim to remove at least 50 % of the volume of drug to be injected.

Injecting

Once CSF collection is completed, the needle hub should be connected to the chemotherapy syringe and a tight seal obtained. The needle should be stabilized with the non-dominant hand to ensure that its position is not altered during this maneuver, as seen in Fig. 15.2. Slowly inject the chemotherapy. Resistance usually increases as the injection proceeds. However, if excessive resistance is felt, cease administration and remove the syringe to ensure that CSF is still free flowing.

Reinserting the Stylet

One study [37] found that reinserting the stylet after a diagnostic LP was associated with reduced rates of PDPH. The authors hypothesized that strands of dura may enter the needle bore during CSF sampling and be threaded back during removal of the needle, producing a larger dural defect and allowing longer leakage of CSF. Replacing the stylet may allow the strands to be pushed out, reducing the risk of prolonged leakage.

If this postulated mechanism is correct, then it is reasonable to assume that injecting medication through the needle may achieve the same desired effect. Therefore, if IT chemotherapy was injected, the needle and syringe can be removed as a unit without reinserting the stylet. However, if the LP was done for diagnostic sampling only, the stylet should always be reinserted prior to removing the needle [38].

After withdrawing the needle, manual pressure using gauze should be applied for a few minutes, with longer times preferred in those with lower platelet counts or traumatic procedures.

After the Procedure

Bed Rest

In patients who have received intrathecal chemotherapy, lying supine for 1–2 h is advisable as it facilitates distribution of chemotherapy throughout the CSF. However, in patients who have received a diagnostic LP only no specific bed rest is required and patients may ambulate once they have recovered from the effects of sedation [39].

Documentation

As for all procedures, proper documentation of consent, orders, and the procedure details should be carefully documented. The operator should properly document any problems encountered, the number of attempts, and chemotherapy administration. Standardized procedure forms or templates can be useful to allow efficiency in this regard.

Figures 15.3, 15.4, 15.5, and 15.6 show samples of standardized documentation used at our institution for LPs and bone marrow aspirates/biopsies. Figure 15.3 is a standardized consent form; Fig. 15.4 is a preprinted orderset for intrathecal chemotherapy; Fig. 15.5 is a procedure

SickKids
THE HOSPITAL FOR SICK CHILDREN

Barcode

LAST NAME (FIRST)

DATE OF BIRTH YY – MM – DD SEX MRN

ADDRESS

IMPRINT OR ENTER DETAILS BY HAND

Haematology/Oncology/BMT

CONSENT TO TREATMENT FORM

Patients and their families
If you want help reading this form, or have questions, please ask your doctor or nurse. When we use the word treatment on this form, we mean treatment, test or operation.
Please complete all appropriate sections on page 1 & 2.

Name of the Patient (please print) ______________________________

I agree to the treatment *Check all that apply*: ❑Lumbar Puncture, ❑Lumbar Puncture with intrathecal chemotherapy
______________________ ❑Bone Marrow Aspirate, ❑Bone Marrow Biopsy, ❑Unilateral ❑Bilateral

I agree that ______________________________
(Name of doctor or health care practitioner [HCP])
And I have talked about why this treatment is necessary and what will happen during the treatment. He / she has explained the chances of the treatment not working and the medical problems that might happen with the treatment. I also agree to other treatments that may be needed while the doctor or HCP is doing this treatment. I understand that my doctor or HCP may ask other doctors, residents, fellows or HCPs to do all or part of this treatment. I understand the information on this form and have had the opportunity to ask the doctor or HCP questions about the treatment.

______________________ ______________________
Signature of Parent or substitute decision maker Date/Time

______________________ ______________________
Name of substitute decision maker (if signature above) Relationship to the patient

(A) PHYSICIAN'S, SURGEON'S OR HEALTH CARE PRACTITIONER'S STATEMENT

I certify that I have explained the nature of this treatment, its associated risks and benefits and the possible alternatives, including the likely consequences of not having the treatment, to the patient or substitute decision maker, or both.

______________________ ______________________
Signature of physician, surgeon or HCP Date/Time

____
Name of physician, surgeon or HCP (please print)

Summary of Risks:

Please check applicable risks:
☑ Local pain or discomfort
☑ Bleeding
☑ Infection
❑ Headache *These additional risks to be discussed for lumbar punctures only*
❑ Neurological complications

Form #### (Rev. 2012/01) Chart Copy Page 1 of 1

Fig. 15.3 Sample consent to treatment form for lumbar punctures and bone marrow procedures (used with permission from The Hospital for Sick Children © 2012)

SickKids®
THE HOSPITAL FOR
SICK CHILDREN

G120

LAST NAME	(FIRST)	
DATE OF BIRTH (YYYY/MM/DD)	SEX	MRN
Address		
imprint addressograph or enter details by hand		

Haematology/Oncology
Medical Orders

Allergies: ______________________ ☐ **No Allergies Known**
Is the patient on anticoagulants? ☐ Yes ☐ No

Procedure & Intrathecal Chemotherapy Orders

Protocol: ______________________ **Diagnosis**: ______________________

(Cycle/Phase and Day #): ______________ Date of procedure: ______________ (YYYY/MM/DD)

Procedure & Laboratory Orders		
PROCEDURE	☐ Lumbar puncture (diagnostic) ☐ Lumbar puncture with Intrathecal Chemotherapy ☐ Opening pressure: ______ cm H_2O Initials:	
	☐ Bone Marrow Aspirate ☐ Bone Marrow Biopsy	☐ Unilateral ☐ Bilateral
LABORATORY	☐ CSF Chemistry ☐ BM Smears ☐ BM molecular studies ☐ CSF Cell count ☐ BM Flow ☐ CSF Cytology ☐ BM Cytogenetics ☐ Other:__________	
RESEARCH	☐ Bone Marrow Aspirate ☐ CSF ☐ comments:______________________	☐ Notify CRA to collect specimen

Ondansetron

☐ ondansetron 5 mg/m^2 IV prior to IT chemotherapy _____mg

☐ See separate order for other chemotherapy

Intrathecal (IT) Chemotherapy Order ☐ **N/A**				
Age: ________ **yrs** (on date of IT administration)				
INTRATHECAL CHEMOTHERAPY	☐ Single IT ☐ Double IT ☐ Triple IT			
	☐ **methotrexate**: __________ mg intrathecally x 1 dose ☐ **hydrocortisone**: __________ mg intrathecally x 1 dose ☐ **cytarabine**: __________ mg intrathecally x 1 dose			
MEDICATION ADMINISTRATION RECORD	**Date** YYYY-MM-DD	**Time**	**Dose & Volume Checked by**	**Administered by**

______________	________	______________________	______________
Date Ordered (YYYY-MM-DD)	Time (hh:mm)	Signature	Print Name

Procedure & IT ppo Last Revised: 2012/08/21 White to: Chart; Yellow to: Pharmacy; Pink to: Procedure Nurse Page 1 of 1

Fig. 15.4 Sample preprinted orderset for procedure and intrathecal chemotherapy orders (used with permission from The Hospital for Sick Children © 2012)

SickKids
THE HOSPITAL FOR
SICK CHILDREN

Haematology /Oncology
Procedure Documentation Record

LAST NAME (FIRST)

DATE OF BIRTH SEX MRN
YY MM DD

ADDRESS

IMPRINT OR ENTER DETAILS BY HAND

Date of Procedure:________________________(YYYY-MM-DD)

A. Patient Verification Patient Verified by: ______________________________

☐ Patient ☐ Parent/Substitute ☐ Other: ______________________________

Time Out conducted at : ____________________ By: ____________________

B. Procedure Documentation:

☐ 1) Lumbar puncture (diagnostic):
The patient was prepped and draped in the usual sterile fashion. A ___gauge ____inch spinal needle was inserted at the level of L ____.
______mL of (clear/blood tinged/bloody) fluid was obtained on the _____attempt. The needle was removed.

☐ 2) Lumbar puncture with Intrathecal (IT) chemotherapy:
The patient was prepped and draped in the usual sterile fashion. A ___gauge ____inch spinal needle was inserted at the level of L ____.
______mL of (clear/blood tinged/bloody) fluid was obtained on the _____attempt. IT chemotherapy administered. The needle was removed.

☐ 3) Bone marrow aspirate:
The patient was prepped and draped in the usual sterile fashion. A ___gauge ____cm bone marrow aspirate needle was inserted in the (right posterior iliac crest/ other_______). _____mL of bone marrow was obtained with ______placements of the needle. The needle was removed.
☐ The procedure was repeated on the contralateral side).

☐ 4) Bone marrow biopsy:
Patient was prepped and draped in the usual sterile fashion. A ___gauge ____cm bone marrow biopsy needle was inserted in the (right posterior iliac crest/other________). A core of bone marrow tissue was removed on the ______attempt. The needle was removed.
☐ The procedure was repeated on the contralateral side.

Additional notes:

____________________ ____________________ ____________________
Print Name Signature Date Time (YYYY-MM-DD hh:mm)

Form # 55909(Rev. 2012/05) Chart Copy Page 1 of 1

Fig. 15.5 Sample procedure documentation form (used with permission from The Hospital for Sick Children © 2012)

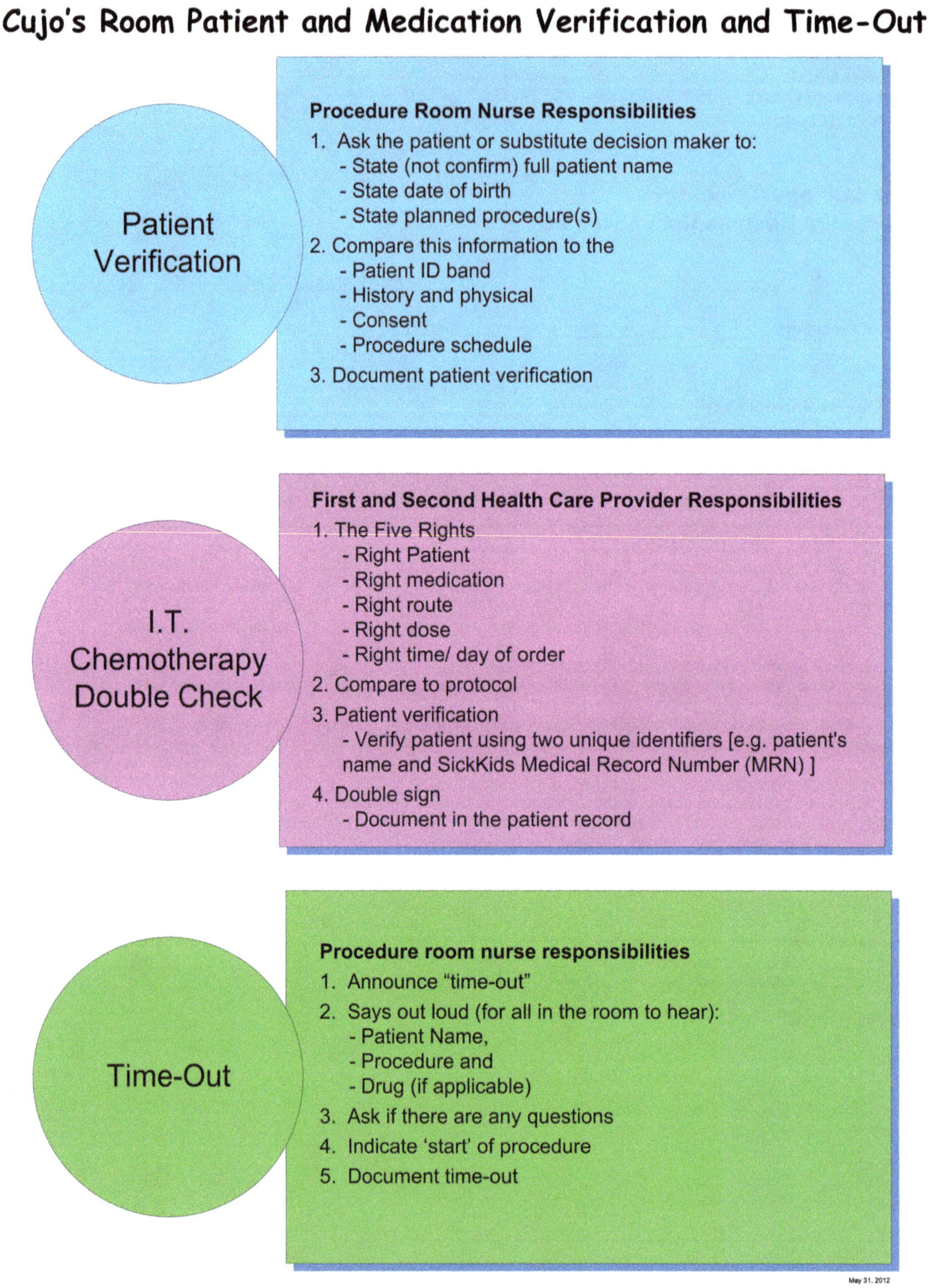

Fig. 15.6 Sample wall poster for patient and medication safety reminders

documentation form; and Fig. 15.6 is a wall poster used for "time-out" safety checking. The use of such template documentation instruments can help facilitate the efficiency and quality of care in the procedure room.

Complications

Headache

The most common complication of an LP is PDPH. It can be defined as any headache after an LP that worsens within 15 min of sitting or standing and is relieved within 15 min of lying down. Most PDPHs occur within 3 days of the procedure. They are believed to be caused by a puncture in the dura that allows CSF leakage. The reported rate of PDPH varies across studies from 2 to 60 %, depending on the setting [2]. As mentioned, the rates of PDPH have been shown to decrease with atraumatic needles, smaller gauge needles, maintaining the needle bevel direction parallel to the dural fibers, and reinserting the stylet in diagnostic LPs. Bed rest and fluid supplementation do not prevent PDPH [40]. For the management of PDPH, the reader is referred to recent Cochrane systematic reviews [41, 42].

Other Complications

The most significant complications include cerebral herniation, spinal hematomas, and inadvertent administration of incorrect IT chemotherapy. Other complications include backache, subdural fluid collections, epidermoid cysts, and infectious complications such as cellulitis, skin abscess, discitis [43], and epidural abscess [44].

Bone Marrow Aspiration and Trephine Biopsy

Indications

Bone marrow aspirations (BMA) are used for the diagnostic investigation or monitoring of patients with abnormal blood counts, hematologic disorders, suspected malignancies, or metabolic, infiltrative, or infectious diseases that can involve the bone marrow. Additionally, bone marrow trephine biopsies (BMB) are performed when an assessment of bone marrow cellularity, architecture, or focal lesions is required, when there is inadequate marrow aspiration, and for the staging of lymphomas and small round blue cell tumors of childhood [45]. The bone marrow aspirate and trephine biopsy are complementary procedures and are usually performed together (BMAT).

Contraindications

When performed by a trained operator, BMATs are generally safe procedures and adverse events are uncommon [46]. The most frequent complications are bleeding and pain. Rare cases of severe bleeding with large hematomas [47], anemia, and death [48] have been reported. Hemorrhagic disorders, severe thrombocytopenia, and anticoagulation may be considered relative contraindications and their correction should be considered before the procedure whenever feasible [49]. Local skin or bone infections should exclude the use of that particular site for the procedure.

Methods

Before the Procedure

Many of the principles of preparing for the BMAT are similar to those outlined above for LPs. A full patient assessment and informed consent should be performed and documented. The patient's identity, indications, and contraindications for the procedure and allergies should be reviewed. The BMAT is a painful procedure and conscious sedation or general anesthesia should always be used when it is performed on children. In addition, infiltration of local anesthetic such as lidocaine into the periosteum should be used, as it can help reduce post-procedure pain.

Ensure all equipment is prepared (see Table 15.2). BMA needles are generally available in 18 gauge or 15 gauge. BMB or Jamshidi needles are generally available in adult (11 gauge, 4 in.), pediatric (13 gauge, 3.5 in.), or infant (13 gauge, 2 in.) sizes.

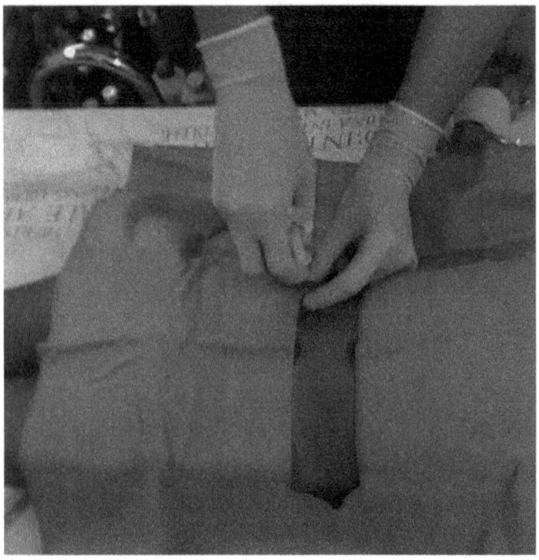

Fig. 15.7 Insertion of a bone marrow aspirate needle into the anterior iliac crest

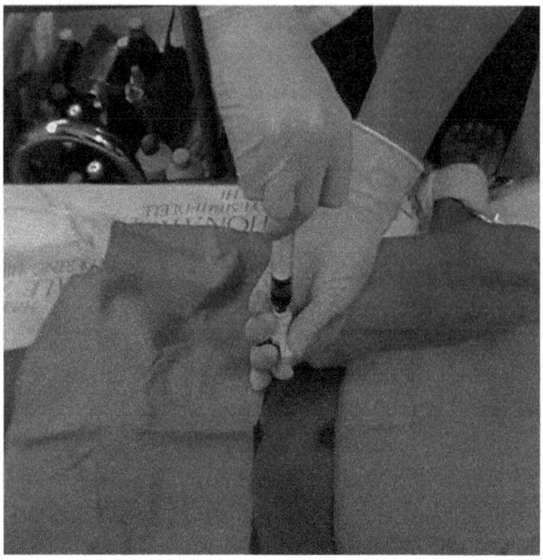

Fig. 15.8 Aspiration of bone marrow

Ensure that all slides and tubes needed for the various required samples are available.

During the Procedure

The optimal site for the procedure should be palpated and identified. The posterior superior iliac crest is a common site of this procedure for most children [50]. It can be accessed with the patient in the lateral decubitus position. The anterior iliac crest may also be used and, in obese patients, may be easier to palpate. In infants, the tibial tuberosity can also be used. The sternum is generally best avoided.

Wearing sterile gloves, gown, and mask, the operator should cleanse the puncture site and apply sterile drapes. The iliac crest is palpated to locate the desired site for the procedure. Local anesthetic, such as 1 or 2 % lidocaine, is injected intradermally and into the periosteum.

The skin is punctured with the BMA needle and advanced to the bone. Then a twisting motion with firm pressure is applied to penetrate the bone, and the needle is advanced until it is firmly anchored (see Fig. 15.7). The stylet is removed, a syringe is connected, and strong suction is applied to obtain a few drops of bone marrow aspirate. Excess aspiration should be avoided as it will result in dilute smears. Smears from the aspirate should immediately be made (the sample will clot within a few seconds) and the presence of particles must be ensured.

Thereafter, using a new syringe, additional samples are aspirated as needed (see Fig. 15.8). For suspected leukemia, ≥2 mL each is collected in EDTA tubes for flow cytometry and molecular studies. The needle is relocated; then ≥3 mL is collected for cytogenetic studies (in a heparinized tube). Additionally, any samples for infectious, metabolic, or research studies can be obtained as needed.

The BMB is generally performed after the BMA. While the sequence is probably unimportant, the two procedures should be performed at slightly different sites along the bone and using separate needles. Obtaining a biopsy from the same spot as the aspirate can result in a denuded or distorted biopsy sample [51]. However, although the bone entry site is changed, all the needle insertions and relocations should be carried out through the same single skin incision.

With the obturator locked securely in place, the biopsy needle is held with the hub in the palm and the index finger close to the tip to allow control. With steady pressure and a rotatory motion, the needle is advanced through the soft tissues, the cortical bone, and into the marrow

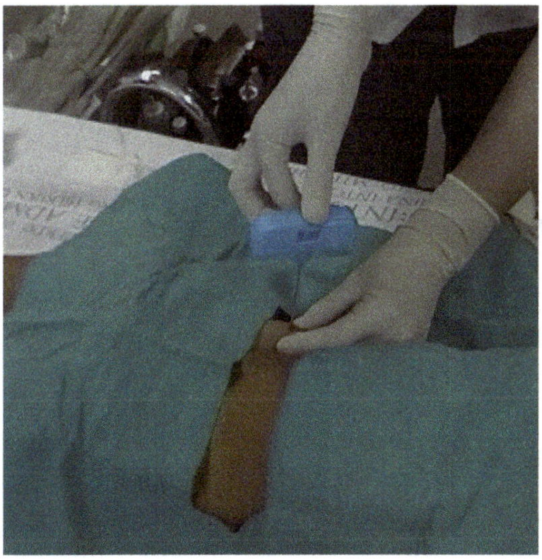

Fig. 15.9 Insertion of a bone marrow biopsy needle into the anterior iliac crest

cavity (see Fig. 15.9). When the needle is firmly anchored, the obturator is removed and the needle is advanced another 1–2 cm. The biopsy specimen in the needle core should be broken from the surrounding bone by vigorously rotating the needle several times in both directions [50]. The needle should be withdrawn slowly. Using a probe inserted from the distal end of the needle, the biopsy specimen is dropped into a formalin specimen bottle. Manual pressure is held until bleeding stops, and a pressure bandage is applied.

After the Procedure

The operator should again document the details of the procedure. Adequate analgesics should be provided and the patient should be instructed to remove the bandage the next day. No specific bed rest is required; patients may ambulate once they have recovered from the effects of sedation.

Thoracentesis (Pleural Tap)

This invasive procedure is used to obtain fluid from the pleural space.

Indications

In conditions such as pneumonia, tuberculosis, congestive cardiac failure, and malignancies such as lymphoma and Kaposi sarcoma, a pleural effusion may be present. In some instances a pneumothorax or haemothorax may develop. The pleural tap can be used for diagnosis of malignant disease as well as for therapeutic purposes. The fluid removed should be sent for cytology, microscopy, culture and sensitivity, and biochemistry.

Contraindications

The contraindications to a pleural tap include an uncorrected bleeding disorder and local infection such as cellulitis. Relative contraindications include mechanical ventilation or the presence of only one functioning lung [52].

Methods

A chest X-ray or ultrasound may be performed to confirm the clinical suspicion of a pleural effusion. The level of the fluid as seen on sonar should be marked on the patient's chest. The procedure must be explained to the child and his/her caregivers. The equipment required for a pleural tap is shown in Table 15.2.

The pleural tap can be performed at the bedside. The patient should be in a sitting position with his or her back toward the person performing the tap. The patient should lean forward on a hospital table or pillow with arms folded and neck flexed forward. The chest should be percussed to determine the upper level of fluid (if not already marked by the sonographer). Make a mark along the sixth or seventh rib interspace along the posterior axillary line [52, 53]. Clean the area with either iodine or chlorhexidine. When the skin is dry, infiltrate the skin and subcutaneous tissue with 2–5 mL lidocaine 1 % using a 25 gauge needle. The entry point of the needle should be just above the upper border of the rib to avoid the artery and nerve which run below the rib. A 21-gauge needle attached to a

50 mL syringe should then be inserted in the same spot. Aspirate slowly while advancing the needle. The aspirate should be sent for microbiology, biochemistry, lactate dehydrogenase, and cytology.

Monitor the patient carefully during the procedure. If the patient experiences discomfort, it may be due to a vasovagal reaction [54]. If cough occurs, this may be due to needle contact with the visceral pleura and aspiration should be stopped. A small amount of blood in the aspirate could be from the cutaneous blood vessels while introducing the needle. However, if the aspirate continues to be bloody this could suggest a haemothorax. Aspirate due to haemothorax does not clot. If the aspirate clots, stop the procedure as this may mean that the liver or spleen has been punctured. Monitor the patient for signs of internal hemorrhage.

In the majority of patients there is no need for a chest X-ray after thoracentesis. In a study of 231 thoracenteses performed in 199 patients, complications were suspected in 30 patients and only 9 were confirmed by a chest X-ray [55]. A small amount of air need not be aspirated but a significant pneumothorax necessitates chest tube insertion.

Complications

These include pneumothorax, bleeding at the site of entry, haemothorax, internal hemorrhage, and hypotension.

Abdominal Paracentesis

Abdominal paracentesis is used to drain ascitic fluid from the abdominal cavity.

Indications

A paracentesis is performed in children whose cardiorespiratory and/or gastrointestinal functions are compromised by ascites, and to ascertain the etiology of ascites.

Contraindications

Include an uncorrected coagulopathy and pregnancy (second and third trimesters).

Methods

The patient and caregivers should be informed about the procedure. The bladder must be emptied. In children, sedation may be needed. Ultrasonography of the abdomen must be performed to exclude abdominal mass(es). The radiologist may mark a suitable point for paracentesis, usually in the midline. The patient should lie in a lateral position if there is a smaller of fluid or supine if there is substantial ascites.

Sterilize the area with antiseptic solution and use a sterile drape. Once the area is dry, infiltrate the area of the skin with lidocaine 1 %. Insert an 18-gauge needle/cannula at 90° to the skin at the designated point slowly until the ascitic fluid starts to flow. Collect samples for microbiology, cytology, and biochemistry. Thereafter connect the cannula to a tube to drain the rest of the ascites into a container. When the ascitic fluid has stopped flowing, remove the cannula, clean the area, and apply gauze and adhesive tape.

Complications

Hypotension can develop if too much ascitic fluid is removed. Fluid may leak from the puncture site. Pulling the skin downwards from the aspiration site and releasing the skin when the needle is in the peritoneal cavity—the "Z technique"—can minimize this. The leak can be closed with a suture. Using aseptic technique can prevent infection.

Intravenous Lines

Venous cannulas or catheters are widely used for the administration of medications, chemotherapy, fluids, and blood products. Children with cancer also undergo various investigative procedures which also require venous access.

In all procedures for intravenous cannulation, strict antiseptic methods should be employed. As before, the operator should have the necessary skills and knowledge. Extra care should be exercised when carrying out the procedure in patients with a bleeding diathesis.

Peripheral Vein Catheterization

Additional equipment required for this procedure are tourniquet, tape, and 18- to 25-gauge cannulas.

The following veins are commonly used: cephalic, median basilica, median antecubital, fifth interdigital, saphenous, and the veins of the dorsalateral aspect of the foot. An assistant should preferably be available to hold and stabilize the extremity. The site of cannulation should be cleaned with antiseptic solution such as alcohol or chlorhexidine. A tourniquet is applied to the limb above the site of puncture. The vein is punctured at an angle of 15–45°. Once blood is seen, advance a further 1–2 mm. While holding the needle still, thread the cannula into the vein. Release the tourniquet and remove the needle. Attach the cannula to the IV line. Apply adhesive tape to hold the cannula in place. The intravenous fluid should run freely if the IV is in a proper position.

Scalp Vein Catheterization

This procedure will require a razor, a 25- to 27-gauge butterfly needle, 2–5 mL syringe with sterile normal saline, and alcohol swabs.

Identify the visible veins on the scalp such as the superficial temporal, posterior auricular, or occipital veins. Shave the selected area and clean with alcohol. Attach the butterfly needle to a 2 ml syringe with normal saline and flush to remove air. Puncture the vein at 15–30° until blood is seen in the butterfly tubing. Then advance the needle into the vein. Secure the butterfly needle with tape and push normal saline in the syringe to test the patency of the vein.

External Jugular Cannulation

A 21- to 22-gauge cannula, intravenous line flushed with normal saline, iodine or alcohol swabs, sterile gauze, and an assistant are required for this procedure. Turn the head of the patient to the left so that the head touches the left shoulder. Insert the needle into the external jugular vein. When blood is seen, advance the cannula and remove the needle. Attach the cannula to the intravenous line [53].

Venous cannulation may cause phlebitis at the insertion site, catheter-related blood stream infection, and endocarditis. The risk of infection is markedly reduced when the lines are inserted in the upper limbs rather than the lower limbs.

Central Venous Catheter Insertion

A central venous catheter (CVC, see Fig. 15.10) is inserted into the central veins and the tip is situated in the superior vena cava. CVCs can be described by the way they are introduced into the patient. They can be described by the site of insertion (e.g., subclavian, internal jugular, or femoral). A peripherally inserted central catheter (PICC) is

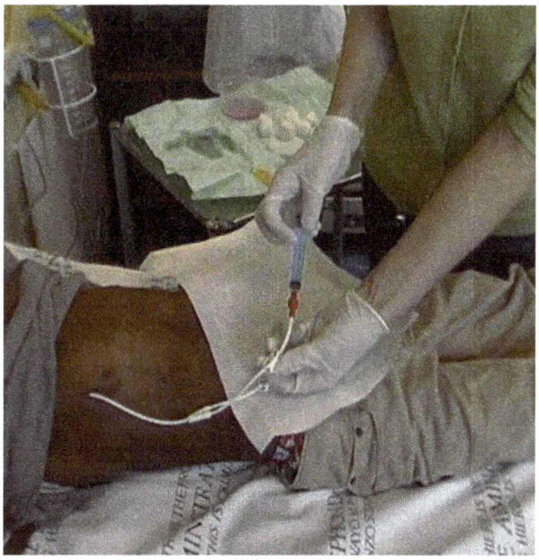

Fig. 15.10 A central venous catheter being used to draw blood

a CVC that is inserted via the antecubital vein [56]. CVCs can also be classified as tunneled or non-tunneled catheters. A tunneled catheter is a long-term device that is buried in a subcutaneous tunnel before it enters the central vein [57]. An implanted catheter is a tunneled catheter that ends in a subcutaneously implanted port. Catheters are made of various materials and may be impregnated with antimicrobial or anticoagulant agents. Some catheters may have more than one lumen.

If long-term venous access is planned then a tunneled or implanted device should be used. Multi-lumen catheters are associated with increased risk of infection compared to single lumen catheters, so should be used only when the use of multiple lumens is a necessity.

Indications

CVCs are indicated in children with cancer who have limited accessible veins, particularly after prolonged use of peripheral veins, and who require long-term chemotherapy, blood products, antibiotics, fluids, and frequent phlebotomy.

Methods

The indication for a CVC, the insertion procedure, potential complications, and care should be explained to the patient and caregivers. Informed consent must be obtained.

The insertion of a CVC must be performed by a skilled health professional in an operating theatre, intensive care unit, or radiology unit. Before insertion the coagulation status of the patient should be ascertained. Aseptic methods should be employed to avoid infection. These include hand washing, sterile gloves and gowns, a cap mask, and a sterile drape with a fenestration. The insertion site should be cleaned with an antiseptic such as chlorhexidine and allowed to dry. Insertion can be guided by ultrasound. As CVC insertion is an advanced technique, the details of the insertion or tunneling procedures are beyond the scope of this chapter. Once inserted, the catheter should be firmly anchored with sutures to prevent movement. Before use, the position of the tip should be confirmed by X-ray or echocardiogram.

Complications

Early complications include bleeding, malpositioning of the catheter, pneumothorax, and air embolism. Late complications include infections, thrombosis, and malfunctioning of the catheter [58].

Studies have noted that cancer patients with implanted port systems [55] have a median of 0.2 infections per 1,000 catheter days, while those with subcutaneous tunneled CVCs have a range of 1.4–2.2 infections per 1,000 catheter days [59, 60].

The type of catheter and whether it is impregnated with antibiotics and/or anticoagulants play a role in the risk of infection. Infections can also occur during routine use or care of the catheter such as during flushing with saline/heparin and injection of drugs.

The catheter-related incidence of thrombosis in children, both symptomatic and asymptomatic, can be as high as 50 %. The incidence varies depending upon methods of diagnosis of thrombosis by ultrasonography or venogram. With improvements in the design of catheters, the incidence is likely to decrease.

References

1. Pui C-H, Thiel E. Central nervous system disease in hematologic malignancies: historical perspective and practical applications. Semin Oncol. 2009;36(4 Suppl 2):S2–16.
2. Pui CH, Campana D, Pei D, Bowman WP, Sandlund JT, Kaste SC, et al. Treating childhood acute lymphoblastic leukemia without cranial irradiation. N Engl J Med. 2009;360(26):2730–41.
3. Straus SE, Thorpe KE, Holroyd-Leduc J. How do I perform a lumbar puncture and analyze the results to diagnose bacterial meningitis? JAMA. 2006;296(16): 2012–22.
4. Rennick G, Shann F, de Campo J. Cerebral herniation during bacterial meningitis in children. BMJ. 1993;306(6883):953–5.
5. Gopal AK, Whitehouse JD, Simel DL, Corey GR. Cranial computed tomography before lumbar puncture: a prospective clinical evaluation. Arch Intern Med. 1999;159(22):2681–5.
6. Greig PR, Goroszeniuk D. Role of computed tomography before lumbar puncture: a survey of clinical practice. Postgrad Med J. 2006;82(965): 162–5.
7. Hasbun R, Abrahams J, Jekel J, Quagliarello VJ. Computed tomography of the head before lumbar

puncture in adults with suspected meningitis. N Engl J Med. 2001;345(24):1727–33.
8. Baer ET. Post-dural puncture bacterial meningitis. Anesthesiology. 2006;105(2):381–93.
9. Kelly S, Malhotra R. Infection control measures taken during lumbar punctures: a survey of current practice. J Hosp Infect. 2010;76:S53.
10. Ruff RL, Dougherty Jr JH. Complications of lumbar puncture followed by anticoagulation. Stroke. 1981; 12(6):879–81.
11. Kreppel D, Antoniadis G, Seeling W. Spinal hematoma: a literature survey with meta-analysis of 613 patients. Neurosurg Rev. 2003;26:1–49.
12. Heppner PA, Monteith SJ, Law AJJ. Spontaneous spinal hematomas and low-molecular-weight heparin. Report of four cases and review of the literature. J Neurosurg Spine. 2004;1(2):232–6.
13. Horlocker TT, Wedel DJ, Rowlingson AJ, Enneking K, Kopp SL, Benzon HT, et al. Regional anesthesia in the patient receiving antithrombotic or thrombolytic therapy: American Society of Regional Anesthesia and Pain Medicine Evidence-Based Guidelines (third edition). Reg Anesth Pain Med. 2010;35:64–101.
14. Das P, Carcao M, Hitzler J. Use of recombinant factor VIIa prior to lumbar puncture in pediatric patients with acute leukemia. Pediatr Blood Cancer. 2006; 47(2):206–9.
15. Silverman R, Kwiatkowski T, Bernstein S, Sanders N, Hilgartner M, Cahill-Bordas M, et al. Safety of lumbar puncture in patients with hemophilia. Ann Emerg Med. 1993;22(11):1739–42.
16. Caruso V, Iacoviello L, Castelnuovo AD, Storti S, Mariani G, de Gaetano G, et al. Thrombotic complications in childhood acute lymphoblastic leukemia: a meta-analysis of 17 prospective studies comprising 1752 pediatric patients. Blood. 2006;108:2216–22.
17. Howard SC, Gajjar A, Ribeiro RC, Rivera GK, Rubnitz JE, Sandlund JT, et al. Safety of lumbar puncture for children with acute lymphoblastic leukemia and thrombocytopenia. JAMA. 2000;284(17): 2222–4.
18. The C17 Council. Guideline for platelet transfusion thresholds for pediatric hematology/oncology patients. Edmonton. 2010. www.c17.ca. Accessed Apr 2013.
19. Gajjar A, Harrison PL, Sandlund JT, Rivera GK, Ribeiro RC, Rubnitz JE, et al. Traumatic lumbar puncture at diagnosis adversely affects outcome in childhood acute lymphoblastic leukemia. Blood. 2000;96(10):3381–4.
20. Burger B, Zimmermann M, Mann G, Kuhl J, Loning L, Riehm H, et al. Diagnostic cerebrospinal fluid examination in children with acute lymphoblastic leukemia: significance of low leukocyte counts with blasts or traumatic lumbar puncture. J Clin Oncol. 2003;21(2):184–8.
21. Rech A, de Carvalho GP, Meneses CF, Hankins J, Howard S, Brunetto AL. The influence of traumatic lumbar puncture and timing of intrathecal therapy on outcome of pediatric acute lymphoblastic leukemia. Pediatr Hematol Oncol. 2005;22(6):483–8.
22. Te Loo DM, Kamps WA, Van Der Does-Van Den Berg A, Van Wering ER, De Graaf SS. Prognostic significance of blasts in the cerebrospinal fluid without pleocytosis or a traumatic lumbar puncture in children with acute lymphoblastic leukemia: Experience of the Dutch Childhood Oncology Group. J Clin Oncol. 2006;24(15):2332–6.
23. Howard SC, Gajjar AJ, Cheng C, Kritchevsky SB, Somes GW, Harrison PL, et al. Risk factors for traumatic and bloody lumbar puncture in children with acute lymphoblastic leukemia. JAMA. 2002;288(16): 2001–7.
24. Maurizi P, Russo I, Chiaretti A, Coccia P, Rizzo D, Lazzareschi I, et al. Procedural analgo-sedation role in reducing the incidence of traumatic lumbar puncture in children with acute lymphoblastic Leukemia. Eur J Cancer. 2011;47:S291.
25. Chiaretti A, Ruggiero A, Barbi E, Pierri F, Maurizi P, Fantacci C, et al. Comparison of propofol versus propofol-ketamine combination in pediatric oncologic procedures performed by non-anesthesiologists. Pediatr Blood Cancer. 2011;57(7):1163–7.
26. Mantadakis E, Katzilakis N, Foundoulaki E, Kalmanti M. Moderate intravenous sedation with fentanyl and midazolam for invasive procedures in children with acute lymphoblastic leukemia. J Pediatr Oncol Nurs. 2009;26(4):217–22.
27. Nagel K, Willan AR, Lappan J, Korz L, Buckley N, Barr RD. Pediatric oncology sedation trial (POST): a double-blind randomized study. Pediatr Blood Cancer. 2008;51(5):634–8.
28. Hollman GA, Schultz MM, Eickhoff JC, Christenson DK. Propofol-fentanyl versus propofol alone for lumbar puncture sedation in children with acute hematologic malignancies: propofol dosing and adverse events. Pediatr Crit Care Med. 2008;9(6):616–22.
29. Cechvala MM, Christenson D, Eickhoff JC, Hollman GA. Sedative preference of families for lumbar punctures in children with acute leukemia: propofol alone or propofol and fentanyl. J Pediatr Hematol Oncol. 2008;30(2):142–7.
30. World Health Organization. Vincristine (and other vinca alkaloids) should only be given intravenously via a minibag. 2007. http://www.who.int/patientsafety/activities/technical/vincristine/en/. Accessed Apr 2013.
31. Fisher A, Lupu L, Gurevitz B, Brill S, Margolin E, Hertzanu Y. Hip flexion and lumbar puncture: a radiological study. Anaesthesia. 2001;56(3):262–6.
32. Tarkkila PJ, Heine H, Tervo RR. Comparison of Sprotte and Quincke needles with respect to post dural puncture headache and backache. Reg Anesth. 1992;17(5):283–7.
33. Richman JM, Joe EM, Cohen SR, Rowlingson AJ, Michaels RK, Jeffries MA, et al. Bevel direction and postdural puncture headache: a meta-analysis. Neurologist. 2006;12(4):224–8.

34. Bruccoleri RE, Chen L. Needle-entry angle for lumbar puncture in children as determined by using ultrasonography. Pediatrics. 2011;127(4):e921–6.
35. Abualenain J, Ranniger C, Jacobs D. Measurement of CSF opening pressure during lumbar puncture in the sitting position in the emergency department. Acad Emerg Med. 2011;1:S244–5.
36. Avery RA, Shah SS, Licht DJ, Seiden JA, Huh JW, Boswinkel J, et al. Reference range for cerebrospinal fluid opening pressure in children. N Engl J Med. 2010;363(9):891–3.
37. Basurto Ona X, Martinez Garcia L, Sola I, Bonfill Cosp X. Drug therapy for treating post-dural puncture headache. Cochrane Database Syst Rev. 2011;8:CD007887.
38. Strupp M, Brandt T. Should one reinsert the stylet during lumbar puncture? N Engl J Med. 1997;336(16):1190.
39. Thoennissen J, Herkner H, Lang W, Domanovits H, Laggner AN, Mullner M. Does bed rest after cervical or lumbar puncture prevent headache? A systematic review and meta-analysis. CMAJ. 2001;165(10):1311–6.
40. Boonmak P, Boonmak S. Epidural blood patching for preventing and treating post-dural puncture headache. Cochrane Database Syst Rev. 2010;1:CD001791.
41. Yazici N, Yalcin B, Cila A, Alnay A, Buyukpamukcu M. Discitis following lumbar puncture in non-Hodgkin lymphoma. Pediatr Hematol Oncol. 2005;22(8):689–94.
42. Reihsaus E, Waldbaur H, Seeling W. Spinal epidural abscess: a meta-analysis of 915 patients. Neurosurg Rev. 2000;23(4):175–204. discussion 5.
43. Orazi A, O'Malley D, Arber D. Illustrated pathology of the bone marrow. Cambridge: Cambridge University Press; 2006.
44. Bain BJ. Bone marrow biopsy morbidity and mortality. Br J Haematol. 2003;121:949–51.
45. Sarigianni M, Vlachaki E, Chissan S, Klonizakis F, Vetsiou E, Anastasiadou KI, et al. Haematoma caused by bone marrow aspiration and trephine biopsy. Hematol Rep. 2011;3(3):e25.
46. Le Dieu R, Luckit J, Saundarasun M. Complications of trephine biopsy. Br J Haematol. 2003;121:822.
47. Malempati S, Joshi S, Lai S, Braner DA, Tegtmeyer K. Videos in clinical medicine: bone marrow aspiration and biopsy. N Engl J Med. 2009;361:e28.
48. Abla O, Friedman J, Doyle J. Performing bone marrow aspiration and biopsy in children: recommended guidelines. Paediatr Child Health. 2008;13(6):499–501.
49. Islam A. Bone marrow aspiration before bone marrow core biopsy using the same bone marrow biopsy needle: a good or bad practice? J Clin Pathol. 2007;60(2):212–5.
50. http://note3.blogspot.com/2004/02/thoracentesis-procedure-guide.html. Accessed 28 May 2013.
51. Abla O, Friedman J, Doyle J. Performing bone marrow aspiration and biopsy in children: Recommended guidelines. Pediatr Child Health. 2008;13(6):499–501.
52. Islam A. Bone marrow aspiration before bone marrow core biospy using the same bnoe marrow biopsy needle: a good or bad practice? J Clin Pathol. 2007;60(2):212–5.
53. Hospital for sick children handbook of pediatrics. 11th ed.
54. www.studentconsult.com/spleen/procedures/pleural tap.cfm. Accessed 28 May 2013.
55. Pertersen WG, Zimmerman R. Limited utility of chest radiology after thoracentesis. Chest. 2000;117(4):1038–42.
56. Infusion of Nurses Society. Infusion nursing standards of practice. Cambridge, MA: INS and Becton Dickinson; 2006 (111).
57. Dougherty L, Watson J. Vascular access devices. In: Dougherty L, Lister S, editors. The Royal Marsden Hospital manual of clinical nursing procedures. 7th ed. Oxford: Blackwell Publishing; 2008.
58. Shiffer CA, Manga PB, et al. Central venous catheter care for the patient with cancer: American society of Clinical Oncology, clinical practice guideline. J Clin Oncol. 2013;31(10):1357–70. htt://jco.ascopubs.org/cgi/doi/10.1200/JCO
59. Safdar N, Maki DG. Use of vancomycin containing lock of flush solutions for prevention of blood stream infection associated with central venous access devices: a meta-analysis of prospective randomized trials. Clin Infect Dis. 2006;43:474–84.
60. Maki DG, Kluger DM, Crnich CK. The risk of blood stream infection in adults with different intravascular devices: a Systematic review of 200 prospective studies. Mayo Clin Proc. 2006;81:1159–71.

Acute Lymphoblastic Leukemia 16

Stephen P. Hunger and Federico G. Antillon

Overview

Acute lymphoblastic leukemia (ALL) is the most common form of cancer in children in high income countries (HIC). The incidence rate of ALL in the United States is about 35 cases/million among children <15 years old and 13 cases/million among adolescents 15–19 years old, and these rates increased steadily between 1975 and 2006 at a rate of 0.8 % average annual percentage change [1, 2]. In the United States, ALL accounts for 25 % of cancers occurring at age 0–14.99 years and 20 % of cases that occur before 20 years [1]. Due to the lack of tumor registries, data regarding the incidence of pediatric ALL in low income countries (LIC) is much less robust than data available from HIC, but the available data suggest that incidence rates for childhood leukemia in LIC are about half those reported in middle income countries (MIC) and HIC [3].

There are several reasons that might explain the apparently lower incidence of ALL in LIC as opposed to MIC and HIC. There likely are true differences in incidence rate. In HIC there is a dramatic peak in ALL incidence rates (~80 cases/million) at 2–3 years of age [1]. This peak is not seen in LIC and emerges in countries as they industrialize [4]. Several explanations have been proposed to explain this peak, including population mixing and an abnormal immune response to a common infection that is delayed in HIC due to lack of exposure in early life [5]. It is also highly likely that many cases of ALL are not diagnosed in LIC, particularly the lowest income countries, due to the similarity in symptoms to those of infectious diseases with rapid onset of symptoms and frequent death from infectious complications. Supporting this, childhood leukemia incidence is lowest in the countries with the lowest gross national income and the highest under 5-year mortality rates [3].

Childhood ALL is universally and rapidly fatal without effective therapy. Treatment of this disease in HIC is one of the major success stories in modern medicine. The first cures of childhood ALL occurred about 50 years ago; today over 85 % of children that develop ALL in HIC will be cured and recent reports show 5-year survival rates exceeding 90 % [6–9]. Treatment of relapsed ALL is much less effective than treatment of newly diagnosed ALL, and the chance of cure following relapse is related to site of relapse,

---

SPH is the Ergen Family Chair in Pediatric Cancer.

S.P. Hunger, M.D. (✉)
Children's Hospital Colorado and the Department of Pediatrics, Center for Cancer and Blood Disorders, University of Colorado School of Medicine, 13123 East 16th Avenue, Box B115, Aurora, CO 80045, USA
e-mail: Stephen.Hunger@childrenscolorado.org

F.G. Antillon, M.D.
Unidad Nacional de Oncología Pediátrica, Guatemala City, Guatemala

D.C. Stefan and C. Rodriguez-Galindo (eds.), *Pediatric Hematology-Oncology in Countries with Limited Resources: A Practical Manual*, DOI 10.1007/978-1-4614-3891-5_16,

ALL genetic features, and time between initial diagnosis and relapse [10].

However, most children that develop ALL don't live in the HIC of North America and Western Europe, but in rapidly developing countries such as India and China and in LIC and MIC (LMIC) in Africa, Asia, and Central and South America with large populations of children less than 20 years old. Although the estimates are imperfect, if one projects US incidence rates onto these countries China and India are predicted to have 4–5 times as many pediatric ALL cases as the United States, and Indonesia, Pakistan, and Nigeria to have about the same number of cases as the United States. Because of this, it is essential to develop ways to improve the diagnosis and treatment of childhood ALL in LMIC throughout the world.

Twinning Between HIC and LMIC

While this seems a daunting task, there is a clear pathway to success. There are multiple examples of partnerships (twinning) between centers in LMIC and those in HIC that have led to major improvements in ALL survival rates in LMIC within 5–10 years [11–13]. In many instances this has involved adoption of intact or modified HIC treatment regimens in LMIC, which requires health care systems that can provide relatively intensive chemotherapy and supportive care. A prime example of this approach is provided by the AHOPCA (Central American Association of Pediatric Hematology Oncology) group in Central America. Beginning 15–20 years ago collaborations were established between pediatric cancer programs in Nicaragua, El Salvador, and Guatemala and those in Monza and Milan, Italy and St. Jude Children's Research Hospital in the United States. Treatment plans were implemented in dedicated units in Nicaragua, El Salvador, and Guatemala with intensive training and provision of financial resources by the HIC centers, leading to rapid improvements in survival. These efforts expanded to include other Central American countries and AHOPCA now conducts their own clinical trials. In Guatemala, survival rates for pediatric ALL now range from 50 % (high risk) to 90 % (low risk) [14]. This strategy is possible in countries with reasonably well-developed health care systems, with infant mortality rates less than 40–50/1,000 live births serving as a good surrogate marker. In HIC, a substantial majority of ALL treatment failures are due to relapse and/or disease resistance. In contrast, the major causes of treatment failure in LMIC, particularly when treatment programs are first established, are abandonment of therapy (almost unheard of in HIC) and treatment-related mortality (TRM) [15]. High rates of TRM can be a major problem associated with implementing intensive HIC ALL regimens in LMIC [16]. In HIC, contemporary ALL treatment regimens are typically associated with TRM rates less than 5 %, but TRM can be 5–10 times higher with the same regimens in LIC, particularly those with infant mortality rates greater than 50/1,000 live births.

One potential way to address treatment of pediatric ALL in countries not able to deliver intensive therapy safety is to first implement less intensive treatment regimens similar to those used in HIC in North America and Western Europe in the 1970s and 1980s and increase treatment intensity only when these therapies are shown to be safe and effective in the LIC center [17]. This strategy also has advantages, particularly when health care resources are limited, as it starts with treatments that are less costly, less toxic, and do not require sophisticated diagnostic tests, but has the potential to cure 40–50 % of children with ALL if TRM can be kept low and abandonment minimized. While this cure rate may seem low, it is likely at least 4–5 times as high as current cure rates in many LIC and successful implementation of this strategy sets the stage for further improvements in cure rates through use of more effective contemporary HIC ALL therapies.

Diagnosis of ALL

Children with ALL are commonly brought to medical attention for symptoms caused by ineffective production of normal blood cells due to

Table 16.1 Common symptoms seen in children with ALL

Symptom/exam finding	Laboratory finding and/or cause
Hematological	
Pallor	Anemia due to decreased red blood cells
Fatigue	Anemia due to decreased red blood cells
Bruising	Thrombocytopenia due to decreased platelets
Bleeding (nose, GI tract, CNS)	Thrombocytopenia due to decreased platelets
Petechiae (tiny red spots that don't blanch with pressure)	Pinpoint hemorrhages in the skin due to decreased platelets
Fever	Infectious or noninfectious; often resolves quickly with onset of ALL therapy
Infection	Decreased neutrophils and/or impaired neutrophil function
Non-hematological	
Bone pain	Expansion of marrow space due to replacement by leukemia; may manifest as irritability and refusal to walk in young children
Joint pain or swelling	Infiltration with leukemia cells; may lead to misdiagnosis as juvenile rheumatoid arthritis and/or rheumatic fever
Hepatomegaly and/or splenomegaly	Infiltration with leukemia cells
Lymphadenopathy	Infiltration with leukemia cells
Testicular enlargement	Infiltration with leukemia cells; typically rock-hard, painless, lumpy
Somnolence	CNS involvement and increased ICP
Headache and/or neck pain	CNS involvement and increased ICP
Vomiting	CNS involvement and increased ICP
Cranial nerve palsies	CNS involvement
Seizures	CNS involvement
Respiratory and/or cardiac compromise	Mediastinal mass obstructing airway and/or pleural or pericardial effusions; most common with T-cell ALL
Elevated LDH	Rapidly proliferative leukemia; seen especially with high WBC count, infant ALL, T-cell ALL, or Burkitt's leukemia
Renal dysfunction	Kidney injury due to tumor lysis and/or infiltration of kidney with leukemia cells; seen especially with high WBC count, infant ALL, T-cell ALL, or Burkitt's leukemia
Rash (raised blue lesions)	Skin infiltrations; seen particularly in young infants where may be confused with congenital cytomegalovirus infection

GI gastrointestinal, *CNS* central nervous system, *ICP* intracranial pressure, *WBC* white blood cell

replacement of the bone marrow (BM) by leukemia, and leukemic involvement of other organs (Table 16.1). A high index of suspicion is required to diagnose ALL because most of these symptoms are nonspecific, and can also be seen with a variety of other disorders, especially infectious diseases that are quite prevalent in many LMIC such as Dengue fever. Because of this, the differential diagnosis is quite broad (Table 16.2).

Simple laboratory tests readily available at most hospitals are needed to establish a diagnosis of ALL including a complete blood cell count with microscopic examination of a peripheral blood smear. In most cases a bone marrow (BM) aspirate/biopsy with microscopic examination is performed to establish the diagnosis. The peripheral blood or BM smear, or biopsy touch preparation is generally stained with Wright's stain (or a variant such as the Wright-Giemsa stain) to identify the different types of blood cells. In some cases additional cytochemical stains are used to distinguish ALL from acute myeloid leukemia (AML), including Sudan black, myeloperoxidase, and nonspecific esterase. In HIC flow cytometry is almost always used to definitively establish the diagnosis of leukemia, the subtype (ALL vs. AML), and immunophenotype (B-cell precursor vs. T-cell ALL). While this information is very useful, particularly when therapy may be tailored to immunophenotype in HIC, it is not required

Table 16.2 Differential diagnosis of ALL

Disease(s)	Important distinctions
Hematologic and oncologic disorders	
Acute myeloid leukemia (AML)	Symptoms similar; morphology of blasts in PB and/or BM is different; cytochemical staining of PB/BM samples may be required to differentiate ALL and AML blasts
Non-Hodgkin's lymphoma (NHL)	T-NHL and T-ALL may have very similar symptoms and findings; usually treated in same manner
Metastatic solid tumors	May see marrow replacement with small round blue cell tumors such as neuroblastoma, rhabdomyosarcoma, or Ewing sarcoma; primary solid tumor usually, but not always, present on physical exam or X-rays studies; special stains of BMA/Bx may be required
Idiopathic thrombocytopenic purpura (ITP)	Isolated thrombocytopenia in ITP; typically otherwise healthy with sudden onset of bruising/bleeding; BM morphology shows abundant megakaryocytes and normal other cells in ITP
Severe aplastic anemia (SAA)	Pancytopenia may be seen in both ALL and SAA; BMA/Bx is severely hypocellular/empty in SAA but packed in ALL. ALL sometimes presents with pancytopenic phase and serial BMA/Bx may be needed to establish diagnosis
Myelodysplastic (MDS) and/or myeloproliferative (MPD) disorders	Pancytopenia may be seen in both ALL and MDS/MPD; BMA/Bx +/− special stains needed to establish distinction
Hemophagocytic lymphohistiocytosis (HLH)	HLH can present with fever, systemic illness, pancytopenia, hepatosplenomegaly, and lymphadenopathy. BMA/Bx may be required to establish correct diagnosis
Non-hematological disorders	
Juvenile rheumatoid arthritis (JRA)	Small percentage of ALL cases present with prominent joint symptoms and fever and can be confused with JRA; BMA/Bx should establish correct diagnosis
B_{12} or folate deficiency	B_{12} and folate deficiency primarily cause anemia with characteristic red blood cell morphology; B_{12} deficiency may be associated with neurological symptoms
Infections	
Viral infections EBV, CMV, etc.)	Can present with fever, hepatosplenomegaly, generalized lymphadenopathy, and elevated white blood cell count with marked lymphocytosis; lymphocyte morphology can help distinguish from ALL but BMA/Bx may be needed to establish diagnosis
Dengue fever	Dengue associated with fever, headache, muscle and joint pains, and frequently with measles-like rash. Some cases have low white blood cell and platelet counts with bleeding; Dengue endemic in many areas of tropics and subtropics; may need BMA/Bx to establish correct diagnosis

PB peripheral blood, *BMA/Bx* bone marrow aspirate/biopsy, *EBV* Epstein Barr virus, *CMV* cytomegalovirus

for the diagnosis and effective treatment of ALL. The flow cytometry machines and reagents are typically very expensive and not usually available in resource-limited settings present in many LMIC. However, if present, simplified algorithms have been established that can facilitate diagnosis and monitoring of ALL treatment response (minimal residual disease) at relatively low cost [18].

There are several systems that have been used to classify ALL based on morphology and/or immunophenotype. For many years the French–American–British (FAB) system that classified cases as L1, L2, or L3 based on morphology was used [19]. This classification is useful mainly for the recognition of the distinctive L3 morphology of Burkitt's leukemia. This subtype comprises only 1–2 % of childhood ALL cases in HIC, but requires very different treatment, similar or identical to that used for advanced stage Burkitt's lymphoma, than other

ALL cases [20]. Other than this, the FAB classification of ALL does not provide significant clinical utility and has been supplanted by the 2008 World Health Organization (WHO) classification [21]. However, neither WHO nor FAB classification is needed to treat ALL in LMIC.

Important Issues in the Initial Medical Management of Children with ALL

The specific approaches to ALL treatment are discussed below. Induction chemotherapy typically lasts 4 weeks and consists of three or four drugs administered orally, intramuscularly, or intravenously including a corticosteroid (prednisone [PRED] or dexamethasone [DEX]), vincristine (VCR), and an asparaginase (ASNase) preparation with or without an anthracycline. A simple 2-drug 4-week PRED/VCR regimen with or without intrathecal chemotherapy will induce complete remission in about 85 % of children with ALL, and this rate can be increased to 95 % or higher with the addition of ASNase [22]. Even this simple regimen produced TRM rates of 3–5 % when first introduced in HIC in the 1970s. Thus, vigorous supportive care is essential.

Metabolic derangements and supportive care: Children with ALL can present with high white blood cell (WBC) counts and lymphoblasts can undergo lysis either spontaneously or after treatment is begun. Dying WBC release intracellular contents including potassium, phosphorus, and DNA that is metabolized via the uric acid pathway [23]. Acute tumor lysis syndrome (TLS) is characterized by hyperkalemia, hyperuricemia, hyperphosphatemia, and secondary hypocalcemia. It is classified as laboratory TLS if only metabolic abnormalities are present and clinical TLS when this is accompanied by clinical symptoms including renal dysfunction manifested as increased creatinine, cardiac rhythm disturbances (due to hyperkalemia), seizures, or death. The risk of TLS is highest in children with high and/or rapidly increasing WBC and/or bulky extramedullary disease; thus, major risk factors for TLS include WBC >100,000/μL, infant ALL, T-cell ALL, and Burkitt's leukemia. The risk can be exacerbated by dehydration and/or malnutrition, and delayed diagnosis, all of which are common in LMIC.

Symptoms of TLS are caused by the metabolic derangements listed above. The problems are often exacerbated by formation of calcium phosphate and/or uric acid crystals in the kidney that cause acute renal injury leading to further impairment in urine output and increased metabolic abnormalities. Measures used to prevent TLS include vigorous intravenous hydration where possible, usually at twice maintenance fluid requirement rates or 3,000 mL/m^2/day. Urine output should be at least 2 cc/kg/h and preferably 3–5 cc/kg/h. Loop diuretics such as furosemide may be needed to insure adequate urine output and to make sure that fluid input and urine output are matched. Because higher urine pH increases the solubility of uric acid, bicarbonate (40–80 mEq/L) is usually added to intravenous fluids to prevent uric acid precipitation in renal tubules. However, higher urine pH promotes calcium phosphate crystallization, so caution must be used. Allopurinol, which inhibits the enzyme xanthine oxidase needed for uric acid formation, is administered 50–100 mg orally three times/day to prevent TLS. Ideally hydration, urinary alkalinization, and allopurinol should be given for 12–48 h prior to the start of chemotherapy and continued for the first 3–7 days of treatment. This may not be possible in patients that present with very high WBC and signs/symptoms due to leukostasis.

In the worst cases, TLS can be fatal due to renal failure and/or cardiac dysrhythmias. However, clinically significant TLS can be prevented or managed successfully in the overwhelming majority of children with ALL using the measures discussed above, even with oral hydration when necessary due to local conditions.

Transfusion support: Children with ALL frequently present with or develop symptomatic anemia and/or thrombocytopenia. Prior to the advent of effective ALL therapy, death due to anemia and/or bleeding was common, and this remains a major concern in LMIC. In HIC that almost always have well-established blood banks and ready access to red blood cells and platelets for transfusion, this problem is relatively simple to manage and transfusions are typically provided to treat symptoms of anemia or thrombocytopenia, or prophylactically when blood values fall below certain levels (typically 7–8 g/dL of hemoglobin or hematocrit <20 %, and platelet count <10–20,000/μL). In contrast, access to and the safety of blood components for transfusion are major problems in LMIC. Even when transfusions are feasible, they are often very expensive and available only if the family is able to pay. In the absence of a volunteer blood banking system as present in most HIC, family members and friends may need to be recruited to provide blood for transfusion to children with ALL and testing for blood-borne infectious agents such as Hepatitis B and C and HIV may not be readily available. Development of an effective blood banking system is often a major barrier that must be overcome as ALL treatment programs are established at LMIC centers. When possible, blood products should be irradiated to decrease the risk of transfusion-acquired graft versus host disease.

Treatment and prevention of infections: Another major cause of morbidity and mortality in children with ALL is infections. Bacterial and fungal infections are particularly problematic during induction therapy or during intensive phases of post-induction therapy. Because prolonged corticosteroid use is associated with oral and vaginal yeast infections, especially candida albicans or other candida species, most children with ALL receive oral nystatin (or similar agents) during induction or other periods of prolonged corticosteroid use. Fluconazole and itraconazole may be more effective than nystatin, but are much more expensive, can be associated with hepatotoxicty, and alter the pharmacokinetics of vincristine.

Bacterial infections occur commonly in children with ALL, particularly in association with neutropenia. Intravenous antibiotics should be given when fever develops and the absolute neutrophil count (ANC) is <500/μL or if there is concern about systemic infection based on other clinical considerations. The choice of antibiotics will vary based upon the local experience regarding the type of organisms that are prevalent in the population and the pattern of local antibiotic resistance. In general, treatment should include coverage for enteric gram negative organisms such as *E. coli* and *Pseudomonas aeruginosa* and gram positive organisms such as *Staphylococcus aureus*.

A unique problem for children with ALL is the risk of *Pneumocystis carinii* (now termed *Pneumocystis jiroveci*) pneumonia (PCP). Prior to the advent of effective prophylaxis, 20–25 % of children treated for ALL developed PCP, often with fatal consequences [24]. Prophylaxis with trimethoprim-sulfamethoxazole (TMP/SMX) is highly effective [24, 25], and children with ALL should receive PCP prophylaxis with TMP/SMX at a dose of TMP 5 mg/kg/day in two divided doses given on 2–3 consecutive days each week starting soon after diagnosis and continuing until 3 months after ALL therapy is completed. Those unable to tolerate TMP/SMX can be treated with Dapsone (1–2 mg/kg/day; maximum dose 100 mg/day) or atovaquone (30–45 mg/kg/day). Aerosolized pentamidine given every 4 weeks is also an option, but this is less likely to be available in LMIC.

Venous access: Because ALL treatment involves multiple doses of intravenous chemotherapy with drugs that are vesicants (vincristine, anthracyclines) and can cause significant injury to the skin and tissue if they extravasate, almost all children with ALL in HIC have an indwelling central venous catheter. These are almost never available in LIC and variably available in MIC. Hence, most children will receive ALL chemotherapy through peripheral intravenous catheters (IVs) inserted specifically to administer the chemotherapy. Significant care must be taken to insure proper IV placement before administration of vesicant agents.

Varicella: Another significant concern in children with ALL is development of a primary varicella infection or reactivation of the varicella-zoster virus (VZV) causing shingles. In the United States, primary varicella infection in children with ALL is now rare due to near universal vaccination against VZV. However, VZV vaccination is uncommon in LMIC and primary varicella infection occurs frequently and can cause significant morbidity including visceral and CNS involvement, secondary bacterial infection, and post-VZV inflammatory complications [26]. Without effective antiviral therapy and supportive care, primary VZV infection during ALL treatment is associated with a 5–10 % risk of mortality [27]. With effective therapy, death is uncommon; a recent review of primary varicella infection in HIC showed only 20 deaths among over 35,000 children with ALL, with 14 of these 20 deaths occurring in the first year of therapy [27]. Following a documented exposure to VZV in a nonimmune patient varicella-zoster immune globulin (VZIG) can be given if available. It is essential to isolate exposed patients from other patients for 21 days following exposure (28 days if VZIG is administered) to prevent nosocomial outbreaks. If clinical varicella develops, treatment with intravenous acyclovir 500 mg/m^2/dose three times daily (or related antivirals) should be given immediately and therapy should be continued until all lesions are scabbed and no new lesions have developed for 24 h. Renal dysfunction can develop with IV acyclovir treatment, so patients should receive IV fluids and creatinine levels should be monitored closely. It is reasonable to transition to oral therapy after 3 days of IV therapy if the patient is responding well. Chemotherapy, particularly corticosteroids, is generally suspended during treatment of active infection, but this may not be possible if a patient develops varicella in the first few months of therapy. Good data do not exist regarding acyclovir treatment at the time of exposure, but this practice is common in many LMIC. For example, in Guatemala, if a patient has been exposed and has had no varicella in the past, acyclovir is given orally at 30 mg/kg/day for 7 days, starting 10 days after the exposure. Results are good with this approach (Melgar M, Antillon F, personal communication). Development of shingles during ALL therapy can also be associated with significant complications and treatment with an appropriate antiviral is indicated (IV acyclovir is usually given at half the dose used for treatment of primary VZV). Because immunocompromised patients can have viremia and shed virus via aerosol routes, ALL patients with shingles should be isolated until the infection is resolved.

Nutritional assessment and support: The incidence of malnutrition in LMIC children can be as high as 50 % and the presence of malnutrition can have a major impact on the tolerance, effectiveness, and safety of ALL treatment [28]. Simple anthropomorphic measurements, including triceps skin fold thickness (TSFT) and mid upper arm circumference (MUAC), can be used to assess nutritional status. Antillon and colleagues recently reported that more than 50 % of children diagnosed with ALL in Guatemala had moderate or severe nutritional deprivation at the time of initial diagnosis, that severe nutritional deprivation was associated with an increased risk of treatment abandonment and relapse, but that the risk of death was decreased significantly in children that improved their nutritional status in the first 6 months of therapy [28]. Algorithms have been developed to guide nutritional interventions in AHOPCA that should be widely applicable to other LMIC [29]. A major focus of support efforts for the families of children with ALL in LMIC is often the provision of food baskets that can provide nutritional support to the patient, siblings, and other family members, thereby decreasing financial pressures that may lead to abandonment.

Antiemetic therapy: Nausea and vomiting secondary to chemotherapy can be prevented in most cases. Every effort should be made to prevent this side effect and to provide adequate antiemetic drugs. Preventive treatment should start before chemotherapy is given and should continue as long as nausea and vomiting are likely to be produced. Scheduled antiemetic doses should be given regardless of symptoms. Nevertheless, drug costs for 5-HT3 receptor agonists may be a limiting factor in LMIC. If cost is an issue the use of metoclopramide, diphenhydramine, and dexamethasone is useful if chemotherapy has a mild or moderately emetogenic potential. If the emetogenic potential is high, 5-HT3 receptor agonists should be used if possible.

Abandonment of therapy: Abandonment of therapy is a major cause of treatment failure in most LMIC affecting 40–60 % cases [30, 31]. The AHOPCA group defines abandonment as an interruption of 4 or more weeks of scheduled therapy; this has been suggested as a uniform definition by the SIOP Abandonment Working Group [32]. Successful interventions have been used to prevent abandonment in different countries. At the National Pediatric Cancer Unit in Guatemala, abandonment has decreased from the historic 42 % before opening of the cancer center to less than 2 % in 2011 for all types of pediatric cancer through the establishment of a psychosocial team including both social workers and psychologists whose aim is to support families throughout the cancer experience, and provide funds for transportation, lodging, and food baskets when necessary (Silvia Rivas F and Antillon F, unpublished observations). In Recife, Brazil, through the provision of lodging, social work, transportation, and food subsidies, and the establishment of a parent group, a fundraising foundation, and a patient tracking system, abandonment among children with ALL decreased from 16 % in 1980 to 1 % in 2002 [12].

General Concepts of Pediatric ALL Treatment

Treatment for ALL in HIC consists of complex combination chemotherapy regimens that last about 2.5–3 years, with 6–8 months of relatively intensive therapy followed by 1.5–2 years of low intensity maintenance therapy during which most children can resume normal activities and attend school. A core set of chemotherapy drugs needed for treatment of childhood ALL has been defined (Table 16.3) with additional information available regarding drugs needed for pediatric oncology treatment in LMIC [33, 34]. These drugs have been widely available in HIC for many years; most are readily available in LMIC and relatively inexpensive, with the exception of asparaginase preparations, which can be extremely expensive in both LMIC and HIC.

When remissions of childhood ALL first began to be achieved consistently in the 1960s, a major cause of treatment failure was isolated central nervous system (CNS) relapse. Aur and colleagues showed that the rate of CNS relapse could be decreased substantially and survival increased by adding prophylactic or presymptomatic cranial irradiation (2,400 cGy) plus five doses of intrathecal methotrexate [35]. Later studies showed that cranial irradiation could be eliminated for most good risk patients with

Table 16.3 Drugs used to treat pediatric acute lymphoblastic leukemia

Class	Specific drugs	Phase of therapy	Route of administration
Corticosteroids	Prednisone, dexamethasone	Induction, reinduction, maintenance	PO, IV
Vinca alkaloids	Vincristine	Throughout therapy	IV
Asparaginase preparations	*E. coli* asparaginase, PEG-asparaginase, *erwinia* asparaginase	Induction, reinduction	IM, IV
Anthracyclines	Doxorubicin, daunorubicin	Induction, reinduction	IV
Alkylating agents	Cyclophosphamide	Consolidation, reconsolidation	IV
Antimetabolites	Cytarabine	Consolidation, reconsolidation	IV, SC, IT
	Methotrexate	Intensification, maintenance	IV, IM, PO, IT
	6-Mercaptopurine, 6-thioguanine	Consolidation, reconsolidation, and maintenance	PO

PO oral, *IV* intravenous, *IM* intramuscular, *SC* subcutaneous, *IT* intrathecal intensive intrathecal chemotherapy and better systemic therapy [36, 37]. The use of cranial irradiation has been greatly reduced in most contemporary HIC regimens, and some have completely eliminated this treatment modality [38–40].

As discussed earlier, over 80–85 % of children diagnosed with ALL in HIC can be cured. The development of large cooperative treatment groups that conduct clinical trials, which often include 70 % or more of children with ALL in a given country, has been critical to improvements in survival for pediatric ALL in HIC [9]. There is near universal access to effective treatments for pediatric ALL in most HIC and widespread availability of knowledge about the specifics of effective treatment regimens. Although children with ALL have a significant risk of short- and long-term toxicity, most children that are cured will go on to lead healthy and productive lives. Thus it is essential to develop ways to deliver appropriate therapy to children with ALL in LMIC.

Specifics of Pediatric ALL Treatment Regimens and Their Implementation in LMIC

One strategy that has been very effective in some MIC is twinning partnerships that implement contemporary HIC treatment regimens. This approach is resource-intensive, both in terms of costs and the need for substantial investment of time from the HIC partner. Oncologists from both the MIC and HIC play a key role in this process, but it is critical not to overlook or underestimate the importance of education and assistance of MIC nurses, social workers, data managers, and physicians that provide diagnostic support and supportive care such as pathologists and specialists in pediatric surgery, infectious disease, and intensive care medicine. With this approach, substantial improvements in cure rates can be obtained in a relatively short time [12].

It is very important not to despair if sufficient resources are not available to pursue this approach. Many children with ALL can be cured with less intensive and less expensive treatment regimens similar to those used in HIC in the 1970s and 1980s [36, 41, 42], and some can be cured with even less therapy especially if cranial irradiation can be given. A very simple regimen that includes only induction and maintenance should be feasible in most LIC (Table 16.4). The rate of CNS relapse will be high with this regimen, and cranial irradiation should be administered if possible. This regimen is similar to that used in many HIC in the 1960s and 1970s and

Table 16.4 A simple ALL treatment regimen

Agent	Dose/route	Days
Induction (4 weeks)		
Prednisone	60 mg/m^2/day PO in three divided doses	1–28
Vincristine	1.5 mg/m^2 IV (max dose 2 mg)	1, 8, 15, 22
Methotrexate	Age-specific[a] given IT	Days 1, 15
Consolidation (4 weeks); start when ANC >1,000/μl and platelets >100,000/μL		
6-Mercaptopurine	50–75 mg/m^2/day PO	1–28
Vincristine	1.5 mg/m^2 IV (max dose 2 mg)	1
Methotrexate	Age-specific[a] given IT	Days 1, 8, 15, 22
Maintenance (continue for 3 years from diagnosis); start when ANC >1,000/μL and platelets >100,000/μL. Adjust doses of 6-MP and MTX to maintain ANC >1,000/μL and platelets >100,000/μL		
Repeat 12 weeks cycles		
6-Mercaptopurine (6-MP)	50–75 mg/m^2/day PO	1–84
Methotrexate (MTX)	20 mg/m^2 PO or IM/IV	8, 15, 22, 29, 36, 43, 50, 57, 64, 71, 78
Vincristine	1.5 mg/m^2 IV (max dose 2 mg)	1, 8, 15
Prednisone	40 mg/m^2/day PO in three divided doses	1–21
Methotrexate	Age-specific[a] given IT	Day 1

Perform bone marrow aspirate at end induction, start maintenance, and periodically during maintenance

Cranial irradiation (2,400 cGy given as 200 cGy/day Monday through Friday for 12 days) should be given between consolidation and maintenance if possible

PO oral, *IV* intravenous, *IM* intramuscular, *IT* intrathecal, *ANC* absolute neutrophil count

[a]Age-specific intrathecal methotrexate: 1–2 years 8 mg; 2–3 years 10 mg; 3+ years 12 mg

Table 16.5 Modified CCG 105 standard treatment regimen

Agent	Dose/route	Days
Induction (4 weeks)		
Prednisone	40 mg/m²/day PO in three divided doses	1–28
Vincristine	1.5 mg/m² IV (max dose 2 mg)	1, 8, 15, 22
E. coli asparaginase	6,000 units/m² IM	3 times/week (Mon, Wed, Fri) starting at day 3; weeks 1, 2, and 3
Methotrexate	Age-specific[a] given IT	Days 1, 15
Consolidation (4 weeks); start when ANC >1,000/μL and platelets >100,000/μL		
6-Mercaptopurine	50–75 mg/m²/day PO	1–28
Vincristine	1.5 mg/m² IV (max dose 2 mg)	1
Methotrexate	Age-specific[a] given IT	Days 1, 8, 15, 22
Maintenance (continued for 2 years for girls and 3 years for boys from day 1 of phase); start when ANC >1,000/μL and platelets >100,000/μL. Adjust doses of 6-MP and MTX to maintain ANC >1,000/μL and platelets >100,000/μL		
Repeat 12 weeks cycles		
6-Mercaptopurine (6-MP)	50–75 mg/m²/day PO	1–84
Methotrexate (MTX)	20 mg/m² PO or IM/IV	8, 15, 22, 29, 36, 43, 50, 57, 64, 71, 78
Vincristine	1.5 mg/m² IV (max dose 2 mg)	1, 29, 57
Prednisone	40 mg/m²/day PO in three divided doses	1–5, 29–33, 57–61
Methotrexate	Age-specific[a] given IT	Day 1

Perform bone marrow aspirate at end induction, start maintenance, and periodically during maintenance

Possible substitutions: replace prednisone with dexamethasone 6 mg/m²/day PO in three divided doses; add a prednisone prophase (60 mg/m²/day PO in three divided doses on days 1–7 with IT MTX on day 1) prior to starting induction therapy

PO oral, *IV* intravenous, *IM* intramuscular, *IT* intrathecal

[a]Age-specific intrathecal methotrexate: 1–2 years 8 mg; 2–3 years 10 mg; 3+ years 12 mg

can cure 20–30 % of children with ALL (fewer without cranial irradiation) if rates of TRM and abandonment can be minimized.

Several regimens exist that can be implemented in most settings and should be able to cure about 50 % of children with ALL if TRM can be kept low and abandonment minimized; once these are implemented successfully, treatment intensity can be increased gradually with careful monitoring of TRM [17]. A modified version of the baseline treatment regimen used by the Children's Cancer Group (CCG 105) for low and intermediate risk ALL patients until the late 1980s is shown in Table 16.5 [41]. This regimen produced a 16-year event-free survival (EFS) rate of 59 % [43]. Without cranial irradiation, the rate of CNS relapse with this regimen was 20–25 % [37]. The subsequent CCG 1922 study showed that substitution of dexamethasone for prednisone significantly improved EFS and decreased CNS relapse rate [44]. Based on this, it would be very reasonable to modify the regimen shown in Table 16.5 to use dexamethasone during induction and maintenance rather than prednisone. The Berlin–Frankfurt–Muenster (BFM) group adopted a 1-week prednisone prophase consisting of 7 days of prednisone 60 mg/m²/day with a dose of IT methotrexate on day 1 in the early 1980s [45]. This phase was introduced to give time to stabilize the patient and minimize the risk of TLS before multi-agent therapy began, and it would also be reasonable to modify this regimen to include a prophase.

A key finding of the CCG 105 study was that outcomes were improved by either adoption of the intensive induction/consolidation regimen pioneered by the BFM group or addition of a delayed intensification (DI) reinduction/

reconsolidation phase [41, 43, 45, 46]. Because introducing intensive phases of treatment after remission is achieved is safer, once the Table 16.5 regimen is implemented successfully with low TRM, a DI phase can be introduced [17]. If dexamethasone is used, this regimen would mimic that used in CCG 1922 which achieved an 85 % 6-year EFS rate in children with standard risk (see below) ALL (Table 16.6) [44]. A prednisone prophase could also be used with this regimen, but addition of the DI phase obviates the need for cranial irradiation in most patients.

Additional treatment intensifications that are commonly used in HIC ALL protocols include a 4-drug induction that includes an anthracycline and intensive consolidation (the BFM Ia and Ib phases), and use of escalating dose IV methotrexate without leucovorin rescue or high dose IV methotrexate plus leucovorin rescue during the interim maintenance phase. Once these are implemented the regimen starts to recapitulate a HIC regimen, as has been shown to be effective in AHOPCA [14, 47].

As is true for HIC, treatment of relapsed ALL is less effective than treatment of newly diagnosed ALL in LMIC. However, data from the AHOPCA group show that 20–30 % of children with ALL that relapse in MIC can survive at least 3 years following treatment with chemotherapy (without stem cell transplantation) and that this rate is about 50 % in good risk subsets [48]. Thus, relapse should not be viewed as hopeless and rational treatment strategies can be developed guided by simple clinical prognostic factors.

Prognostic Factors

Simple factors predictive of outcome include age (younger is better, except for infants less than 1 year) and initial WBC count (lower is better). They are combined in the NCI/Rome risk classification syndrome that divides non-infant ALL patients (B-cell precursor only) into standard (SR; age 1.00–9.99 years and initial WBC <50,000/μL) and high-risk subsets (HR; age ≥10 years or initial WBC ≥50,000/μL) [49]. Immunophenotying to determine cell lineage is performed in most HIC, but is not readily available in most LMIC and is not essential. About 80–85 % of children with ALL have B-cell precursor (BCP; previously termed common) ALL, 10–15 % have T-cell ALL, and 1–2 % have mature B-cell ALL or Burkitt's leukemia. Children with T-ALL have an inferior outcome to those with BCP ALL [9]. Because T-ALL is more common in blacks, the frequency of T-ALL will vary according to the racial composition of the population. As noted earlier, Burkitt's leukemia is treated completely differently than ALL.

Other more sophisticated and often very expensive diagnostic tests readily available in HIC include cytogenetic or molecular genetic studies to define sentinel abnormalities, many of which have important prognostic implications. These tests are generally not available in LMIC, and are not essential to delivering effective therapy. A major prognostic factor is the rapidity of response to single agent or multi-agent therapy, which can be measured simply and inexpensively by peripheral blood or bone marrow morphology, or in a complicated and expensive manner using advanced flow cytometry and/or molecular genetic techniques. The response to the prednisone prophase is perhaps the easiest prognostic factor. In HIC, about 90 % are good responders (<1,000 lymphoblasts/μL at the end of the prophase) and have a dramatically better outcome than 10 % of patients with a poor response (≥1,000 lymphoblasts/μL at the end of the prophase) [50]. The CCG showed the BM morphology after 7–14 days of multi-agent chemotherapy was a very strong prognostic factor, with patients that have ≥25 % marrow blasts after 7–14 days of therapy having a particularly poor outcome [51].

Summary

ALL is the most common pediatric cancer. Five-year survival rates exceed 90 % in HIC, and, through twinning, centers in LIC with infant mortality rates less than 40–50/1,000 live births have attained cure rates of 50–70 %.

Table 16.6 Modified CCG 1922 treatment regimen

Agent	Dose/route	Days
Induction (4 weeks)		
Dexamethasone	6 mg/m^2/day PO in three divided doses	1–28
Vincristine	1.5 mg/m^2 IV (max dose 2 mg)	1, 8, 15, 22
E. coli asparaginase	6,000 units/m^2 IM	3 times/week (Mon, Wed, Fri) starting at day 3; weeks 1, 2, and 3
Methotrexate	Age-specific[a] given IT	Days 1, 15
Consolidation (4 weeks); start when ANC >1,000/μL and platelets >100,000/μL		
6-Mercaptopurine	50–75 mg/m^2/day PO	1–28
Vincristine	1.5 mg/m^2 IV (max dose 2 mg)	1
Methotrexate	Age-specific[a] given IT	Days 1, 8, 15, 22
Interim maintenance (8 weeks); start when ANC >1,000/μL and platelets >100,000/μL		
6-Mercaptopurine	50–75 mg/m^2/day PO	1–49
Methotrexate	20 mg/m^2 PO or IM/IV	1, 8, 15, 22, 29, 36, 43, 50
Vincristine	1.5 mg/m^2 IV (max dose 2 mg)	1, 29
Dexamethasone	6 mg/m^2/day PO in three divided doses	1–5, 29–33
Methotrexate	Age-specific[a] given IT	Day 29
Delayed intensification (8 weeks); start when ANC >1,000/μL and platelets >100,000/μL; use same parameters to start day 29 therapy		
Dexamethasone	10 mg/m^2/day PO in three divided doses	1–7 and 15–21
Vincristine	1.5 mg/m^2 IV (max dose 2 mg)	1, 8, 15
E. coli asparaginase	6,000 units/m^2 IM	3 times/week (Mon, Wed, Fri) starting at day 3; weeks 1 and 2
Doxorubicin	25 mg/m^2 IV	1, 8, 15
Cyclophosphamide	1,000 mg/m^2 IV	29
6-Thioguanine	60 mg/m^2/day PO	29–42
Cytarabine	75 mg/m^2 IV or SQ	29–32 and 36–39
Methotrexate	Age-specific[a] given IT	Days 1, 29
Maintenance (continued for 2 years for girls and 3 years for boys from day 1 of phase); start when ANC >1,000/μL and platelets >100,000/μL. Adjust doses of 6-MP and MTX to maintain ANC >1,000/μL and platelets >100,000/μL		
Repeat 12 weeks cycles		
6-Mercaptopurine (6-MP)	50–75 mg/m^2/day PO	1–84
Methotrexate (MTX)	20 mg/m^2 PO or IM/IV	8, 15, 22, 29, 36, 43, 50, 57, 64, 71, 78
Vincristine	1.5 mg/m^2 IV (max dose 2 mg)	1, 29, 57
Dexamethasone	6 mg/m^2/day PO in three divided doses	1–5, 29–33, 57–61
Methotrexate	Age-specific[a] given IT	Day 1

Perform bone marrow aspirate at end induction, start maintenance, and periodically during maintenance

Possible substitution: add a prednisone prophase (60 mg/m^2/day PO in three divided doses on days 1–7 with IT MTX on day 1) prior to starting induction therapy

[a]Age-specific intrathecal methotrexate: 1–2 years 8 mg; 2–3 years 10 mg; 3+ years 12 mg

PO oral, *IV* intravenous, *IM* intramuscular, *SC* subcutaneous, *IT* intrathecal

Outcomes for relapsed ALL are much worse, stressing the need for effective therapy at initial diagnosis. Graduated intensity regimens have the promise to decrease TRM and improve survival and may be particularly effective in LIC with infant mortality rates greater than 50/1,000 live births.

References

1. Ries LA, Smith MA, Gurney JG, et al. Cancer incidence and survival among children and adolescents: United States SEER Program 1975–1995, National Cancer Institute. Bethesda, MD; 1999.
2. Smith MA, Seibel NL, Altekruse SF, et al. Outcomes for children and adolescents with cancer: challenges for the twenty-first century. J Clin Oncol. 2010;28: 2625–34.
3. Howard SC, Metzger ML, Wilimas JA, et al. Childhood cancer epidemiology in low-income countries. Cancer. 2008;112:461–72.
4. Greaves M. A natural history for pediatric acute leukemia. Blood. 1993;82:1043–51.
5. Greaves M. Infection, immune responses and the aetiology of childhood leukaemia. Nat Rev Cancer. 2006;6:193–203.
6. Gaynon PS, Angiolillo AL, Carroll WL, et al. Long-term results of the children's cancer group studies for childhood acute lymphoblastic leukemia 1983-2002: a Children's Oncology Group Report. Leukemia. 2010;24:285–97.
7. Moricke A, Zimmermann M, Reiter A, et al. Long-term results of five consecutive trials in childhood acute lymphoblastic leukemia performed by the ALL-BFM study group from 1981 to 2000. Leukemia. 2010;24:265–84.
8. Salzer WL, Devidas M, Carroll WL, et al. Long-term results of the pediatric oncology group studies for childhood acute lymphoblastic leukemia 1984-2001: a report from the Children's Oncology Group. Leukemia. 2010;24:355–70.
9. Hunger SP, Lu X, Devidas M, et al. Improved survival for children and adolescents with acute lymphoblastic leukemia between 1990 and 2005: a report from the Children's Oncology Group. J Clin Oncol. 2012;30: 1663–9.
10. Nguyen K, Devidas M, Cheng SC, et al. Factors influencing survival after relapse from acute lymphoblastic leukemia: a Children's Oncology Group study. Leukemia. 2008;22:2142–50.
11. Masera G, Baez F, Biondi A, et al. North-South twinning in paediatric haemato-oncology: the La Mascota programme, Nicaragua. Lancet. 1998;352:1923–6.
12. Howard SC, Pedrosa M, Lins M, et al. Establishment of a pediatric oncology program and outcomes of childhood acute lymphoblastic leukemia in a resource-poor area. JAMA. 2004;291:2471–5.
13. Veerman AJ, Sutaryo, Sumadiono. Veerman AJ, Sutaryo, Sumadiono. Twinning: a rewarding scenario for development of oncology services in transitional countries. Pediatr Blood Cancer. 2005;45: 103–6.
14. Antillon-Klussmann F, Valverde P, Garrido C, et al. Treatment of acute lymphoblastic leukemia in limited income country: the experience of the Unidad Nacional de Oncologis Pediatrica (UNOP) of Guatemala. Pediatr Blood Cancer. 2010;55:861 (abstr.).
15. Metzger ML, Howard SC, Fu LC, et al. Outcome of childhood acute lymphoblastic leukaemia in resource-poor countries. Lancet. 2003;362:706–8.
16. Gupta S, Antillon FA, Bonilla M, et al. Treatment-related mortality in children with acute lymphoblastic leukemia in Central America. Cancer. 2011;117(20): 4788–95.
17. Hunger SP, Sung L, Howard SC. Treatment strategies and regimens of graduated intensity for childhood acute lymphoblastic leukemia in low-income countries: a proposal. Pediatr Blood Cancer. 2009;52: 559–65.
18. Coustan-Smith E, Ribeiro RC, Stow P, et al. A simplified flow cytometric assay identifies children with acute lymphoblastic leukemia who have a superior clinical outcome. Blood. 2006;108:97–102.
19. Bennett JM, Catovsky D, Daniel MT, et al. The morphological classification of acute lymphoblastic leukaemia: concordance among observers and clinical correlations. Br J Haematol. 1981;47:553–61.
20. Miles RR, Arnold S, Cairo MS. Risk factors and treatment of childhood and adolescent Burkitt lymphoma/ leukaemia. Br J Haematol. 2012;156:730–43.
21. Campo E, Swerdlow SH, Harris NL, et al. The 2008 WHO classification of lymphoid neoplasms and beyond: evolving concepts and practical applications. Blood. 2012;117:5019–32.
22. Ortega JA, Nesbit Jr ME, Donaldson MH, et al. L-Asparaginase, vincristine, and prednisone for induction of first remission in acute lymphocytic leukemia. Cancer Res. 1977;37:535–40.
23. Howard SC, Jones DP, Pui CH. The tumor lysis syndrome. N Engl J Med. 2011;364:1844–54.
24. Hughes WT, Kuhn S, Chaudhary S, et al. Successful chemoprophylaxis for Pneumocystis carinii pneumonitis. N Engl J Med. 1977;297:1419–26.
25. Hughes WT, Rivera GK, Schell MJ, et al. Successful intermittent chemoprophylaxis for Pneumocystis carinii pneumonitis. N Engl J Med. 1987;316:1627–32.
26. Feldman S, Hughes WT, Daniel CB. Varicella in children with cancer: seventy-seven cases. Pediatrics. 1975;56:388–97.
27. Caniza MA, Hunger SP, Schrauder A, et al. The controversy of varicella vaccination in children with acute lymphoblastic leukemia. Pediatr Blood Cancer. 2012;58:12–6.
28. Antillon F, Rossi E, Molina AL, et al. Nutritional status of children during treatment for acute lymphoblastic leukemia in Guatemala. Pediatr Blood Cancer. 2013;60(6):911–5.
29. Sala A, Antillon F, Pencharz P, et al. Nutritional status in children with cancer: a report from the AHOPCA workshop held in Guatemala City, August 31-September 5, 2004. Pediatr Blood Cancer. 2005;45:230–6.
30. Luna-Fineman S, Slowing K, Valverde P, et al. Pediatric cancer in Guatemala: a retrospective study. Med Pediatr Oncol. 1997;229:353 (abstr.).
31. Arora RS, Eden T, Pizer B. The problem of treatment abandonment in children from developing countries with cancer. Pediatr Blood Cancer. 2007;49:941–6.

32. Mostert S, Arora RS, Arreola M, et al. Abandonment of treatment for childhood cancer: position statement of a SIOP PODC Working Group. Lancet Oncol. 2011;12:719–20.
33. Masera G, Eden T, Schrappe M, et al. Statement by members of the Ponte di Legno Group on the right of children to have full access to essential treatment for acute lymphoblastic leukemia. Pediatr Blood Cancer. 2004;43:103–4.
34. Barr RD, Sala A, Wiernikowski J, et al. A formulary for pediatric oncology in developing countries. Pediatr Blood Cancer. 2005;44:433–5.
35. Aur RJ, Simone J, Hustu HO, et al. Central nervous system therapy and combination chemotherapy of childhood lymphocytic leukemia. Blood. 1971;37:272–81.
36. Pullen J, Boyett J, Shuster J, et al. Extended triple intrathecal chemotherapy trial for prevention of CNS relapse in good-risk and poor-risk patients with B-progenitor acute lymphoblastic leukemia: a Pediatric Oncology Group study. J Clin Oncol. 1993;11:839–49.
37. Tubergen DG, Gilchrist GS, O'Brien RT, et al. Prevention of CNS disease in intermediate-risk acute lymphoblastic leukemia: comparison of cranial radiation and intrathecal methotrexate and the importance of systemic therapy: a Childrens Cancer Group report. J Clin Oncol. 1993;11:520–6.
38. Pui CH, Campana D, Pei D, et al. Treating childhood acute lymphoblastic leukemia without cranial irradiation. N Engl J Med. 2009;360:2730–41.
39. Pui CH, Howard SC. Current management and challenges of malignant disease in the CNS in paediatric leukaemia. Lancet Oncol. 2008;9:257–68.
40. Veerman AJ, Kamps WA, van den Berg H, et al. Dexamethasone-based therapy for childhood acute lymphoblastic leukaemia: results of the prospective Dutch Childhood Oncology Group (DCOG) protocol ALL-9 (1997-2004). Lancet Oncol. 2009;10:957–66.
41. Tubergen DG, Gilchrist GS, O'Brien RT, et al. Improved outcome with delayed intensification for children with acute lymphoblastic leukemia and intermediate presenting features: a Childrens Cancer Group phase III trial. J Clin Oncol. 1993;11:527–37.
42. van Eys J, Berry D, Crist W, et al. A comparison of two regimens for high-risk acute lymphocytic leukemia in childhood. A Pediatric Oncology Group Study. Cancer. 1989;63:23–9.
43. Hunger SP, Winick NJ, Sather HN, et al. Therapy of low-risk subsets of childhood acute lymphoblastic leukemia: when do we say enough? Pediatr Blood Cancer. 2005;45:876–80.
44. Bostrom BC, Sensel MR, Sather HN, et al. Dexamethasone versus prednisone and daily oral versus weekly intravenous mercaptopurine for patients with standard-risk acute lymphoblastic leukemia: a report from the Children's Cancer Group. Blood. 2003;101:3809–17.
45. Riehm H, Gadner H, Henze G, et al. Results and significance of six randomized trials in four consecutive ALL-BFM studies. Haematol Blood Transfus. 1990;33:439–50.
46. Schrappe M. Evolution of BFM trials for childhood ALL. Ann Hematol. 2004;83 Suppl 1:S121–3.
47. Antillon F, Baez FL, Barr R, et al. AMOR: a proposed cooperative effort to improve outcomes of childhood cancer in Central America. Pediatr Blood Cancer. 2005;45:107–10.
48. Marjerrison S, Antillon F, Fu L, 6, et al. Outcome of children treated for relapsed acute lymphoblastic leukemia in Central America. Cancer. 2013;119(6):1277–83.
49. Smith M, Arthur D, Camitta B, et al. Uniform approach to risk classification and treatment assignment for children with acute lymphoblastic leukemia. J Clin Oncol. 1996;14:18–24.
50. Schrappe M, Reiter A, Riehm H. Cytoreduction and prognosis in childhood acute lymphoblastic leukemia. J Clin Oncol. 1996;14:2403–6.
51. Gaynon PS, Desai AA, Bostrom BC, et al. Early response to therapy and outcome in childhood acute lymphoblastic leukemia: a review. Cancer. 1997;80:1717–26.

Acute Myeloid Leukemia 17

Miguel Bonilla and Raul C. Ribeiro

Abbreviations

6-MP	6-Mercaptopurine
6-TG	6-Thioguanine
ADE	Cytarabine + daunorubicin + etoposide
AHOPCA	Central America Pediatric Hematology Oncology Association
AIE	Cytarabine + idarubicin + etoposide
AMKL	Acute megakaryoblastic leukemia
AML	Acute myeloid leukemia
APL	Acute promyelocytic leukemia
APL-DS	Acute promyelocytic leukemia differentiation syndrome
ARAC	Cytarabine
ATO	Arsenic trioxide
ATRA	all-*trans*-retinoic acid
BFM	The Berlin/Frankfurt/Muenster Study Group
BM	Bone marrow
CNS	Central nervous system
CNS-2	Low number of blasts in CSF (<5)
CNS-3	Blasts in LCR ≥5
CR	Complete remission
CR1	Initial complete remission
CSF	Cerebrospinal fluid
DAT	Daunorubicin + cytarabine + 6-thioguanine
DAUNO	Daunorubicin
DS	Down syndrome
EFS	Event-free survival
FAB	French-American-British
GIMEMA	Gruppo Italiano Malattie Ematologiche
HAM	High-dose cytarabine + mitoxantrone
HIC	High-income countries
HSCT	Hematopoietic stem cell transplantation
ICU	Intensive care unit
IDA	Idarubicin
LIC	Low-income countries
M3v	Hypogranular or microgranular variant form of M3 myeloid leukemia
MAE	Mitoxantrone + cytarabine + etoposide
ML	Myeloid leukemia
ML-DS	Myeloid leukemia of Down syndrome
MRC	The Medical Research Council
MTZ	Mitoxantrone
NOPHO	Nordic Society for Pediatric Hematology and Oncology
OS	Overall survival
PB	Peripheral blood

M. Bonilla, M.D.
International Outreach Program, St. Jude Children's Research Hospital, Memphis, TN, USA
e-mail: miguel.bonilla@stjude.org

R.C. Ribeiro, M.D. (✉)
Department of Oncology, Leukemia and Lymphoma Division and International Outreach Program, St. Jude Children's Research Hospital, Memphis, TN, USA
e-mail: raul.ribeiro@stjude.org

D.C. Stefan and C. Rodriguez-Galindo (eds.), *Pediatric Hematology-Oncology in Countries with Limited Resources: A Practical Manual*, DOI 10.1007/978-1-4614-3891-5_17,

PETHEMA	Programa Español de Tratamientos en Hematologia
TMD	Transient myeloproliferative disorder
TRM	Treatment-related mortality
VP-16	Etoposide
WBC	White blood cells
WHO	World Health Organization

Introduction

In low-income countries (LIC), the treatment of children with cancer is influenced by unique circumstances that restrict improvement in cure rates. The management of acute myeloid leukemia (AML) demands a multidisciplinary teamwork approach as the treatment intensity required to decrease the disease-associated mortality may actually contribute to increased mortality because of toxicity. Assuring rapid access to medical facilities, providing appropriate medications and blood products, developing a core of trained health care professionals and laboratory personnel, improving diagnostic methods, and balancing the intensity of treatment and the quality of supportive care are all necessary for improved treatment results.

This chapter describes some of the important features of the commonly used therapeutic strategies that have been proved effective in treating children with AML in high-income countries (HIC). Included are approaches for particular subtypes, such as acute promyelocytic leukemia (APL) and myeloid leukemia of Down syndrome (ML-DS). Strategies to adapt effective treatment for use in LIC are also described.

Furthermore, this chapter highlights the importance of improved supportive care measures and the barriers to and challenges in implementing them in LIC.

Acute Myeloid Leukemia in Children: Overview

AML represents approximately 15–20 % of acute leukemias in children; a similar incidence has been reported in LIC [1, 2].

Table 17.1 Frequent signs and symptoms of AML

- Anemia, manifested by pallor and weakness
- Fever, resulting from infection or leukemia itself
- Hepatosplenomegaly
- Adenopathy
- Petechiae, ecchymosis, epistaxis, gingival bleeding
- Severe hemorrhage or disseminated intravascular coagulation, most common in APL
- Gum infiltration
- Leukemic skin infiltration
- Granulocytic sarcoma or chloroma found in orbital, paranasal sinuses, or paraspinal areas

The signs and symptoms of AML result from the diffuse leukemic infiltration of the bone marrow and extramedullary sites (Table 17.1). Pallor, petechiae, and fever are the most common presenting signs and symptoms. Fever can result from leukemia itself or an associated infection. Hepatosplenomegaly and generalized adenopathy can be present in AML but are less common than in acute lymphoblastic leukemia. Skin involvement and subcutaneous involvement are relatively common, and deposits of myeloid cells (chloroma, myeloblastoma) can occur in any organ or tissue. Gingival swelling typically is seen in cases of monoblastic leukemia. Anemia and thrombocytopenia reflect the suppression of normal hematopoiesis by leukemia-induced bone marrow suppression. The white blood cell (WBC) count is variable and depends on the proliferative capacity of the leukemic cells. Coagulopathy, a hallmark of APL, can occur in other AML subtypes, particularly in those with hyperleukocytosis. Hemorrhage and thrombosis may occur and represent final events of a combination of thrombocytopenia, hypofibrinogenemia, infection, inflammation, and prothrombotic substances released by the leukemic cells.

Diagnosis and Classification

The diagnosis and classification of AML relies on morphologic, cytochemical, immunophenotypic, cytogenetic, and molecular features of the leukemic cells. The presence of Auer rods is a specific but not sensitive marker of AML. Arrangement of Auer rods in bundles (faggot cells)

Table 17.2 Comparison of FAB and WHO classifications of AML

FAB classification	–	Classifies into 8 subtypes, from M0 to M7, determined by morphologic, immunophenotypic, and cytogenetic features
WHO classification	–	Incorporates genetic, morphologic/cytochemical, and immunophenotypic information into subtypes of AML with clinical and prognostic relevance
	–	Allows the AML diagnosis to be made regardless of the blast cell count in cases associated with specific genetic abnormalities

Table 17.3 Frequent subtypes of pediatric AML in the WHO classification

- Acute myeloid leukemia with recurrent genetic abnormalities
  - AML with t(8;21)
  - AML with abnormal bone marrow eosinophils and inv(16)
  - APL with t(15;17) (PML/RAR) and variants
  - AML with t(9;11)
  - AML (megakaryoblastic) with t(1;22)
- Therapy-related myeloid neoplasms
- Acute myeloid leukemia, not otherwise specified
  - Acute myelomonocytic leukemia
  - Acute monoblastic/monocytic leukemia
  - Acute erythroid leukemia
  - Acute megakaryoblastic leukemia
- Myeloid sarcoma (Previously known as granulocytic sarcoma or chloroma, it should be considered as AML)
- Myeloid proliferation related to Down syndrome
  - Transient abnormal myelopoiesis
  - Myeloid leukemia associated with Down syndrome

(Comprising: transient abnormal myelopoiesis, myelodysplastic syndrome, and myeloid leukemia associated with Down syndrome)

is very suggestive of APL. Cytochemical studies (myeloperoxidase, Sudan Black, nonspecific esterase), immunophenotyping, cytogenetic studies, and molecular studies provide further evidence of the AML subtype and yield information critical to prognosis and selection of risk-adapted therapies.

In LIC, the diagnosis of AML is commonly based on morphology and variably supported by cytochemical and immunophenotypic analysis. For this reason, AML is classified according to the French-American-British (FAB) criteria. Only highly specialized cancer units can perform cytogenetics and molecular biology studies. Lacking the information such studies can offer, many LIC institutions are prevented from implementing optimized therapy based on an accurate characterization of AML subtypes.

The current World Health Organization (WHO) classification of the myeloid neoplasms incorporates morphologic, immunophenotypic, cytogenetic, molecular, and clinical information to reach a final classification (Table 17.2) [3]. The WHO scheme is the standard for uniform characterization of AML and should be used for treatment comparisons among different collaborative groups (Table 17.3).

Treatment of Pediatric AML

Modern treatment of pediatric of AML is similar to that proposed in adult AML protocols. Treatment guidelines have been established for more than 3 decades. Attempts to treat pediatric AML using ALL guidelines were unsuccessful. Improvement in pediatric AML outcome has been essentially a result of improved supportive care, risk-stratification, and effective management of infections, particularly fungal infection. Clinical trials that incorporated these elements, including judicious indications for hematopoietic stem cell transplantation (HSCT), have yielded the best results [4, 5].

In general, complete remission (CR) rates of around 95 % and overall survival (OS) rates of up to 70 % are reported in HIC (Table 17.4) [6–9]. Treatment failures are mainly due to AML relapse and, to a lesser extent, treatment-related mortality (TRM).

In contrast with the progress made in pediatric AML in HIC, the outcomes in LIC have not improved significantly [10, 11]. Lack of expeditious access to tertiary care centers for opportune diagnosis and treatment, scarcity of resources needed for diagnosis and treatment, disparities between the increase in chemotherapy intensity and the quality of supportive care,

Table 17.4 Examples of treatment regimens used in AML

AML-BFM Study Group	*Induction*: AIE (ARAC+IDA+VP-16)
AML-BFM 93 [26]	*Consolidation*:
	High-risk patients: HD-ARAC+ MTZ (HAM) + 6-week consolidation with 6-TG + prednisone + vincristine + doxorubicin + ARAC + cyclophosphamide
	Standard-risk patients: 6-week consolidation (see above) without HAM
	Intensification: HD-ARAC + VP-16 (HAE)
	CNS prophylaxis: Intrathecal ARAC + cranial irradiation
	HSCT: allogeneic HSCT in high-risk patients if matched related donor is available
	Maintenance: 6-TG daily + ARAC monthly for a total of 12 months
	CR 82 %, 5-year OS 57 %
Medical Research Council	*Induction I*: ARAC+DAUNO+VP-16 (ADE) versus MTZ+ARAC+VP-16 (MAE)
MRC AML12 Trial [8]	*Induction II*: same as induction I but with ARAC shortened from 10 to 8 days
	Consolidation 1: Amsacrine+ARAC+VP-16
	Consolidation 2: HD-ARAC+ L-asparaginase
	Consolidation 3–4: HD-ARAC+MTZ
	CNS prophylaxis: Triple intrathecal methotrexate + ARAC+ hydrocortisone
	HSCT: allogeneic HSCT in standard or poor risk patients with matched related donor available
	CR 90 %, 10-year OS 61 %
NOPHO-AML 93 [7]	*Induction I*: ARAC+ 6-TG+VP-16+DOXO
	Induction II: same as induction I for good responders, or ARAC+MTZ for poor responders
	Consolidation 1: HD-ARAC+MTZ
	Consolidation 2: HD-ARAC+VP-16
	Consolidation 3: HD-ARAC
	Consolidation 4: HD-ARAC+VP-16
	CNS prophylaxis: Intrathecal methotrexate
	HSCT: allogeneic HSCT recommended to all patients with matched family donor
	CR 92 %, 5-year OS 65 %

6-TG 6-thioguanine, *ARAC* cytarabine, *CNS* central nervous system, *DAUNO* daunorubicin, *DOXO* doxorubicin, *HD-ARAC* high-dose cytarabine, *HSCT* hematopoietic stem cell transplantation, *IDA* idarubicin, *MTZ* mitoxantrone, *VP-16* etoposide

and a high prevalence of abandonment of treatment hamper the outcomes (Table 17.5) [10, 12–14]. Furthermore, high mortality rates before or during induction reaching 18 %, with overall TRM higher than 20 %, and relapse reaching 35 % impose additional obstacles to better cure rates [10, 15–17]. All of these factors come together in a scenario where malnutrition is present in more than half of children with cancer [12, 18, 19]. These circumstances along with the high prevalence of severe acute and chronic infections at the time of diagnosis constitute major issues that

Table 17.5 Principal barriers in treating AML in LIC

- Scant development of local multidisciplinary team and laboratory facilities
- Insufficient financial support for pediatric oncology units
- Lack of rapid access to medical facilities
- Scarce development of supportive care measures, which results in inadequate balance between intensity of chemotherapy and supportive care
- High rate of abandonment of treatment
- Lack of information that hinders learning from treatment strategies in LIC that have either succeeded or failed. Few published reports from LIC's experiences

negatively influence the outcomes of children with AML in LIC [20].

For APL, the introduction of therapy with all-trans-retinoic acid (ATRA) and arsenic trioxide (ATO) has been an important breakthrough in reducing the risk of early mortality related to coagulopathy, increasing CR rate, and reducing relapse, thereby improving the outcomes of this subtype of myeloid leukemia. Overall survival in APL is greater than 90 % in HIC, but in LIC the difficulties noted above limit the overall survival of patients [14, 21–23].

Induction Therapy

The main objective in AML treatment is to achieve a complete remission. Complete morphological remission is defined as less than 5 % blast cells in bone marrow (BM) with evidence of normal myelopoiesis recovery, and without extramedullary disease. The use of molecular and immunophenotypic markers has revealed that meaningful remission is achieved after the leukemia burden is less than 0.1 % [24, 25]. An intensive induction schedule is instrumental in achieving the treatment objective.

Currently, the combination of cytarabine and anthracycline with etoposide or thioguanine is considered the mainstay of induction treatment in AML, inducing remission rates of up to 90 % in pediatric patients [8, 26].

Various strategies have been implemented to intensify the induction treatment and are intended to increase the CR rates and positively affect the outcomes. Some examples are increasing cytarabine dosage, utilizing diverse anthracycline drugs, and shortening the intervals between initial cycles of chemotherapy (i.e., intensive timing). However, in some trials higher intensity negatively affected the CR rate because of an increased number of deaths related to toxicity [4], corroborating the importance of an optimal balance between intensive chemotherapy and a supportive care.

Results from earlier studies demonstrated that cytarabine and anthracycline, both used as single agents, were effective in inducing initial CR in at least one third of the patients.

Improvements in CR rates were achieved by increasing the total dosage of chemotherapy drugs during induction, or by shortening the time between the initial blocks of treatment (intensive timing) without increasing the cumulative dose of chemotherapy.

The intensification of cytarabine therapy achieved by increasing the number of cytarabine days resulted in an improvement in CR rate [27–29]. It has been demonstrated that increasing the doses of cytarabine overcomes some resistance mechanisms of leukemic cells [30, 31]. The combination of cytarabine with daunorubicin (DAUNO) (7 days of cytarabine + 3 days of DAUNO) in induction therapy resulted in improved CR and OS rates [27, 29, 32].

An alternative strategy to intensify the induction therapy is the addition of a third drug such as etoposide or purine analogs to the 7 + 3 regimen. This addition resulted in better CR and OS rates; however, no significant evidence of superiority was found when etoposide versus purine analog regimens were compared [33].

Likewise, anthracyclines at higher doses have improved the outcomes in patients with AML, with optimal results related to a cumulative dose of 375–550 mg/m^2, when administered in the context of treatment with high-dose cytarabine as postremission therapy [34, 35]. Nevertheless, use of this dose intensification has been limited because of its cardiotoxicity, associated with either high peak serum concentrations or cumulative dosages >300 mg/m^2 [36]. To reduce cardiotoxicity it has been proposed to split the daily dose or prolong the infusion of anthracyclines; other options are the use of liposomal anthracyclines or cardioprotectant agents. However, there is concern about a possible higher rate of secondary malignancies in pediatric cancer patients treated with a cardioprotectant [37].

Several different anthracycline drugs have been prospectively evaluated. Idarubicin (IDA), mitoxantrone (MTZ) (an anthracenedione), and other agents have been studied as substitutes for DAUNO, but it appears that no anthracycline agent has any advantage over another in terms of improving the outcome [35, 38].

The Medical Research Council (MRC) AML12 trial compared the efficacy and toxicity during induction therapy of DAUNO and MTZ, each agent in a combination with similar doses of cytarabine and etoposide (ADE regimen versus MAE regimen, respectively). With an approximate dose ratio of 4:1 for daunorubicin:mitoxantrone, no significant difference in CR rate or event-free survival (EFS) was found; additionally, MTZ was associated with increased myelosuppression [8].

IDA is frequently used as part of the induction treatment with a dose ratio of 5:1 for daunorubicin:idarubicin [26]. The Berlin/Frankfurt/Muenster (BFM) Study Group compared the induction with cytarabine, idarubicin, and etoposide (AIE) versus ADE. With the AIE regimen there was better reduction of blast cells in the bone marrow at day 15 in high-risk patients. However, both treatment groups had a similar OS [26]. An additional advantage of IDA is its main metabolite idarubicinol, which has a prolonged plasma half-life and exerts antileukemic activity in the cerebrospinal fluid (CSF) [39].

Doxorubicin appears to increase the incidence of moderate and severe mucosal toxicity: stomatitis and typhlitis were more frequent in patients treated with doxorubicin than with DAUNO [40].

Purine nucleoside analogs such as clofarabine, cladribine, and fludarabine, which were initially tested and found effective in relapsed AML [41–43], have been also incorporated in induction treatment of de novo AML, but their impact on CR rates and OS have not been determined.

The most common induction regimens include cytarabine and anthracycline. A third agent, usually etoposide or purine analogs, is sometimes added to the cytarabine/anthracycline regimen. In settings with limited resources, two courses of induction with cytarabine, an anthracycline, and a third drug, usually etoposide, are used to induce remission. Seven days of cytarabine with 3 days of anthracycline seem to be an adequate and practical schedule in settings with high early mortality rates. For patients with leukocytosis, cytarabine (usually 100 mg/m^2 every 12 h for 48–72 h administered intravenously via bolus injection or continuous infusion) can reduce the WBC count and allow for support measures to stabilize patients with concurrent infectious, hemorrhagic, or metabolic complications. Alternatively, hydroxyurea (25–50 mg/kg/day) can be used for the same purpose.

Considering its therapeutic advantages and toxicity profile, DAUNO seems to be better suited for induction in LIC because it is associated with less mucosal toxicity, including mucositis and typhlitis, than doxorubicin.

In LIC, the lack of the optimal supportive care found in HIC prevents the delivery of the second induction treatment in a shorter time interval (i.e., use of an intensive timing strategy). For this reason, the rapid clearance of blasts exerted by IDA likely does not represent a practical advantage that can outweigh the risks associated with intensive timing that are encountered in LIC.

Implementing a three-drug induction strategy (ADE or DAT: DAUNO, cytarabine, 6-thioguanine) requires a careful evaluation of the actual supportive resources that are available locally to assure an optimal balance between intensity of treatment and supportive care. Key issues to define this optimal balance are the magnitude of the early mortality rate and the duration of myelosuppression. High TRM rates represent a negative impact on survival that surpasses the advantages of a three-drug induction regimen.

Postremission: Consolidation Therapy

Postremission therapy is necessary to eradicate any residual disease and prevent relapse in patients with AML. In this regard, different AML cooperative groups have implemented several strategies. Evidence from AML trials has demonstrated that intensification of postremission therapy, with or without HSCT, is an effective strategy to improve outcomes [4, 5, 26, 44]. A number of trials in children and adults demonstrated that postremission therapy with high-dose cytarabine ($\leq$1 g/m^2/dose) played a key role in improving the outcome in children with AML [45].

Currently, in most of the pediatric AML trials, the standard consolidation treatment is based on a total of two to five courses of high-dose cytarabine, combined with non-cross-resistant agents similar to what was previously given during the induction [7, 46–48]. However, there is no clear evidence that more than three consolidation courses after two courses of induction leads to better outcomes [8, 49].

The combination of high-dose cytarabine with mitoxantrone (HAM) when given as a consolidation block may provide the advantage of enhancing the cytotoxic activity by introducing a non-cross-resistant agent (mitoxantrone) [26].

The use of etoposide as part of the postremission intensification strategy has contributed to the improvement of outcomes in AML [50]. Treatment with HSCT as a consolidation strategy has been studied, but recommendations for HSCT in first CR remain controversial [34, 51]. There is evidence that HSCT improves the outcomes in children with high-risk AML but not in those with favorable cytogenetic findings [25, 26, 52–54].

A meta-analysis found no benefit in relapse rate and OS for autologous HSCT versus chemotherapy alone. Additionally, it appears that there is an increased risk of death during first remission for patients treated with autologous HSCT. Consequently, autologous HSCT should not be recommended as the first-line postremission therapy for AML children in first CR (CR1) [55].

Data from MRC showed that allogeneic HSCT in CR1 failed to show a survival advantage because of an increase in procedure-related deaths. Furthermore, autologous HSCT did not improve the long-term survival, not because of increased procedure-related deaths, but because of inferior survival after relapse [8]. Therefore, accurately diagnosing patients who have predictors of poor response to chemotherapy can be benefited by allogeneic HSCT in CR1.

With the exception of APL, a maintenance therapy has not proved to be effective for AML patients when treated with intensified therapy [32, 46, 56]. Therefore, the prolonged maintenance treatment has been omitted in most of the contemporary clinical trials [8, 46–48].

CNS-Directed Therapy

The incidence of central nervous system (CNS) leukemia in pediatric AML at the time of diagnosis ranges from 3 to 30 % [35, 51, 57]. CNS leukemia is associated with young age, hyperleukocytosis/leukostasis, monocytic leukemia (FAB M4 or M5) including acute myelomonocytic leukemia with bone marrow eosinophilia (M4eo) with inv(16), and MLL gene rearrangement [51, 57].

Previously, for AML patients without CNS involvement, the CNS prophylaxis was either single or triple intrathecal drug delivery, given alone or combined with cranial irradiation. Currently, there is evidence that treatment with repeated courses of intensive chemotherapy combined with intrathecal therapy, even omitting cranial irradiation, may prevent CNS relapse [51]. Furthermore, in the context of intensive treatment comprising high-dose cytarabine, which crosses the blood–brain barrier, CNS leukemic infiltration at diagnosis is not an adverse prognostic factor, and these patients can be cured without cranial irradiation [51, 58, 59]. Therefore, at present, most clinical trials have abandoned the cranial irradiation, even for patients who presented with CNS involvement [47, 48, 60]. An additional reason to omit cranial irradiation is its late sequelae, including secondary malignancies [61, 62]. The BFM Study Group, however, continues using cranial irradiation because of the reduction in systemic relapses observed in patients receiving CNS irradiation in their studies [26].

At relapse, the incidence of CNS involvement appeared to be less in patients who received CNS prophylaxis as part of the initial treatment than in those who did not [63].

There are no data comparing the efficacy of single drug (either methotrexate or cytarabine) versus triple drug (methotrexate, cytarabine, and hydrocortisone) intrathecal therapy. However, evidence from clinical trials revealed that the triple intrathecal regimen is associated with low rates of CNS leukemia relapse [8, 51, 60]. Currently, CNS prophylaxis with single or triple intrathecal chemotherapy at age-adjusted doses is commonly used for most pediatric clinical trials.

Total doses range from 4 to 12, but the optimal number remains unknown [4, 57].

It appears that in pediatric AML a small number of blasts in the CSF (CNS-2 status) do not represent a risk factor for CNS relapse in patients treated with intensive chemotherapy [58, 59]. Moreover, there is evidence that in the context of intensive chemotherapy combined with intrathecal treatment, CNS positive status (CNS-3 status) at the time of diagnosis does not affect OS [58, 59]. Patients with CNS3 status require intensified CNS-directed therapy. The accepted treatment approach is to administer weekly intrathecal therapy until the CSF is clear of leukemic cells, not less than four doses, and then monthly doses until the end of therapy, without cranial irradiation [8, 57, 59, 60].

Acute Promyelocytic Leukemia in Children

APL is a particular subtype of AML with distinct clinical features, genetic abnormality, and excellent outcomes when treated appropriately. In many series, APL constitutes 5–10 % of childhood AML [8, 46, 48] with a higher incidence in some ethnic groups as reported in Hispanic and Mediterranean populations [2, 64–67].

APL is characterized by an increased risk of life-threatening hemorrhagic complications, an abnormal promyelocytes morphology (M3 FAB) strongly associated with the t(15;17), and a high sensitivity to ATRA and ATO that leads to favorable outcomes.

APL is a medical emergency because of the increased risk of life-threatening hemorrhagic complications occurring at the time of diagnosis or during the initial treatment. The risk of early hemorrhagic death, mainly intracranial hemorrhage, is higher in patients with WBC count $>10\times10^9$/L and with the M3 variant morphology [4].

Commonly, the diagnosis of APL has been based on the leukemic cells morphology complemented with the confirmatory demonstration of the t(15;17).

The FAB morphological classification describes two subtypes of APL: the classical M3 form (M3-AML) and the hypogranular or microgranular variant form (M3v-AML). The M3-AML form is characterized by hypergranular promyelocytes with heavy azurophilic granules, bundles of Auer rods (faggot cells), and bilobed nuclei. By contrast, in the M3v-AML form, the majority of blast cells have bilobed, multilobed, or reniform nuclei, with few or no azurophilic granules; still, in M3v-AML at least a few cells with features of classical M3-AML morphology can be found [4, 68].

A characteristic, but not diagnostic, immunophenotypic profile has been described, namely, the consistent expression of CD117 and the lack of CD34 and HLA-DR expression. The presence of these findings, in the context of myeloperoxidase-positive blast cells, and myeloid antigen expression as CD13 and/or CD33 make APL diagnosis possible [69].

Cytogenetics and molecular analysis identify either APL with the classical t(15;17) or the variant forms; also molecular methods allow subsequent molecular minimal residual disease (MRD) monitoring.

In the current WHO classification, APL is classified in the subgroup of AML with recurrent genetic abnormalities (see Table 17.3). According to this classification, the demonstration of the t(15;17) is sufficient for the diagnosis of AML, regardless of the blast cell percentage in peripheral blood (PB) or BM [3]. The WHO classification also recognizes three *RARalpha* variant translocations, two of them with t(11;17), and one with t(5;17). Each of these variants has a different response to ATRA, with t(11;17) being the most resistant to this treatment [3, 70].

The therapy with ATRA should be initiated immediately in children with leukemia presenting with peripheral blood blasts with APL cell morphology.

Currently, up to 80 % of children with APL are cured when their treatment protocol combines ATRA and anthracycline (Table 17.6) [71–74]. The unique sensitivity of APL blast cells to ATRA and to ATO has contributed to the achievement of CR rates around 95 % by reducing the risk of early mortality related to hemorrhagic disorders. ATRA induces the differentiation of the

Table 17.6 Examples of treatment regimens used in APL

GIMEMA APL-AIDA 2000 [99]	*Induction*: ATRA+IDA (AIDA regimen)
	Consolidation: 3 monthly courses
	High-risk patients: HD-ARAC+IDA+ATRA (course 1); MTZ+VP-16+ATRA (course 2); ARAC+IDA+6-TG+ATRA (course 3)
	Low-/intermediate-risk patients: omitting ARAC from courses 1 and 3, and omitting VP-16 from course 2
	CNS prophylaxis: methotrexate + methylprednisolone before each consolidation cycle
	Maintenance: low-dose chemotherapy with 6-MP+methotrexate; alternating with ATRA for 15 days every 3 months, during 2 years
	CR 94 %, 6-year OS 87 %
PETHEMA LPA 2005 [21]	*Induction*: ATRA+IDA (AIDA regimen)
	Consolidation: 3 monthly courses
	High-risk patients: HD-ARAC+IDA+ATRA (course 1); MTZ+ATRA (course 2); ARAC+IDA+ATRA (course 3)
	Low-/intermediate-risk patients: omitting ARAC from courses 1 and 3, and reducing dose of MTZ
	CNS prophylaxis: not given
	Maintenance: low-dose chemotherapy with 6-MP+methotrexate; alternating with ATRA for 15 days every 3 months, during 2 years
	CR 92 %, 4-year OS 88 %
AML-BFM Study Group AML-BFM 2004 for APL [79]	*Induction*: ATRA+AIE (ARAC+IDA+VP-16)
	Consolidation: 3 courses: intermediate-dose ARAC+IDA (course 1); intermediate dose ARAC+MTZ (course 2); HD-ARAC+VP-16 (course 3)
	CNS prophylaxis: Intrathecal ARAC (in a total of 11) + cranial irradiation
	Maintenance: low-dose chemotherapy with 6-TG+ARAC; alternating with ATRA for 15 days every 3 months during 18 months
	CR 94 %, 5-year OS 94 %

6-MP 6-mercaptopurine, *6-TG* 6-thioguanine, *ARAC* cytarabine, *ATRA* all-*trans* retinoic acid, *CNS* central nervous system, *DAUNO* daunorubicin, *GIMEMA* Gruppo Italiano Malattie Ematologiche dellAdulto, *HD-ARAC* high-dose cytarabine, *IDA* idarubicin, *MTZ* mitoxantrone, *PETHEMA* Programa Español de Tratamientos en Hematologia, *VP-16* etoposide

leukemic blasts into mature granulocytes and consequently induces apoptosis without acute lyses of the leukemic blasts, thus preventing the release of fibrinolytic and procoagulant factors from the cytoplasmic granules of the leukemic promyelocytes.

Despite this beneficial action, ATRA can cause considerable, but manageable toxicity by producing severe complications by inducing and increasing the WBC count and in some cases causing APL-differentiation syndrome (APL-DS) [75, 76]. The pathogenesis of APL-DS appears to be related with an excessive inflammatory response; it is characterized by fever, weight gain, respiratory distress, pulmonary infiltrates, pleural or pericardial effusion, and renal failure [57, 75, 76].

As a single agent, ATRA was shown to be highly effective in inducing CR, but with a high rate of relapse [72, 77]. ATRA combined with chemotherapy improved the outcomes. Additionally, the combined use of ATRA and chemotherapy decreased the incidence of the APL-DS in patients with WBC counts greater than 10×10^9/L [78].

Currently, the concomitant use of ATRA and anthracycline is considered the optimal induction treatment [4, 72, 74, 78]. An ATRA dose of 25 mg/m^2/day appears to produce outcomes similar to that achieved with the higher dose of 45 mg/m^2/day commonly used in adults [72, 74, 78]. For patients with non-ATRA-sensitive AML-M3, the therapeutic approach must be based on a standard intensive AML protocol.

Anthracyclines are commonly used to obtain better results in APL treatment, but the cardiotoxicity associated with a high cumulative dose limits their use. Alternatively, it appears that it can be equally effective to combine reduced doses of anthracycline with cytarabine and ATRA during consolidation treatment [79].

APL is the only subtype of AML in which maintenance therapy has proven benefit. Treatment with 6-mercaptopurine and methotrexate, combined with intermittent courses of ATRA (15 days every 3 months) has improved the results [74]. Additionally, HSCT in CR1 is not indicated because of the good results obtained with chemotherapy alone.

In countries with limited resources, treating children with APL can be challenging but could yield encouraging results, since the outcomes can be positively influenced by better supportive measures [23, 66].

The risk of fatal hemorrhage is higher in centers with difficulties in maintaining adequate supplies of blood components for transfusion support. Therefore, the early recognition of the diagnosis may prompt the adoption of immediate actions: initiation of treatment with ATRA at 25 mg/m^2, early onset of intense plasma and platelet transfusional support, and avoidance of procedures with an intrinsic risk of bleeding, e.g., spinal taps, placement of central venous catheters, leukapheresis.

In settings with suboptimal availability of blood products, prophylactic/preemptive transfusion of platelet and plasma products, rather than therapeutic transfusion, can increase the CR rate and lead to better outcomes. Therefore, increasing the threshold for platelet transfusion in order to maintain platelet counts $\geq 50 \times 10^9$/L emerges as a mandatory practice in centers with inadequate supplies of products for transfusion support. Similarly, fibrinogen levels should be maintained above 1.5–2 g/L with fresh frozen plasma or cryoprecipitate [72, 73, 78, 80]. Additionally, because of its rapid impact on both fibrinolytic and procoagulant aspects of the coagulopathy, adequate access to ATRA is critical to pediatric oncology units in LIC.

Leukocytosis is associated with an increased incidence of APL-DS. Therefore, anthracycline should be started with ATRA therapy on the first day of induction for patients with high WBC counts ($>10 \times 10^9$/L). Patients with high WBC are also at high risk of developing APL-DS. For this reason, dexamethasone (0.5–1.0 mg/kg every 12 h), should also be given to these patients at the beginning of therapy. If patients progress to severe APL-DS, ATRA should be discontinued for 72 h and carefully reintroduced [72, 78]. Similarly, the reduction of ATRA dose (from 45 to 25 mg/m^2) can reduce the incidence of APL-DS and pseudo tumor cerebri [66, 72, 78].

Down Syndrome: Transient Myeloproliferative Disorder and Myeloid Leukemia

Myeloid leukemia (ML) in Down syndrome (DS) is a unique form of leukemia because of distinctive clinical and biological features. DS-associated AML is very responsive to standard AML chemotherapy regimens [81].

Down Syndrome: Transient Myeloproliferative Disorder

Infants with DS are also at risk of developing a transient myeloproliferative disorder (TMD), a condition with a presentation often indistinguishable from leukemia.

TMD may be diagnosed in 5–10 % of newborns with DS. It is characterized by the presence of circulating megakaryoblasts in the PB with various degrees of leukocytosis, abnormal platelet count, and hepatomegaly/splenomegaly in a newborn with DS [4, 82–84]. Most of the patients with TMD will have spontaneous remission within 3–6 months. About 25 % of TMD patients will develop myeloid leukemia 1–3 years after the resolution of the TMD phase. In addition, this transient disorder can occur in phenotypically normal newborns with mosaic DS. Almost all cases of TMD have megakaryoblasts with a mutation in the *GATA1* gene located on chromosome X. The same mutation is found in megakaryoblastic leukemia occurring in children with DS younger than 4 years. There is evidence that the *GATA1* mutation occurs in utero, in hematopoietic cells in the fetal liver, having spontaneous resolution when hematopoiesis in fetal liver ceases [4, 85, 86].

Unless complications occur, no chemotherapy is indicated for TMD. A short course of low-dose cytarabine, e.g., 1–1.5 mg/kg/day for 3–12 days, is usually indicated in patients with hepatic or pulmonary dysfunction, hemorrhagic disorder, or hyperleukocytosis [4, 83, 87, 88].

In patients with TMD, the causes of death are related to organ failure secondary to hyperviscosity affecting the liver, heart, lungs, and kidney, and causing bowel ischemia with necrotizing enterocolitis.

In countries with limited resources, the opportune identification of TMD and its appropriate treatment is a feasible option, given that the diagnosis can be reliably based on clinical and hematological findings in infants with DS. Therefore, to define the criteria for the initiation of an early chemotherapeutic treatment may be of significant benefit for the outcomes.

Currently, the early onset of treatment with low-dose cytarabine is recommended for patients with WBC count $>100 \times 10^9$/L, progressive organomegaly, evidence of liver dysfunction, bleeding diatheses, multiple effusions (pleural, pericardial ascites or hydrops), preterm delivery, low birth weight (<3 kg), or failure of spontaneous remission [83, 87, 88].

Close monitoring in the next 4 years, given the increased risk for the development of leukemia during this period, would allow for opportune diagnosis of myeloid leukemia with megakaryoblastic features and consequently improve the outcomes. Thus, DS patients with persistent thrombocytopenia, or any other blood count abnormality, whether or not previously treated for TMD, should be evaluated to rule out myeloid leukemia.

Down Syndrome: Myeloid Leukemia

Children with DS younger than 4 years have a 500-fold higher incidence of acute megakaryoblastic leukemia (AMKL) than non-DS children [82, 89]. Furthermore, AMKL represents the predominant AML subtype in children with DS [89], although other morphological subtypes can occur.

According to the current WHO classification scheme, the diagnosis of myeloid leukemia in children with DS should be made regardless of the blast count in BM or PB (see Table 17.3) [3, 57]. It has been proposed that in DS patients, myelodysplasia and ML-DS be considered as successive stages of a single entity named myeloid leukemia associated with Down syndrome [3, 90]. Both entities share similar biological features and high sensitivity to chemotherapy; additionally, about 20 % of patients with ML-DS had a variable period of myelodysplasia before their diagnosis [89].

With reduced treatment regimens and prolonged intervals of recovery between each course of therapy, younger children with ML-DS respond well, with long-term survival rates of about 80 % [81, 83, 91, 92]. Regardless of the reduction in treatment intensity, the relapse rates have stayed low at about 5 % [81, 91, 92]. Older pediatric patients, particularly those older than 4 years, with ML-DS tend to have inferior outcomes with increasing age at diagnosis [81], and they should be treated on the same pediatric AML regimens for non-DS.

The increased risk for severe cardiotoxicity related to anthracycline in children with AML-DS appears to be related to the augmented quantity of genes located on chromosome 21, which predisposes to anthracycline-related cardiomyopathy [4, 93]. Consequently, the recommended cumulative dose of anthracycline in children with DS is 220–240 mg/m^2 [81].

Because of the increased risk of severe toxicity without therapeutic benefit, HSCT is not indicated as frontline therapy in DS with AML [81].

Supportive Care

Implementing more intensive AML treatment protocols in LIC requires synchronously advancing key supportive care components such as prevention and treatment of infectious complications, accessibility to intensive care units (ICU), and efficient transfusional and nutritional support.

The disparity in cure rates between HIC and LIC can be reasonably attributed in part to the scarce development of supportive care measures together with a high rate of abandonment of therapy. Therefore, strategies to improve cure rates should focus on those factors, considering that these interventions must be designed based on understanding of the characteristic settings in LIC.

Treatment of Infection: Overview

Bacterial and fungal infections during neutropenia after chemotherapy are the main cause of mortality during treatment in developing countries [10, 14–16, 94]. The strategies for managing and preventing infectious diseases occurring during leukemia treatment have helped increase the cure rate. Patients with febrile neutropenia or with clinically/microbiologically documented infections should be hospitalized and treated with broad-spectrum antibiotics and antifungal agents. The diagnostic workup and therapeutic decisions should be based on guidelines with clearly defined timely decisions.

Antibiotic Prophylaxis

Antibiotic prophylaxis is defined as the use of antimicrobial agents at the onset of neutropenia without fever or any sign of infection.

It is cost-effective to implement antibiotic prophylaxis strategies in LIC for two key reasons: first, its potential impact on reducing the complications and mortality rate commonly encountered when treating rather than preventing infections and, second, the lower cost of prophylaxis compared with the cost of the therapeutic treatment, which often requires ICU support [95].

The intensity of the chemotherapy and the prolonged severe neutropenia are factors directly associated with severe infections and treatment-related death. Additionally, patients with AML are more susceptible to severe infections due to the utilization of chemotherapy regimens associated with higher mucosal injury. The impact of these factors can be exacerbated in settings where the time of initiation of antibiotics is usually delayed because of the lack of immediate access to hospital beds, including access to ICU, along with the scarcity of antimicrobial and antifungal supplies that often occurs in LIC.

In HIC, antimicrobial prophylaxis has been shown to reduce the incidence of severe infection. Given the limitations on care of patients with AML in LIC, antimicrobial prophylaxis may provide a benefit thereby reducing the rate of severe infection and consequently decreasing the high mortality rate.

Recent studies from the AHOPCA group (Central America Pediatric Hematology Oncology Association) reported an increased risk of microbiologically documented infections associated with a longer length of time between the last chemotherapy and the initial sign or symptom of infection. This situation can be a reflection of the prolonged neutropenia, which is well known to be associated with adverse outcome in children with cancer [96]. Furthermore, parental illiteracy was found to be associated with delay in the decision to seek care after the onset of fever; also, more deaths occurred in patients with a long travel time to the hospital and in families with a low annual household income [97].

In such circumstances, antimicrobial prophylaxis seems to be a reasonable approach to reduce the impact of infectious complications. Its advantage may come either from the benefit provided by antimicrobial agents in preventing severe infections or the simple gain added by maintaining the patient under close surveillance (a short-time travel away from the cancer unit), thus facilitating prompt attention to any complication, including noninfectious complications such as hemorrhagic events.

The design of the prophylactic regimen should be based on knowledge and evidence from centers at developed countries, but adapted to the local epidemiology of infectious diseases and accessibility to antimicrobial agents. There is a recognized benefit of prophylaxis with cefepime or vancomycin-containing regimen in patients with AML treated with high-dose cytarabine who are at increased risk of developing sepsis and pneumonia for viridians group streptococci [95]. The same recognition of benefit applies to fluoroquinolone prophylaxis in reducing the risk of infection-related mortality, trimethoprim-sulfamethoxazole in patients with prolonged periods of neutropenia who are at increased risk of *Pneumocystis jirovecii* infection, and voriconazole for antifungal prophylaxis [98].

Transfusional Support

In AML, hemorrhage can occur at the time of diagnosis or during treatment; this complication can be related to thrombocytopenia and/or deficiency of coagulation factors. Particularly in APL, bleeding in the CNS is the leading cause of early death. The risk of death related to coagulopathy can be reduced with intensive fresh frozen plasma and platelet transfusion [80].

Shortage of blood product supply is a recurrent situation in blood banks in LIC. A practical approach to this situation would be the adoption of defined guidelines for transfusion, e.g., setting the threshold for platelet transfusion at a higher value in anticipation of the blood bank's delay in meeting the patient's requirements. In addition, as described in the APL section, intensive prophylactic (instead of therapeutic) transfusion support with platelet and fresh-frozen plasma may increase the CR rate by preventing the early mortality related to hemorrhagic events.

Beside treatment and prevention of infectious complications and transfusional support, safety of indwelling venous catheters, early dental intervention to restore oral health, and improvement of nutritional status, among others, are areas of care where improvement is feasible and would have great effectiveness in reducing the risk of severe complications.

In summary, various significant factors influence survival: some are associated with the medical field per se, while others are related to the patient's social, cultural, and economic setting. Although efforts to address the sociodemographic factors are necessarily multidisciplinary and require an extended time for their implementation, measures to address the medical issues can be implemented in a shorter time within the clinical setting.

References

1. Valsecchi MG, Tognoni G, Bonilla M, Moreno N, Baez F, Pacheco C, et al. Clinical epidemiology of childhood cancer in Central America and Caribbean countries. Ann Oncol. 2004;15(4):680–5.
2. Mejia-Arangure J, Bonilla M, Lorenzana R, Juarez-Ocana S, de Reyes G, Perez-Saldivar M, et al. Incidence of leukemias in children from El Salvador and Mexico City between 1996 and 2000: population-based data. BMC Cancer. 2005;5(1):1–9.
3. Vardiman JW, Thiele J, Arber DA, Brunning RD, Borowitz MJ, Porwit A, et al. The 2008 revision of the World Health Organization (WHO) classification of myeloid neoplasms and acute leukemia: rationale and important changes. Blood. 2009;114(5):937–51.
4. Gibson B, Perentesis J, Alonzo T, Kaspers G. Treatment of acute myeloid leukemia. In: Reaman GH, Smith FO, editors. Childhood leukemia. Berlin: Springer; 2011. p. 121–60.
5. Gorman MF, Ji L, Ko RH, Barnette P, Bostrom B, Hutchinson R, et al. Outcome for children treated for relapsed or refractory acute myelogenous leukemia (rAML): a Therapeutic Advances in Childhood Leukemia (TACL) Consortium study. Pediatr Blood Cancer. 2010;55(3):421–9.
6. Pui CH. Childhood leukemias. N Engl J Med. 1995; 332(24):1618–30.
7. Lie SO, Abrahamsson J, Clausen N, Forestier E, Hasle H, Hovi L, et al. Long-term results in children with AML: NOPHO-AML Study Group—report of three consecutive trials. Leukemia. 2005;19(12): 2090–100.
8. Gibson BES, Webb DKH, Howman AJ, De Graaf SSN, Harrison CJ, Wheatley K, et al. Results of a randomized trial in children with acute myeloid leukaemia: Medical Research Council AML12 trial. Br J Haematol. 2011;155(3):366–76.
9. Creutzig U, Zimmermann M, Lehrnbecher T, Graf N, Hermann J, Niemeyer CM, et al. Less toxicity by optimizing chemotherapy, but not by addition of granulocyte colony-stimulating factor in children and adolescents with acute myeloid leukemia: results

of AML-BFM 98. J Clin Oncol. 2006;24(27): 4499–506.
10. Yadav SP, Ramzan M, Lall M, Sachdeva A. Pediatric acute myeloid leukemia: final frontier for pediatric oncologists in developing world. Pediatr Hematol Oncol. 2011;28(8):647–8.
11. Perez-Cuevas R, Doubova SV, Zapata-Tarres M, Flores-Hernandez S, Frazier L, Rodriguez-Galindo C, et al. Scaling up cancer care for children without medical insurance in developing countries: the case of Mexico. Pediatr Blood Cancer. 2013;60(2): 196–203.
12. Antillon F, Rossi E, Molina AL, Sala A, Pencharz P, Valsecchi MG, et al. Nutritional status of children during treatment for acute lymphoblastic leukemia in Guatemala. Pediatr Blood Cancer. 2013;60:911–5.
13. Bonilla M, Rossell N, Salaverria C, Gupta S, Barr R, Sala A, et al. Prevalence and predictors of abandonment of therapy among children with cancer in El Salvador. Int J Cancer. 2009;125(9):2144–6.
14. Xu XJ, Tang YM, Song H, Yang SL, Shi SW, Wei J. Long-term outcome of childhood acute myeloid leukemia in a developing country: experience from a children's hospital in China. Leuk Lymphoma. 2010;51(12):2262–9.
15. Gallegos-Castorena S, Medina-Sanson A, Gonzalez-Ramella O, Sanchez-Zubieta F, Martínez-Avalos A. Improved treatment results in Mexican children with acute myeloid leukemia using a Medical Research Council (MRC)-acute myeloid leukemia 10 modified protocol. Leuk Lymphoma. 2009;50(7):1132–7.
16. Gupta S, Bonilla M, Fuentes SL, Caniza M, Howard SC, Barr R, et al. Incidence and predictors of treatment-related mortality in paediatric acute leukaemia in El Salvador. Br J Cancer. 2009;100(7): 1026–31.
17. Gupta S, Antillon FA, Bonilla M, Fu L, Howard SC, Ribeiro RC, et al. Treatment-related mortality in children with acute lymphoblastic leukemia in Central America. Cancer. 2011;117(20):4788–95.
18. Sala A, Rossi E, Antillon F, Molina AL, de Maselli T, Bonilla M, et al. Nutritional status at diagnosis is related to clinical outcomes in children and adolescents with cancer: a perspective from Central America. Eur J Cancer. 2012;48(2):243–52.
19. Israels T, Chirambo C, Caron HN, Molyneux EM. Nutritional status at admission of children with cancer in Malawi. Pediatr Blood Cancer. 2008;51(5):626–8.
20. Stefan DC, Dippenaar A, De Bruin G, Uys R, van Toorn R. Challenges to treatment of leukemia in HIV-positive children. J Trop Pediatr. 2012;58:521–2.
21. Sanz MA, Montesinos P, Rayon C, Holowiecka A, de la Serna J, Milone G, et al. Risk-adapted treatment of acute promyelocytic leukemia based on all-trans retinoic acid and anthracycline with addition of cytarabine in consolidation therapy for high-risk patients: further improvements in treatment outcome. Blood. 2010;115(25):5137–46.
22. Kelaidi C, Ades L, Fenaux P. Treatment of acute promyelocytic leukemia with high white cell blood counts. Mediterr J Hematol Infect Dis. 2011;3(1): e2011038.
23. Ribeiro RC, Rego E. Management of APL in developing countries: epidemiology, challenges and opportunities for international collaboration. Hematology Am Soc Hematol Educ Program. 2006;162–8.
24. Coustan-Smith E, Ribeiro RC, Rubnitz JE, Razzouk BI, Pui CH, Pounds S, et al. Clinical significance of residual disease during treatment in childhood acute myeloid leukaemia. Br J Haematol. 2003;123(2): 243–52.
25. Rubnitz JE, Inaba H, Dahl G, Ribeiro RC, Bowman WP, Taub J, et al. Minimal residual disease-directed therapy for childhood acute myeloid leukaemia: results of the AML02 multicentre trial. Lancet Oncol. 2010;11(6):543–52.
26. Creutzig U, Zimmermann M, Ritter J, Reinhardt D, Hermann J, Henze G, et al. Treatment strategies and long-term results in paediatric patients treated in four consecutive AML-BFM trials. Leukemia. 2005; 19(12):2030–42.
27. Vormoor J, Boos J, Stahnke K, Jurgens H, Ritter J, Creutzig U. Therapy of childhood acute myelogenous leukemias. Ann Hematol. 1996;73(1):11–24.
28. Rai KR, Holland JF, Glidewell OJ, Weinberg V, Brunner K, Obrecht JP, et al. Treatment of acute myelocytic leukemia: a study by cancer and leukemia group B. Blood. 1981;58(6):1203–12.
29. Wells RJ, Woods WG, Lampkin BC, Nesbit ME, Lee JW, Buckley JD, et al. Impact of high-dose cytarabine and asparaginase intensification on childhood acute myeloid leukemia: a report from the Childrens Cancer Group. J Clin Oncol. 1993;11(3):538–45.
30. Hubeek I, Stam RW, Peters GJ, Broekhuizen R, Meijerink JP, van Wering ER, et al. The human equilibrative nucleoside transporter 1 mediates in vitro cytarabine sensitivity in childhood acute myeloid leukaemia. Br J Cancer. 2005;93(12):1388–94.
31. Gale RP. Advances in the treatment of acute myelogenous leukemia. N Engl J Med. 1979;300(21): 1189–99.
32. Rees JK, Gray RG, Swirsky D, Hayhoe FG. Principal results of the Medical Research Council's 8th acute myeloid leukaemia trial. Lancet. 1986;2(8518): 1236–41.
33. Stevens RF, Hann IM, Wheatley K, Gray RG, on behalf of the MRC Childhood Leukaemia Working Party. Marked improvements in outcome with chemotherapy alone in paediatric acute myeloid leukaemia: results of the United Kingdom Medical Research Council's 10th AML trial. Br J Haematol. 1998;101(1): 130–40.
34. Kaspers GJL, Creutzig U. Pediatric acute myeloid leukemia: international progress and future directions. Leukemia. 2005;19(12):2025–9.
35. Rubnitz JE, Gibson B, Smith FO. Acute myeloid leukemia. Hematol Oncol Clin North Am. 2010; 24(1):35–63.
36. Kremer LCM, van der Pal HJH, Offringa M, van Dalen EC, Voûte PA. Frequency and risk factors of

subclinical cardiotoxicity after anthracycline therapy in children: a systematic review. Ann Oncol. 2002; 13(6):819–29.
37. Tebbi CK, London WB, Friedman D, Villaluna D, De Alarcon PA, Constine LS, et al. Dexrazoxane-associated risk for acute myeloid leukemia/myelodysplastic syndrome and other secondary malignancies in pediatric Hodgkin's disease. J Clin Oncol. 2007;25(5): 493–500.
38. AML Collaborative Group. A systematic collaborative overview of randomized trials comparing idarubicin with daunorubicin (or other anthracyclines) as induction therapy for acute myeloid leukaemia. Br J Haematol. 1998;103(1):100–9.
39. Reid JM, Pendergrass TW, Krailo MD, Hammond GD, Ames MM. Plasma pharmacokinetics and cerebrospinal fluid concentrations of idarubicin and idarubicinol in pediatric leukemia patients: a Childrens Cancer Study Group report. Cancer Res. 1990;50(20): 6525–8.
40. Yates J, Glidewell O, Wiernik P, Cooper MR, Steinberg D, Dosik H, et al. Cytosine arabinoside with daunorubicin or adriamycin for therapy of acute myelocytic leukemia: a CALGB study. Blood. 1982; 60(2):454–62.
41. Inaba H, Stewart CF, Crews KR, Yang S, Pounds S, Pui CH, et al. Combination of cladribine plus topotecan for recurrent or refractory pediatric acute myeloid leukemia. Cancer. 2010;116(1):98–105.
42. Miano M, Pistorio A, Putti MC, Dufour C, Messina C, Barisone E, et al. Clofarabine, cyclophosphamide and etoposide for the treatment of relapsed or resistant acute leukemia in pediatric patients. Leuk Lymphoma. 2012;53(9):1693–8.
43. Locatelli F, Testi AM, Bernardo ME, Rizzari C, Bertaina A, Merli P, et al. Clofarabine, cyclophosphamide and etoposide as single-course re-induction therapy for children with refractory/multiple relapsed acute lymphoblastic leukaemia. Br J Haematol. 2009;147(3):371–8.
44. Tsukimoto I, Tawa A, Horibe K, Tabuchi K, Kigasawa H, Tsuchida M, et al. Risk-stratified therapy and the intensive use of cytarabine improves the outcome in childhood acute myeloid leukemia: the AML99 trial from the Japanese Childhood AML Cooperative Study Group. J Clin Oncol. 2009;27(24):4007–13.
45. Roboz GJ. Novel approaches to the treatment of acute myeloid leukemia. ASH Educ Program Book. 2011; 2011(1):43–50.
46. Perel Y, Auvrignon A, Leblanc T, Michel G, Reguerre Y, Vannier JP, et al. Treatment of childhood acute myeloblastic leukemia: dose intensification improves outcome and maintenance therapy is of no benefit–multicenter studies of the French LAME (Leucemie Aigue Myeloblastique Enfant) Cooperative Group. Leukemia. 2005;19(12):2082–9.
47. Pession A, Rondelli R, Basso G, Rizzari C, Testi AM, Fagioli F, et al. Treatment and long-term results in children with acute myeloid leukaemia treated according to the AIEOP AML protocols. Leukemia. 2005;19(12): 2043–53.
48. Ravindranath Y, Chang M, Steuber CP, Becton D, Dahl G, Civin C, et al. Pediatric Oncology Group (POG) studies of acute myeloid leukemia (AML): a review of four consecutive childhood AML trials conducted between 1981 and 2000. Leukemia. 2005; 19(12):2101–16.
49. Kaspers GJ. Pediatric acute myeloid leukemia. Expert Rev Anticancer Ther. 2012;12(3):405–13.
50. Bishop JF, Lowenthal RM, Joshua D, Matthews JP, Todd D, Cobcroft R, et al. Etoposide in acute nonlymphocytic leukemia. Australian Leukemia Study Group. Blood. 1990;75(1):27–32.
51. Pui CH, Schrappe M, Ribeiro RC, Niemeyer CM. Childhood and adolescent lymphoid and myeloid leukemia. Hematology Am Soc Hematol Educ Program 2004;118–45.
52. Lange BJ, Smith FO, Feusner J, Barnard DR, Dinndorf P, Feig S, et al. Outcomes in CCG-2961, a children's oncology group phase 3 trial for untreated pediatric acute myeloid leukemia: a report from the children's oncology group. Blood. 2008;111(3): 1044–53.
53. Gassas A, Afzal S, Ishaqi MK, Finkelstein-Shechter T, Rojas M, Dupuis A, et al. Pediatric standard-risk AML with fully matched sibling donors: to transplant in first CR or not? Bone Marrow Transplant. 2008; 42(6):393–6.
54. Yanada M, Matsuo K, Emi N, Naoe T. Efficacy of allogeneic hematopoietic stem cell transplantation depends on cytogenetic risk for acute myeloid leukemia in first disease remission: a metaanalysis. Cancer. 2005;103(8):1652–8.
55. Wang J, Ouyang J, Zhou R, Chen B, Yang Y. Autologous hematopoietic stem cell transplantation for acute myeloid leukemia in first complete remission: a meta-analysis of randomized trials. Acta Haematol. 2010;124(2):61–71.
56. Perel Y, Auvrignon A, Leblanc T, Vannier JP, Michel G, Nelken B, et al. Impact of addition of maintenance therapy to intensive induction and consolidation chemotherapy for childhood acute myeloblastic leukemia: results of a prospective randomized trial, LAME 89/91. Leucamie Aique Myeloide Enfant. J Clin Oncol. 2002;20(12):2774–82.
57. Creutzig U, van den Heuvel-Eibrink MM, Gibson B, Dworzak MN, Adachi S, de Bont E, et al. Diagnosis and management of acute myeloid leukemia in children and adolescents: recommendations from an international expert panel. Blood. 2012;120(16): 3187–205.
58. Abbott BL, Rubnitz JE, Tong X, Srivastava DK, Pui CH, Ribeiro RC, et al. Clinical significance of central nervous system involvement at diagnosis of pediatric acute myeloid leukemia: a single institution's experience. Leukemia. 2003;17(11):2090–6.
59. Johnston DL, Alonzo TA, Gerbing RB, Lange BJ, Woods WG. The presence of central nervous system

disease at diagnosis in pediatric acute myeloid leukemia does not affect survival: a Children's Oncology Group study. Pediatr Blood Cancer. 2010;55(3):414–20.
60. Ribeiro RC, Razzouk BI, Pounds S, Hijiya N, Pui CH, Rubnitz JE. Successive clinical trials for childhood acute myeloid leukemia at St Jude Children's Research Hospital, from 1980 to 2000. Leukemia. 2005;19(12):2125–9.
61. Walter AW, Hancock ML, Pui CH, Hudson MM, Ochs JS, Rivera GK, et al. Secondary brain tumors in children treated for acute lymphoblastic leukemia at St Jude Children's Research Hospital. J Clin Oncol. 1998;16(12):3761–7.
62. Loning L, Zimmermann M, Reiter A, Kaatsch P, Henze G, Riehm H, et al. Secondary neoplasms subsequent to Berlin-Frankfurt-Munster therapy of acute lymphoblastic leukemia in childhood: significantly lower risk without cranial radiotherapy. Blood. 2000;95(9):2770–5.
63. Johnston DL, Alonzo TA, Gerbing RB, Lange BJ, Woods WG. Risk factors and therapy for isolated central nervous system relapse of pediatric acute myeloid leukemia. J Clin Oncol. 2005;23(36):9172–8.
64. Zubizarreta PA, Rose AB, Felice MS, Alfaro E, Delfino S, Cygler AM, et al. Childhood acute promyelocytic leukemia: no benefit of all-trans-retinoic acid administered in a short-course schedule. Pediatr Hematol Oncol. 2000;17(2):155–62.
65. Malta CA, Pacheco EC, Cantu RA, Conter V, Lietti G, Masera G, et al. Childhood acute promyelocytic leukemia in Nicaragua. Ann Oncol. 1993;4(10):892–4.
66. Jeddi R, Ghedira H, Ben AY, Kacem K, Ben AR, Aissaoui L, et al. ATRA and anthracycline-based chemotherapy in the treatment of childhood acute promyelocytic leukemia (APL): a 10-year experience in Tunisia. Med Oncol. 2011;28(4):1618–23.
67. Zhang L, Zhu X. Epidemiology, diagnosis and treatment of acute promyelocytic leukemia in children: the experience in China. Mediterr J Hematol Infect Dis. 2012;4(1):e2012012.
68. Sainty D, Liso V, Cantu-Rajnoldi A, Head D, Mozziconacci MJ, Arnoulet C, et al. A new morphologic classification system for acute promyelocytic leukemia distinguishes cases with underlying PLZF/RARA gene rearrangements. Blood. 2000;96(4):1287–96.
69. Dong HY, Kung JX, Bhardwaj V, McGill J. Flow cytometry rapidly identifies all acute promyelocytic leukemias with high specificity independent of underlying cytogenetic abnormalities. Am J Clin Pathol. 2011;135(1):76–84.
70. Grimwade D, Biondi A, Mozziconacci MJ, Hagemeijer A, Berger R, Neat M, et al. Characterization of acute promyelocytic leukemia cases lacking the classic t(15;17): results of the European Working Party. Groupe Francais de Cytogenetique Hematologique, Groupe de Francais d'Hematologie Cellulaire, UK Cancer Cytogenetics Group and BIOMED 1 European Community-Concerted Action "Molecular Cytogenetic Diagnosis in Haematological Malignancies". Blood. 2000;96(4):1297–308.
71. Sanz MA, Montesinos P, Vellenga E, Rayon C, de la Serna J, Parody R, et al. Risk-adapted treatment of acute promyelocytic leukemia with all-trans retinoic acid and anthracycline monochemotherapy: long-term outcome of the LPA 99 multicenter study by the PETHEMA Group. Blood. 2008;112(8):3130–4.
72. Masetti R, Vendemini F, Zama D, Biagi C, Gasperini P, Pession A. All-trans retinoic acid in the treatment of pediatric acute promyelocytic leukemia. Expert Rev Anticancer Ther. 2012;12(9):1191–204.
73. Li EQ, Xu L, Zhang ZQ, Xiao Y, Guo HX, Luo XQ, et al. Retrospective analysis of 119 cases of pediatric acute promyelocytic leukemia: comparisons of four treatment regimes. Exp Ther Med. 2012;4(1):93–8.
74. Testi AM, Biondi A, Lo CF, Moleti ML, Giona F, Vignetti M, et al. GIMEMA-AIEOPAIDA protocol for the treatment of newly diagnosed acute promyelocytic leukemia (APL) in children. Blood. 2005;106(2):447–53.
75. Montesinos P, Sanz MA. The differentiation syndrome in patients with acute promyelocytic leukemia: experience of the pethema group and review of the literature. Mediterr J Hematol Infect Dis. 2011;3(1):e2011059.
76. Rego EM, De Santis GC. Differentiation syndrome in promyelocytic leukemia: clinical presentation, pathogenesis and treatment. Mediterr J Hematol Infect Dis. 2011;3(1):e2011048.
77. Adamson PC. All-trans-retinoic acid pharmacology and its impact on the treatment of acute promyelocytic leukemia. Oncologist. 1996;1(5):305–14.
78. Sanz MA, Grimwade D, Tallman MS, Lowenberg B, Fenaux P, Estey EH, et al. Management of acute promyelocytic leukemia: recommendations from an expert panel on behalf of the European LeukemiaNet. Blood. 2009;113(9):1875–91.
79. Creutzig U, Zimmermann M, Dworzak M, Urban C, Henze G, Kremens B, et al. Favourable outcome of patients with childhood acute promyelocytic leukaemia after treatment with reduced cumulative anthracycline doses. Br J Haematol. 2010;149(3):399–409.
80. Tallman MS, Altman JK. How I treat acute promyelocytic leukemia. Blood. 2009;114(25):5126–35.
81. Creutzig U, Reinhardt D, Diekamp S, Dworzak M, Stary J, Zimmermann M. AML patients with Down syndrome have a high cure rate with AML-BFM therapy with reduced dose intensity. Leukemia. 2005;19(8):1355–60.
82. Seewald L, Taub JW, Maloney KW, McCabe ER. Acute leukemias in children with Down syndrome. Mol Genet Metab. 2012;107(1–2):25–30.
83. Bruwier A, Chantrain CF. Hematological disorders and leukemia in children with Down syndrome. Eur J Pediatr. 2012;171(9):1301–7.
84. Roy A, Roberts I, Vyas P. Biology and management of transient abnormal myelopoiesis (TAM) in children

with Down syndrome. Semin Fetal Neonatal Med. 2012;17(4):196–201.
85. Malinge S, Izraeli S, Crispino JD. Insights into the manifestations, outcomes, and mechanisms of leukemogenesis in Down syndrome. Blood. 2009;113(12): 2619–28.
86. Ahmed M, Sternberg A, Hall G, Thomas A, Smith O, O'Marcaigh A, et al. Natural history of GATA1 mutations in Down syndrome. Blood. 2004;103(7):2480–9.
87. Klusmann JH, Creutzig U, Zimmermann M, Dworzak M, Jorch N, Langebrake C, et al. Treatment and prognostic impact of transient leukemia in neonates with Down syndrome. Blood. 2008;111(6):2991–8.
88. Massey GV, Zipursky A, Chang MN, Doyle JJ, Nasim S, Taub JW, et al. A prospective study of the natural history of transient leukemia (TL) in neonates with Down syndrome (DS): Children's Oncology Group (COG) study POG-9481. Blood. 2006;107(12):4606–13.
89. Zipursky A, Thorner P, De Harven E, Christensen H, Doyle J. Myelodysplasia and acute megakaryoblastic leukemia in Down's syndrome. Leuk Res. 1994;18(3):163–71.
90. Hasle H, Niemeyer CM, Chessells JM, Baumann I, Bennett JM, Kerndrup G, et al. A pediatric approach to the WHO classification of myelodysplastic and myeloproliferative diseases. Leukemia. 2003;17(2): 277–82.
91. Rao A, Hills RK, Stiller C, Gibson BE, De Graaf SSN, Hann IM, et al. Treatment for myeloid leukaemia of Down syndrome: population-based experience in the UK and results from the Medical Research Council AML 10 and AML 12 trials. Br J Haematol. 2006;132(5):576–83.
92. Zeller B, Gustafsson G, Forestier E, Abrahamsson J, Clausen N, Heldrup J, et al. Acute leukaemia in children with Down syndrome: a population-based Nordic study. Br J Haematol. 2005;128(6):797–804.
93. Xavier AC, Taub JW. Acute leukemia in children with Down syndrome. Haematologica. 2010;95(7): 1043–5.
94. Gupta S, Bonilla M, Valverde P, Fu L, Howard SC, Ribeiro RC, et al. Treatment-related mortality in children with acute myeloid leukaemia in Central America: incidence, timing and predictors. Eur J Cancer. 2012;48(9):1363–9.
95. Kurt B, Flynn P, Shenep JL, Pounds S, Lensing S, Ribeiro RC, et al. Prophylactic antibiotics reduce morbidity due to septicemia during intensive treatment for pediatric acute myeloid leukemia. Cancer. 2008;113(2):376–82.
96. Gupta S, Bonilla M, Gamero M, Fuentes SL, Caniza M, Sung L. Microbiology and mortality of pediatric febrile neutropenia in El Salvador. J Pediatr Hematol Oncol. 2011;33(4):276–80.
97. Gavidia R, Fuentes SL, Vasquez R, Bonilla M, Ethier MC, Diorio C, et al. Low socioeconomic status is associated with prolonged times to assessment and treatment, sepsis and infectious death in pediatric fever in El Salvador. PLoS One. 2012;7(8):e43639.
98. Gafter-Gvili A, Fraser A, Paul M, Leibovici L. Meta-analysis: antibiotic prophylaxis reduces mortality in neutropenic patients. Ann Intern Med. 2005;142(12 Pt. 1):979–95.
99. Lo-Coco F, Avvisati G, Vignetti M, Breccia M, Gallo E, Rambaldi A, et al. Front-line treatment of acute promyelocytic leukemia with AIDA induction followed by risk-adapted consolidation for adults younger than 61 years: results of the AIDA-2000 trial of the GIMEMA Group. Blood. 2010; 116(17):3171–9.

Hodgkin Lymphoma

18

Monika Metzger and Mhamed Harif

Introduction

Hodgkin lymphoma (HL) in children and adolescents is one of the success stories in the quest to cure childhood cancer, and, at least in high income countries (HIC), has excellent outcomes. This success, however, has not translated to all low and middle income countries (LMIC), where patients present with a long history of symptoms, in poor clinical condition with malnutrition, infections, signs of chronic illness, and advanced stages. Survival in LMIC is also hampered by lack of adequate diagnosis, staging, drug shortages, inadequate access to radiotherapy, delays in therapy, and social hardship leading to abandonment of therapy. The cost of HL therapy is largely driven by pathology evaluation, radiation therapy, and diagnostic imaging studies; chemotherapy and supportive care comprise only a smaller portion of the costs. The minimum necessary supportive care consists of antibiotics and antiemetics; blood products are rarely needed, and therapy can be administered in the outpatient setting without the need for growth factor support. In a study evaluating the cost of therapy in Africa for a child with stage II disease and followed for 2 years the cost was above USD 6,500 in a continent where the annual gross domestic product per inhabitant is usually less than USD 2,000 [1]. These costs can possibly be reduced by carefully choosing the minimal necessary diagnostic imaging studies required for staging, and chemotherapy regimens that will permit omitting radiotherapy. Another hidden cost of therapy though is the loss of income parents have to incur while visiting the pediatric oncology unit for their child to receive therapy, or even worse, their child is admitted to the hospital due to toxicity of therapy. Families with multiple kids need to also consider the cost of investment to cure a child with cancer in view of other healthy children at home. However, because HL is curable, easily diagnosed, and comprises an important portion of children with cancer, every child presenting to medical attention with suspected diagnosis of HL should be given a chance of cure. The cost of relapse should be avoided upfront, and the cost to society of loosing a child to cancer ought to be avoided altogether.

M. Metzger, M.D. (✉)
Department of Oncology, St Jude Children's Research Hospital, University of Tennessee Health Sciences Center, Memphis, TN, USA
e-mail: monika.metzger@stjude.org

M. Harif
Centre Hospitalier Universitaire Mohammed VI, Marrakech, Morocco

Epidemiology

In HIC, HL has a bimodal distribution with the first prominent peak in young adult and the second peak after the age of 50. In most reported studies in LMIC HL occurs in younger age

D.C. Stefan and C. Rodriguez-Galindo (eds.), *Pediatric Hematology-Oncology in Countries with Limited Resources: A Practical Manual*, DOI 10.1007/978-1-4614-3891-5_18,

with a peak incidence at 5–9 years of age [2, 3]. This is considered to be due to poor socioeconomic conditions with earlier exposure to infectious agents. Histopathology distribution is also different with mixed cellularity subtype being the most frequent histology in this setting while in HIC nodular sclerosis HL is the most common subtype of HL.

Epstein-Barr virus (EBV) seems to play an important role in HL, particularly in LMIC where it has been shown that more than 90 % of tumors have EBV markers. In HIC it is found in only about 50 % of the tumors. It has been shown that EBV-infected B cells are transformed into lymphoblastoid cell lines that are considered as a prerequisite for malignant transformation [4]. The main markers of EBV-infected cells are the nuclear antigens EBNA and latent membrane proteins (LMP). LMP1 and EBNA1 which are expressed in most EBV-infected cells are a good marker of chronic infection. EBV markers are mainly found in mixed cellularity subtype and in children less than 10 years old [5].

Pathology

Clinical presentation is most frequently a painless cervical or supraclavicular lymphadenopathy. Mediastinal lymphadenopathies are usually discovered at chest X-ray or CT scan. They are rarely compressive, associated with nonproductive cough, dyspnea, or superior vena cava syndrome. Infradiaphragmatic HL is very rare (less than 5 %) as initial symptoms [6]. In about 30 % of patients cytokine production is responsible for nonspecific systemic symptoms including fever, weight loss, or drenching night sweats. These symptoms are usually associated with more aggressive disease.

Pathology confirmation is mandatory to establish the diagnosis of HL. It is best done when a good lymph node biopsy is made. The biopsy should be done on the most representative enlarged lymph node since sometimes satellite reactive lymph nodes can be misleading. HL is a lymphoid neoplasm composed of Hodgkin and multinucleated cells called Reed-Sternberg (HRS) cells surrounded by immuno-reactive cells (lymphocytes, plasmocytes, eosinophiles, etc.) and various amount of fibrosis. WHO recognizes two major subtypes of Hodgkin lymphoma, classical HL and nodular lymphocyte predominant HL. Histopathology classification of HL is based on proportion of HRS and the pattern of reactive background (Table 18.1).

Immunophenotyping is recommended as a routine diagnostic tool. In LMIC where this technique is not available for all patients, it should be done when clinical and/or pathological morphological findings are not clearly consistent with HL. The most common phenotype of HRS cells is expression of CD30 and CD15 and negativity of CD45. CD30 is the most frankly expressed marker but is not specific as it may also be expressed in anaplastic large cell lymphoma; CD15 is less frequently and less intensely expressed. EBV marker LMP1 may also be helpful in establishing the diagnosis [7].

Staging and Response Evaluation

Staging of Hodgkin lymphoma is performed according to the Ann Arbor staging classification as detailed in Table 18.2 [8]. It is desirable to carefully document signs and symptoms at presentation as well as all sites of involvement at diagnosis in order to better follow up response to therapy. Furthermore, a proper staging is important in determining adequate risk category of the patient to help decide on the appropriate management. Table 18.3 lists all evaluations for presenting new patients. A thorough medical history focusing on unexplained fevers, drenching night sweats, or more than 10 % unintentional weight loss in the last 6 months will confirm the presence of B symptoms, an important prognostic factor and indicator of more advanced disease. In countries with prevalent malnutrition and endemic malaria, these symptoms may often be difficult to attribute to the lymphoma versus general health conditions, but given the often late presentation and bulk of the disease, it is best to err on the side of caution and attribute them to the lymphoma. Signs of superior vena cava syndrome (dyspnea, facial

Table 18.1 Histopathology subtype of Hodgkin lymphoma (RS: Reed-Sternberg)

Pathology classification		Clinical features
Classical Hodgkin lymphoma		
Nodular sclerosis	RS cells set in a background of reactive lymphocytes, eosinophils, and plasma cells with varying degrees of collagen fibrosis/sclerosis	Most frequent in adolescent and young adult
		Slight female predominance
		Mediastinal involvement (80 %)
Mixed cellularity	RS cells admixed with numerous inflammatory cells including lymphocytes, histiocytes, eosinophils, and plasma cells without sclerosis	EBV association (75 %)
		Male predominant
		Young age
		Peripheral lymph node involvement
		Advanced stage
Lymphocyte-rich	Few RS cells. Many B cells. Fine sclerosis	Rare
		Localized stages
		Good prognostic
Lymphocyte-depleted	Pleomorphic RS cells with only few reactive lymphocytes	Rare
		Advanced stages (bone marrow, retroperitoneal, and abdominal organ involvement)
		Sometime HIV-associated
Nodular lymphocyte predominant Hodgkin lymphoma		
		Very rare
		Young age
		Good prognostic

Table 18.2 Ann Arbor staging system with Cotswold modifications for Hodgkin lymphoma [8]

Stage	
I	Involvement of a single lymph node region or lymphoid structure, e.g., spleen, thymus, or Waldeyer's ring
II	Involvement of two or more lymph node regions on the same side of the diaphragm
III	Involvement of lymph node regions on both sides of the diaphragm (III), which may be accompanied by involvement of the spleen (III_S)
IV	Diffuse or disseminated involvement of one or more extranodal organs or tissues, with or without associated lymph node involvement
Symptoms	
A	Absence of B symptoms
B	Fever (temperature >38 °C), drenching night sweats, unexplained loss of >10 % of body weight within the preceding 6 months
Disease bulk and extension	
X	Bulky disease (a widening of the mediastinum by more than one-third or the presence of a nodal mass with a maximal dimension >6 cm)
E	Involvement of a single extranodal site that is contiguous from a known nodal site

swelling, cough, orthopnea, and headache) or of tracheal and/or bronchial compression (cough, dyspnea, and orthopnea) should immediately alert the medical practitioner of a possible large mediastinal mass and prompt a chest radiograph for evaluation. Careful physical examination of all peripheral lymph node groups, documenting site and size, as well as evaluation for hepatosplenomegaly should be part of the initial staging work-up. While laboratory tests are desirable to determine adequate organ function prior to starting therapy, and can also contribute to inform on the prognosis, these are not required for risk classification and unavailability should not be an obstacle to therapy. In regard to diagnostic imaging, chest radiographs can inform about bulk of a chest mass (mediastinal to thoracic ratio greater than 33 %), as well as the presence of obvious pulmonary nodules. When CT or MRI is not available for a full anatomic localization of disease, an abdominal ultrasound can be used to evaluate infradiaphragmatic

Table 18.3 Diagnostic evaluation for newly diagnosed Hodgkin lymphoma

Diagnostic evaluation	Important elements	Comments
Medical history	"B" symptoms	Unexplained fever with temperatures above 38.0 °C orally, unexplained weight loss ≥10 % within 6 months preceding diagnosis, and drenching night sweats
	Symptoms of a mediastinal mass	Superior vena cava syndrome: dyspnea, facial swelling, cough, orthopena, and headache
		Tracheal or bronchial compression: cough, dyspnea, and orthopnea
Physical examination	Lymph nodes	Location and size of all abnormal lymph nodes should be documented
	Tonsils	Symmetry, size, and nodular infiltration
	Lung auscultation	Stridor is heard when tracheal compression is significant and wheezing when smaller airways are compressed by hilar lymphadenopathy
	Liver and spleen	Hepatomegaly splenomegaly is common, even if the spleen does not have macroscopic lymphoma infiltration
	Blood pressure and cardiac auscultation	A friction rub indicates pericardial effusion; pulsus paradoxus implies cardiac tamponade
Laboratory tests	Complete blood count	Anemia and leukocytosis have been associated with a poor prognosis
	Biochemistry profile	Lactate dehydrogenase and low albumin have been associated with a poor prognosis. Creatinine and bilirubin measurement are necessary prior to chemotherapy administration to determine whether dose adjustments are needed. Elevated alkaline phosphatase is associated with bone involvement, and a bone scan or skeletal survey is warranted if it is significantly elevated
	Erythrocyte sedimentation rate, C-reactive protein	Elevation of these and other markers of inflammation have been associated with a poor prognosis and can be followed for response
Diagnostic imaging, anatomic	Chest radiograph	To determine mediastinal to thoracic ratio and evaluate tracheal compression, look for obvious pulmonary nodules
	Skeletal survey	To evaluate suspected sites of bony involvement for patients with localized symptoms and/or elevated alkaline phosphatase
	US abdomen and pelvis	Useful to assess infradiaphragmatic disease when CT or MRI is not available
	CT of neck, chest	Lymph node size and location, and to evaluate for pulmonary involvement and extranodal extension
	CT or MRI of abdomen, and pelvis	Lymph node size and location, lymphomatous involvement of the spleen and/or liver
Diagnostic imaging, functional	Gallium-67 scintigraphy	Metabolic activity of involved nodes and organs. Lower sensitivity than PET, but helpful in assessing response in residual masses
	^{99}T bone scintigraphy	Useful to detect bone lesions in patients with an elevated alkaline phosphatase when PET/CT is not available
	^{18}FDG-PET	Metabolic activity of involved nodes and organs. Requires expertise due to high sensitivity but low specificity
Biopsy	Lymph node	Excisional, not fine needle, in order to confirm the diagnosis prior to initiation of therapy
	Bone marrow	In patients that are not already high risk and in whom involvement would change risk assignment and therapy

disease like liver and spleen involvement as well as inform about para-aortic and iliac nodal involvement. Currently, the gold standard as far as functional imaging is the ^{18}Fluoro-deoxyglucose positron emission tomography (PET scan) which can reveal metabolic activity in involved nodal groups and extralymphatic organs, as well as indicate bone and bone marrow involvement. In the absence of this modality, a ^{99}Technetium bone scan can be performed in patients with suspected bony disease due to localized pain or elevated alkaline phosphatase; however, a localized skeletal radiograph of the involved bones showing destruction will also suffice. Bone marrow biopsies are painful and expensive, so that unless the information gained by this procedure will change the patient's therapy, it shall be omitted [9].

Response assessment after the first two cycles of therapy should include the same modalities utilized at the time of diagnosis and should be performed according to the guidelines of the adopted treatment regimen. At the off-therapy evaluation all extranodal disease should have disappeared; most lymph nodes will have returned to a normal size (≤1 cm) and be soft and mobile. In case of nodular sclerosing HL, a large mediastinal mass may not have completely involuted at the end of therapy, given the nature of the pathology, but should be followed by regular chest radiographs to make sure it continues to regress over time. Frequent imaging is not required for follow-up; careful physical examination and evaluation will be more informative in raising concern of relapse [10].

Frontline Therapy

As previously discussed in the staging section a correct risk classification is very important when selecting the right treatment approach. Every protocol or treatment guideline will have its own risk classification so that the medical practitioner choosing a treatment approach needs to carefully review the risk definitions prior to deciding on therapy (Tables 18.4 and 18.5). In most places the choice of regimen (Table 18.6) will be dictated by drug availability and the experience of the treating physician, as well as supportive care resources. As has recently and dramatically been shown, drug substitutions need to be carefully evaluated [11]. In Central America, AHOPCA (Central American Association of Pediatric Hematology-Oncology), a modified Stanford V regimen, was used for high risk patients in whom they substituted mechlorethamine by cyclophosphamide given that the former was not available. The disappointing result of only 55 % 3-year event-free survival was originally attributed to the bulky and advanced stages at presentation [12]; however, this may not be a sufficient explanation, as the same substitution carried out by the St Jude-Stanford-Dana-Farber consortium during a National shortage also led to poorer outcomes [11]. It is therefore best to choose a proven regimen that utilizes available drugs than to assume one can substitute an unavailable drug. The choice of whether or not to choose a regimen that includes radiotherapy will be determined by the available infrastructure, but also the experience and willingness of often adult radiation oncologists in treating children.

The more sophisticated the staging evaluation can be performed, the more fine-tuned a treatment can be chosen. A risk-stratified approach can only be given if one has complete confidence on the accurate disease evaluation at presentation. This is particularly true in case of a response-adapted regimen in which early response evaluation will dictate escalation or de-escalation of therapy. Furthermore, in case of only gross disease staging, where not all sites can be excluded confidently, the medical practitioner has to rely more on the intensity of the chemotherapy to eliminate all disease. In view of limited access to a complete staging work-up, it makes more sense to only risk-stratify into localized versus advanced disease, or treat all children the same as shown in Table 18.4, whereas when radiotherapy is also incorporated into treatment, as seen in Table 18.5, a risk classification into three risk groups is more often performed and radiotherapy often chosen according to response to chemotherapy. In a setting with very limited resources, 4–6 cycles of ABVD could be given to

Table 18.4 Treatment results for pediatric Hodgkin lymphoma of chemotherapy only trials in middle and low income countries

		Outcome (years)			
Chemotherapy	Stage	No. of patients	Event-free survival	Disease-free survival	Overall Survival
AHOPCA [24]					
6 COPP	I, IIA, IIIA	216	63 (5)	–	–
8 COPP/ABV	IIB, IIIB, IV		60 (5)	–	–
Argentina (GATLA) [25]					
3 CVPP	IA, IIA	10	86 (7)	–	–
6 CVPP	IB, IIB	16	87 (7)	–	–
Chennai, India [26]					
6 COPP/ABV	All stages	129	–	87 (5)	93 (5)
Egypt [27]					
8 OAP	All stages	60	–	53 (6)	60 (6)
8 COMP	All stages	59	–	70 (6)	76 (6)
Jordan [28]					
4–6 MOPP	I, II	14	92 (3)		100 (3)
6–8 MOPP	III, IV	16		–	
Nicaragua [29]					
6 COPP	I, IIA	14	100 (3)	–	100 (3)
8–10 COPP/ABV	IIB, III, IV	34	75 (3)	–	–
Madras, India [30]					
6 COPP/ABV	I–IIA	10	89 (5)	–	–
6 COPP/ABV	IIB–IVB	43	90 (5)	–	–
Mali (GFAOP) [31]					
4–6 COPP/ABV	I, IIA	0	–	–	–
6–10 COPP/ABV	IIB, III, IV	7	–	–	5/7 alive
New Delhi, India [32]					
6 COPP	All stages	34	–	80 (5)	–
New Delhi, India [33]					
8 COPP/ABVD	All stages	148	88 (5)	–	92 (5)
Saudi Arabia [34]			81 (5)	–	86 (5)
4–6 ABVD	All stages	35			
MOPP	All stages	20			
Uganda [35]					
6 MOPP	I–IIIA	38	–	75 (5)	–
6 MOPP	IIIB–IV	10	–	60 (5)	–

GATLA grupo Argentino del tratamiento de la leucemia; *ABVD* doxorubicin (Adriamycin), bleomycin, vinblastine, dacarbazine; *COPP* cyclophosphamide, vincristine (Oncovin), procarbazine, prednisone; *CVPP* cyclophosphamide, vincristine, procarbazine, prednisone; *MOPP* mechlorethamine (Mustargen), vincristine (Oncovin), procarbazine, prednisone

Table 18.5 Treatment results for pediatric Hodgkin lymphoma of combined modality trials in middle and low income countries

			Outcome (years)			
Chemotherapy	Radiation	Stage	No. of patients	Event-free survival	Disease-free survival	Overall Survival
AHOPCA [12, 36]						
4 ABVD	None or 25 Gy IFRT	IA, IIA	80	91 (3)	–	100 (3)
6 ABVD	20–25 Gy IFRT	IA, IIA (≥4 nodal sites, bulk)	162	85 (3)	–	94 (3)
Stanford V[a]	20–25 Gy IFRT	IIB, IIIB, IV	206	55 (3)		75 (3)
Brazil (IMIP) [37]						
4 VAMP+	15–20 Gy IFRT	IA, IIA	28	96 (5)	–	100 (5)
6 VAMP/COP	15–20 Gy IFRT	IB, IIB, III, IV	34	60 (5)	–	72 (5)
Brazil [38]						
6 MOPP/ABV	±EFRT	All stages	71	–	82 (5)	90 (5)
6 ABVD	±IFRT	All stages	115	–	86 (5)	94 (5)
China [39]						
4 COMP/ABV	±IFRT	I, IIA (no bulk, no hila, <4 sites)	8	100 (4)	–	100 (4)
6 COMP/ABV	±IFRT	I–III	32	80 (4)	–	97 (4)
3 COMP/ABV—EA—CHOP	±IFRT	IV	16	63 (4)	–	69 (4)
Egypt [40]						
2 O(E/P)PA	30 Gy IFRT	IA, IIA	121	–	92 (5)	96 (5)
2 O(E/P)PA +2 COPP	25 Gy IFRT	IIB, IIIA		–	81 (5)	96 (5)
2 O(E/P)PA +4 COPP	20 Gy IFRT	IIIB, IV		–	80 (5)	93 (5)
Iran [41]						
2–4 O(E/P)PA	±20–25 Gy IFRT	IA, IIA	12	79 (5)	–	94 (5)
2 OPPA+4 COPDac	±20–15 Gy IFRT	IIB, III, IV	28			
Morocco [42]						
4 VBVP	20 Gy IFRT	All stages	114	43 (7)	–	–
Morocco [43]						
VAMP	25.5 Gy IFRT	IA, IIA (no bulk, no E)	22	69 (5)	–	88 (5)
2 OPPA/4 COPP	25.5 Gy IFRT	I, II, III, IV	138	74 (5)	–	
New Delhi, India [43]						
4 ABVD	25–40 Gy IFRT	I–IIA	79	–	91 (5)	86 (5)
6–8 ABVD	25–40 Gy to bulk	IIB, III, IV	183	–	73 (5)	
Saudi Arabia [34]						
ABVD	15–30 Gy IFRT	All stages	12	–	91 (5)	100 (5)

(continued)

Table 18.5 (continued)

Chemotherapy	Radiation	Stage	Outcome (years) No. of patients	Event-free survival	Disease-free survival	Overall Survival
Turkey [44]						
6 COPP	30–40 Gy IFRT	All stages	148	–	–	66 (10)
Turkey [46]						
3 COPP	20–25 Gy IFRT	I, II (nLP and MC)	132	82 (5)		94 (5)
3 ABVD	20–25 Gy IFRT	I, II (NS and LD)				
6 COPP	15–25 Gy IFRT	III, IV	78	55 (5)		86 (5)

ABVD doxorubicin (Adriamycin), bleomycin, vinblastine, dacarbazine; *COPP* cyclophosphamide, vincristine (Oncovin), procarbazine, prednisone; *CVPP* cyclophosphamide, vincristine, procarbazine, prednisone; *MOPP* mechlorethamine (Mustargen), vincristine (Oncovin), procarbazine, prednisone

Table 18.6 Selected frontline chemotherapy regimens

Agent (cycle length)	Dose (mg/m^2)	Route	Schedule	Maximum dose
ABVD (28 days)				
Doxorubicin	25	IV	Days 1 and 15	
Bleomycin	10	IV	Days 1 and 15	
Vinblastine	6	IV	Days 1 and 15	
Dacarbazine	375	IV	Days 1 and 15	
COPP/ABVD (57 days)				
Cyclophosphamide	650	IV	Days 1 and 8	
Vincristine	1.4	IV	Days 1 and 8	2 mg
Procarbazine	100	PO	Days 1 through 14	
Prednisone	40	PO	Days 1 through 14	
Doxorubicin	25	IV	Days 29 and 43	
Bleomycin	10	IV	Days 29 and 43	
Vinblastine	6	IV	Days 29 and 43	
Dacarbazine	375	IV	Days 29 and 43	
COP(P/Dac)[b] (28 days)				
Cyclophosphamide	500	IV	Days 1 and 8	
Vincristine	1.5	IV	Days 1 and 8	2 mg
Prednisone	40	PO	Days 1 through 15	
Procarbazine[b]	100	PO	Days 1 through 15	
Dacarbazine[b]	250	IV	Days 1 through 3	
MOPP (28 days)				
Mechlorethamine	6	IV	Days 1 and 8	
Vincristine	1.4	IV	Days 1 and 8	2 mg
Procarbazine	100	PO	Days 1 through 15	
Prednisone	40	PO	Days 1 through 15	

(continued)

Table 18.6 (continued)

Agent (cycle length)	Dose (mg/m^2)	Route	Schedule	Maximum dose
O(E/P)PA[a] (28 days)				
Vincristine	1.5	IV	Days 1, 8, and 15	2 mg
Etoposide[a]	125	IV	Days 1 through 5	
Procarbazine[a]	100	PO	Days 1 through 15	
Prednisone	60	PO	Days 1 through 15	
Doxorubicin	40	IV	Days 1 and 15	
VAMP (28 days)				
Vinblastine	6	IV	Days 1 and 15	
Doxorubicin	25	IV	Days 1 and 15	
Methotrexate	20	IV	Days 1 and 15	
Prednisone	40	PO	Days 1 through 14	20 mg TID

[a] Choose either etoposide or procarbazine, both regimens effective (etoposide more toxic)
[b] Choose either procarbazine or dacarbazine, both regimens effective

patients with localized disease and 6–8 cycles of COPP/ABVD to patients with advanced disease with or without consolidative radiotherapy. Particularly if chemotherapy is given two cycles beyond remission, radiotherapy can be omitted.

Finally, it is very important to instruct patients and families upfront about the curability of the disease and give as much support as necessary to prevent abandonment of therapy. Timely administration of therapy without undue delays is very important to prevent relapses. Most chemotherapy regimens can be given in an ambulatory setting and will not require hospitalization, though in cases of patients with an already compromised general clinical status, significant anemia, and infections due to neutropenia will require careful attention and treatment.

Refractory or Relapsed Disease

Before a relapse can be declared all effort must be made to rebiopsy the suspected site of disease. This is very important, especially where PET scans are not available to evaluate metabolic activity, as residual masses can represent residual scar tissue, or a reactive lymph node or transformation into a non-Hodgkin lymphoma. Adverse prognostic factors after relapse include inadequate response to initial second-line therapy [13], the presence of B symptoms [14], and early relapse [15, 16] (occurring between 3 and 12 months from the end of therapy). In HIC, more than 50 % of patients can still be cured after relapse with intensive cytoreduction, and consolidative radiotherapy with or without autologous stem cell transplant [13, 16]. Many patients in LMIC often only have one opportunity at being cured from their disease and this is at presentation. As can be seen in Tables 18.4 and 18.5, there are no significant differences between disease- or event-free survival and overall survival, since once a patient has relapsed cure is rarely possible in those settings. Most patients in LMIC will have received a rather intensive frontline regimen given the questionable adequacy of staging upfront and often would require intensive chemo-radiotherapy with or without autologous stem cell transplant for cure in a setting where this is not possible. There are no data in the literature on salvage regimens utilized successfully in LMIC. In Central America, AHOPCA has used ICE (ifosfamide, carboplatinum, and etoposide) or a "modified ICE" for two cycles beyond complete response followed by radiotherapy with moderate success (data not published). Table 18.7 depicts the doses and routes of administration for effective regimens in relapsed pediatric Hodgkin

Table 18.7 Selected retrieval chemotherapy regimens

Agent (variable)	Dose (mg/m^2)	Route	Schedule	Maximum dose
ICE				
Ifosfamide*	1670	IV	Days 1, 2, and 3	
Carboplatin	AUC=5	IV	Day 2	800 mg
Etoposide	100	IV	Days 1, 2, and 3	
Modified ICE				
Cyclophosphamide	440	IV	Days 1 through 5	
Etoposide	100	IV	Days 1 through 5	
Alternating after count recovery with				
Carboplatinum	500	IV	Day 1	
Etoposide	100		Days 1 through 3	
IV				
Ifosfamide[a]	3000	IV	Days 1 through 4	
Vinorelbine	25	IV	Days 1 and 5	
IGV				
Ifosfamide[a]	2000	IV	Days 1 through 4	
Gemcitabine	800	IV	Days 1 and 4	
Vinorelbine	20	IV	Day 1	
Prednisone	50	PO	Days 1 through 4	
GV				
Gemcitabine	1200	IV	Days 1 and 8	
Vinorelbine	25	IV	Days 1 and 8	

[a]MESNA given every time ifosfamide is given according to institutional guidelines and experience

lymphoma, as well as the other very effective and less toxic regimens and combinations including gemcitabine and vinorelbine [17–20] but which are often, unfortunately, not available in LMIC.

Long-Term Follow-up

As the survival rates are exceeding 90 % in HIC and are increasing significantly in the rest of the world, treatment-related late effects are becoming an important issue. Preventive approaches are designed in order to reduce those late effects. Long-term follow-up is aiming at evaluating and treating side effects when possible at due time.

Adverse effects are variable according to the dose and field of radiation therapy and to chemotherapy regimen and also according to the age of exposure. The main issues are fertility, heart problems and secondary cancers (Table 18.8).

Table 18.8 Main long-term side effects and their causes

Involved organ	Agents	Side effects
Cardiac	Anthracyclines	Cardiomyopathy
	Radiotherapy	Arythmias
		Pericarditis
		Coronaropathy
Pulmonary	Bleomycin	Fibrosis
	Radiotherapy	
Gonadal	Alkylating agents	Delayed puberty
	Radiotherapy	Azoospermia
		Hypogonadism
Bone	Steroids	Osteopenia
	Radiotherapy	Osteonecrosis
		Hypoplasia
Second malignancies	Alkylating agents	Leukemia
	Topoisomerase II inhibitors	Sarcomas
	Radiotherapy	Breast cancer
Thyroid	Radiotherapy	Hypothyroidism
		Thyroid cancer

One of the objectives of multimodality treatment is to reduce cummulative doses of each drug and radiation therapy in order to reduce toxicity without losing efficacy [21, 22].

However, in LMIC follow-up is a real problem since most patients cannot afford the cost of follow-up and sometimes are not aware of its importance. Lost to follow-up can reach up to 50 % of patients. It is important to have the parents and the patients aware of the importance of long-term follow-up. Optimal guidelines have been recommended by the Children's Oncology Group [23].

Summary

Proper education of primary health care providers into signs and symptoms of cancer, in this particular case of chronic enlarged cervical, axillary, or inguinal lymph nodes, as well as mediastinal mass is fundamental. Diagnosis of HL can be confirmed with basic histology; a simple staging work-up is all that is necessary prior to starting live-saving chemotherapy that can mostly be given in an outpatient setting. The incidence of HL across geographic regions varies, but it is curable even in countries with very limited resources with outcomes varying between 60 and 90 % survival. Outcomes for relapsed HL in LMIC are much worse than in HIC given the limitations of intensive cytoreduction and unavailability of autologous stem cell transplant and therefore the aim should be to achieve cure with frontline therapy. As more children become cancer survivors also in LMIC, awareness of long-term effects of therapy becomes more and more important.

References

1. Stefan DC, Stones D. How much does it cost to treat children with Hodgkin lymphoma in Africa? Leuk Lymphoma. 2009;50:196–9.
2. Harif M, Trachli A, Quessar A, et al. Hodgkin's disease in the very young child. Apropos of 11 cases. Bull Cancer. 1996;83:937–9.
3. Stiller CA, Parkin DM. Geographic and ethnic variations in the incidence of childhood cancer. Br Med Bull. 1996;52:682–703.
4. Tanner J, Weis J, Fearon D, et al. Epstein-Barr virus gp350/220 binding to the B lymphocyte C3d receptor mediates adsorption, capping, and endocytosis. Cell. 1987;50:203–13.
5. Gandhi MK, Tellam JT, Khanna R. Epstein-Barr virus-associated Hodgkin's lymphoma. Br J Haematol. 2004;125:267–81.
6. Maity A, Goldwein JW, Lange B, et al. Mediastinal masses in children with Hodgkin's disease. An analysis of the Children's Hospital of Philadelphia and the Hospital of the University of Pennsylvania experience. Cancer. 1992;69:2755–60.
7. Kurtin PJ, Pinkus GS. Leukocyte common antigen–a diagnostic discriminant between hematopoietic and nonhematopoietic neoplasms in paraffin sections using monoclonal antibodies: correlation with immunologic studies and ultrastructural localization. Hum Pathol. 1985;16:353–65.
8. Carbone PP, Kaplan HS, Musshoff K, et al. Report of the Committee on Hodgkin's Disease Staging Classification. Cancer Res. 1971;31:1860–1.
9. Hines-Thomas MR, Howard SC, Hudson MM, et al. Utility of bone marrow biopsy at diagnosis in pediatric Hodgkin's lymphoma. Haematologica. 2010;95:1691–6.
10. Vose JM, Link BK, Grossbard ML, et al. Long term follow-up of a phase II study of Rituximab in combination with CHOP chemotherapy in patients with previously untreated aggressive non-Hodgkin's lymphoma (NHL). Blood. 2002;100:361A.
11. Metzger ML, Billett A, Link MP. The impact of drug shortages on children with cancer–the example of mechlorethamine. N Engl J Med. 2012;367:2461–3.
12. Castellanos EM, Metzger M, Baez LF, et al. A risk-adapted, response-based therapeutic regimen using a modified Stanford V approach for the treatment of children with high risk Hodgkin lymphoma, AHOPCA LH 2004, a therapeutic regimen from the Central America and Dominican Republic Association of Pediatric Oncology. In ASH Annual Meeting Abstracts Vol. 114; 2009. p. 718.
13. Metzger ML, Hudson MM, Krasin MJ, et al. Initial response to salvage therapy determines prognosis in relapsed pediatric Hodgkin lymphoma patients. Cancer. 2010;116:4376–84.
14. Moskowitz CH, Nimer SD, Zelenetz AD, et al. A 2-step comprehensive high-dose chemoradiotherapy second-line program for relapsed and refractory Hodgkin disease: analysis by intent to treat and development of a prognostic model. Blood. 2001;97:616–23.
15. Gorde-Grosjean S, Oberlin O, Leblanc T, et al. Outcome of children and adolescents with recurrent/refractory classical Hodgkin lymphoma, a study from the Societe Francaise de Lutte contre le Cancer des Enfants et des Adolescents (SFCE). Br J Haematol. 2012;158:649–56.
16. Schellong G, Dorffel W, Claviez A, et al. Salvage therapy of progressive and recurrent Hodgkin's disease: results from a multicenter study of the pediatric DAL/GPOH-HD study group. J Clin Oncol. 2005;23:6181–9.

17. Bonfante V, Viviani S, Devizzi L, et al. High-dose ifosfamide and vinorelbine as salvage therapy for relapsed or refractory Hodgkin's disease. Eur J Haematol Suppl. 2001;64:51–5.
18. Cole PD, Schwartz CL, Drachtman RA, et al. Phase II study of weekly gemcitabine and vinorelbine for children with recurrent or refractory Hodgkin's disease: a children's oncology group report. J Clin Oncol. 2009;27:1456–61.
19. Santoro A, Bredenfeld H, Devizzi L, et al. Gemcitabine in the treatment of refractory Hodgkin's disease: results of a multicenter phase II study. J Clin Oncol. 2000;18:2615–9.
20. Santoro A, Magagnoli M, Spina M, et al. Ifosfamide, gemcitabine, and vinorelbine: a new induction regimen for refractory and relapsed Hodgkin's lymphoma. Haematologica. 2007;92:35–41.
21. Donaldson SS, Link MP. Combined modality treatment with low-dose radiation and MOPP chemotherapy for children with Hodgkin's disease. J Clin Oncol. 1987;5:742–9.
22. Hudson MM, Neglia JP, Woods WG, et al. Lessons from the past: opportunities to improve childhood cancer survivor care through outcomes investigations of historical therapeutic approaches for pediatric hematological malignancies. Pediatr Blood Cancer. 2012;58:334–43.
23. Landier W, Bhatia S, Eshelman DA, et al. Development of risk-based guidelines for pediatric cancer survivors: the Children's Oncology Group Long-Term Follow-Up Guidelines from the Children's Oncology Group Late Effects Committee and Nursing Discipline. J Clin Oncol. 2004;22:4979–90.
24. Castellanos EM, Barrantes JC, Baez LF, et al. A chemotherapy response based therapeutic approach to pediatric Hodgkin lymphoma using COPP regimen for favorable and COPP/ABV for unfavorable Hodgkin lymphoma in children and adolescents. An Association of Pediatric Hematology Oncology of Central America (AHOPCA) protocol: AHOPCA LH 1999. Pediatr Blood Cancer. 2013 (in press).
25. Sackmann-Muriel F, Zubizarreta P, Gallo G, et al. Hodgkin disease in children: results of a prospective randomized trial in a single institution in Argentina. Med Pediatr Oncol. 1997;29:544–52.
26. Sagar TG, Chandra A, Raman SG. Childhood Hodgkin disease treated with COPP/ABV hybrid chemotherapy: a progress report. Med Pediatr Oncol. 2003;40:66–9.
27. Al-Tonbary Y, Sarhan MM, El-Ashry RA, et al. Comparative study of two mechlorethamine, vincristine, procarbazine, and prednisone derived chemotherapeutic protocols for the management of pediatric Hodgkin lymphoma (HL): single-center 5-year experience. Leuk Lymphoma. 2010;51:656–63.
28. Madanat FF. MOPP therapy in children with Hodgkin's disease. Am J Pediatr Hematol Oncol. 1989;11:407–10.
29. Baez F, Ocampo E, Conter V, et al. Treatment of childhood Hodgkin's disease with COPP or COPP-ABV (hybrid) without radiotherapy in Nicaragua. Ann Oncol. 1997;8:247–50.
30. Sripada PV, Tenali SG, Vasudevan M, et al. Hybrid (COPP/ABV) therapy in childhood Hodgkin's disease: a study of 53 cases during 1989–1993 at the Cancer Institute, Madras. Pediatr Hematol Oncol. 1995;12:333–41.
31. Togo B, Traore F, Togo AP, et al. Hodgkin lymphoma at the paediatric oncology unit of gabriel toure teaching hospital, Bamako, Mali: 5-year experience. Adv Hematol. 2011;2011:327237.
32. Chandra J, Naithani R, Singh V, et al. Developing anticancer chemotherapy services in a developing country: Hodgkin lymphoma experience. Pediatr Blood Cancer. 2008;51:485–8.
33. Arya LS, Dinand V, Thavaraj V, et al. Hodgkin's disease in Indian children: outcome with chemotherapy alone. Pediatr Blood Cancer. 2006;46:26–34.
34. Belgaumi A, Al-Kofide A, Joseph N, et al. Hodgkin lymphoma in very young children: clinical characteristics and outcome of treatment. Leuk Lymphoma. 2008;49:910–6.
35. Olweny CL, Katongole-Mbidde E, Kiire C, et al. Childhood Hodgkin's disease in Uganda: a ten year experience. Cancer. 1978;42:787–92.
36. Castellanos EM, Metzger ML, Fuentes S, et al. A Response-based ABVD regimen with or without radiotherapy for pediatric low and intermediate risk Hodgkin lymphoma in Central America and Dominician Republic. A report from AHOPCA. Pediatr Blood Cancer. 2012;59:977–8.
37. Hsu SC, Metzger ML, Hudson MM, et al. Comparison of treatment outcomes of childhood Hodgkin lymphoma in two US centers and a center in Recife, Brazil. Pediatr Blood Cancer. 2007;49(2):139–44.
38. Souza EM, Baiocchi OC, Zanichelli MA, et al. Comparison between hybrid MOPPABV and ABVD chemotherapy protocols for Hodgkin's lymphoma in public hospitals of the largest South American city: a retrospective 14-year study. Ann Hematol. 2009;88:633–7.
39. Gao YJ, Tang JY, Pan C, et al. Risk-adapted chemotherapy without procarbazine in treatment of children with Hodgkin lymphoma. World J Pediatr. 2013;9:32–5.
40. El-Badawy S, Aboulnaga S, Abou GA, et al. Risk adapted combined modality treatment in children with Hodgkin's disease: NCI, Cairo. J Egypt Natl Canc Inst. 2008;20:99–110.
41. Alebouyeh M, Moussavi F, Haddad-Deylami H, et al. Successful ambulatory treatment of Hodgkin's disease in Iranian children based on German-Austrian DAL-HD 85–90: single institutional results. Ann Oncol. 2005;16:1936–40.
42. Hessissen L, Oulhiane N, Elkhorassani M, et al. Pediatric Hodgkins disease in Morocco. Pediatr Blood Cancer. 2005;44:199.

43. Hessissen L, Khtar R, Madani A, et al. Improving the prognosis of pediatric Hodgkin lymphoma in developing countries: a Moroccan Society of Pediatric Hematology and Oncology study. Pediatr Blood Cancer. 2013;60(9):1464–9.
44. Ganesan P, Kumar L, Raina V, et al. Hodgkin's lymphoma–long-term outcome: an experience from a tertiary care cancer center in North India. Ann Hematol. 2011;90:1153–60.
45. Buyukpamukcu M, Varan A, Akyuz C, et al. The treatment of childhood Hodgkin lymphoma: improved survival in a developing country. Acta Oncol. 2009; 48:44–51.
46. Buyukpamukcu M, Atahan L, Caglar M, et al. Hodgkin's disease in Turkish children: clinical characteristics and treatment results of 210 patients. Pediatr Hematol Oncol. 1999;16:119–29.

Non-Hodgkin Lymphoma

19

David K. Stones and Biobele J. Brown

Introduction

Non-Hodgkin lymphoma (NHL) is a malignant disease that arises from the lymphocytic lineage. It is a group of diverse diseases and essentially includes all lymphomas that are not classified as Hodgkin lymphoma. As the cells of the immune system are diverse and malignant transformation can occur in any of these cells line at any stage, there is a wide diversity of types of NHL. They all differ in their aetiologies, pathogenesis, genetics, clinical manifestations, patterns of spread as well as response to treatment and survival. Although they generally arise in the lymph nodes and the spleen they have a high propensity to be wide spread at diagnosis. The extent at diagnosis, rate and manner of progression and response to chemotherapy and radiotherapy is very different to that of Hodgkin lymphoma. Childhood NHL is a very different disease to the NHL in adults and the sites, staging and treatment as well as the subtypes of disease are different. This group of diseases has a propensity to progress rapidly and most children have extensive disease at presentation and this is probably due to the fact that the lymphoid cells traffic throughout the body. This makes them very much like the leukemia in certain aspects of presentation and disease extent as well as treatment options. In the 1970s the survival rate was <20 % and practically all these were localized stage disease; long-term survival of widespread disease was poor with most demising in the first 2 years after diagnosis. The prognosis in general is now very good and in the developed world almost 80 % will become long-term survivors with the rate slightly lower in the adolescents [1, 2]. These advances in survival rates have come about because of better understanding of the disease entity, more rational staging systems, marked improvements in supportive care for the complications of NHL as well as the therapy-related toxicities. New drug regimens have been developed using old drugs that have been available for many years.

Incidence and Epidemiology

The NHL is classified essentially into T and B cell NHL based on the histological characteristics and then further classified according to the clinical features.

In adults most common type seen is diffuse large B cell which has an incidence between 30 and 40 % followed by the follicular T cell with an incidence of 20–30 % [3].

D.K. Stones (✉)
Department of Paediatrics and Child Health, University of the Free State, PO Box 339(G69), Bloemfontein 9300, South Africa
e-mail: stonesdk@UFS.ac.za

B.J. Brown, M.D.
Department of Paediatrics, College of Medicine, University of Ibadan, Ibadan, Nigeria

D.C. Stefan and C. Rodriguez-Galindo (eds.), *Pediatric Hematology-Oncology in Countries with Limited Resources: A Practical Manual*, DOI 10.1007/978-1-4614-3891-5_19,

Table 19.1 Incidence and age distribution of specific types of NHL[a]

	Incidence of NHL per million person-years							
	Males				Females			
Age (years)	<5	5–9	10–14	15–19	<5	5–9	10–14	15–19
Burkitt	3.2	6	6.1	2.8	0.8	1.1	0.8	1.2
Lymphoblastic	1.6	2.2	2.8	2.2	0.9	1.0	0.7	0.9
DLBCL	0.5	1.2	2.5	6.1	0.6	0.7	1.4	4.9
Other (mostly ALCL)	2.3	3.3	4.3	7.8[b]	1.5	1.6	2.8	3.4[b]

ALCL anaplastic large cell lymphoma, *DLBCL* diffuse large B-cell lymphoma, *NHL* non-Hodgkin lymphoma
[a]*Source*: Adapted from Percy et al. [3]
[b]In older adolescents, indolent and aggressive histologies (more commonly seen in adult patients) are beginning to be found

In children the incidence and subtypes are very different. It is the third most common malignancy seen in the developed world and accounts for 15 % of cancers in children less than 20 years of age with an incidence of about ten cases per million [1, 2]. The incidence in certain areas of the world, especially in Uganda and Nigeria in Africa, is much higher and figures of 150 per million are seen in children between 5 and 10 years of age [4].

NHL is more common in children under 10 years of age, but as the adolescent peak of Hodgkin disease (HD) commences, the incidence of NHL becomes less.

The incidence in children depends on the age, histology, gender and race. There is no specific age peak but it is seldom seen in children below 3 years of age. There is some evidence that the incidence is slowly increasing especially in children over the age of 15 but below this age the incidence has remained constant [1]. NHL is more common in males than females except for the primary mediastinal B-cell lymphoma (PBML) in which the sex ratio is almost equal. The incidence and age distribution of the specific types of NHL according to the gender is described in Table 19.1.

The incidence of the NHL also varies according to the histological subtype and there are very definite subgroups of patients who develop specific types on NHL. NHL is much more common in males in all age groups as well as the subtypes. Burkitt lymphoma (BL) is more prevalent in children between 5 and 15 years of age while lymphoblastic lymphoma (LL) is spread evenly over all the age groups. The other subtypes, anaplastic large cell lymphoma (ALCL) and diffuse large B-cell lymphoma (DLBCL), tend to occur in older patients and are seldom seen in younger children.

The incidence of lymphoma also varies in different areas of the world and in Africa there is a high incidence of BL and in Nairobi almost 52 % of childhood cancers are lymphoma with BL making up 34 % of these cases [5]. Similar high incidences are also seen in Uganda.

A paper from Pakistan [6] showed that median age for their patients with NHL was just over 8 years of age; there was a male predominance of 3:1 and 78 % of their children had BL.

A similar study from Baghdad [7] showed that NHL accounted for 19 % of all their childhood cancer cases: 90 % were non-lymphoblastic and treated on B-cell protocols. Again there was a male predominance of 2:1 while their age was lower between 5 and 7 years. More than 90 % of their patients had stage 3 or 4 disease.

In South America [8] it was shown that they also had a male predominance while they had a lower incidence of BL, 50 %, while LL accounted for 30 % of the cases. The majority of their patients had high-stage disease.

The aetiology of NHL is largely unknown but certain agents have been implicated in the aetiology. The best known is the link between Epstein–Barr virus (EBV), malaria and climate and BL that was elucidated by Denis Burkitt and Anthony Epstein who then discovered the EBV virus which bears his name. Other suggested agents have included toxins, pesticides and previous chemotherapy. The human deficiency virus (HIV) is associated with an increased incidence of lymphoma and a 100-fold increase in NHL is seen in HIV-infected persons [2].

Immunodeficiency, whether on a genetic basis or post transplant, has also been associated with an increase in NHL.

In Africa most of the cases are due to endemic BL and a high incidence is seen in equatorial areas of Africa.

Pathological Classification

The 2008 World Health Organization (WHO) Classification of Tumours of Haematopoietic and Lymphoid Tissues is shown in Table 19.2 [6]. However, NHL in childhood is usually classified based on morphologic, immunophenotypic, genetic features and clinical presentation. The main histological subtypes in pediatric patients are Burkitt and Burkitt-like lymphoma, DLBCL, lymphoblastic lymphoma and ALCL [10–12]. Their distribution in the United Kingdom is as follows:

Burkitt and Burkitt-like lymphoma/leukemia	42.2 %
Lymphoblastic lymphoma	27.2 %
ALCL	15 %
Others	15.6 %

Most of the other NHLs in the various classifications are not common in Pediatrics. The most recent WHO classification has identified pediatric follicular lymphoma and pediatric nodal marginal zone lymphoma as unique entities.

Burkitt Lymphoma

Microscopically, BL is characterized by a diffuse infiltrative pattern, and the medium- to small-sized cells are homogenous with round to ovoid nuclei, 1–3 prominent basophilic nucleoli and basophilic cytoplasm that usually contain fat vacuoles. BL is histologically characterized by a "starry sky"

Table 19.2 WHO classification of lymphoid neoplasms (2008)

Precursor lymphoid neoplasms
B lymphoblastic leukemia/lymphoma
B lymphoblastic leukemia/lymphoma, NOS
B lymphoblastic leukemia/lymphoma with recurrent genetic abnormalities
B lymphoblastic leukemia/lymphoma with t (9; 22) (q34;q11.2); BCR-ABL1
B lymphoblastic leukemia/lymphoma with t (v; 11q23); MLL rearranged
B lymphoblastic leukemia/lymphoma with t (12:21) (p13;q22); TEL-AML1 (ETV6-RUNX1
B lymphoblastic leukemia/lymphoma with hyperploidy
B lymphoblastic leukemia/lymphoma with hypodiploidy (hypodiploidy ALL)
B lymphoblastic leukemia/lymphoma with t (5; 14) (q31;q32); IL3-IGH
B lymphoblastic leukemia/lymphoma with t (1; 19) (q23;p13.3); E2A-PBX1 (TCF3-PBX1)
B lymphoblastic leukemia/lymphoma
T lymphoblastic leukemia/lymphoma
Mature B-cell neoplasms
Chronic lymphocytic leukemia/small lymphocytic lymphoma
B-cell prolymphocytic leukemia
Splenic marginal zone lymphoma
Hairy cell leukemia
Splenic lymphoma/leukemia, unclassifiable
Splenic diffuse red pulp small B-cell lymphoma[a]
Hairy cell leukemia-variant[a]
Lymphoplasmacytic lymphoma
Waldenström macroglobulinemia
Heavy chain diseases
Alpha heavy chain disease
Gamma heavy chain disease
Mu heavy chain disease
Plasma cell myeloma
Solitary plasmacytoma of bone
Extraosseous plasmacytoma
Extranodal marginal zone B-cell lymphoma of mucosa-associated
lymphoid tissue (MALT lymphoma)
Nodal marginal zone B-cell lymphoma (MZL)
Pediatric type nodal MZL
Follicular lymphoma
Pediatric type follicular lymphoma
Primary cutaneous follicle centre lymphoma
Mantle cell lymphoma
Diffuse large B-cell lymphoma (DLBCL), not otherwise specified

(continued)

Table 19.2 (continued)

T cell/histiocyte-rich large B-cell lymphoma
DLBCL associated with chronic inflammation
Epstein–Barr virus (EBV)+DLBCL of the elderly
Lymphomatoid granulomatosis
Primary mediastinal (thymic) large B-cell lymphoma
Intravascular large B-cell lymphoma
Primary cutaneous DLBCL, leg type
ALK+ large B-cell lymphoma
Plasmablastic lymphoma
Primary effusion lymphoma
Large B-cell lymphoma arising in HHV8-associated multicentric
Castleman disease
Burkitt lymphoma
B-cell lymphoma, unclassifiable, with features intermediate between diffuse large B-cell lymphoma and Burkitt lymphoma
B-cell lymphoma, unclassifiable, with features intermediate between
diffuse large B-cell lymphoma and classical Hodgkin lymphoma
Hodgkin lymphoma
Nodular lymphocyte-predominant Hodgkin lymphoma
Classical Hodgkin lymphoma
Nodular sclerosis classical Hodgkin lymphoma
Lymphocyte-rich classical Hodgkin lymphoma
Mixed cellularity classical Hodgkin lymphoma
Lymphocyte-depleted classical Hodgkin lymphoma
The mature T-cell and NK-cell neoplasms
T-cell prolymphocytic leukemia
T-cell large granular lymphocytic leukemia
Chronic lymphoproliferative disorder of NK-cells[a]
Aggressive NK-cell leukemia
Systemic EBV+ T-cell lymphoproliferative disease of childhood (associated with chronic active EBV infection)
Hydroa vacciniforme-like lymphoma
Adult T-cell leukemia/lymphoma
Extranodal NK/T-cell lymphoma, nasal type
Enteropathy-associated T-cell lymphoma
Hepatosplenic T-cell lymphoma
Subcutaneous panniculitis-like T-cell lymphoma
Mycosis fungoides
Sézary syndrome
Primary cutaneous CD30+ T-cell lymphoproliferative disorder
Lymphomatoid papulosis
Primary cutaneous anaplastic large cell lymphoma
Primary cutaneous aggressive epidermotropic CD8+ cytotoxic
T-cell lymphoma[a]

(continued)

Table 19.2 (continued)

Primary cutaneous gamma-delta T-cell lymphoma
Primary cutaneous small/medium CD4+ T-cell lymphoma[a]
Peripheral T-cell lymphoma, not otherwise specified
Angioimmunoblastic T-cell lymphoma
Anaplastic large cell lymphoma (ALCL), ALK+
Anaplastic large cell lymphoma (ALCL), ALK–[a]

Source: Swerdlow SH, Campo E, Harris NL, et al. WHO Classification of Tumours of Haematopoietic and Lymphoid Tissues. Lyon, France: IARC Press; 2008

Diseases shown in italics are newly included in the 2008 WHO classification

[a]These represent provisional entities or provisional subtypes of other neoplasms

appearance, representing scattered macrophages that have phagocytosed cell debris among proliferating lymphoma cells. The malignant cells show a mature B-cell phenotype and are negative for the enzyme deoxy nucleotidyl transferase (TdT). The cells express surface immunoglobulin, most bearing surface immunoglobulin M with either kappa or lambda light chains. Cell markers that are usually present include CD20+, BCL6+, CD10+ and BCL2–. Expression of the proliferation antigen Ki-67 is observed in virtually all the tumour cells. BL/leukemia expresses a characteristic chromosomal translocation, usually t(8:14) or t(8:22) or t(2;8) [10]. Each of these translocations juxtaposes the c-myc oncogene and immunoglobulin locus regulatory elements, resulting in the inappropriate expression of c-myc, a gene involved in cellular proliferation. Cytogenetic evidence of c-myc rearrangement is the gold standard for diagnosis of BL. The 2008 WHO classification eliminated the variant category of "atypical BL," which had been included in the 2001 classification. Thus, a case with the typical BL phenotype (CD20+, BCL6+, CD10+, BCL2–) and genotype (so-called *MYC*-simple or *MYC/IG* in the absence of other major cytogenetic anomalies) may be classified as BL, even if there is some cytological variability in the morphology of the neoplastic cells [6, 9]. For cases in which cytogenetic analysis is not available, the WHO has recommended that the Burkitt-like diagnosis be reserved for lymphoma resembling BL or with more pleomorphism, large cells and a proliferation fraction (i.e. Ki-67[+] of ≥99 %) [11].

Table 19.3 Common clinical features of childhood non-Hodgkin's lymphoma

Clinical feature	Cause
General features	
Fever	Release of cytokines, infections
Weight loss	Inflammatory cytokine production, acute phase protein response, anorexia
Peripheral lymphadenopathy	Malignant transformation, metastasis
Abdomen	
Abdominal pain and swelling	Ovarian, retroperitoneal, kidney and intestinal masses
Nausea, vomiting, constipation	Intussusception, infections
Hepatosplenomegaly	
Chest	
Respiratory distress/cough	Mediastinal masses with airway compression, pleural effusion
Swelling of the neck, face and arms	Superior vena obstruction by masses
Skin and soft tissue infiltration	Tumour infiltration
Jaw	
Jaw swelling with intra-oral extension, "dental anarchy" (misalignment)	Maxilla more affected than mandible in Burkitt lymphoma
Proptosis	Orbital tumour
Nervous system	
Paraplegia—usually flaccid	Spinal cord invasion
Cranial nerve palsies	Central nervous system involvement

Diffuse Large B-Cell Lymphoma

These are proliferations of large lymphoid cells of B-cell lineage with nuclei at least twice the size of small lymphocytes [14]. The normal architecture of the nodal or extranodal tissue is diffusely replaced with frequent extension into perinodal soft tissues. The malignant cells express pan-B markers including CD19, CD20, CD22 and CD79a with surface immunoglobulin expression in more than half of the cases [14]. The vast majority of pediatric diffuse large B-cell lymphoma cases have a germinal centre B-cell phenotype, as assessed by immunohistochemical analysis of selected proteins found in normal germinal centre B cells, such as the BCL6 gene product and CD10 [15]. About 20 % of pediatric diffuse large B-cell lymphoma presents as primary mediastinal disease (primary mediastinal B-cell lymphoma.

Lymphoblastic Lymphoma

In lymphoblastic lymphomas, the cells are homogenous with scant cytoplasm, round to oval nuclei, with finely stippled chromatin and inconspicuous nucleoli. Lymphoblastic lymphomas are usually positive for TdT, with more than 75 % having a T-cell immunophenotype and the remainder having a precursor B-cell phenotype [10, 16].

Anaplastic Large Cell Lymphoma

The tumours appear as a proliferation of cohesive large, bizarre, pleomorphic cells with abundant cytoplasm (more than most lymphomas) with eccentric horseshoe-shaped nuclei with multiple or single prominent nucleoli [14]. While the predominant immunophenotype of ALCL is mature T-cell, null-cell disease (i.e. no T-cell, B-cell or NK-cell surface antigen expression) does occur. All ALCL cases are CD30+ and more than 90 % of pediatric ALCL cases have a chromosomal rearrangement involving the ALK gene [17]. The category of ALCL in the 2001 WHO classification included both ALK+ and ALK− tumours and excluded primary cutaneous-ALCL. The 2008 classification concluded that current evidence warranted delineation of ALK+ ALCL as a distinct entity. ALK+ ALCL occurs mainly in pediatric and young age groups, has a better prognosis than ALK− ALCL, and exhibits differences in genetics [18].

Clinical Features

The clinical features of NHL depend on the site affected and the histological subtype. Although, low- and intermediate-grade malignant tumours predominate in adults, more than 90 % of children with NHL have high-grade malignant tumours with a propensity for malignant dissemination [19]. At least 60 % of children have advanced disease (stage III or IV) at diagnosis (Table 19.3) [10, 19]. Childhood NHL is predominantly an extranodal disease with primary sites involving the abdomen in 31 % of cases, mediastinum in 26 % of cases, head and neck region (including Waldeyer's ring and cervical nodes) in 29 % of cases. Only 6.5 % present with peripheral nodes outside the neck [20]. While most of the abdominal tumours are B-cell lymphomas, most mediastinal tumours are T-cell lymphomas [19]. Manifestations of abdominal tumour include pain, abdominal masses, nausea and vomiting resulting from intestinal obstruction caused by direct compression of the bowel lumen or by intussusceptions. NHL is the commonest cause of intussusceptions in children older than 6 years of age. Patients with large abdominal masses are at risk for the tumour lysis syndrome on initiation of chemotherapy [10]. Common clinical features of non-Hodgkin's lymphoma are shown in Table 19.3.

Lymphoblastic Lymphoma

This is mostly of a T-cell immunophenotype and typically presents as a mediastinal mass, often with an associated pleural effusion. Large mediastinal masses may manifest as severe respiratory distress resulting from airway compression or swelling of the neck, face and arms due to obstruction of the superior vena cava [10]. Lymphoblastic lymphoma may also affect the liver and spleen although isolated primary involvement of the abdomen is rare [10]. Patients may also present with peripheral lymphadenopathy and infiltration of the skin and soft tissues [13].

Anaplastic Large Cell Lymphoma

ALCL may affect nodal as well as extranodal sites. As much as 70 % of patients present with peripheral lymphadenopathy, the commonest site being cervical. Other sites involved include bones, soft tissue or skin, mediastinum or lungs [13]. The skin is the commonest extranodal site [21]. B symptoms such as fever and weight loss are also common in ALCL but relatively uncommon in other forms of NHL.

Burkitt Lymphoma

Burkitt lymphoma (BL) is characterized by a very short doubling time of 24 h and the interval from initiating or promoting events to diagnosis may be comparatively short. There are three clinico-epidemiologic forms of BL namely endemic, sporadic and HIV-associated types.

The jaw is the most commonly affected site in endemic BL; in high-incidence areas up to 90 % of patients may have clinical or subclinical jaw (radiographic abnormalities) involvement [22]. After the jaw the abdomen is the second commonest site of involvement of endemic BL; intra-abdominal structures are involved in 50–60 % of cases. Some parts of Nigeria like Ibadan have however reported a predominance of abdominal sites above jaw in endemic BL [23]. Other sites affected in the endemic tumour include the orbit, ovaries, retroperitoneal structures, kidneys, omentum, bowel wall and the central nervous system. CNS involvement includes cranial nerve palsies, paraplegia (usually flaccid) and malignant CSF pleocytosis. Only 25 % of patients with cranial nerve palsies have CSF pleocytosis. Invasion of the brain parenchyma is rare. Other sites that may be affected in endemic BL are pleura, endocrine and salivary glands, testes, bone and skin [22].

Unlike endemic BL which peaks at 7 years, a recent study on sporadic BL in the United States has showed two separate peaks among males and females, around the ages 10 and 75 years, and a 3rd peak around the age 40 years among males [24]. Previous reports had indicated that the predominant primary site of sporadic BL was the abdomen [20, 22]. A study in the United States that covered the period 1992–2005 revealed that BL tumours most frequently arose in the lymph nodes (56 %); the abdomen (21 %, primarily in the small or large intestine) is now the second most common site [25]. Other sites of involvement of sporadic BL are bone marrow (14 %, also called Burkitt cell leukemia), the oral cavity and the oropharynx [25]. While central nervous system involvement tends to be more common in endemic BL, bone marrow involvement is more common in the sporadic form.

In Uganda where BL is endemic, the frequency of jaw tumours in HIV-positive children is similar to that in HIV-negative children at presentation [26]. However in addition HIV-positive children presented significantly more often with extra-facial disease (lymphadenopathy 67 %, hepatic masses 51 % and thoracic masses 10 %). HIV-associated BL also present more frequently with advanced stage disease than HIV-negative cases [26].

Diffuse Large B-Cell Lymphoma

DLBCL presents similarly to BL with abdominal presentation being common. However, compared to BL patients, children with DLBCL more frequently present with localized disease, focal lesions in liver, spleen, lung and a mediastinal mass. Bone marrow and central nervous system involvement is also less common in DLBCL compared with other NHL entities [27].

Staging

The most widely used staging scheme for childhood non-Hodgkin lymphoma is that of the St. Jude Children's Research Hospital also known as Murphy Staging [19].

Bone marrow involvement has been defined as 5 % malignant cells in an otherwise normal bone marrow with normal peripheral blood counts and smears. Patients with lymphoblastic lymphoma with more than 25 % malignant cells in the bone marrow are usually considered to have leukemia and may be appropriately treated on leukemia protocols.

CNS disease in lymphoblastic lymphoma is defined by criteria similar to that used for acute lymphocytic leukemia (i.e. white blood cell count of at least 5/μL and malignant cells in the cerebrospinal fluid [CSF]). For any other NHL, the definition of CNS disease is any malignant cell present in the CSF regardless of cell count.

However, the St. Jude's staging classification is unclear on the definition of extensive primary disease and considers all primary abdominal and thoracic tumours as extensive stage III disease, despite original surgical debulking, which may occur at diagnosis. Subsequently, a new French, American and British (FAB) staging classification was developed (Table 19.4) that better defines the staging of childhood B large cell and BL of childhood [28]. This system recognizes the common dissemination to either the central nervous system or bone marrow and the fact that this is indicative of a poor prognosis (Table 19.5).

BL constitutes the majority of NHL in equatorial Africa. BL in Africa is frequently staged according to a staging system previously described by Magrath et al. [29] based on survival in patients with BL at the Lymphoma Treatment Centre (LTC) in Uganda. This system has recently been used in a multicentre study of African BL by the International Network for Cancer treatment and Research (INCTR) and renamed the LTC system (Table 19.6) [30]. It is useful in resource-constrained places like Africa where the Murphy system cannot be applied due to lack of expertise and facilities for performance of bone marrow aspiration cytology and cerebrospinal fluid examination.

Differential Diagnosis

A number of childhood conditions including infections like tuberculosis might mimic non-Hodgkin lymphoma in their presentation (Table 19.7).

Table 19.4 Murphy staging of childhood non-Hodgkin lymphoma

Stage I
A single tumour (extranodal) or single nodal area is involved, with the exclusion of the abdomen and mediastinum
Stage II
A single tumour with regional node involvement
Two or more nodal areas involved on same side of the diaphragm
Two single (extranodal) tumours with or without regional node involvement on same side of diaphragm
A primary gastrointestinal tract tumour (completely resected) with or without regional node involvement
Stage III
Two single tumours (extranodal) on both sides of the diaphragm
Two or more nodal areas on both sides of the diaphragm
All primary intrathoracic (mediastinal, pleural or thymic) disease, extensive primary intra-abdominal disease, or any paraspinal or epidural tumours, regardless of other tumour site(s).
Stage IV
Any of the above with initial involvement of the bone marrow and/or central nervous system (CNS)

Source: Murphy SB, Fairclough DL, Hutchison RE, et al.: Non-Hodgkin's lymphomas of childhood: an analysis of the histology, staging, and response to treatment of 338 cases at a single institution. J Clin Oncol 7 (2): 186–93, 1989

Table 19.5 FAB[a] staging system for childhood B large and Burkitt lymphoma

Group A
Completely resected Stage I (St. Jude)
Completely resected abdominal Stage II (St. Jude)
Group B
All patients not eligible for Group A or Group C
Group C
Any CNS involvement[b] and/or bone marrow involvement (≥25 % blasts)

Source: Cairo MS, Gerrard M, Patte C. A new protocol for treatment of mature B-cell lymphoma/leukaemia (BCLL): FAB LMB 96, a SFOP LMB 96/CCG-5961/UKCCSG NHL 9600 international cooperative study. Med Pediatr Oncol 1997;29:320a

[a]FAB French, American, British

[b]CNS: Any L3 blast, cranial nerve palsy or compression, intracerebral mass and/or parameningeal compression

Table 19.6 LTC staging system for Burkitt lymphoma

Stage A: a single extra-abdominal tumour
Stage B: multiple extra-abdominal tumours (including CNS involvement, i.e. CSF pleocytosis or cranial nerve palsies)
Stage C: abdominal tumour with or without facial tumours
Stage D: abdominal tumour with tumour at any other site or sites, except the face alone

Source: Ngoma T, et al. Treatment of Burkitt lymphoma in equatorial Africa using a simple three-drug combination followed by a salvage regimen for patients with persistent or recurrent disease. Br J Haematol. 2012 Sep; 158(6):749–62

Therefore a high grade of suspicion and appropriate laboratory investigations are required to confirm the diagnosis.

Diagnostic Work Up

The following investigations are required for the diagnostic work up of children with non-Hodgkin lymphoma.

Laboratory Tests

Complete blood count

Serum electrolytes, blood urea nitrogen, creatinine, calcium, phosphorus, uric acid

Liver function tests (serum bilirubin, ALT, AST, alkaline phosphates, serum albumin and total protein)

Lactic dehydrogenase level

Viral studies: Hepatitis B and C serology, HIV antibody, HSV antibody, CMV antibody, varicella antibody

Confirmatory Tests

Pathological diagnosis is required for confirmation of diagnosis.

Table 19.7 Differential diagnoses of non-Hodgkin's lymphoma in childhood

Disease	Important similarities and distinctions
Hodgkin lymphoma	May present with lymphadenopathy most commonly cervical, mediastinal masses, hepatosplenomegaly, fever, weight loss similar to NHL. May also cause superior vena caval syndrome
Rhabdomyosarcoma	May present with orbital, jaw and abdominal swellings, paraplegia similar to Burkitt lymphoma
Neuroblastoma	May present with proptosis, jaw swelling, abdominal swelling and paraplegia similar to NHL. However, more often affects children under 5 years of age, associated with scalp swellings and proptosis usually bilateral
Nephroblastoma	May present with abdominal swelling and respiratory symptoms due to pulmonary metastasis but mostly affects children under 5 years of age
Tuberculosis	May present with cough, fever, drenching night sweats, weight loss and lymphadenopathy. Abdominal distension may be present. Paraplegia when present is usually spastic and associated with a gibbus. Chest radiograph may show parenchymal opacities, cavities, effusion, hilar adenopathy
Human immunodeficiency virus infection	May present with fever, cough, weight loss, respiratory symptoms and signs, generalized lymphadenopathy, hepatosplenomegaly. HIV test will be positive but may coexist with lymphoma so tissue biopsy is necessary to exclude lymphoma

Surgical tissue biopsy for histology, immunologic, cytogenetic and molecular studies

Needle aspirate for cytology (tissue biopsy is usually more informative and preferred to needle aspirate [32].

Bilateral bone marrow aspirate and biopsy

Cerebrospinal, pericardial fluid, peritoneal, pleural fluids examination for immunologic and cytogenetic studies

Radiologic Tests

Chest radiograph

Abdominal and pelvic ultrasound scans

Computerized tomography scans of the chest, abdomen and pelvis

Positron emission tomography scans when available (for initial staging and measurement of tumour response)

Magnetic resonance imaging (MRI) when indicated especially for suspected vertebral involvement

A bone marrow examination may be diagnostic in the evaluation of a child with mediastinal mass because bone marrow involvement is frequently found in patients with mediastinal precursor T-cell lymphoblastic lymphoma and because T-cell lymphoblastic lymphoma is often presents with associated mediastinal masses. If bone marrow aspirate is diagnostic, the need for anaesthesia and surgical biopsy may be avoided. In patients with mediastinal masses associated with respiratory distress, the pre-biopsy use of irradiation or steroids may result in rapid shrinkage of the mass but jeopardize establishing a tissue diagnosis. Up to 48 h of prednisolone (40–60 mg/m^2) may be given with rapid clinical improvement and preservation of diagnostic tissue [32, 33].

Treatment of NHL

The treatment of NHL has progressed over the years and there are now very good and established chemotherapy protocols that are able to cure a large number of children. The prognosis of this group of tumours improved once the concept that they are a diffuse disease entity and that treatment needs to be systemic rather than localized was recognized. The survival rate in the early 60s was dismal but with the modern therapy regimes used currently almost 75 % of patients

Table 19.8 Drugs used in treatment of NHL in children

Drug	Dose	Comments
Vincristine	1 mg–2 mg/m^2	IVI push, not for IT use
Doxorubicin	60 mg/m^2	IVI infusion, cardiac toxicity at high doses, need cardiac evaluations
Cyclophosphamide	From 250 to 1,200 mg/m^2 IVI 40–60 mg/kg per os	Needs hydration, given as IVI infusion over 30 min but sometimes as IVI push, also used orally
Methotrexate	75 mg–8 g/m^2	IVI infusion over 3–4 h, needs hydration, alkalinization of urine as well as MTX levels at higher doses, Leucovorin rescue needed
Cytarabine	50 mg–2,000 mg/m^2	IVI push, IVI infusion at higher doses, subcut at times
Ifosfamide	1,500 mg/m^2	IVI infusion over 3 h, needs hydration, MESNA rescue
Etoposide	100 mg/m^2	IVI infusion over 1 h
Prednisone/Prednisolone	60 mg/m^2	IVI or orally, be careful of gastritis
Asparaginase	6,000 μg/m^2	IMI, used in ALL protocols for LL
6-Mercaptopurine	75 mg/m^2	Orally, used in ALL protocols for LL
Methotrexate	20 mg/m^2	Orally, used in ALL protocols for LL
Decadron	6 mg/m^2	Orally, used in ALL protocols for LL
IT therapy		
Methotrexate	8–15 mg IT	Dose is age dependent
Hydrocortisone	8–15 mg IT	Dose is age dependent
Cytarabine	15–30 mg IT	Dose is age dependent

will become long-term survivors [34]. The initial treatments involved excision of localized disease followed by radiotherapy in some cases and the addition of single drugs did, in most cases, not result in significant improvement of the cure rates. The exception to this premise is Burkitt lymphoma in which almost 50 % can be cured with the use of cyclophosphamide alone [35]. It is accepted today that the treatment of NHL is chemotherapy-based.

The current regimes are based on the protocols that are utilized for acute lymphoblastic leukemia and the agents/drugs used are the same. Prednisone, L-asparaginase, vincristine and methotrexate, in various dose regimes, with mercaptopurine are utilized for the treatment of NHL. There are protocols that also use the anthracyclines, cyclophosphamide as well as cytarabine and epipodophyllotoxins. All these protocols give very similar results and are comparable in their survival results as well as the complication and toxicity from the agents used (Table 19.8).

Surgery plays a limited role in the treatment of NHL and is usually reserved to a biopsy of the lymph nodes or of other tissues. Radiotherapy does play a limited role in treatment and has specific indications but long-term studies have shown that it is significantly associated with the late deaths in NHL [2].

As NHLs are a group of aggressive disease prompt and adequate treatment is required. Initial evaluation should be rapid and expedited so that the investigations for staging are done rapidly and the patient prepared for chemotherapy. NHL patients should be treated within the multidisciplinary team framework as there are many elements involved in the treatment. An experienced pediatric oncologist should be the main member but other subspecialties may be co-opted as needed. The pediatric surgeon may be required for biopsy of the nodes, resection of involved intestine when the NHL is localized, for placement of central lines and to treat surgically related complications of treatment. The radiotherapist is seldom involved in the treatment of NHL except in very specific circumstances such as emergency radiation for airway obstruction and central nervous system disease in certain subtypes of NHL. The radiologist should also be consulted early to decide which and in what order the radiological evaluation should be done.

As NHL are among the most rapidly growing tumours adequate measures need to be in place to prevent and treat tumour lysis syndrome (TLS) (Chapter 9: Oncologic Emergencies) before the chemotherapy is commenced. Recognition of TLS and the successful prevention and treatment has resulted in improvement in survival rates. Close attention to the biochemical abnormalities (raised urea, potassium, phosphate and uric acid levels) are paramount to prevent this potentially lethal complication. Prevention entails the used of intravenous fluids, alkalinization of the urine, control of the uric acid levels with either Allopurinol or, where/if available, Rasburicase and close and frequent monitoring of urine output and biochemistry. This complication is seen with higher stage NHL usually of T cell, diffuse large B cell and Burkitt subtypes. The use of a cyto-reduction chemotherapy pre-phase in a significant number of protocols also allows for a more controlled breakdown of the tumour and limits the development of TLS [2].

In developing countries, BL is basically diagnosed through morphology, and the appropriate protocol is then chosen for treatment (see below). However, in many of these countries, facilities for classification of other NHLs into B- and T-cell immunophenotypes are lacking but they still need to be treated. The CHOP regime is efficacious in most cases of NHL and is a useful first-line treatment under these circumstances [36].

The chemotherapy of the various subtypes is different and each will be discussed separately and as localized disease is rare in low- and middle-income countries discussion of protocols in this chapter will be restricted to widespread disease, essentially stage 3 and 4 disease. Protocols for the odd cases of localized disease can be referenced from Pizzo and Poplack [2].

B-Cell Non-Hodgkin Lymphoma

This group of NHL is divided into a number of types of which Burkitt lymphoma (BL) is extremely important but other subtypes are also sometimes seen.

Burkitt Lymphoma

Burkitt lymphoma is probably the most common type of lymphoma seen in sub-Saharan Africa and has a wide distribution. The treatment of this NHL varies from very intensive treatment regimes to very simple but effective treatments for resource-poor countries. There are a large number of very good protocols available and they include the FAB/LMB96 [37], CHOP, BFM 90 protocols which can be used for all stages of BL. Some of these protocols are very intensive and good supportive care is needed for the patients as neutropenia, sepsis and low platelets counts are often seen and may need to be treated aggressively (Tables 19.9 and 19.10).

Survival rates for these protocols are well over 90 % for both localized and non-resected localized disease. Survival rates for extensive or widespread disease, which would need more aggressive treatment, are still between 70 and 90 %.

There are less intensive protocols [35, 38, 39] with single drugs and short courses which have given survival rates that are over 50 % (Tables 19.11 and 19.12). These protocols also have a low-dose regime for the more advanced BL which, although not as effective as the LMB and other protocols, still give a reasonable survival rate. These protocols need minimal supportive care and can be used in low-resourced countries and give reasonable results especially in localized disease but unfortunately, in advanced disease, they are not as effective as the more aggressive regimes. Another limited protocol described [23] has a three-drug protocol for the treatment of BL. It gave very good results with their first-line treatment approach. Their suggested approach for late relapses gave reasonable results with an overall survival rate of >65 % (Table 19.13).

Table 19.9 LMB Group C protocol modified: For BL and DLBCL overall survival rates >90 %

1 BM > 25 % blasts/CNS negative: COP(X 1 or 2): COPADM × 2: CYVE × 2: M1–4

2 BM > 25% balsts/CNS positive: COP(X 1or 2): COPADM × 2: CYVE + MTX: CYVE: M1–4

	Drug	Dose	Regime
Induction (COP × 1 or 2)			
Give second COP for very ill children	Vincristine	1 mg/m^2 (max 2 mg) IVI push	Day 1 (and 8 if second COP)
	Cyclophosphamide	300 mg/m^2 over 30 min IVI infusion	Day 1 (and 8 if second COP)
	Prednisone	60 mg/m^2 PO 12 hourly	Days 1–8 (or 15 if second COP)
	IT Triple therapy (MTX +HYD +CYT)	See below	Days 1, 3, 5 (8, 10, 12 if second COP)
	Leucovorin	15 mg/m^2 PO 12 hourly	Days 2, 4 (9, 11 if second COP)
COPADM × 2 Cycles			
First starts day 8 (15) after COP	21–28 day cycle if ANC >1 × 10^9/L and platelets >100 × 10^9/L		
	Vincristine	2 mg/m^2 (max 2 mg) IVI push	Day 1
	Prednisone	60 mg/m^2 PO 12 hourly	Days 1–5 then taper over 3 days
	Methotrexate	8 g/m^2 over 4 h in 500 mL 5%DW	Day 1
	Leucovorin	15 mg/m^2 PO or IVI 6 hourly × 12 doses	Days 2–4 (Blood level MTX <0.2 mmol to stop Leucovorin)
	Cyclophosphamide	250 mg/m^2 over 30 min IVI infusion 12 hourly	Days 2–4
	Doxorubicin	60 mg/m^2 over 6 h after cyclophosphamide	Day 2
	IT Triple therapy (MTX +HYD +CYT)	See below	Days 2, 4, 6
CYVE × 2 IF CNS NEG			
	21–28 day cycle if ANC >1 × 10^9/L and platelets >100 × 10^9/L		
	Cytarabine	50 mg/m^2 in 200–500 mL DW over 12 h (20H00–08H00)	Days 1–5
	Cytarabine (high dose)	2,000 mg/m^2 200–500 mL rehydration fluid over 2 h (08H00–10H00)	Days 2–5
	VP 16 (Etoposide)	100 mg/m^2 in 200 mL saline over 2 h (14H00-16H00)	Days 2–5
CYVE with MTX (CNS POS)			
	21–28 day cycle if ANC >1 × 10^9/L and platelets >100 × 10^9/L		
	Cytarabine	50 mg/m^2 in 200–500 mL DW over 12 h (20H00-08H00)	Days 1–5
	Cytarabine (high dose)	2,000 mg/m^2 200–500 mL rehydration fluid over 2 h (08H00-10H00)	Days 2–5
	VP 16 (Etoposide)	100 mg/m^2 in 200 mL saline over 2 h (14H00-16H00)	Days 2–5
	Methotrexate (NB only start if ANC >0.5,PLTS >50 000: transaminases <10 normal)	8,000 mg/m^2 in 500 mL saline over 4 h	Day 18 (about)
	Leucovorin	15 mg/m^2 IVI or PO 6 hourly × 12 doses	Days 19–21 (Blood level MTX <0.2 mmol to stop Leucovorin)
	IT Double therapy (HYD +CYT)	See below (6 h prior to Cytarabine)	Day 1
	IT Triple therapy (MTX +HYD +CYT)	See below	Day after MTX

(continued)

Table 19.9 (continued)

1 BM > 25 % blasts/CNS negative: COP(X 1 or 2): COPADM × 2: CYVE × 2: M1–4			
2 BM > 25% balsts/CNS positive: COP(X 1or 2): COPADM × 2: CYVE + MTX: CYVE: M1–4			
	Drug	Dose	Regime
CYVE 2			
	21–28 day cycle if ANC >1 × 10^9/L and platelets >100 × 10^9/L		
	Cytarabine	50 mg/m² in 200–500 mL DW over 12 h (20H00-08H00)	Days 1–5
	Cytarabine high dose	2,000 mg/m² 200–500 mL rehydration fluid over 2 h (08H00-10H00)	Days 2–5
	VP 16 (Etoposide)	100 mg/m² in 200 mL saline over 2 h (14H00-16H00)	Days 2–5
	IT Double therapy (HYD +CYT)	See below (6 h prior to Cytarabine)	Day 1
Maintenance 1			
	21–28 day cycle if ANC >1 × 10^9/L and platelets >100 × 10^9/L		
	Vincristine	2 mg/m² (max 2 mg) IVI push	Day 1
	Prednisone	60 mg/m² PO 12 hourly	Days 1–5 then taper over 3 days
	Methotrexate	8 g/m² over 4 h in 500 mL 5%DW	Day 1
	Leucovorin	15 mg/m² PO or IVI 6 hourly × 12 doses	Days 2–4 (Blood level MTX <0.2 mmol to stop Leucovorin)
	Cyclophosphamide	500 mg/m² over 30 min IVI infusion	Days 2, 3
	Doxorubicin	60 mg/m² over 6 h after cyclophosphamide	Day 2
	IT Triple therapy (MTX + HYD + CYT)	See below	Day 2
Maintenance 2 and 4			
	21–28 day cycle if ANC >1 × 10^9/L and platelets >100 × 10^9/L		
	Cytarabine	50 mg/m² subcut 12 hourly	Days 1–5
	VP 16 (Etoposide)	150 mg/m² over 90 min	Days 1–5
Maintenance 3			
	21–28 day cycle if ANC >1 × 10^9/L and platelets >100 × 10^9/L		
	Vincristine	2 mg/m² (max 2 mg) IVI push	Day 1
	Prednisone	60 mg/m² PO 12 hourly	Days 1–5 then taper over 3 days
	Cyclophosphamide	500 mg/m² over 30 min IVI infusion	Days 1, 2
	Doxorubicin	60 mg/m² over 6 h after cyclophosphamide	Day 1
IT therapy	MTX + hydrocortisone (HYD)	Cytarabine (CYT)	
<1 year	8 mg	15 mg	
1–2 years	10 mg	20 mg	
2–3 years	12 mg	25 mg	
>3 years	15 mg	30 mg	

Source: Adapted from [35]
Remember the fluids and medication to prevent tumour lysis
Remember fluids and/or alkalinization of urine for methotrexate and cyclophosphamide
Remember to check all doses, routes, methods of administration and schedules with the original protocol. Reevaluations are done according to protocol schedule

Table 19.10 LMB Group B 96 modified: For BL and DLBCL overall survival rates >90 %

Stage 1–4: non-resected: CNS negative: marrow <25 % blasts: COP(X 1or 2): COPADM × 2: CYM × 2:			
	Drug	Dose	Regime
Induction (COP × 1 OR 2)			
Give second COP for very ill children	Vincristine	1 mg/m^2 (max 2 mg) IVI push	Day 1 (and 8 if second COP)
	Cyclophosphamide	300 mg/m^2 over 30 min IVI infusion	Day 1 (and 8 if second COP)
	Prednisone	60 mg/m^2 PO 12 hourly	Days 1–8 (or 15 if second COP)
	IT Double therapy	See below	Days 1 (8 if second COP)
COPADM × 2 cycles			
First starts day 8 (15) after COP	21–28 day cycle if ANC >1 × 10^9/L and platelets >100 × 10^9/L		
	Vincristine	2 mg/m^2 (max 2 mg) IVI push	Day 1
	Prednisone	60 mg/m^2 PO 12 hourly	Days 1–5 then taper over 3 days
	Methotrexate	3 g/m^2 over 3 h in 500 mL 5%DW	Day 1
	Leucovorin	15 mg/m^2 PO or IVI 6 hourly × 12 doses	Days 2–4
	Cyclophosphamide	250 mg/m^2 over 30 minutes IVI infusion 12 hourly	Days 2–4
	Doxorubicin	60 mg/m^2 over 6 h after cyclophosphamide	Day 2
	IT Double therapy (MTX + HYD)	See below	Days 2, 6
CYM × 2			
	21–28 day cycle if ANC >1 × 10^9/L and platelets >100 × 10^9/L		
	Methotrexate	3 g/m^2 over 3 h in 500 mL 5%DW	Day 1
	Leucovorin	15 mg/m^2 PO or IVI 6 hourly × 12 doses	Days 2–4
	Cytarabine	100 mg/m^2 in 1,000 mL/m^2 DW over 12 h (20H00–08H00)	Days 2–6
	IT double therapy (MTX + HYD)	See below	Day 2
	IT double therapy (CYT + HYD)	See below	Day 7
IT therapy			
	MTX + hydrocortisone (HYD) (mg)	Cytarabine (CYT) (mg)	
<1 year	8	15	
1–2 years	10	20	
2–3 years	12	25	
>3 years	15	30	

Source: Adapted from [35]
Remember the fluids and medication to prevent tumour lysis
Remember fluids and/or alkalinization of urine for methotrexate and cyclophosphamide
Remember to check all doses, routes, methods of administration and schedules with the original protocol. Reevaluations are done according to protocol schedule

As expected the patients who were non-responders or had early relapse did worse, even with a reasonably aggressive protocol.

Reports from other developing countries show a variety of protocols are used, that vary in intensity, as well as survival rates [6, 7, 8, 38]. The survival rates from these protocols vary from 50 to 60 %. Some countries use the LMB/FAB protocol while others have modified the original protocol to suit their particular needs [6, 7].

Table 19.11 Other protocols: For BL and DLBCL

	Drug	Dose	Regime
GFAOP [38] (overall survival rate 50 %)			
All patients			
	Cyclophosphamide	1,200 mg/m^2 IVI bolus	Days 1, 8, 15
	IT Methotrexate	15 mg	Days 1, 8, 15
	IT Hydrocortisone	15 mg	Days 1, 8, 15
Evaluation day 21			
Complete response Stage 1, 2	No further treatment		
Complete response Stage 3, 4	Cyclophosphamide	1,200 mg/m^2 IVI bolus	Days 1, 15, 28
	IT Methotrexate	15 mg	Days 1, 15, 28
	IT Hydrocortisone	15 mg	Days 1, 15, 28
No CR, refractory/relapsed patients			
	18 day cycle if ANC>1 × 10^9/L and platelets >100 × 10^9/L		
COPM × 2 cycles			
	Vincristine	2 mg/m^2 (max 2 mg) IVI push	Day 1
	Prednisone	60 mg/m^2 PO or IVI daily	Days 1–5 then taper over 3 days
	Methotrexate	3 g/m^2 over 2 h in 500 mL 5%DW	Day 1
	Leucovorin	15 mg/m^2 PO or IVI 6 hourly × 12 doses	Days 2–4
	Cyclophosphamide	250 mg/m^2 IVI infusion 12 hourly with pre-hydration	Days 2–4
	IT Methotrexate	15 mg	Days 2, 6
	IT Hydrocortisone	15 mg	Days 2, 6
CYM × 2 cycles			
	Methotrexate	3 g/m^2 over 2 h in 500 mL 5%DW	Day 1
	Cytarabine	50 mg/m^2 SC 12 hourly	Days 2–6
	IT Methotrexate	15 mg	Day 2
	IT Hydrocortisone	15 mg	Day 2
	IT Cytarabine	30 mg	Day 7
	IT Hydrocortisone	15 mg	Day 7

Source: Adapted from [37]
Remember the fluids and medication to prevent tumour lysis
Remember fluids and/or alkalinization of urine for Methotrexate, Ifosfamide and cyclophosphamide
Remember to check all doses, routes, methods of administration and schedules with the original protocol. Reevaluations are done according to protocol schedule

Nicaragua developed a regime that was based on the local drug supply, availability and affordability [8].

Relapsed and refractory patients pose a major problem in further treatment. Most of the relapses in BL occur within 1 year after the diagnosis (actually close to 90 % if they relapse, relapse in the first 9 months after treatment). Drug resistance is the major problem in these children and unfortunately survival rates of approximately 20 % or less can be expected. Bone marrow transplant (BMT), where available, probably offers the best opportunity for long-term survival. Rituximab, often used by the adults in DLBCL in combination with CHOP, is expensive and has many side effects in children that require aggressive supportive therapy. There are trials underway in pediatric patients to assess its usefulness in relapsed BL.

Table 19.12 Other protocols: For BL and DLBCL

	Drug	Dose	Regime
Hesseling et al. [33] *(Overall survival rate 57 %)*			
	Cyclophosphamide	40 mg/kg IVI with pre-hydration	Day 1
	Cyclophosphamide	60 mg/kg IVI or PO with pre-hydration	Day 8, 18, 28
	IT Methotrexate	12.5 mg	Days 1, 8, 18, 28
	IT Hydrocortisone	12.5 mg	Days 1, 8, 18, 28
Hesseling et al. [36] *(Overall survival rate 60 %)*			
All patients	Cyclophosphamide	40 mg/kg IVI or PO with pre-hydration	Days 1, 8, 15
	IT Methotrexate	12.5 mg	Days 1, 8, 15
	IT Hydrocortisone	12.5 mg	Days 1, 8, 15
Consolidation therapy			
Risk Group 1 (Stage 1, 2 in remission)			
	Cyclophosphamide	60 mg/kg IVI or PO with pre-hydration	Day 29
Risk Group 2 (Stage 3, remission and residual abdominal tumour <30 mL)			
	Cyclophosphamide	60 mg/kg IVI or PO with pre-hydration	Days 29, 43
Risk Group 3 (Stage 3, remission and residual abdominal tumour >30 mL			
	Cyclophosphamide	60 mg/kg IVI or PO with pre-hydration	Days 29, 43, 57
	Vincristine	1.5 mg/m^2 (max 2 mg) IVI push	Days 29, 43, 57
	Methotrexate	1 g/m^2 over 3 h in 200 mL 5%DW	Day 29
	Leucovorin	15 mg PO 6 hourly × 8 doses	Day 30, 31
Bezwoda et al. [34]			
Maximum of 8 cycles	Vincristine	1.4 mg/m^2 (max 2 mg) IVI push	Day 1
CR at cycle 3 had 6 cycles	Prednisone	50 mg/m^2 PO daily	Days 1–5
PR within 3 cycles had 6 cycles	Cyclophosphamide	750 mg/kg IVI with pre-hydration	Day 1
PR or CR only at cycle 6 received another 2 cycles	Doxorubicin	50 mg/m^2	Day 1

Source: Adapted from [33–36]
Remember the fluids and medication to prevent tumour lysis
Remember fluids and/or alkalinization of urine for Methotrexate, Ifosfamide and cyclophosphamide
Remember to check all doses, routes, methods of administration and schedules with the original protocol. Reevaluations are done according to protocol schedule

Diffuse Large B-Cell Lymphoma

The protocols used for this type of lymphoma in children have been the protocols that have been used successfully for BL. The DLBCL in children is an aggressive tumour that resembles BL according to the molecular data that is being gathered [2].

As with BL those children with localized DLBCL do exceptionally well on the protocols, and survival rates are between 90 and 95 %. Children with localized bone lymphoma also do well on these protocols even if the radiotherapy is omitted [2].

Patients with more extensive disease also benefit from the BL-based protocols and survival

Table 19.13 INCTR: for BL and DLBCL overall survival rates of 67 % at 1 year

	Drug	Dose	Regime
First line (FL 1)			
	15 day cycle if ANC >1×10⁹/L and platelets >100×10⁹/L		
All newly diagnosed patients	Vincristine	1.4 mg/m² (max 2 mg) IVI push	Day 1
	Cyclophosphamide	1,200 mg/m² over 30 min IVI infusion	Day 1
	Methotrexate	75 mg/m² IVI	Day 1
	IT Methotrexate	12 mg (<3 years 10 mg)	Day 1, 8
	IT Cytarabine	50 mg (<3 years 40 mg)	Day 4
LR received 3 cycle	Low risk: CNS/Marrow clear, single abdominal mass, 10 cm		
HR received 6 cycles	High risk: All other patients: CNS positive IT in all 6 cycles		
Second line (FL 2)			
	21 day cycle if ANC >1×10⁹/L and platelets >100×10⁹/L		
Failed to respond, relapsed within 6 weeks after FL 1	VP16 (Etoposide)	60 mg/m² IVI infusion	Days 1–3
Patients received 4 cycles	Ifosfamide	1,500 mg/m² over 3 h with pre-hydration	Days 1–3
	MESNA	300 mg/m² with Ifosfamide, then 3 hourly×3 doses	Days 1–3
	Cytarabine	100 mg/m² IVI	Days 1–3
	IT Methotrexate	12 mg (<3 years 10 mg)	Day 1, 8
	IT Cytarabine	50 mg (<3 years 40 mg)	Day 4

Source: Adapted from [28]
Remember the fluids and medication to prevent tumour lysis
Remember fluids and/or alkalinization of urine for Ifosfamide and cyclophosphamide
Remember to check all doses, routes, methods of administration and schedules with the original protocol. Reevaluations are done according to protocol schedule

rates, whichever protocol is used, is between 85 and 90 %. Children with PBML are also treated on these protocols but have an inferior survival rate of between 65 and 70 % and these are very much the same as the rates that are seen in adults with the PBML.

Children that relapse on the protocols used for DLBCL, can in 50 % of cases, be rescued with adult-based protocols with the addition of Rituximab. The ICE protocol (Ifosfamide, Etoposide and Carboplatinum) can be used.

Anaplastic Large Cell lymphoma

There are two variants of ALCL, cutaneous and systemic. Treatment for cutaneous-ALCL (C-ALCL) is not uniform and at the moment most treatment regimes mention surgical excision and then observation alone.

Systemic ALCL (ALK+) is a different disease and there are chemotherapy regimes for the treatment of this NHL. Treatments have included modified ALL or T-cell lymphoma protocols as well as the BFM 90 NHL protocol. Stage 1 has a good survival approaching 90 % while the more extensive stages have lower survival rates of around 75 %

Precursor T-Cell Lymphoma (LL)

There have been many trials done in America that have shown very convincingly that the use of ALL protocol, either high risk or T cell, is necessary for the treatment and cure of children with LL. These protocols should be used for all stages including stage 1 and 2. In the earlier studies of primary mediastinal NHL, although having a good initial response they tended to relapse in marrow and CNS unless the intensive protocols used today were employed in these children. Radiotherapy does appear to be a necessary component of the treatment in certain instances and may play a role in those with CNS disease at presentation. The use of systemic high-dose methotrexate and intra-thecal chemotherapy may be used to avoid the use of cranial irradiation.

Relapsed or refractory disease is difficult to treat and most relapses occur within 1 year of diagnosis. BMT is an option in developed countries but in developing countries palliative care is probably the only alternative.

Other Types of NHL in Children

There are a number of other subtypes of NHL that do occur in children. They are not common and the treatment regimens are not well developed and usually based on the adult literature.

Follicular lymphoma (FL) is rare in children and the treatment varies from conservative [40] to the use of CHOP for a variable number of cycles [41]. Adult patients with FL are often treated with Rituximab but there are few trials in pediatric patients.

Pediatric NMZL is more common than extranodal disease and as the prognosis is excellent treatment varies from surgical excision alone to local irradiation therapy.

Peripheral T-cell lymphoma (PTCL) is rare in children and recent retrospective studies from POG [41] and UKCCSG [42] have been published showing those with localized disease do better and had a survival rate of 50 % at 5 years. It appears that T-cell ALL regimes maybe a better option than the B-cell-orientated protocols [42, 43].

Primary central nervous system lymphoma (PCNSL) is a rare extranodal site for lymphoma and accounts for <5 % of extranodal lymphoma. Of these <1 % occur in patients under 19 years of age, they are usually B-cell lineage (often DLBCL) and may occur at an earlier age in children with immune deficiency, either acquired or inherited. Treatment is problematic and varies from use of BL- to DLBCL-based protocols without use of radiotherapy [2].

What Would We Suggest?

As can be seen from above there are a number of protocols available to treat children with NHL. Some of them are intensive and need adequate resources and support from the laboratories and allied medical staff: on the other hand there are a number of low-intensity protocols available that need limited resources and medications and, although they give inferior results, there are still a significant number of children that can be saved with these low-intensity protocols.

For middle-income countries with adequate resources we feel that the LMB-based protocols [37] are an option, intensive, fairly short and give a good survival rate. The protocol from Ngoma et al. is also an acceptable alternative [30]. These two protocols would probably also be acceptable for all patients with any subtype of B-cell lymphoma. If the resources allow it then appropriate protocols for the subtypes of NHL can be utilized, but most of these protocols are fairly intensive. The children with T-cell lymphoma we would treat with an ALL-based protocol. If the NHL is only diagnosed on morphology the CHOP regime would be an acceptable alternative.

For low-income countries the options are a little different. The approach is to cure as many children as possible with as little toxicity and expense as possible. There are guidelines for use of chemotherapy with suggestions for making the treatment of these children as safe as possible with some basic precautions (Table 19.14). We would suggest any of the protocols developed in Cameroon and Malawi for the Burkitt lymphoma patients [35, 38, 44]. For those patients with other subtypes of B-cell lymphomas the options are limited as most will need aggressive therapy which would mean a drain on the limited resources. We feel that in a lot of these countries these subtypes would be in the minority and that the occasional case could be treated with the appropriate protocol (Tables 19.11 and 19.12).

Table 19.14 Some practical notes

If possible chemotherapy should be given on week days when trained staff available
Check the neutrophil count (or total white cell count) before administering chemotherapy, should be $>1\times10^9$/L and platelets $>100\times10^9$/L
Delay chemotherapy if child has fever, until such time as the infection is under control and patient stable
Remember to monitor urine output as well as intake, BP and other vital signs when the chemotherapy commences
Make sure you have supportive drugs needed before chemotherapy commences, i.e. anti-emetics, allopurinol and IVI fluids
Make sure you have adequate supplies of chemotherapy and rescue medications to complete all the cycles
Check the surface area, weight before each chemotherapy cycle, make sure of the dose to be given (per m^2 or per kg), recalculate if unsure or dose seems inappropriate
Make sure you know how to give chemotherapy, i.e. IVI push, infusion, mix with what fluids, what other supportive measures needed
Chemotherapy should be mixed by an experienced person (physician/pharmacist) in a separate area with a laminar flow unit if available, if not then an extractor hood above mixing surface. The person mixing chemotherapy should be clothed appropriately
For new patients, even with abnormal blood counts or those who are critically ill, the chemotherapy is commenced with appropriate supportive measures
Vincristine causes a fatal encephalopathy if given via the intra-thecal route. Always make sure that the intra-thecal medication is given at a different time to the vincristine
If possible share drugs between patients, this will decrease costs to the hospital, parents or the supplier of the medication
Develop protocol sheets that are easy to understand and sign off the medication as it is given
Photographs make a good clinical record of progress for doctor, patients and parents
Cost of treatment should be guaranteed when treatment starts
Be caring, compassionate, truthful and dedicated, even if you cannot do much, the patients/parents will appreciate it

Source: Adapted from [38]

References

1. Childhood non-Hodgkin lymphoma treatment. www.cancer.gov/cancertopics/pdq/treatment/child-non-hodgkins/Healthprofessional/ Accessed 07/2012
2. Pizzo PA, Poplack DG. Principles and practice of pediatric oncology. 6th ed. Philadelphia: Lippincott Williams & Wilkins; 2011 (Chapter 23: Malignant non-Hodgkin lymphomas in children).
3. Alexander D, Mink P, Adami H, et al. The non-Hodgkin lymphomas: A review of the epidemiologic literature. Int J Cancer. 2007;120:1–39.
4. Lanzkowsky P. Manual of pediatric hematology and oncology. 3rd ed. San Diego: Academic; 2000. (Chapter 13).
5. Wakabi W. Special report: Kenya and Uganda grapple with Burkitt lymphoma. Lancet Oncol. 2008;9(4):319.
6. Ahmad N, Zaidi A, Badar F, et al. Clinical characteristics and outcome analysis of pediatric B-cell non-Hodgkin's lymphoma. Experience with FAB-LMB 96 and UKCCSG B-cell NHL guidelines in a developing country. Asia Pac J Clin Oncol. 2010;6:49–56.
7. Moleti M, Al-Hadad S, Al-Jadiry M, et al. Treatment of children with B-cell non-Hodgkin lymphoma in a low-income country. Pediatr Blood Cancer. 2011;56:560–7.
8. Baez F, Pillon M, Manfredini L, et al. Treatment of pediatric non-hodgkin lymphomas in a country with limited resources: Results of the First National Protocol in Nicaragua. Pediatr Blood Cancer. 2011;56: 560–7.
9. Swerdlow SH, Campo E, Harris NL, et al. WHO classification of tumours of haematopoietic and lymphoid tissues. Lyon: IARC Press; 2008.
10. Sandlund JT, Downing JR, Crist WM. Non-Hodgkin's lymphoma in childhood. N Engl J Med. 1996;334(19): 1238–48.
11. Leoncini L, Raphael M, Stein H. BL. In: Swerdlow SH, Campo E, Harris NL, et al., editors. WHO classification of tumours of haematopoietic and lymphoid tissues. 4th ed. International Agency for Research on Cancer: Lyon; 2008. p. 262–4.
12. Percy CL, Smith MA, Linet M, et al. Lymphomas and reticuloendothelial neoplasms. In: Ries LA, Smith MA, Gurney JG, et al., editors. Cancer incidence and survival among children and adolescents: United States SEER Program 1975–1995. Bethesda, MD: National Cancer Institute, SEER Program, 1999. NIH Pub. No. 99-4649, p. 35–50. Also available online. Last accessed Oct 5, 2012.
13. Wright D, McKeever P, Carter R. Childhood non Hodgkin lymphomas in the United Kingdom; findings from the UK Children's Cancer Study Group. J Clin pathol. 1997;50:128–34.
14. Jaffe ES, Harris NL, Stein H, Vardiman JW. Pathology and genetics of tumours of haematopoietic and lymphoid tissues. Lyon, France: IARC Press; 2001.
15. Oschlies I, Klapper W, Zimmermann M, et al. Diffuse large B-cell lymphoma in pediatric patients belongs predominantly to the germinal-center type B-cell lymphomas: a clinicopathologic analysis of cases included in the German BFM (Berlin-Frankfurt-Munster) Multicenter Trial. Blood. 2006;107(10):4047–52.
16. Neth O, Seidemann K, Jansen P, et al. Precursor B-cell lymphoblastic lymphoma in childhood and adolescence: clinical features, treatment, and results in trials NHL-BFM 86 and 90. Med Pediatr Oncol. 2000;35(1):20–7.

17. Savage KJ, Harris NL, Vose JM, et al. ALK- anaplastic large-cell lymphoma is clinically and immunophenotypically different from both ALK+ ALCL and peripheral T-cell lymphoma, not otherwise specified: report from the International Peripheral T-Cell Lymphoma Project. Blood. 2008;111(12):5496–504.
18. Salaverria I, Bea S, Lopez-Guillermo A, et al. Genomic profiling reveals different genetic aberrations in systemic ALK-positive and ALK-negative anaplastic large cell lymphomas. Br J Haematol. 2008;140(5):516–26.
19. Samuelsson BO, Ridell B, Röckert L, et al. Non-Hodgkin lymphoma in children: a 20-year population-based epidemiologic study in western Sweden. J Pediatr Hematol Oncol. 1999;21:103–10.
20. Murphy SB, Fairclough DL, Hutchison RE, et al. Non-Hodgkin's lymphomas of childhood: an analysis of the histology, staging, and response to treatment of 338 cases at a single institution. J Clin Oncol. 1989;7(2):186–93.
21. Greer JP, Kinney MC, Collins RD, et al. Clinical features of 31 patients with Ki-1 anaplastic large-cell lymphoma. J Clin Oncol. 1991;9(4):539–47.
22. Magrath IT. African Burkitt's lymphoma. history, biology, clinical features and treatment. Am J Pediatr Hematol Oncol. 1991;13(2):222–46.
23. Aderele WL, Antia AU. Burkitt's lymphoma in Ibadan: a review of 133 cases. Nig J Paediatr. 1979;6:1–14.
24. Mbulaiteye SM, Anderson WF, Bhatia K, et al. Trimodal age-specific incidence patterns for BL in the United States, 1973–2005. Int J Cancer. 2010;126(7): 1732–9.
25. Mbulaiteye SM, Biggar RJ, Bhatia K, et al. Sporadic childhood Burkitt lymphoma incidence in the United States during 1992-2005. Pediatr Blood Cancer. 2009;53(3):366–70. doi:10.1002/pbc.22047.
26. Orem J, Maganda A, Mbidde EK, et al. Clinical characteristics and outcome of children with BL in Uganda according to HIV infection. Pediatr Blood Cancer. 2009;52(4):455–8. doi:10.1002/pbc.21769.).
27. Reiter A, Klapper W. Recent advances in the understanding and management of diffuse large B-cell lymphoma in children. Br J Haematol. 2008;142(3): 329–47.
28. Cairo MS, Gerrard M, Patte C. A new protocol for treatment of mature B-cell lymphoma/leukaemia (BCLL): FAB LMB 96, a SFOP LMB 96/CCG-5961/ UKCCSG NHL 9600 international cooperative study. Med Pediatr Oncol. 1997;29:320a.
29. Magrath IT, Lwanga S, Carswell W, et al. Surgical reduction of tumour bulk in the management of abdominal Burkitt's lymphoma. Br Med J. 1974;2:308–12.
30. Ngoma T, Adde M, Durosinmi M, et al. Treatment of BL in equatorial Africa using a simple three-drug combination followed by a salvage regimen for patients with persistent or recurrent disease. Br J Haematol. 2012;158(6):749–62.
31. Ensani F, Mehravaran S, et al. Fine-needle aspiration cytology and flow cytometric immunophenotyping in diagnosis and classification of non-Hodgkin lymphoma in comparison to histopathology. Diagn Cytopathol. 2012;40(4):305–10. doi:10.1002/dc.21561.
32. Loeffler JS, Leopold KA, Recht A, et al. Emergency prebiopsy irradiation for mediastinal masses: impact on subsequent pathologic diagnosis and outcome. J Clinc Oncol. 1986;4:716–21.
33. Boreintein SH, Gerstle T, Malkin D, et al. The effect of prebiopsy corticosteroid treatment on the diagnosis of mediastinal lymphoma. J Pediatr Surg. 2000;35: 973–6.
34. Nathan and Oski's Hematology of Infancy and Childhood. Nathan DG, Ginsburg D, Orkin SH, Look AT (editors). 6th Edition. Saunders, Philadelphia 2003 (Chapter 33).
35. Hesseling P, Molyneux E, Kamiza S, et al. Endemic Burkitt Lymphoma: a 28 day treatment schedule with cyclophosphamide and intrathecal methotrexate. Ann Trop Med. 2009;29:29–34.
36. Bezwoda W, Rastogi R, Valla A, et al. Long-term results of a multicentre randomised, comparative phase III trial of CHOP versus CNOP regimes in patients with intermediate and high grade non-Hodgkin's lymphoma. Eur J Cancer. 1995;31A(6):903–11.
37. Patte C, Auperin A, Gerrard M, et al. Results of the randomized international FAB/LMB96 trial for intermediate risk B-cell non-Hodgkin lymphoma in children and adolescents: Is it possible to reduce treatment for the early responding patients? Blood. 2007;109(7): 2773–80.
38. Hesseling P, Njume E, Kouya F, et al. The Cameroon 2008 Burkitt Lymphoma Protocol: improved event free survival with treatment adapted to disease stage and response to induction therapy. Pediatr Hematol Oncol. 2012;29:119–29.
39. Traore F, Coze C, Atteby J, et al. Cyclophosphamide monotherapy in children with Burkitt lymphoma: a study from the French-African Paediatric oncology Group (GFAOP). Pediatr Blood Cancer. 2011; 56:70–6.
40. Atra A, Meller S, Steven R, et al. Conservative management of follicular non-Hodgkin lymphoma in children. Br J Haematol. 1998;103:220–3.
41. Lorsbach R, Shay-Seymore D, Moore J, et al. Clinicopathological analysis of follicular lymphoma occurring in children. Blood. 2002;99(6): 1959–64.
42. Hutchinson R, Laver J, Chang M, et al. Non-anaplastic peripheral T-cell lymphoma in childhood and adolescence: a children's oncology group study. Pediatr Blood Cancer. 2008;51:29–33.
43. Landman E, Oschlies I, Zimmermann M, et al. Secondary non-Hodgkin lymphoma (NHL) in children and adolescents after cancer other than NHL. Br J Haem. 2008;143:387–94.
44. Hesseling P, Israels T, Harif M, et al. Practical recommendations for the management of children with endemic Burkitt lymphoma (BL) I a resource limited setting. Pediatr Blood Cancer. 2013;60:357–62.

20 Retinoblastoma

Guillermo L. Chantada and Carlos Leal Leal

Introduction

Retinoblastoma is a malignant tumor arising from the embryonic neural retina and it is the most frequent intraocular tumor of childhood occurring in about 1 in 14,000–18,000 live births. Out of an estimated 8,000 children developing retinoblastoma each year worldwide, more than 5,000 [1] are diagnosed in developing countries and a high proportion of them would die of disease dissemination [2]. It is currently unknown if there is an increased incidence of retinoblastoma in some developing countries. Despite some studies reported incidence rates that are up to 3–7 times higher than the reported figures for Western Europe, there are no conclusive population-based studies supporting this probable increased incidence [3]. However, there is no doubt that pediatric oncologists practising in developing countries see more patients with retinoblastoma in their practice. The reason for this phenomenon is probably related to the higher frequency of disseminated retinoblastoma in that setting. There are wide differences in the prevalence of extraocular dissemination and survival in developing countries that are related to socioeconomical indicators [2]. In developed countries, survival rates over 90 % have been achieved decades ago, but as opposed to acute leukemias for example, this successful story is not dependant on highly intensive treatments but in early diagnosis, making intensive treatments not necessary. In middle-income countries, where most children present with advanced disease but still limited to the eye or microscopically disseminated, the cure rate is over 80 % but multimodality treatment is needed [4]. In most lower-income countries, where retinoblastoma presents with metastatic disease less than 30 % of the children survive [5].

Presenting Signs and Symptoms

Retinoblastoma presents in two distinct clinical forms:

1. Heritable form (40 % of the total) which is bilateral in 90 % of the cases or unilateral usually with multifocal tumors in the remaining 10 %. In these cases there is a germline mutation of the *RB1* gene, which has been identified within the chromosome 13q14 [6]. In developed countries, these are usually the result of a new germline mutation in the 75 % or it may be inherited from an affected parent in the remaining 25 % of the cases. However, in developing countries, especially in those

G.L. Chantada, M.D. (✉)
Department of Hemato-Oncology, Hospital JP Garrahan, Buenos Aires, Argentina
e-mail: gchantada@yahoo.com

C.L. Leal, M.D.
Mexican Retinoblastoma Group, Instituto Nacional de Pediatría, Mexico DF, Mexico

D.C. Stefan and C. Rodriguez-Galindo (eds.), *Pediatric Hematology-Oncology in Countries with Limited Resources: A Practical Manual*, DOI 10.1007/978-1-4614-3891-5_20,

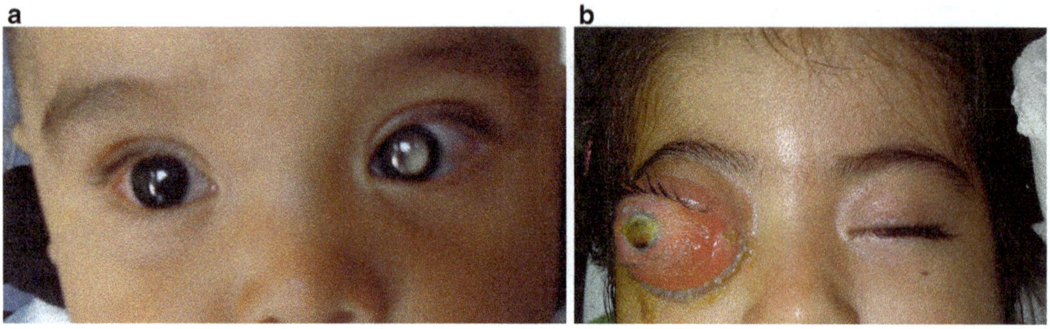

Fig. 20.1 Clinical presentation of retinoblastoma (**a**) leukocoria (**b**) massive orbital dissemination

where survival from retinoblastoma in the previous generation is unlikely, familial cases are much less common. Knudson proposed the "two-hit hypothesis," in order to interpret mutational events in a developing retinal cell leading to the development of retinoblastoma [7]. The Rb1 gene product is crucial in regulating the transition of the cell through the G1 phase of the cell cycle and its inactivation seen in retinoblastoma cases result in deregulated cell proliferation. Mutations at this gene are responsible for retinoblastoma and they have been described in almost every exon of the gene without hot-spots.

2. Sporadic form (60 % of the total): These cases are always unilateral and as such are not heritable. In this form, the *RB1* mutation is only present in tumor cells in the affected retina.

Retinoblastoma is a tumor of the young child and occurs in a narrow age range [8]. The age at presentation correlates with laterality and also with socioeconomical factors that are influenced by late diagnosis. Patients with bilateral retinoblastoma present earlier, usually before 1 year of age, but in developing countries, it is not uncommon to see children with bilateral disease at 1 year or older. Those with unilateral disease often present in the second or third year of life. Familial cases are usually diagnosed by screening usually during the first months of life. However, in developing countries, screening of affected individuals is performed less frequently [9].

The typical presenting sign of retinoblastoma is leukocoria (abnormal white pupillary reflex) (Fig. 20.1a). Leukocoria is usually detected by the parents, who usually seek medical attention reporting this sign to the primary care physician. On rare occasions, the physicians are the ones that detect leukocoria in a physical examination. The detection of leukocoria through a flash photograph is becoming increasingly recognized in the medical practice. Leukocoria is a relatively specific sign with few differential diagnoses which always needs an expert evaluation by an ophthalmologist with a dilated examination of the retina under anesthesia. It is important to note that children with retinoblastoma presenting at this stage, usually look healthy, with no pain and adequate growth, so the pediatrician often tends to underestimate this complaint. Most children at the stage of leukocoria have poor or no vision in the affected eye, but since young children are not able to report decreased vision, this complaint is not common in retinoblastoma. Older children may complain of poor vision. Leukocoria may be difficult to detect in a regular examination done by the primary care physician because it may sometimes be visible when the child looks sideways or with low lighting conditions that lead to pupil dilation. Children presenting with leukocoria are still salvageable in most of the cases if diagnosed timely, so they should be promptly referred to experienced ophthalmologists. When children with leukocoria are not diagnosed timely, the disease invariably progresses to glaucoma leading to buphthalmia (increased eye size). These children usually complain of pain, irritability, or sometimes low-grade fever.

Some of these cases are misdiagnosed as inflammatory eye conditions such as cellulitis, endophthalmitis or uveitis, and retinoblastoma may not be detected since leukocoria may not be easily noticeable in a severely swollen eye. If the diagnosis is not done, the disease progresses to rupture of the eye caused by tumoral invasion of the orbit leading to severe proptosis resulting in an orbital mass (Fig. 20.1b). In these situations, metastatic dissemination may have already occurred and the child usually looks severely sick and emaciated. Unfortunately, in developing countries, children are usually diagnosed at these later stages. In developed countries, parents usually seek medical attention after noticing leukocoria or because strabismus, which is an earlier presenting sign. Strabismus as a presenting sign of retinoblastoma is seldom considered in developing countries.

Biology and Patterns of Spread

Regardless of the specific mutation, the tumor grows from the nuclear layer of the retina either in an endophytic pattern seeding the vitreous or in an exophytic form into the subretinal space and to the choroid in more advanced states. Retinoblastoma usually produces a retinal detachment, and usually eyes with advanced disease show features of both exophytic and endophytic tumors. After filling the eye, retinoblastoma may disseminate to other organs. It usually does so after involving severely the eye structures, so metastatic dissemination is virtually not existent in cases with small tumors limited to the retina. Thus, extension inside the eye is usually a requisite before metastatic dissemination. The tumor can extend through the optic nerve and/or the subarachnoid space to the chiasm, the brain, and later to the meninges. Exophytic tumors may invade the choroid and later the sclera. The tumor usually remain into the eyeball for some period of time, but if left untreated, it eventually invades the orbit and beyond it to the surrounding structures. The metastatic pattern of retinoblastoma include the CNS and hematogenous metastasis involving the bone, bone marrow, or less frequently any other organ.

Histology

The diagnosis of retinoblastoma is usually made by an experienced ophthalmologist without needing pathological confirmation. However, after the eye is enucleated, it is extremely important that the eyeball is evaluated by an experienced pathologist in order to estimate with accuracy the degree and extent of tumoral dissemination in the eye structures. Retinoblastoma usually presents with small undifferentiated anaplastic cells with scanty cytoplasm and large nuclei, occasionally showing photoreceptor features. Calcification is a frequent finding. Retinoblastoma is a tumor of neuroepithelial origin and presents some similar characteristics to other neuroectodermic pediatric tumors. Thus tumor cells often express photoreceptor-differentiation antigens, neuron-specific enolase, and the ganglioside GD2. Retinoblastoma usually stains negative to CD99. However, immunohistochemistry is not vital to the diagnosis of retinoblastoma. Immunocytological evaluation is nevertheless important in cases of extraocular dissemination where tumoral cells should be readily identified by these techniques. The use of immunocytology for GD2 or for the transcription factor CRX has been reported effective for this goal [10]. The likelihood of extraocular relapse is directly correlated with microscopical invasion to critical eye structures such as the optic nerve in its orbital portion beyond the lamina cribrosa, the choroid when is massively invaded and the sclera that implies always a later stage of choroidal invasion [11].

Diagnostic and Extent of Disease Evaluation

When a child is diagnosed with retinoblastoma, it is important to assess the extent of the disease in two levels: (a) intraocular extension, which will predict eye salvage and (b) extraocular dissemination, which will predict patient survival.

Intraocular extension of retinoblastoma is assessed by the ophthalmologist using the indirect ophthalmoscope in a full examination with pupillary dilation under anesthesia. The extent of intraocular disease evaluation should consider the size of the tumors, their location especially their relationship to the macula and the presence of seeding to the vitreous or the subretinal space. On occasions, the tumor causes retinal detachment, which was previously regarded as a poor prognosis feature. Different systems were proposed to group these findings in order to predict eye salvage. The Reese-Ellsworth (R-E) grouping system was used for many years and proved to be effective in predicting eye salvage with radiotherapy treatment. More recently, an international system was proposed to predict eye salvage with modern chemotherapy treatments (Table 20.1) [12].

The evaluation of extraocular extension is usually done by the pediatric oncologist. For a proper extent of extraocular disease evaluation it is important to consider the prevalence of extraocular disease in a given patient population. Since extraocular retinoblastoma is very uncommon in developed countries, most authors recommend that no other staging procedure other than CNS imaging should be done for staging [13]. The low prevalence dissemination in the CSF or in the bone marrow makes evaluation of these sites of low yield and most authors in developed countries do not perform these evaluations routinely in their patients. However, in developing countries with high prevalence of these complications, a full extent of disease evaluation may be needed in most patients [14]. Because extraocular disease is so uncommon in developed countries, there has not been a consensus staging system for extraocular disease for years. However, in recent years, a group of international retinoblastoma experts developed a staging system by consensus that articulates with the intraocular grouping system proposed for the eye-conserving therapies with chemoreduction (Table 20.2) [15]. The TNM system has been recently updated in order to include patients with extraocular dissemination. So, each retinoblastoma program in developing countries should chose the staging system that better accommodates with their patient population, but it is

Table 20.1 The International Grouping System for intraocular disease

Group A
Small tumors away from foveola and disc
• Tumors ≤3 mm in greatest dimension confined to the retina
• Located at least 3 mm from the foveola and 1.5 mm from the optic disc
Group B
All remaining tumors confined to the retina
• All other tumors confined to the retina not in Group A
• Subretinal fluid (without subretinal seeding) ≤3 mm from the base of the tumor
Group C
Local subretinal fluid or seeding
• Local subretinal fluid alone >3 to ≤ 6 mm from the tumor
• Vitreous seeding or subretinal seeding ≤3 mm from the tumor
Group D
Diffuse subretinal fluid or seeding
• Subretinal fluid alone >6 mm from the tumor
• Vitreous seeding or subretinal seeding >3 mm from tumor
Group E
Presence of any or more of these poor prognosis features
• Tumor in anterior segment
• Tumor in or on the ciliary body
• Iris neovascularization
• Neovascular glaucoma
• Opaque media from hemorrhage
• Tumor necrosis with aseptic orbital cellulitis
• Phthisis bulbi

Table 20.2 The International Staging for Retinoblastoma

Stage 0: Patients treated conservatively (subject to presurgical ophthalmologic classifications)
Stage I: Eye enucleated, completely resected histologically
Stage II: Eye enucleated, microscopic residual tumor
Stage III: Regional extension
(a) Overt orbital disease
(b) Preauricular or cervical lymph node extension
Stage IV Metastatic disease
(a) Hematogenous metastasis: (1) single lesion, (2) multiple lesions
(b) CNS extension: (1) prechiasmatic lesion, (2) CNS mass, (3) leptomeningeal disease

important to be consistent in the use of a specific staging system over time in order to be able to compare the results.

Work-Up for Metastatic Disease

Regardless of the disease extension and the setting, all children with retinoblastoma should undergo a head and orbital, gadolinium-enhanced MRI. MRI is preferred to CT scan because it allows for a better estimation of the invasion to the optic nerve [16]. Guidelines for the evaluation of retinoblastoma with MRI have been recently published [16], but it is important to know that in order to obtain a detailed evaluation of the optic nerve or the choroid, it is necessary to use a high-resolution MRI with orbital coils, which are seldom available in developing countries. In addition, MRI is helpful to evaluate the pineal area where it avoids the exposure to radiation in these susceptible patients. However, many centers in developing countries would have only CT scan available for staging of their retinoblastoma patients. In these cases, CT may be useful to identify obvious optic nerve or orbital involvement and CNS extension. Thus, the first step in the initial evaluations in children with retinoblastoma includes a full ophthalmological evaluation and CNS imaging. After this first step, the treating group is able to determine if an eye salvage therapy is possible, if enucleation of the affected eye is needed or if the disease has already spread outside the eye and neoadjuvant therapy is required. At this point, clinical findings are also important to take a decision since children who can only be evaluated with low resolution CT scans and present with massive buphthalmia or glaucoma but imaging studies fail to disclose extension beyond the eyeball may be better treated with preoperative chemotherapy. In these children and in those in whom extraocular disease is present, further staging evaluations are necessary before starting neoadjuvant chemotherapy. These include bilateral bone marrow aspirates and biopsies and lumbar puncture with examination of the cytospin (in those without risks related to the procedure) [14]. A full bone marrow evaluation including bilateral biopsies and aspirates may improve the yield of these procedures, but they need to be done under general anesthesia, which is not always available or recommended in children with advanced disease in developing countries. In situations where children present with obvious extraocular disease, a single bone marrow aspiration could be done, and if the results are positive, no other bone marrow study would be needed. However, a more exhaustive bone marrow evaluation should be done when a single aspiration fails to show malignant cells, especially if no other metastatic site is present. Since retinoblastoma cells may adhere to the tube, the examination of the cytocentrifugate of the CSF specimen, should be always be done regardless of the cell count in order to improve the yield of this procedure. Bone scintigraphy is only recommended in children with confirmed metastatic disease or those with bone pain. This extensive work-up is only necessary at diagnosis in children with clinically advanced disease in whom preoperative enucleation is considered. In cases where enucleation of the affected eye was decided as initial therapy, staging procedures should be done only if high risk of metastatic disease is probably based on the pathological examination. Enucleation should not be delayed because of extent of disease evaluation other than CNS imaging. Children in whom conservative therapy is undertaken do not need any other staging procedure than CNS imaging.

Treatment

The treatment of retinoblastoma in developing countries poses significant and unique challenges for the treating physicians given the paucity of publications, the impact of socioeconomical factors and the influence of the availability of resources. It is important that children with retinoblastoma should be treated in centers with experience in the management of these tumors which on occasions would need the participation of eye hospitals in association with children or cancer centers in order to provide the best possible care. In order to provide tools for treating physicians in these settings, the SIOP-PODC (International Society of Pediatric Oncology-Pediatric Oncology in Developing Countries) published a consensus guideline for graduated-intensity therapy [17].

The Challenges in the Treatment of Unilateral Retinoblastoma: When Is Chemotherapy Indicated?

Initial enucleation of the affected eye is the treatment of choice for children with intraocular unilateral retinoblastoma [18]. It is the simplest and safest therapy for retinoblastoma; however, in some developing countries it is not widely accepted by the affected families. It is important to procure a prosthetic eyeball which can even be fitted in the operating room after the procedure to minimize cosmetic effects. Enucleation should be performed by an experienced pediatric ophthalmologist in order to obtain a long optic nerve stump and avoid eye rupture.

Eyes with secondary glaucoma, invasion of anterior segment (anterior chamber, iris), rubeosis iridis, hyphema, pseudohypopyon, and history of orbital cellulitis or those with affection of more than 2/3 of the retina or massive vitreous or subretinal seeding should be enucleated initially without delay. In some developing countries, as many as two-thirds of children present with enlarged eyeballs, that have a higher risk of microscopic extraocular dissemination [19–21]. These eyes may be difficult to enucleate and are at high risk of rupture [22], which would cause tumor seeding in the orbit. Occasionally, the tumor may be left behind in the resection margin of the optic nerve. These cases are at high risk of death if no further treatment is given and they need intensive chemotherapy and orbital radiotherapy to have a chance for cure. In many of these settings, radiotherapy and intensive chemotherapy are unfortunately not available. In these cases, pre-enucleation chemotherapy may theoretically reduce the tumoral volume in severely buphthalmic eyes, thereby reducing these risks [22]. If pre-enucleation chemotherapy is used, these children should be considered at higher risk for extraocular relapse and adjuvant chemotherapy should be given in all cases, regardless of the pathologic findings upon examination of the enucleated eye [23, 24]. It is important to enucleate these eyes no later than two or three chemotherapy cycles, because chemotherapy resistance may ensue, and the child may die of disseminated disease [25]. Enucleation is always needed in these cases, even when tumor response to neoadjuvant chemotherapy is spectacular, and no local therapy should be done.

After enucleation is done, the affected eyeball should be examined by an expert pathologist. Guidelines for uniform processing of enucleated eyes and for definition of involvement of the different eye structures have been published [26]. These guidelines are applicable in most centers since they do not imply any sophisticated procedure [26]. Centers managing cases where invasion to ocular coats is common should give priority to obtain a high-quality pathology examination. The pediatric oncologist uses this information to decide the need for adjuvant chemotherapy after enucleation. It is essential to identify invasion to the optic nerve, especially when it is beyond the lamina cribrosa paying particular attention to the status of the resection margin, the presence and extent of choroidal invasion, and any degree of scleral involvement. These children benefit from adjuvant chemotherapy but its use in children with other risk factors is controversial and it should be balanced with the potential toxicity of chemotherapy and the availability of second-line therapy in a given setting [11]. So, as a general rule, the use of adjuvant chemotherapy in a given setting should consider the following local scenarios (Table 20.3):

1. The risk of toxicity-related death during a neutropenic episode or other toxic event. Some pathology risk factors such as isolated choroidal invasion or anterior segment invasion are associated to a relatively low risk of extraocular relapse if no adjuvant therapy is given (5–7 %). In centers with limited capacity for managing the side effects of chemotherapy or when

Table 20.3 Use of chemotherapy and radiotherapy in different situations for the treatment of retinoblastoma in developing countries

Clinical situation	Chemotherapy	Radiotherapy	Comments
Adjuvant therapy for enucleated patients with high risk histology (Stages I and II)	Carboplatin 500 mg/m^2/day 1+ Etoposide 100–150 mg/m^2/ days 1 and 2 + Vincristine 1.5 mg/m^2/day 1	Only indicated for patients with tumor invasion to the resection margin of the optic nerve Dose: 4,500 cGy to the orbit, including the chiasm	Higher dose regimens including Cyclophosphamide 65 mg/kg/day 1 with MESNA Vincristine 1.5 mg/m^2/day 1 Idarubicin 10 mg/m^2/day 1 (may be replaced by doxorubicin 30 mg/m^2/day 1) may be more effective in higher risk patients
Orbital retinoblastoma (Stage III)	Carboplatin 500 mg/m^2/day 1+ Etoposide 100–150 mg/m^2/ days 1 and 2+ Vincristine 1.5 mg/m^2/day 1	Dose: 4,500 cGy to the orbit, including the chiasm	Chemotherapy is usually given as neoadjuvant followed by secondary enucleation and adjuvant chemo and radiotherapy. Higher dose regimens including Cyclophosphamide 65 mg/kg/ day 1 with MESNA Vincristine 1.5 mg/m^2/day 1 Idarubicin 10 mg/m^2 day 1 (may be replaced by doxorubicin 30 mg/m^2/day 1)
Metastatic retinoblastoma (uni and bilateral) (Stage IV)	Option 1: Carboplatin 500 mg/ m^2/days 1 and 2+ Etoposide 100 mg/m^2/days 1–3 Alternating with Cyclophosphamide 65 mg/kg/ day 1+ Vincristine 1.5 mg/m^2/day 1+ Idarubicin 10 mg/m^2/day 1 (may be replaced by doxorubicin 30 mg/m^2/day 1) Option 2: Ifosfamide (1.8 g/m^2/ days 1–5)+Etoposide (100 mg/ m^2/days 1–5) (+/–carboplatin)	As palliative treatment and for the treatment of bulk disease persisting after high dose chemotherapy	When high dose chemotherapy and stem cell transplantation is not available palliative therapy may be considered. Regimens useful for conservative therapy are usually well tolerated. For children in extremely poor condition, oral chemotherapy with etoposide or cyclophosphamide may be used
Conservative therapy for bilateral retinoblastoma	Carboplatin 500 mg/m^2/day 1+ Etoposide 100–150 mg/m^2/ days 1 and 2+ Vincristine 1.5 mg/m^2/day 1	To be avoided when tumor can be controlled by local therapy. If used: 3,600–4,500 cGy to the whole eye depending on tumor extension.	Some eyes with less advanced disease may be treated omitting etoposide. Children younger than 3 months should be given carboplatin alone or periocular topotecan

patients with compliance problems are treated, the risk of a chemotherapy-associated death may outweigh the benefit of adjuvant chemotherapy in children with low-risk disease.

2. The need of high-quality pathology assessments. This is essential, especially when withdrawal of adjuvant therapy is considered because unrecognized high-risk children may have an extraocular relapse that might have been avoided with adjuvant chemotherapy. Examples of this include omission of scleral invasion in cases with massive choroidal invasion, which is typically seen when an insufficient number of slides have been reviewed. Postlaminar optic nerve involvement may be missed when slides of insufficient quality are analyzed. When expert pathology examination is not available, better results may be

obtained with the use of adjuvant chemotherapy in all patients when the prevalence of high-risk features is high.

3. The availability of rescue therapy with high-dose chemotherapy and stem cell rescue. Extraocular relapse of retinoblastoma is seldom curable with conventional therapy (except of isolated orbital relapse) [27]. So, if this treatment modality is not available, all efforts should be done to prevent extraocular relapse, even when it is possible that some children would be over-treated with adjuvant chemotherapy.
4. The choice of the chemotherapy regimen for adjuvant therapy. There is some evidence coming from non-randomized studies that intensive regimens including alkylating agents and occasionally anthracyclines are more effective in preventing extraocular relapse than moderate dose carboplatin-based regimens. However, this difference may be seen only in higher risk children and they are conceivably associated to higher risk of fatal toxicity and increased supportive care needs, so this small benefit will be lost in setting with less than optimal supportive care facilities. A list of published chemotherapy regimens is given in Table 20.3.

Bilateral Retinoblastoma and the Challenge of Conservative Therapy in Developing Countries

The indications for enucleation of affected eyes in bilateral retinoblastoma are essentially the same than for unilateral disease. Adjuvant therapy for enucleated eyes in cases of bilateral retinoblastoma should follow the same guidelines as those for cases of unilateral disease. However, there are specific challenges in developing countries. A variable proportion of children in developing countries present with one or both eyes with advanced intraocular disease, which are considered as Group D in the original International Classification. These cases present a dilemma in developing countries. It is necessary to remember that chemoreduction with systemic chemotherapy, the current standard conservative therapy of retinoblastoma originated from developed countries, where adequate supportive care measures and high technology resources operated by highly qualified teams. It is important to identify the local capabilities for conservative therapy in each setting. In low-income settings, usually conservative therapy is not available and since most children present with advanced disease, it is usually not a priority. It should be considered that enucleation would cure a high proportion of children with bilateral retinoblastoma in those settings; however, bilateral enucleation is seldom accepted by affected families. Hence, treating physicians often embark on conservative therapy using systemic chemotherapy when limited focal therapies are available. It is important that patients with intraocular disease not be exposed to treatments with conservative intent in a setting that has no facilities or experience in localized therapy. Conservative therapy of retinoblastoma is only feasible where an experienced ophthalmologist is available for evaluating these children under general anesthesia with adequate safety, focal therapies such as lasers and cryotherapy are available and patients are able to comply with frequent follow-up examinations over long periods of time. In some developing countries, centers of excellence for conservative treatment have been created. So, chemoreduction followed by focal therapy to avoid external-beam radiotherapy (EBRT) may not be feasible in some developing countries and may lead to poorer results when done in inadequate settings. This treatment is particularly dangerous in settings with a high rate of abandonment of follow-up, because children may die as a consequence of chemotherapy toxicity or partially treated tumors may reactivate and disseminate. As a general rule, conservative therapy of Group D eyes should not be considered routinely in centers with limited resources and enucleation is preferred, especially when the contralateral eye has less advanced disease. For eyes with less advanced disease, conservative therapies may achieve good results even in settings with limited resources. However, in developing countries, very few children present with less advanced disease and often EBRT is needed for tumor control. However, this modality is seldom available and it is not uncommon to see patients treated with several rounds of chemotherapy with a conservative intent that have progressive disease needing EBRT which is not available. In a proportion of these cases, especially in those with a single remaining eye, extraocular disease develops, as a consequence of family refusal of enucleation, but also because reluctance of treating physicians to consider enucleation when there is still time to save the child's life. It should be always remembered that chemotherapy does not cure intraocular retinoblastoma [28]. Its only benefit is avoiding or delaying EBRT, which is associated with 6–17 % increased risk of mortality caused by radiation-induced second tumors during adulthood in developed countries. Avoidance of EBRT also results in improved cosmesis and lower probability of ocular side effects. However, there is no proven benefit in terms of ocular salvage. Therefore in developing countries with high prevalence of advanced disease, especially in those where compliance for follow-up examinations is not optimal, physicians leading a retinoblastoma program may consider developing EBRT facilities for conservative therapy. The advantages of such approach would be that children treated with EBRT need less-intensive follow-up and most those with Groups B and C may be cured with 2-month course of radiotherapy, whereas children treated with chemoreduction and local therapy usually need a more detailed and longer follow-up to consolidate tumor response and treat later relapses [29]. However, the limitation of such approach includes the need for qualified cataract surgery for repairing radiation-induced cataracts that occur in almost all irradiated patients, the need of safe anesthesia, and of course the availability of a linear accelerator for EBRT operated by qualified personnel.

The Challenge of Treating Overt Extraocular Disease

Children with overt extraocular retinoblastoma, regardless of the laterality, are at high risk of mortality. In developing countries, it is critical to differentiate those children with distant metastatic disease to those with only macroscopical dissemination to the orbit or regional lymph nodes since the latter are curable with moderately intense chemotherapy. Even though children with metastatic disease are not curable with conventional chemotherapy, they may benefit from it since it may help resolve severe pain caused by an orbital mass or emaciation caused by tumor dissemination [30]. Newly diagnosed retinoblastoma is a chemosensitive tumor that responds well to many chemotherapeutic agents, even at low doses. Thus, standard or low-dose chemotherapy with an intention of life prolongation should be given to children with metastatic disease. If high-dose chemotherapy followed by autologous stem cell rescue is available, it should be considered, especially for children with no CNS involvement.

Upfront surgery should not be attempted in children with massive orbital invasion and mutilating surgeries such as orbital exenteration should be avoided. Secondary surgery with a limited exenteration or resection of the residual mass is usually enough for tumor control if followed by adjuvant chemotherapy and radiotherapy [30].

The Challenge of Treatment of Patients Whose Parents Refuse Recommended Therapy

Enucleation of an affected eye may not be acceptable to some affected families and consent may not be given for this life-saving procedure [31]. This parental decision is influenced by many and complex socioeconomical, cultural, and religious factors that may be different in each setting. If left untreated, retinoblastoma is uniformly fatal; so every strategy to try to save these children should be employed. Centers where compliance is a substantial problem should establish a comprehensive program to approach these families [32]. Successful experiences have been reported in Central America [33], where multidisciplinary teams give support to high-risk families. There is no uniformly effective approach for this problem and each center should establish a culturally sensitive program to approach holistically this problem.

Some centers use chemotherapy for the treatment of children whose families do not consent initial enucleation [34]. Even though this may give time to approach the families to reconsider their decision it should be done at the last resort, when other strategies have failed and definitive drop out is imminent. In these situations, the clinician must balance the risks and benefits of this approach. This strategy is associated with risks related to the possibility of chemotherapy-related toxicity, including death, in these high-risk families. In these situations, the clinicians should be convinced that enucleation is the only treatment with a curative intent and conservation of those eyes is not an option. If these eyes are not enucleated, extraocular relapse would be inevitable. These risks must be weighed against the fact that if no chemotherapy is given, the family will drop out and the child will die of disease dissemination. When pre-enucleation chemotherapy is used, and the eye is enucleated secondarily, the pathological evaluation of the enucleated eye may not be adequate for risk assignment. In these cases, adjuvant chemotherapy should be given.

The Challenge of Early Diagnosis: Are Media Campaigns Useful?

Theoretically, retinoblastoma would be the ideal tumor for screening since it occurs in a narrow age range, it is curable if diagnosed early, its natural history is well known from familial cases which prove the efficacy of early diagnosis in terms of ocular and patient survival [8]. However, retinoblastoma is a rare disease and the diagnosis can only be confirmed with a relatively invasive procedure such as ocular examination under anesthesia. Nevertheless many groups and organizations worldwide launched awareness campaigns directed to the public in order to disseminate information about leukocoria as a presenting sign of retinoblastoma [35]. The impact of these campaigns is difficult to estimate and to be more efficient they should also target doctors who are usually not aware of the possibility of cancer in children with leukocoria either [36]. These campaigns may be effective where disease presents with metastatic disease in a high proportion of children since they would not impact the possibility of ocular survival. Targeting treatment refusal is probably more cost-effective in these settings since usually the same countries that have high proportion of metastatic disease at presentation are the same that have compliance problems. There, the few children who are diagnosed timely may not be cured because their families would not consent enucleation.

Second Malignancies in Retinoblastoma Survivors

Children with the germline mutations of the *RB1* gene are at increased risk of secondary non-retinoblastoma malignancies [37]. The occurrence of these malignancies is determined by the mutation but it is also influenced by treatment received [38]. The use, dose, and possibly the age when radiation therapy was administered increase the risk of secondary tumors in the irradiated field [39]. Typically the most common secondary tumors are sarcomas which may occur in the irradiation field or elsewhere in the body, including soft tissue tumors or osteogenic sarcoma, skin tumors such as melanoma and also epithelial tumors. It is probable that children with germline mutations for the Rb1gene do not have an increased susceptibility for secondary leukemias; so when this complication occurs, it is usually related to the use of chemotherapy [40]. Survival from a second tumor is higher when early diagnosis is achieved; so some authors recommend specific surveillance to detect these tumors earlier. Mortality for secondary acute leukemia is high. Overall, the prevalence of secondary malignancies is reported to increase steadily with age, leading to a mortality rate of 25–50 years of age [41], although with modern therapies, it may be much less [42]. Osteosarcoma and melanoma are more frequent in adolescents and young adults, whereas epithelial tumors are more frequent in older adults. Patients with non-hereditary retinoblastoma are not inherently at an increased risk of second malignancies [41].

Trilateral retinoblastoma differs to other secondary malignancies since it arises from the same putative progenitor cell, so the term refers to the association of bilateral retinoblastoma with an asynchronous intracranial primitive neuroectodermal tumor. The exact incidence of this malignancy is not known. Previous studies suggested that up to 3–9 % of patients with the genetic form would develop trilateral disease [43]. However, more recent series show a decreased prevalence and there is indirect evidence that it is less common in developing countries [44]. Occasionally a pineal mass is detected in a follow-up MRI in an asymptomatic child. In these cases, it is important to rule out pineal cysts which have been reported in children with retinoblastoma and always do not progress to malignant tumors [45]. Some authors suggested that the use of chemotherapy may reduce the incidence of trilateral retinoblastoma but these results were not based from population-based studies and included a low number of cases [46]. The prognosis has until recently been almost uniformly fatal, but when high-dose chemotherapy and autologous stem cell rescue is available, some children may be cured.

References

1. Kivela T. The epidemiological challenge of the most frequent eye cancer: retinoblastoma, an issue of birth and death. Br J Ophthalmol. 2009;93(9):1129–31.
2. Canturk S, Qaddoumi I, Khetan V, Ma Z, Furmanchuk A, Antoneli CB, et al. Survival of retinoblastoma in less-developed countries impact of socioeconomic and health-related indicators. Br J Ophthalmol. 2010; 94(11):1432–6.
3. BenEzra D, Chirambo MC. Incidence of retinoblastoma in Malawi. J Pediatr Ophthalmol. 1976;13(6): 340–3.
4. Leal-Leal C, Flores-Rojo M, Medina-Sanson A, Cerecedo-Diaz F, Sanchez-Felix S, Gonzalez-Ramella O, et al. A multicentre report from the Mexican Retinoblastoma Group. Br J Ophthalmol. 2004;88(8): 1074–7.
5. Kazadi Lukusa A, Aloni MN, Kadima-Tshimanga B, Mvitu-Muaka M, Gini Ehungu JL, Ngiyulu R, et al. Retinoblastoma in the democratic republic of congo: 20-year review from a tertiary hospital in kinshasa. J Cancer Epidemiol. 2012;2012:920468.
6. Dryja TP, Rapaport JM, Epstein J, Goorin AM, Weichselbaum R, Koufos A, et al. Chromosome 13 homozygosity in osteosarcoma without retinoblastoma. Am J Hum Genet. 1986;38(1):59–66.
7. Knudson Jr AG, Hethcote HW, Brown BW. Mutation and childhood cancer: a probabilistic model for the incidence of retinoblastoma. Proc Natl Acad Sci U S A. 1975;72(12):5116–20.
8. Abramson DH, Beaverson K, Sangani P, Vora RA, Lee TC, Hochberg HM, et al. Screening for retinoblastoma: presenting signs as prognosticators of patient and ocular survival. Pediatrics. 2003;112(6 Pt 1):1248–55.
9. Chantada GL, Dunkel IJ, Qaddoumi I, Antoneli CB, Totah A, Canturk S, et al. Familial retinoblastoma in developing countries. Pediatr Blood Cancer. 2009; 53(3):338–42.
10. Terry J, Calicchio ML, Rodriguez-Galindo C, Perez-Atayde AR. Immunohistochemical expression of CRX in extracranial malignant small round cell tumors. Am J Surg Pathol. 2012;36(8):1165–9.
11. Chantada GL, Dunkel IJ, de Davila MT, Abramson DH. Retinoblastoma patients with high risk ocular pathological features: who needs adjuvant therapy? Br J Ophthalmol. 2004;88(8):1069–73.
12. Linn Murphree A. Intraocular retinoblastoma: the case for a new group classification. Ophthalmol Clin North Am. 2005;18(1):41–53, viii.
13. Azar D, Donaldson C, Dalla-Pozza L. Questioning the need for routine bone marrow aspiration and lumbar puncture in patients with retinoblastoma. Clin Experiment Ophthalmol. 2003;31(1):57–60.
14. Chantada GL, Rossi J, Casco F, Fandino A, Scopinaro M, de Davila MT, et al. An aggressive bone marrow evaluation including immunocytology with GD2 for advanced retinoblastoma. J Pediatr Hematol Oncol. 2006;28(6):369–73.
15. Chantada G, Doz F, Antoneli CB, Grundy R, Clare Stannard FF, Dunkel IJ, et al. A proposal for an international retinoblastoma staging system. Pediatr Blood Cancer. 2006;47(6):801–5.
16. de Graaf P, Goricke S, Rodjan F, Galluzzi P, Maeder P, Castelijns JA, et al. Guidelines for imaging retinoblastoma: imaging principles and MRI standardization. Pediatr Radiol. 2012;42(1):2–14.
17. Chantada G, Luna-Fineman S, Sitorus RS, Kruger M, Israels T, Leal-Leal C, Bakhshi S, Qaddoumi I, Abramson DH, Doz F. SIOP-PODC recommendations for graduated-intensity treatment of retinoblastoma in developing countries. Pediatr Blood Cancer. 2013;60(5):719–27.
18. Sultan I, Wilson MW, Nawaiseh I, Mehyar M, Kharma S, Al-Qudimat M, et al. Enucleation for retinoblastoma: the experience of a single center in Jordan. Int Ophthalmol. 2010;30(4):407–14.
19. Carrim ZI, Kajaige J, Bowman RJ, Lavy TE, Scanlan P. First-year experience of chemotherapy for advanced retinoblastoma in Tanzania: disease profile, outcomes, and challenges in 2008. J Pediatr Ophthalmol Strabismus. 2012;49(3):176–83.
20. Bhurgri Y, Muzaffar S, Ahmed R, Ahmed N, Bhurgri H, Usman A, et al. Retinoblastoma in Karachi, Pakistan. Asian Pac J Cancer Prev. 2004;5(2):159–63.

21. Kashyap S, Meel R, Pushker N, Sen S, Bakhshi S, Sreenivas V, et al. Clinical predictors of high risk histopathology in retinoblastoma. Pediatr Blood Cancer. 2012;58(3):356–61.
22. Bellaton E, Bertozzi AI, Behar C, Chastagner P, Brisse H, Sainte-Rose C, et al. Neoadjuvant chemotherapy for extensive unilateral retinoblastoma. Br J Ophthalmol. 2003;87(3):327–9.
23. Zhao J, Dimaras H, Massey C, Xu X, Huang D, Li B, et al. Pre-enucleation chemotherapy for eyes severely affected by retinoblastoma masks risk of tumor extension and increases death from metastasis. J Clin Oncol. 2011;29(7):845–51.
24. Chantada G, Leal-Leal C, Brisse H, de Graaf P, Sitorus RS, Qaddoumi I, et al. Is it pre-enucleation chemotherapy or delayed enucleation of severely involved eyes with intraocular retinoblastoma that risks extraocular dissemination and death? J Clin Oncol. 2011;29(24):3333–4; author reply 5–6.
25. Bai S, Ren R, Li B, Xu X, Zhao B, Gao F, et al. Delay in the diagnosis of retinoblastoma in China. Acta Ophthalmol. 2011;89(1):e72–4.
26. Sastre X, Chantada GL, Doz F, Wilson MW, de Davila MT, Rodriguez-Galindo C, et al. Proceedings of the consensus meetings from the International Retinoblastoma Staging Working Group on the pathology guidelines for the examination of enucleated eyes and evaluation of prognostic risk factors in retinoblastoma. Arch Pathol Lab Med. 2009;133(8):1199–202.
27. Leal-Leal CA, Rivera-Luna R, Flores-Rojo M, Juarez-Echenique JC, Ordaz JC, Amador-Zarco J. Survival in extra-orbital metastatic retinoblastoma:treatment results. Clin Transl Oncol. 2006;8(1):39–44.
28. Shields CL, Mashayekhi A, Cater J, Shelil A, Meadows AT, Shields JA. Chemoreduction for retinoblastoma. Analysis of tumor control and risks for recurrence in 457 tumors. Am J Ophthalmol. 2004; 138(3):329–37.
29. Wilson MW, Haik BG, Rodriguez-Galindo C. Socioeconomic impact of modern multidisciplinary management of retinoblastoma. Pediatrics. 2006; 118(2):e331–6.
30. Ali MJ, Reddy VA, Honavar SG, Naik M. Orbital retinoblastoma: where do we go from here? J Cancer Res Ther. 2011;7(1):11–4.
31. Sitorus RS, Moll AC, Suhardjono S, Simangunsong LS, Riono P, Imhof S, et al. The effect of therapy refusal against medical advice in retinoblastoma patients in a setting where treatment delays are common. Ophthalmic Genet. 2009;30(1):31–6.
32. Mostert S, Arora RS, Arreola M, Bagai P, Friedrich P, Gupta S, et al. Abandonment of treatment for childhood cancer: position statement of a SIOP PODC Working Group. Lancet Oncol. 2011;12(8):719–20.
33. Luna-Fineman S, Barnoya M, Bonilla M, Fu L, Baez F, Rodriguez-Galindo C. Retinoblastoma in Central America: report from the Central American Association of Pediatric Hematology Oncology (AHOPCA). Pediatr Blood Cancer. 2012;58(4): 545–50.
34. Luna-Fineman S, Alejos A, Amador G, Barnoya M, Benavides R, Castellanos M, et al. Pre-enucleation chemotherapy in advanced intraocular retinoblastoma. Central American experience: AHOPCA II. [Abstract]. Pediatr Blood Cancer. 2012;59(6):984.
35. Leander C, Fu LC, Pena A, Howard SC, Rodriguez-Galindo C, Wilimas JA, et al. Impact of an education program on late diagnosis of retinoblastoma in Honduras. Pediatr Blood Cancer. 2007;49(6):817–9.
36. Leal-Leal CA, Dilliz-Nava H, Flores-Rojo M, Robles-Castro J. First contact physicians and retinoblastoma in Mexico. Pediatr Blood Cancer. 2011;57(7): 1109–12.
37. Eng C, Li FP, Abramson DH, Ellsworth RM, Wong FL, Goldman MB, et al. Mortality from second tumors among long-term survivors of retinoblastoma. J Natl Cancer Inst. 1993;85(14):1121–8.
38. Marees T, Moll AC, Imhof SM, de Boer MR, Ringens PJ, van Leeuwen FE. Risk of second malignancies in survivors of retinoblastoma: more than 40 years of follow-up. J Natl Cancer Inst. 2008;100(24):1771–9.
39. Moll AC, Imhof SM, Schouten-Van Meeteren AY, Kuik DJ, Hofman P, Boers M. Second primary tumors in hereditary retinoblastoma: a register-based study, 1945–1997: is there an age effect on radiation-related risk? Ophthalmology. 2001;108(6):1109–14.
40. Gombos DS, Hungerford J, Abramson DH, Kingston J, Chantada G, Dunkel IJ, et al. Secondary acute myelogenous leukemia in patients with retinoblastoma: is chemotherapy a factor? Ophthalmology. 2007;114(7): 1378–83.
41. Yu CL, Tucker MA, Abramson DH, Furukawa K, Seddon JM, Stovall M, et al. Cause-specific mortality in long-term survivors of retinoblastoma. J Natl Cancer Inst. 2009;101(8):581–91.
42. Turaka K, Shields CL, Meadows AT, Leahey A. Second malignant neoplasms following chemoreduction with carboplatin, etoposide, and vincristine in 245 patients with intraocular retinoblastoma. Pediatr Blood Cancer. 2012;59(1):121–5.
43. Kivela T. Trilateral retinoblastoma: a meta-analysis of hereditary retinoblastoma associated with primary ectopic intracranial retinoblastoma. J Clin Oncol. 1999;17(6):1829–37.
44. Antoneli CB, Ribeiro Kde C, Sakamoto LH, Chojniak MM, Novaes PE, Arias VE. Trilateral retinoblastoma. Pediatr Blood Cancer. 2007;48(3):306–10.
45. Beck Popovic M, Balmer A, Maeder P, Braganca T, Munier FL. Benign pineal cysts in children with bilateral retinoblastoma: a new variant of trilateral retinoblastoma? Pediatr Blood Cancer. 2006;46(7):755–61.
46. Shields CL, Meadows AT, Shields JA, Carvalho C, Smith AF. Chemoreduction for retinoblastoma may prevent intracranial neuroblastic malignancy (trilateral retinoblastoma). Arch Ophthalmol. 2001;119(9): 1269–72.

21 Soft Tissue Sarcomas

Iyad Sultan, Roberta Ortiz, and Andrea Ferrari

Introduction

Soft tissue sarcomas (STS) are a very heterogeneous group of non-epithelial extraskeletal malignancies that are classified on a histogenic basis according to the adult tissue they resemble. Overall, STS are rare: with an annual incidence around 2–3/100,000, they comprise for less than 1 % of all malignant tumors and account for 2 % of total cancer-related mortality [1]. However, in pediatric age STS are relatively more frequent, accounting for 8 % of tumors.

- Rhabdomyosarcoma (RMS) represents about 50 % of STS of childhood and adolescence:
  - It is one of the typical embryonal tumors of childhood, composed by cells resembling normal fetal skeletal muscle.
  - It is always characterized by high grade of malignancy, local invasiveness, and a marked propensity to metastasize, to the point that all RMS patients should be assumed to have micrometastatic disease at diagnosis.
  - It is generally characterized by good response to chemotherapy (90 % response rate) and radiotherapy.
- The remaining 50 % of pediatric STS are usually grouped under the definition of "non-rhabdomyosarcoma soft tissue sarcomas" (NRSTS); these tumors represent more than three fourths of all STS in patients ages 15–19 years:
  - They are very rare tumors, some of them being peculiar of infants and small children, but most of the entities being really tumors more common in adults than in children.
  - They have a very heterogeneous clinical behavior, related to the different subtypes, but also to the different grade of malignancy;
  - Like their adult counterparts, they tend to be seen as being relatively insensitive to chemotherapy, though treatment strategies have changed to some degree in recent years and multiple-modality treatments including systemic chemotherapy have increasingly been attempted.

I. Sultan, M.D.
Department of Pediatric Oncology, King Hussein Cancer Center, Amman, Jordan

R. Ortiz, M.D.
Department of Pediatric Hematology-Oncology, Manuel de Jesus Rivera, La Mascota Hospital, Managua, Nicaragua

A. Ferrari, M.D. (✉)
Pediatric Oncology Unit, Fondazione IRCCS Istituto Nazionale dei Tumori, Via G. Venezian, 1, Milan 20133, Italy
e-mail: andrea.ferrari@istitutotumori.mi.it

D.C. Stefan and C. Rodriguez-Galindo (eds.), *Pediatric Hematology-Oncology in Countries with Limited Resources: A Practical Manual*, DOI 10.1007/978-1-4614-3891-5_21,

Rhabdomyosarcoma

RMS is a highly malignant mesenchymal tumor with a propensity to undergo myogenesis [2]. RMS can occur at any age, but its incidence declines significantly with increasing age (about three in four cases occur in children under 10 years old, with a first peak incidence in 3- to 5-year-olds and a second, smaller peak in adolescence) [3].

RMS is classically divided into the favorable histologic group of embryonal subtype (including the spindle cell and botryoid variants) and the unfavorable group of alveolar RMS [4]. Genetically, embryonal RMS is associated with loss of heterozygosity at 11p15, involving loss of maternal genetic information; the majority (80–85 %) of the alveolar RMS have the reciprocal chromosomal translocations t(2;13)(q35;q14) or t(1;13)(p36;q14). Recently, an European study demonstrated that fusion negative RMS, with histological aspects resembling alveolar RMS, are clinically and molecularly indistinguishable from embryonal tumors [5].

RMS is not usually associated with genetic syndromes; however, increased incidence has been reported with neurofibromatosis type 1, Li Fraumeni syndrome, Costello syndrome as well as genitourinary congenital anomalies [6].

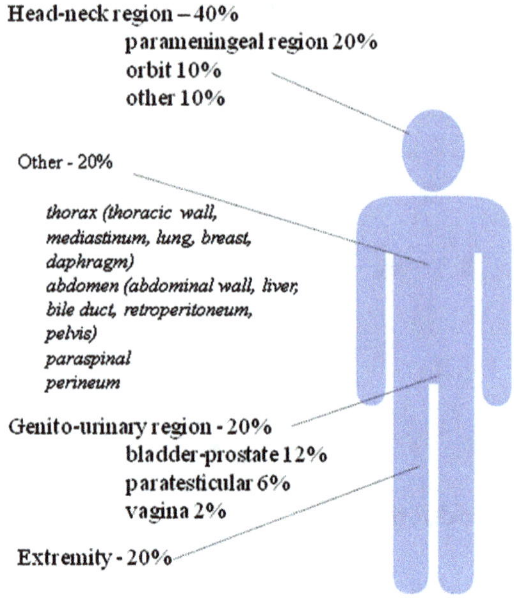

5-year overall survival of RMS by site

Location	5-year OS
Paratesticular-vagina	90-95%
Orbit	85-90%
Bladder/prostate	75-80%
Parameningeal	70%
Other	60-65%
Extremities	55%

Fig. 21.1 Distribution of primary sites of rhabdomyosarcoma and survival according to tumor location

Clinical Presentation

RMS can arise anywhere in the body and it is generally characterized by local aggressiveness and a propensity to metastasize. The most common locations are the head-neck region (i.e., parameningeal and orbital sites) and the genitourinary tract (i.e., bladder and prostate, vagina, paratesticular region) (Fig. 21.1). The most common presentation is a painless mass. Other presenting symptoms depend on the site of origin: pain could arise at any location; proptosis, nasal obstruction, hemorrhagic discharge, and cranial nerve palsies are typical symptoms of head-neck RMS; hematuria, polypoid vaginal extrusion of a mass, and painless scrotal mass are typical presentation of genitourinary RMS; ascites and gastrointestinal, or urinary tract obstruction could be associated to intraabdominal RMS. Symptoms related to distant metastasis depend on the site and size or degree of involvement.

Different tumor sites may be associated to different RMS subtype: botryoid histology is seen commonly in the mucosa of the female genital tract and in the head and neck region of young children, while alveolar RMS is common in the extremities of adolescents.

Regional lymph node dissemination is present in around 20 % of cases (it is higher in alveolar RMS, in adolescents, and in tumor of the extremities). Distant metastasis is present in 15–25 % of newly diagnosed patients, lung being the most common site of hematogenous metastasis (40–50 %), followed by bone marrow (10–20 %) and bone (10 %).

Table 21.1 Approach to patients with rhabdomyosarcoma before initiating treatment

Collect data at diagnosis	*Patient*	*Physical exam*	*Imaging studies*
	Age	Lymph node (special sites: neurological exam to detect cranial nerve palsy in parameningeal RMS)	Local imaging (MRI/CT)
	Nutritional status		*Distant metastases stage*
	Tumor		Chest CT
	Size (< or ≥5 cm)		Bone scan
	Site (see below)		*Other studies*
			Bone marrow biopsies
Tumor site	Favorable	Orbit	
		Head-neck non-parameningeal	
		Genitourinary non-bladder/prostate	
	Unfavorable	Parameningeal	
		Extremities	
		Other sites: trunk, chest, abdominal wall, etc.	
TNM classification	*T1* and *T2* based on local invasiveness	*N0*/*N1* and *M0*/*M1*: absence or presence of nodal and distant involvement	
	A or *B*, i.e., less or more than 5 cm		
Assess regional lymph nodes	Physical exam	All tumors	
	CT/MRI	Important for pelvic and extremity tumors	
	Sentinel node biopsy	Consider for extremity tumors	
	Retroperitoneal sampling	Consider for paratesticular tumors	
Assess resectability	Resectable	Conservative complete excision with negative margins	
	Unresectable	Biopsy only	
Extent of resection	*IRS grouping*		
	Group I	Completely excised tumors with negative microscopic margins	
	Group II	Grossly resected tumors with microscopic residual disease and/or regional lymph nodal spread	
	Group III	Gross residual disease after incomplete resection or biopsy	
	Group IV	Metastases at onset	
Histology	Favorable	Embryonal, spindle cell, botryoid	
	Unfavorable	Alveolar	
Before proceeding to treatment, we should have the following information	1. Imaging of primary tumor (essential for radiotherapy planning)		
	2. Full surgical report		
	3. Pathology data (histology and margins)		
	4. Lymph node assessment if needed		
	5. Metastatic work-up done (chest CT, bone scan, bilateral bone marrow biopsies)		
	6. Stage		

RMS rhabdomyosarcoma, *MRI* magnetic resonance imaging, *CT* computed tomography scan, *TNM* tumor node metastases, *IRS* Intergroup Rhabdomyosarcoma Study

Diagnosis, Risk Stratification, and Prognosis

Table 21.1 describes initial diagnostic work-up and information needed before proceeding to treatment. Ultrasonogram is often the first instrumental assessment to be used. Computed tomography (CT) scan or magnetic resonance imaging (MRI) of the primary site is mandatory for the local extension assessment before any treatment (MRI could be considered superior in defining soft tissue extension). Distant assessment requires chest CT scan,

Table 21.2 Children Oncology Group (COG) risk stratification

Risk	Estimated 5-year EFS (%)	Description	Current treatment
Low risk	90	Nonmetastatic embryonal tumors	Subset 1: VAC × 4 cycles followed by VA for a total of 24 weeks
		Except intermediate risk	Subset 2: VAC
Intermediate risk	65–73	Nonmetastatic embryonal tumors in unfavorable locations (stage 2 or 3) with incomplete resection (clinical group III) *and* All nonmetastatic alveolar	VAC
			ARST0531 study randomizes patients between VAC and VAC + VI
High risk	<30	All metastatic	ARST0431 backbone (benefit with multiagent chemotherapy with interval compression—dose-density: VAC + VDC + VI + IE)

VAC vincristine + actinomycin-D + cyclophosphamide, *VI* vincristine + irinotecan, *VDC* vincristine + doxorubicin + cyclophosphamide, *IE* ifosfamide + etoposide

Technetium bone scan, abdominal ultrasound, and bone marrow aspiration plus trephine biopsy, to identify lung, bone, abdominal, and bone marrow dissemination, respectively. Special sites may require particular evaluations, i.e., cerebrospinal fluid cytology in parameningeal RMS, to assess meningeal dissemination; regional lymph node biopsy in extremity RMS; retroperitoneal lymph node sampling in paratesticular RMS older than 10 years [7–9].

The initial biopsy (incisional biopsy or tru-cut) has the aim to define the histological diagnosis and should be the initial surgical procedure in all patients, also when a subsequent primary excision is planned. Initial biopsy must be carefully planned by experienced surgeons, taking into account the possible subsequent definitive surgery, which must include the scar and the biopsy tract (for example, in RMS of the extremities, the incision must be longitudinal to the limb and not traverse multiple compartment; very careful hemostasis must be ensured to avoid post-surgical hematoma and drains).

The prognosis of RMS depends on multiple factors, including age, primary tumor site and size, lymph node involvement, histology, surgical resection, and distant metastasis. In the past 30 years, the cure rates for RMS have improved dramatically from 25 to 30 % (before the modern chemotherapy-era) to approximately 70 %, due to the development of multidisciplinary and risk-adapted treatment approaches conducted by International cooperative groups. Of course, not all patients with RMS fare well with modern therapies. Patients with alveolar histology continue to have less than optimal outcome. Most patients with distant metastasis do not achieve long-term cure and may benefit of more intensive treatment and are candidates for experimental treatment with novel agents [10].

With the identification of different prognostic factors [11–16], risk assessment has now become more complex, but also more accurate. The approaches of Children Oncology Group (COG) (Table 21.2) and European pediatric Soft Tissue Sarcoma Study Group (EpSSG) (Table 21.3) for risk stratification use similar principles but with different approaches. The EpSSG, for example, identifies low, standard, high, and very high-risk groups (with eight subgroups) for localized RMS, plus the group of metastatic RMS cases; the EpSSG high-risk group grossly corresponds to the COG intermediate-risk group.

Table 21.3 European pediatric Soft Tissue Sarcoma Study Group (EpSSG) RMS 2005 risk stratification

Risk group	Subgroup	Pathology	Postsurgical stage	Site	Node stage	Size and age	therapy
Low risk	*A*	Favorable	I	Any	N0	Favorable	VA
standard risk	*B*	Favorable	I	Any	N0	Unfavorable	IVA + VA or IVA ± XRT
	C	Favorable	II, III	Favorable	N0	Any	
	D	Favorable	II, III	Unfavorable	N0	Favorable	
High risk	*E*	Favorable	II, III	Unfavorable	N0	Unfavorable	*First random*: IVA + XRT vs. IVADo + XRT
	F	Favorable	II, III	Any	N1	Any	*Second random*: maintenance[a] vs. stop therapy
	G	Unfavorable	I, II, III	Any	N0	Any	
Very high risk	*H*	Unfavorable	I, II, III	Any	N1	Any	IVADo + XRT + maintenance

VA vincristine + actinomycin-D, *IVA* ifosfamide + vincristine + actinomycin-D, *IVADo* ifosfamide + vincristine + actinomycin-D + doxorubicin, *XRT* radiotherapy
[a]Maintenance chemotherapy: vinorelbine and low-dose oral cyclophosphamide

Treatment

RMS is a rare tumor and its treatment is necessarily multidisciplinary and complex. The overall multimodality treatment strategy involves surgery, radiotherapy, and chemotherapy, and it is important that the optimal intensity and timing of these treatment modalities should be planned with regard to the patients' risk stratification and late effects of treatment. In particular, radiotherapy needs to be used with caution in children, given the important sequelae of these treatments. For example, survivors after parameningeal RMS (requiring full doses and large volume of radiotherapy) have a high risk of facial growth retardation (bone and soft tissue hypoplasia, facial asymmetry), but also dental abnormalities, neuroendocrine dysfunctions (growth hormone deficiency, hypothyroidism), visual problems, hearing loss.

Chemotherapy

The VAC regimen (vincristine, actinomycin-D, cyclophosphamide, given at 1.2 mg/m^2/cycle) is the gold standard for chemotherapy for RMS in North America. On the other hand, the standard in Europe is considered the IVA regimen (ifosfamide, given at 6 g/m^2/cycle, vincristine, actinomycin-D), which differs only in the choice of alkylating agent—probably producing a slightly different pattern of hematological, renal, and gonadal toxicity. The Intergroup Rhabdomyosarcoma Study (IRS)-IV study found no differences in survival rates in a randomized comparison between VAC and IVA [17]. The duration of treatment is currently 6–12 months according to different protocols.

As mentioned above, the risk stratification as adopted by the collaborative groups directs the treatment direction. In the COG most recent low-risk RMS trial (ARST0331), patients with subset I (Table 21.2) had an excellent outcome (2 year EFS, 88 %; OS, 98 %) with short therapy duration (22 weeks) and a low cumulative dose (4.8 g/m^2) of cyclophosphamide. On the other hand, subset 2 had a 3-year EFS of 66 % using low dose of cyclophosphamide [18]. This group had better outcome on the previous protocols with standard doses of cyclophosphamide.

The COG intermediate-risk/EpSSG high-risk RMS category is currently treated with the standard VAC or IVA regimen. Adding other agents to these regimens by collaborative groups did not result in significant impact to survival, so far. Among other drugs that were tested, camptothecin derivatives (topoisomerase I inhibitors) showed the best outlook. Addition of topotecan to the standard VAC regimen for intermediate-risk

RMS failed to show benefit [19]. Nevertheless, the more promising drug, irinotecan, combined with vincristine is being evaluated in combination with the VAC regimen in the same population of patients.

Doxorubicin is an effective drug in RMS, but the role of anthracyclines as part of a multidrug regimen remains somewhat controversial. For that reason doxorubicin is being evaluated in the current EpSSG trial (Table 21.3). It was also added to the COG high-risk RMS trial ARST0431 which is currently used as a backbone for future trials in high-risk patients [10]. Of note, this regimen incorporated irinotecan/vincristine and ifosfamide/etoposide and used an approach of "dose-compression"—increase of chemotherapy dose intensity and dose density by administering chemotherapy cycles at 2-week interval instead of the usual 3-week interval—similar to that used successfully for Ewing sarcoma [20]. In fact, the prognosis of metastatic RMS remains poor and their management is the subject of ongoing trials. The limited pool of these patients makes it difficult to conduct randomized trials to answer critical questions, but it is agreed that treatment intensification is warranted for this group of patients. High-dose, myeloablative chemotherapy, followed by autologous stem cell rescue, has been variously attempted in metastatic RMS patients. Weigel et al. reviewed 389 patients reported in the literature who underwent myeloablative chemotherapy for metastatic or recurrent RMS [21] and found the outcome much the same as in reports on metastatic patients given conventional therapy [22, 23]. This approach remains experimental and should not be considered as a standard approach for patients with high-risk RMS.

Finally, a potentially interesting option is that of maintenance therapy (metronomic therapy, i.e., regular, frequent administration of low doses of drug with the aim to achieve an anti-angiogenic effect). Currently, the approach of a 6-month maintenance therapy comprising a combination of vinorelbine and low-dose oral cyclophosphamide is under investigation in the EpSSG RMS trial for high-risk patients [24] (Table 21.3).

Possible complications of chemotherapy should be always taken into account. The VAC regimen has serious toxicity that might be exploited in malnourished and very young population. Some of these toxicities are tolerable, including neuropathy that is commonly observed after weekly administration of vincristine. Neutropenia is often observed but is less expected if lower doses of cyclophosphamide are used [25]. A very serious complication is hepatopathy, in the form of veno-occlusive disease (VOD) [26]. This potentially fatal complication is observed mainly in children less than 3 years of age and warrants careful dosing of vincristine and actinomycin-D in this group. Acute and late cardiotoxicity is a known complication of doxorubicin.

Radiotherapy

Radiotherapy is the mainstay of treatment in RMS, since local progression or relapse continues to represent the major cause of treatment failure. Radiotherapy is generally delivered to the pretreatment tumor volume with doses generally ranging between 40 and 55 Gy [17, 27–35]. Three-dimensional conformal radiotherapy—if available—may reduce the long-term toxicity by avoiding unnecessary exposure to vital structures. Similarly, intensity-modulated radiotherapy (IMRT), proton radiotherapy, and interstitial brachytherapy may provide adequate local control with better delineation of the treatment area, and hence, decreased toxicity.

Various issues on radiotherapy in RMS remain to be clarified: should all patients with RMS receive radiotherapy? Can the dose of treatment be modified based on response to treatment and delayed surgical resection? Is it possible to reduce the volume of radiotherapy based on new tumor volume following treatment with chemotherapy and/or surgery?

As for the first question, there is a general consensus that radiotherapy may be omitted in IRS group I patients (initial complete resection) with favorable histology, whereas it must be always required for alveolar histotypes. COG protocols suggest radiotherapy for all RMS patients except for IRS group I embryonal RMS [30], while in European groups it is more debated the indication of radiotherapy in IRS group III patients (patients with initially unresected tumor) after delayed complete surgery or after complete remission to initial chemotherapy, for those tumors arising in particularly favorable sites (i.e., orbit or vagina), especially for young children.

As for the second question, COG recently published its experience with dose reduction (up to 36 Gy) in patients with low-risk embryonal RMS, based on completeness of surgical resection of the primary tumor. Local control was adequate when cyclophosphamide was given (patients treated with VAC regimen), but the analysis suggested that radiotherapy dose reduction should be avoided in patients treated with two drugs only (VA) [34].

The third question remains unanswered: it has been suggested that volume reduction (from the pre-chemotherapy to the post-chemotherapy volume) may be potentially safe (but not for parameningeal cases) [35], but to date the standard treatment volume should remain the pre-chemotherapy one, except for very selected situations (e.g., large pelvic or chest wall tumors where pretreatment volume radiation exposes normal structures to untolerable doses of radiation).

Surgery

Surgery for RMS has evolved over the years from the primary treatment modality (prior to the introduction of effective antineoplastic agents) to one component of a multidisciplinary approach, and from an aggressive surgery to a more conservative organ-sparing procedures, to the point that chemotherapy and radiotherapy may permit in some cases to cure the disease without any surgery (i.e., patients with parameningeal RMS).

Surgery with risk of anatomic or functional impairment is not recommended as first surgical approach and should be considered only as salvage treatment, after the failure of other procedures (special circumstances must be considered, however, e.g., a lower extremity RMS in a toddler, the choice between amputation and radiotherapy, with its long-term effects on limb growth, may pose a difficult dilemma). Tumors considered unresectable at diagnosis can be conservatively and completely resected in a large percentage of cases after tumor shrinkage achieved by primary chemotherapy. Wide resections are generally considered adequate to obtain local control, differently from adult STS that in general should require compartmental resection. In case of primary marginal resection, primary re-operation (prior to any other treatment) is recommended when feasible, hoping to achieve clear margins and proving the absence of microscopic residue in order to avoid radiotherapy [36].

Recently, a possible role for debulking procedure has been suggested for huge retroperitoneal and pelvic RMS [37]. This issue remains, however, controversial, particularly when these surgeries necessitate mutilation. What to do in cases of masses that remain after finishing treatment is debatable; biopsy may cause difficulty in interpreting results, in particular when mature rhabdomyoblasts are detected [38, 39].

Finally, surgery of positive regional lymph nodes is generally considered a diagnostic procedure: any involved lymph nodes warrant radiotherapy, so initial radical lymphadenectomy (which carries a high risk of morbidity) is unnecessary.

Special Situations

Orbital RMS

Orbital RMS carries an excellent outcome, probably reflecting favorable biological behavior combined with early diagnosis because of the location. Embryonal histology is present in approximately 90 % of these cases [40]. The surgical approach to these patients is limited to initial biopsy. Complete resection or exenteration is limited to patients who have local failure following radiotherapy. In a review of pooled data from different studies conducted in Europe and North America, the 10-year EFS and OS were 77 % and 87 %, respectively. Eighty percent of patients received radiotherapy as part of primary therapy. Although more patients who did not receive radiotherapy had local relapse, OS was excellent

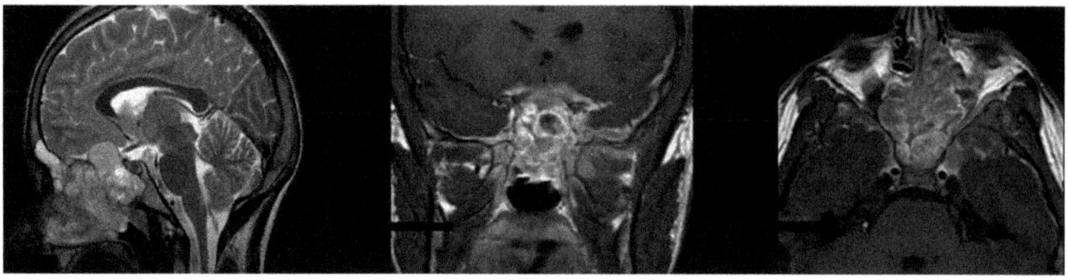

Fig. 21.2 Magnetic resonance imaging of a 13-year-old patient with a huge alveolar rhabdomyosarcoma arising from nasopharynx/nasal cavity and sphenoidal region, with cranial base bone erosion, intracranial extension, and meningeal diffusion

regardless of the use of radiotherapy, since many relapsing cases were salvaged with radiation and more systemic chemotherapy [40]. The current recommendation in COG protocols is to treat these patients with radiotherapy (reduced dose of 45 Gy), while in Europe the use of radiotherapy is left to the discretion of the treating institution (recommended in Italy and not in France).

Parameningeal RMS

This group of tumors arising in middle ear/mastoid, nasopharynx/nasal cavity, parapharyngeal space, paranasal sinuses, pterygopalatine, and infratemporal fossa region represents a special challenge (Fig. 21.2). Complete resection is rarely feasible even after chemotherapy (difficult accessibility parameningeal sites, risk of mutilation) and radiation therapy must imply high-doses and wide fields, with risk of serious sequelae, in particular in young children. Initial attempts to improve survival by cranial radiotherapy or intrathecal chemotherapy were of no proven value [41]. The cornerstone of local control remains well-planned conformal radiotherapy, though recently, IMRT and proton radiotherapy emerged as viable choices for better delivery of radiation without compromising outcome [42, 43]. COG recommend early radiotherapy (<2 weeks after initiating systemic treatment) in patients with meningeal impingement (defined as cranial nerve palsy, cranial base bone erosion with or without intracranial extension). Despite increased long-term morbidity in infants and toddlers, radiotherapy remains necessary to achieve local control [44].

Paratesticular RMS

Paratesticular RMS generally have a good prognosis, in the range of 90 % survival [7]. This is probably due to the peculiar superficial location that allows early diagnosis and complete surgery in most cases, but perhaps also due to a general favorable biology (the adverse prognostic role of alveolar subtype would be counterbalanced by the favorable site, for example) [45].

Paratesticular RMS should be resected, associated to orchidectomy, via an inguinal excision. European groups do not require surgical evaluation of retroperitoneal lymph nodes as routine staging procedure in paratesticular RMS [7], while biopsy is recommended in COG study in patients over 10 years old, considered at major risk to nodal involvement.

Bladder/Prostate RMS

These tumors are typically seen in young patients. Bladder tumors tend to grow intraluminally (Fig. 21.3), in or near the trigon. Prostate tumors usually produce large pelvic masses. Historically, the best approach for local control was believed to be complete excision with margin clearance, which was often pelvic exenteration or aggressive resection with serious complications. However, whether this approach should be always required remains debatable [46], and in some cases a less aggressive surgery with organ preservation may be considered a better option. Brachytherapy may be indicated, providing adequate local control with least morbidity [47].

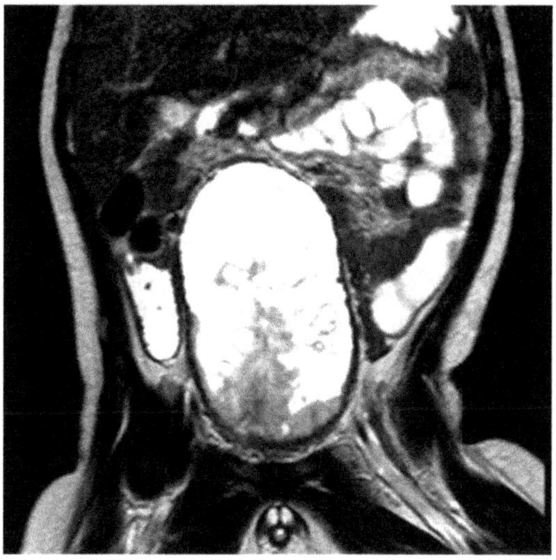

Fig. 21.3 Magnetic resonance imaging of a 2-year-old patient with an embryonal rhabdomyosarcoma of the bladder: the tumor grew intraluminally to completely fill the organ

Young Patients

Patients less than 1 year old at diagnosis continue to have worse prognosis in comparison to older children (1–10 years old). Whether this is the result of different biology of the tumor or treatment modifications that are practiced (e.g., reduction of chemotherapy does, omission of radiotherapy) is not clear yet [48, 49]. Practical general roles in the management of infants with RMS may be the following:

- Careful dosing of chemotherapeutic agents to avoid hepatotoxicity (e.g., VOD).
- In case of initial reduction of chemotherapy doses, these should be increased in subsequent cycles if therapy has been well tolerated.
- Maximum surgical resection to compensate for the high complication related to radiotherapy: amputation may be considered for extremity unresectable tumors since the long-term functional outcome of an irradiated limb may be much worse than amputation.
- Careful planning of radiotherapy; although decreasing treatment volume is not well established based on available data, the decision to decrease volume should lean toward reducing toxicity in this age group.
- When decisions are made to decrease treatment, survival should remain as the main target of treatment. This was shown by the International Society of Pediatric Oncology—Malignant Mesenchymal Tumour Committee (SIOP-MMT) approach to young children with parameningeal tumors, where treatment reduction resulted in unacceptable low survival [44].

Relapsed RMS

Relapsing patients remain one of the greatest challenges in the management of RMS. Approximately, one third of these patients can be expected to be alive at 3 years. Actual long-term cure remains to be possible in a minority of patients, in particular, those who relapse locally and did not receive radiotherapy as part of their initial therapy fare better [50]. Aggressive surgery and second-line drugs should be considered; however, it may be said that in countries with limited resources, treating patients with recurrent metastatic disease may be generally of little value, unless it is directed to proper palliative care.

Challenges in Developing Countries

It is generally considered that the therapeutic standards achieved in developed countries in RMS are unlikely to be reproduced in low-income countries, due to the differences in health infrastructures and training, the limited availability of some active drugs and supportive care to face life-threatening toxicities of modern chemotherapy, and the poor treatment compliance by patients. Nevertheless, the quality of care in developing countries is rapidly increasing.

A limited number of RMS series in developing countries has been published [25, 51–55] (Table 21.4).

Multiple factors seem to have a role in affecting RMS patient outcomes in developing countries. In addition to the general socio-economic factors that adversely affect the care of children with cancer in countries with limited resources, negative factors that may be more specific for RMS include:

Table 21.4 Published rhabdomyosarcoma series by developing countries

Study	Country	Number of pts	Results	Comments
Al-Jumaily et al. [25]	Jordan	45 pts	4-year PFS=61 % 4-year OS=72 %	Improved outcome in more recent years with multidisciplinary care and protocol adjustments
Badr et al. [54]	East Egypt	41 pts	FFS=68 % OS=57 %	Metastatic disease=39 %
Wood et al. [51]	South Africa	49 pts with genitourinary RMS	OS=65 % Better in pts treated after 1992 (80 %)	More advanced tumors compared to the literature
Friedrich et al. [53]	Central America	240 RMS among 785 pts with sarcoma	4-year EFS=33 % 4-year OS=44 %	High rate of metastatic disease at diagnosis; treatment abandonment=25 %
Hessissen L et al. [52]	Morocco	100 pts	10-year EFS=39 % 10-year OS=70 %	Treatment abandonment=37 %
Antillon F et al. [55]	Guatemala	47 pts	3-year EFS=26 % 3-year OS=43 %	Difficulties in local control; abandonment=30 %
Shouman et al. [56]	Egypt	190 pts	5-year FFS=40 % 5-year OS=50 %	No standardized protocols

RMS rhabdomyosarcoma, *PFS* progression-free survival, *OS* overall survival, *FFS* failure-free survival, *EFS* event-free survival *pts* patients

1. The problem of delayed diagnosis and advanced stage of disease at diagnosis, related to the difficulty in referral to specialized centers and the poor access to healthcare in general; delay in diagnosis in RMS has been demonstrated to be a significant prognostic factor [57].
2. The high percentage of abandonment of treatment prior to its completion (particularly when transportation is a challenge), probably due to refusal to radical local control and the need for long treatment plan.
3. Intensive chemotherapy toxicity; patients with malnutrition are at particular risk, and the lack of supportive care including the lack of well-equipped intensive care units and the cost of growth factors make it difficult to provide treatment for high-risk patients.
4. The poor quality of local control, potentially related, in principle, to the quality of radiotherapy techniques, the personal experience of radiotherapists and surgeons, the nonoptimal multimodal interaction between radiotherapists, surgeons, and pediatric oncologists in defining local procedures.

Many initiatives and intervention programs are considered in order to improve early diagnosis and decrease abandonment rates, i.e., public information and education programs to improve awareness at various levels (patient, community, healthcare system) and facilitating early referrals to medical care, social worker program to strongly support the families, including financial assistance, the development of satellite pediatric oncology units to facilitate treatment of patients in rural areas.

The current programs of partnership with groups of healthcare providers in the developed countries may prospectively improve quality of care in countries with limited resources. Establishing a continuous cooperation with international experts to discuss difficult cases may be of great importance. Programs involving telemedicine, in particular tele-pathology, may be considered and can potentially have a major impact on outcome.

Concerning more specifically the management of RMS patients, possible suggestions may be as follow:

- Establish multidisciplinary teams that meet regularly to discuss these patients. Particular attention should be given for the best planning of local treatments. Involve surgeons and radiotherapists in the programs. All RMS cases should be considered as "difficult" case and discussed accordingly.
- Simplify stratification. Use the standard therapy for most cases. Avoid reduction of therapy (e.g., VA chemotherapy in low-risk cases) because of the risk of inadequate staging accuracy.
- Use shorter duration of treatment when possible (e.g., 6 months instead of 12 months) and lower doses of cyclophosphamide (1.2 g/m^2) to prevent unnecessary exposure to higher dose.
- Try to provide definitive therapy in first-line therapies. For example, protocols that try to minimize radiation in upfront treatment rely heavily on close surveillance to identify early local relapses; this might not be practical in places where patients might be lose for follow-up.
- Establish palliative care programs that handle patients with poor outcome, e.g., relapsed patients.

Non-rhabdomyosarcoma Soft Tissue Sarcoma

The term NRSTS describes a group of very heterogeneous malignant tumors with different biology and clinical history, classified on the basis of their differentiation according to the adult tissue they resemble [58]. Whether these tumors originate from a mesenchymal stem cell or from a less primitive precursor committed to a differentiative lineage is still unknown. However, the current WHO classification (WHO 2002) [59] describes soft part tumors as adipocytic tumors (e.g., liposarcoma), fibroblastic/myofibroblastic tumors (e.g., fibrosarcoma), fibrohistiocytic tumors (e.g., pleomorphic sarcoma), smooth muscle tumors (e.g., leiomyosarcoma), perivascular tumors (e.g., the so-called PEComa, perivascular epithelioid cell tumors), skeletal muscle tumors (e.g., rhabdomyosarcoma), vascular tumors (e.g., epithelioid hemangioendothelioma, angiosarcoma), chondro-osseous tumors (e.g., mesenchymal condrosarcoma), and the vast group of tumors of uncertain differentiation (including synovial sarcoma, epithelioid sarcoma, alveolar soft part sarcoma, and many other subtypes). The WHO classification also recognizes three prognostic categories: benign tumors, malignant tumors, and tumors with intermediate prognosis (locally aggressive and rarely metastasizing). NRSTS are malignant tumors by definition. There are often clinical and histologic overlaps between these forms, making their diagnosis particularly challenging and complex. Although the diagnosis is based on morphology, the widespread use of immunohistochemistry with specific lineage markers and the identification of cytogenetic and molecular genetic abnormalities have contributed to a more precise classification and to a better understanding of the mechanisms involved in tumor development and prognosis. A modern view divides STS according to their genomic and expression: (a) sarcomas with specific translocation, (b) sarcomas with specific activating or inactivating mutations, (c) sarcomas with 12q13-15 amplification, and (d) sarcomas with a complex genomic profile [60].

Clinical Presentation

Similarly to RMS, NRSTS can arise anywhere in the soft part of the body: the most common clinical presentation is that of a painless growing mass localized at lower extremities (Fig. 21.4); less frequent sites are the trunk or the head and neck region.

Their destructive local behavior and the propensity to local relapse, as well as their tendency to give distant metastases, may widely vary and are correlated to the different degree of malignancy along histotype and tumor grade. Some NRSTS can grow rapidly and present at diagnosis with

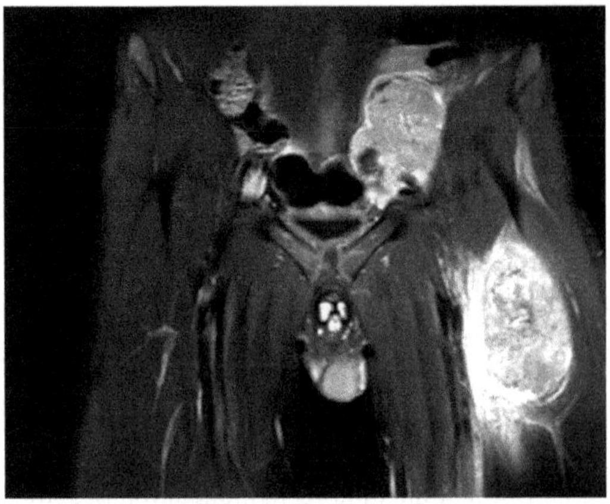

Fig. 21.4 Magnetic resonance imaging of a 16-year-old boy with a malignant peripheral nerve sheath tumor (MPNST) of the thigh, with regional lymph nodal involvement

lung metastases, other tumors may have an indolent course, being diagnosed after removing a small swelling that has existed for several years. Generally, low-grade tumors are often locally aggressive, but unlikely to metastasize, while high-grade tumors are more aggressive and have a strong propensity to metastasize, particularly to the lung [61–64]. The two most widely used grading systems for NRSTS in pediatric age are the POG (Pediatric Oncology Group) system [65] and the FNCLCC (French Fédération Nationale des Centres de Lutte Contre le Cancer) system [66], which identify three grade of malignancy according to tumor resemblance to its normal counterpart, mitotic activity, and necrosis. However, some histotypes (i.e., synovial sarcoma, alveolar sarcoma, angiosarcoma) should be considered high-grade regardless of their morphological parameters, whereas in some cases (i.e., clear cell sarcoma, extraskeletal myxoid chondrosarcoma) the biological course seems impossible to predict from histological features.

In some cases, different histotypes with the same grade of malignancy may display the same clinical behavior. Other histotypes differ significantly for their natural history. As examples, malignant peripheral nerve sheath tumors (MPNST) occur most frequently at axial sites and are characterized by high local aggressiveness and poor prognosis, particularly when associated to neurofibromatosis type 1 (NF1) [67]; epithelioid sarcomas present typical features such as peculiar superficial distal location (i.e., hand, fingers), indolent growth, and tendency for lymph node involvement [68]; desmoplastic small round cell tumors (DSRCT) usually present as a large abdominal mass already disseminated to all the abdomen at the time of diagnosis, and the outcome is extremely poor [69]. Table 21.5 summarizes biological and clinical features of some NRSTS subtypes.

A particular group of mesenchymal tumors of infancy is represented by fibroblastic-myofibroblastic tumors of intermediate prognosis: desmoid-type fibromatoses, infantile fibrosarcoma, and inflammatory myofibroblastic tumor are locally aggressive tumors that rarely metastasize; they often appear as large, rapidly growing tumors infiltrating adjacent structures, but in some cases also spontaneous regressions have been described. They are potentially curable disease, but managing them is often a challenge in terms of their correct diagnosis and appropriate treatment [70]. In the last years, the treatment approach to these tumors has changed to some degree, taking into account the risk of severe iatrogenic anatomical and functional sequelae, i.e., from aggressive surgery to a multidisciplinary approach that involves a minimal-morbidity systemic treatment (e.g., mild chemotherapy containing no alkylating agents or anthracyclines for infantile fibrosarcoma) [71, 72] or also wait-and-see strategy for desmoid-type fibromatosis [73].

Diagnosis, Risk Stratification, and Prognosis

The diagnostic work-up for NRSTS is similar to that of RMS. Children presenting with an atypical soft tissue mass always require prompt attention and a multidisciplinary expert evaluation; the physician who first see the patient (sometimes pediatric dermatologist, vascular surgeon) should consider consulting a pediatric oncologist even before any precise diagnosis has been established. Benign lesions may mimic malignant diseases and vice versa and, for example, no

Table 21.5 Distinctive clinical and biological features of some NRSTS subtypes

Histotypes	Molecular findings	Clinical characteristics and outcome
NRSTS subtypes typical of infants		
Infantile fibrosarcoma	t(12;15;)(p13;q25)	Rapid growth
	ETVG (TEL)-NTRK3 (*as mesoblastic nephroma*)	Relatively high chemosensitiveness (also to alkylating and anthracyclines-free regimens)
		Overall good prognosis (overall survival in the 90 % range)
Extracranial extrarenal rhabdoid tumor	Mutated hSNF5/INI 1 gene	Highly malignant tumor arising in kidney or soft part
		Poor prognosis
		Intensive multiagent chemotherapy
NRSTS subtypes typical of adolescents and young adults		
Synovial sarcoma	t(X;18)(p11;q11)	Most frequent NRSTS subtype in pediatric age
	SYT-SSX1, SYT-SSX2, SYT-SSX4	Extremity site (but it is the most frequent subtype in lung, pleura, and mediastinum)
		60 % Response rate to chemotherapy (ifosfamide-doxorubicin), halfway between adult STS (40 %) and pediatric small round cell sarcomas (RMS) (80 %)
Malignant peripheral nerve sheath tumor (MPNST)	Loss or rearrangement of 10p, 11q, 17q, and 22q	30 % Associated to neurofibromatosis type 1 (NF-1)
		Frequently located in the trunk
		Poor response to chemotherapy, poor prognosis
Dermatofibrosarcoma protuberans	t(17;22) t(2;17)(p23;q23)	Subcutaneous tumor, generally low-grade small lesion with indolent growth
	ALK-CLTC PDGFb-COL1A1	Excellent outcome with surgery
Desmoplastic small round cell tumor	t(11;22) (p13;q12)	Abdominal mass widely disseminated at onset, peritoneal seeding, metastases
	EWS-WT1	Extremely poor outcome
		Need for noval strategy and new drugs
Epithelioid sarcoma		Superficial distant site (fingers)
		Indolent course, but risk of lymph nodal spread
Alveolar soft part sarcoma	t(X;17)(p11.2;q25)	Head and neck and other unusual locations, high risk of metastases
	TFE3-ASPL	Poor response to chemotherapy, poor prognosis
Extra-osseous pPNET/ Ewing's sarcoma	t(11;22)(q24;q12)	Less frequent than bone Ewing's sarcoma, same biology, probably similar clinical history
	FLI1/EWS	High malignant tumors, strong propensity to give metastases
		Need for multimodality strategy including multiagent chemotherapy
Extraskeletal mesenchymal chondrosarcoma	Complex cytogenetic alteration	Head-neck region (orbit); highly aggressive tumor
	t(11;22) (q24;q12) (as Ewing family tumors)	Need for multimodality strategy including multiagent chemotherapy
NRSTS subtypes typical of older adults (very rare in children)		
Clear cell sarcoma	t(12;22)(q13;q12)	Extremity site, deep-seated
	t(9;22)(q22;q12)	Poor response to chemotherapy; poor prognosis
Adult-type fibrosarcoma	t(2,5) and t(7,22)	Tendency to metastatic spread according to tumor grade
Leiomyosarcoma		Retroperitoneum
		Immunocompromised patients

(continued)

Table 21.5 (continued)

Histotypes	Molecular findings	Clinical characteristics and outcome
Liposarcoma	Myxoid liposarcoma:	Different biology and clinical behavior according to the subtype, i.e., well-differentiated, dedifferentiated, or myxoid/round cell subtype
	t(12;16)(q13;p11)	Retroperitoneal location
	t(12;22)(q13;q12)	
	FUS-CHOP	
Angiosarcoma		High grade sarcoma, poor prognosis;
		Associated with lymphedema, after radiotherapy;
		Breast
Extraskeletal myxoid chondrosarcoma	t(9;22)(q22;q12)	Slow-growing tumor of extremity
	t(9;17)(q22;q11.2)	
	EWS-CHN	

NRSTS non-rhabdomyosarcoma soft tissue sarcoma, *STS* soft tissue sarcoma, *RMS* rhabdomyosarcoma, *pPNET* primitive peripheral neuroectodermal tumor

well-defined radiological criteria exist for the differential diagnosis between benign vascular tumors and sarcomas. Growing lesions that are already more than 3–5 cm in size and deeply seated beneath the deep fascia may warrant a biopsy. Needle core or incisional biopsy is indicated, while fine needle aspiration is rarely adequate to provide enough material to allow an adequate histological subtyping of the sarcoma. Excisional biopsy (or initial unplanned resection) should be avoided for the risk violation of tissue planes, resulting in dissemination of the tumor cells throughout the operative field.

MRI or CT scan of the primary site defines the local tumor extension. Since the risk of metastatic spread is definitely lower in NRSTS than in RMS (e.g., around 6 % for synovial sarcoma), and the majority of metastases occur in the lung (in 85 % of cases), some of the investigations generally suggested the distant assessment in RMS may be potentially omitted (e.g., technetium bone scan and bone marrow biopsy), at least for NRSTS other than high grade, to reduce both the burden of ionizing radiation received by pediatric patients and costs [74]. Similarly, chest CT scanning may improve the accuracy of pulmonary staging over X-ray, but requires different ionizing radiation exposures that might have carcinogenic potential. Recent studies showed that tumor diameter represented the major prognostic factor in STS [75], and in synovial sarcoma it may be used as a variable for identifying patients at greater risk of metastases (those with tumor size more than 5 cm) and warranting more accurate radiological investigations; in other words, the risk of metastases is very low in cases with tumor smaller than 5 cm, so CT scan can be omitted for them [74]. Similar considerations might suggest to reduce the indication for radiological investigations also in the patient follow-up.

In pediatric protocols, NRSTS are staged according to the same systems adopted for RMS, i.e., the clinical TNM system and the postsurgical IRS classification (Table 21.1).

The overall cure rate for NRSTS patients is around 70 %, but is strictly correlated to the risk group. Treatment must be planned according to the risk stratification, with the aim to give more intensive therapies to patients with less favorable prognostic factors, while avoiding overtreatment and side effects (without jeopardizing the outcome) in cases with more favorable clinical features.

Prognostic variables in NRSTS are the following [61–64, 67, 76–78]:

Disease extension at diagnosis: survival is very poor in children with metastatic disease (less than 20 % can be cured).

Initial surgery: 5-year overall survival is around 90 % in patients who underwent complete resection at diagnosis (IRS group I), 80 % in those who had marginal resection (group II) and 50 % in initially unresected cases (group III).

Histology: among adult-type NRSTS, MPNST generally have worse prognosis.

Tumor grade: survival around 90 % for G1, 80 % for G2, and 65 % for G3.

Tumor site: survival around 80 % for extremity tumors and 60 % for axial location.

Tumor size: survival around 90 % for tumor < 5 cm, 55 % for size > 5 cm.

Patient's age: 5-year survival of 85 and 70 % for age less than and over than 10 years, respectively.

Tumor invasiveness (T-stage) and superficial/deep location are often associated to tumor size and site and are not commonly used in risk stratification in children. Most of these variables are inter-correlated, i.e., MPNST were often large and axial tumors, unresectable at diagnosis [67].

Treatment

While in the past children with NRSTS were often treated according to the guidelines defined for RMS, in the recent years both the COG and the EpSSG developed specific multimodal risk-adapted protocols focused on pediatric NRSTS (i.e., the COG ARST0332 and the EpSSG NRSTS 2005) [78]. The treatment management of NRSTS is complex and necessarily multidisciplinary. These tumor types are usually considered scarcely sensitive to chemotherapy (tumor response in the range of 40 % or less), and surgery thus remains the unquestionable keystone of treatment. The aim of surgery is that of obtaining adequate surgical margins with limited or no long-term sequelae. The definition of "adequate margins" depends on the quantity of healthy tissues surrounding the tumor (generally considered >1 cm), but also on its quality (periostium, vessel sheath, epineurium, or muscular fascia may act as barriers) [79]. The quality of the surgical operation is crucial since the chances of adjuvant therapies being able to compensate for inadequate surgery are still debatable. Demolitive surgery (e.g., amputation) is not generally considered as a standard procedure for patients at first onset; however, it is a justified option in particular situation, as locally relapsing patients [80] or in those cases with very large tumors presenting with long delay (as may often happen in developed countries).

Radiotherapy plays a well-defined role in local control, after incomplete resection and, according to adult experiences, also after wide excision, especially in case of large tumors. However, the indication for radiotherapy is usually stricter in children, given the higher risk of severe late effects (i.e., the risk of retardation or arrest of irradiated bone growth, the risk of functional impairment and that of second postirradiation tumor).

The role of chemotherapy in NRSTS remains a debated issue, in particular for the large group of adult-type STS histotypes (adult-type fibrosarcoma, MPNST, epithelioid sarcoma, leiomyosarcoma, clear cell sarcoma of soft part, liposarcoma, alveolar soft part sarcoma, undifferentiated polymorphous sarcomas, malignant solitary fibrous tumor/hemangiopericytoma, angiosarcoma, dermatofibrosarcoma). In this heterogenous group of tumors, chemotherapy response rate is generally in the range of 40 %. However, chemotherapy is necessary as front-line treatment in patients with advanced unresectable disease [62–64, 81, 82], with the aim of converting these cases into conservative complete resections, but also for treating any micrometastases promptly. Patients who respond to chemotherapy generally have better chances of survival, as well as those who may undergo complete delayed surgical resection and those treated with radiotherapy, suggesting that intensive multimodal treatment should be recommended in these patients [64].

The possible role of adjuvant chemotherapy in preventing distant recurrences after initial surgery is a further point of controversy. As a matter of fact, the outcome after initial tumor resection is reasonably good in patients with small and low-grade tumor (survival rate up to 90 %), while the prognosis for patients with high-grade and large invasive tumors may be unsatisfactory for the high risk of developing distant metastases (metastases-free survival around 40 %), particularly to the lung [64, 83, 84]. This would suggest,

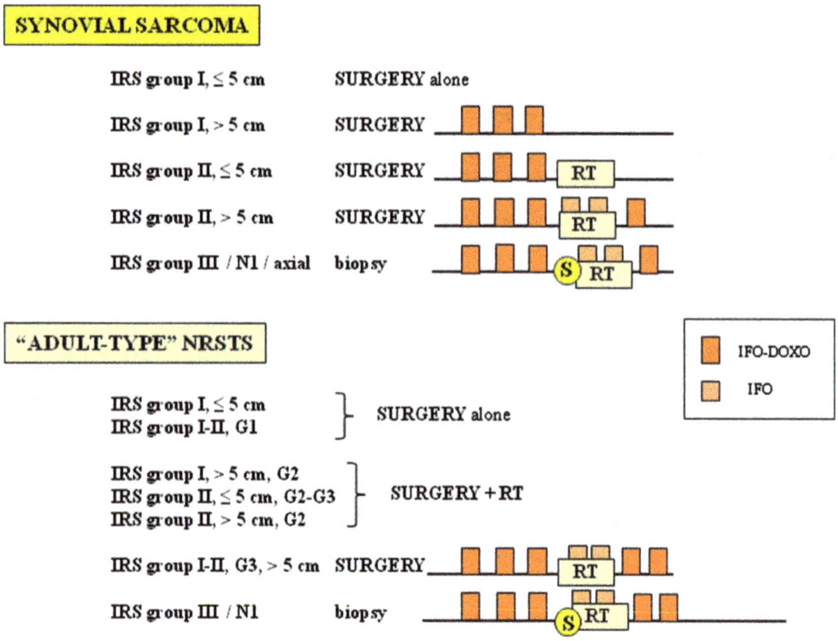

Fig. 21.5 Risk-adapted treatment plan for synovial sarcoma and adult-type soft tissue sarcoma in the European pediatric Soft Tissue Sarcoma Study Group (EpSSG) non-rhabdomyosarcoma soft tissue sarcoma (NRSTS) 2005 protocol. *IRS* Intergroup Rhabdomyosarcoma Study, *N1* invasion of regional lymph nodes, *G* tumor grade, *IFO-DOXO* ifosfamide (9 g/m^2/cycle)—doxorubicin (75 mg/m^2/cycle) chemotherapy, *IFO* ifosfamide (6 g/m^2/cycle) chemotherapy, *RT* radiotherapy (50.4–54 Gy), *S* surgery

in principle, the use of systemic chemotherapy to try to improve survival. Moreover, some studies would advise an efficacy of adjuvant chemotherapy when targeting a selected group of high-risk patients (G3, size >5 cm) most likely to respond to chemotherapy, and when delivering the combinations of drugs currently recognized as the most effective in STS (full-dose ifosfamide plus anthracyclines) [83, 85, 86]. In the EpSSG NRSTS 2005 protocol, ifosfamide-doxorubicin adjuvant therapy is currently recommended in selected patients with high tumor grade and large tumor size (Fig. 21.5).

A tailored discussion should be dedicated to synovial sarcoma: this is the most common NRSTS in adolescents, an high-grade sarcoma crosswise between the pediatric and the adult age groups [87]. The chemosensitivity of synovial sarcoma probably stands midway between that of the most typical adult STS and that of pediatric small round cell tumors, such as RMS. This tumor has been historically treated, in Europe at least, as a "RMS-like" tumor by pediatric oncologists: all children with synovial sarcoma had received chemotherapy, even after the complete excision of very small tumors. An overall survival around 80 % has been reported in pediatric series [87–90]. Further analyses, however, permitted to identify a subset of patients—i.e., completely resected, with tumor smaller than 5 cm—with a very low risk of metastatic spread, for which adjuvant chemotherapy might be omitted, in principle, without jeopardizing the results [91]. The current management of pediatric synovial sarcoma patients has therefore changed to some degree, also taking suggestions from adult experiences and moved towards a treatment concept partially similar to that adopted in the adult setting: the full-dose ifosfamide-doxorubicin chemotherapy is currently adopted as standard regimen, and its indication is given according to the patient's risk stratification, based on tumor size and site and surgical stage (and is omitted in low-risk patients) [78] (Fig. 21.5).

Finally, it is worthwhile to report that in recent years various drugs other than the ifosfamide-doxorubicin combination have proved fairly active against particular STS histotypes, and the next steps of the treatment of NRSTS will go in the direction of histology-driven therapies (i.e., taxanes for angiosarcoma, gemcitabine ± docetaxel for leiomyosarcoma, trabectedine for myxoid/round cell liposarcoma) [92–94]. The improvement in our understanding of the biology of these tumors is paving the way towards the investigation of novel targeted drugs, the products of the specific chromosomal translocations occurring in NRSTS becoming the targets of new molecular agents specifically designed to influence the tumor's biology [95–97].

References

1. Gurney JG, Young GL, Jr, Roffers SD, et al. Soft tissue sarcomas. In: Ries LAG, Smith MA, Gurney JG, et al., editors. Cancer incidence and survival among children and adolescents: United States SEER program 1975–1995, National Cancer Institute, SEER Program. NIH Pub. No. 99–4649. Bethesda, MD; 1999:111. http://seer.cancer.gov/publications/childhood/softtissue.pdf
2. Parham DM, Ellison DA. Rhabdomyosarcomas in adults and children: an update. Arch Pathol Lab Med. 2006;130(10):1454–65.
3. Sultan I, et al. Comparing adult and pediatric rhabdomyosarcoma in the surveillance, epidemiology and end results program, 1973 to 2005: an analysis of 2,600 patients. J Clin Oncol. 2009;27(20):3391–7.
4. Newton Jr WA, et al. Classification of rhabdomyosarcomas and related sarcomas. Pathologic aspects and proposal for a new classification—an Intergroup Rhabdomyosarcoma Study. Cancer. 1995;76(6):1073–85.
5. Williamson D, et al. Fusion gene-negative alveolar rhabdomyosarcoma is clinically and molecularly indistinguishable from embryonal rhabdomyosarcoma. J Clin Oncol. 2010;28(13):2151–8.
6. Ruymann FB, et al. Congenital anomalies associated with rhabdomyosarcoma: an autopsy study of 115 cases. A report from the Intergroup Rhabdomyosarcoma Study Committee (representing the Children's Cancer Study Group, the Pediatric Oncology Group, the United Kingdom Children's Cancer Study Group, and the Pediatric Intergroup Statistical Center). Med Pediatr Oncol. 1988;16(1):33–9.
7. Ferrari A, Bisogno G, Casanova C, et al. Paratesticular rhabdomyosarcoma: report from the Italian and German Cooperative Group. J Clin Oncol. 2002;20:449–55.
8. De Corti F, et al. Sentinel node biopsy in pediatric soft tissue sarcomas of extremities. Pediatr Blood Cancer. 2009;52(1):51–4.
9. Goldfarb B, et al. The role of retroperitoneal lymphadenectomy in localized paratesticular rhabdomyosarcoma. J Urol. 1994;152(2 Pt 2):785–7.
10. Malempati S, Hawkins DS. Rhabdomyosarcoma: review of the Children's Oncology Group (COG) Soft-Tissue Sarcoma Committee experience and rationale for current COG studies. Pediatr Blood Cancer. 2012;59(1):5–10.
11. Crist WM, et al. Prognosis in children with rhabdomyosarcoma: a report of the intergroup rhabdomyosarcoma studies I and II. Intergroup Rhabdomyosarcoma Committee. J Clin Oncol. 1990;8(3):443–52.
12. Joshi D, et al. Age is an independent prognostic factor in rhabdomyosarcoma: a report from the Soft Tissue Sarcoma Committee of the Children's Oncology Group. Pediatr Blood Cancer. 2004;42(1):64–73.
13. Meza JL, et al. Analysis of prognostic factors in patients with nonmetastatic rhabdomyosarcoma treated on intergroup rhabdomyosarcoma studies III and IV: the Children's Oncology Group. J Clin Oncol. 2006;24(24):3844–51.
14. Neville HL, et al. Preoperative staging, prognostic factors, and outcome for extremity rhabdomyosarcoma: a preliminary report from the Intergroup Rhabdomyosarcoma Study IV (1991–1997). J Pediatr Surg. 2000;35(2):317–21.
15. Rodary C, et al. Prognostic factors in 951 nonmetastatic rhabdomyosarcoma in children: a report from the International Rhabdomyosarcoma Workshop. Med Pediatr Oncol. 1991;19(2):89–95.
16. Rodary C, et al. Prognostic factors in 281 children with nonmetastatic rhabdomyosarcoma (RMS) at diagnosis. Med Pediatr Oncol. 1988;16(2):71–7.
17. Crist WM, et al. Intergroup Rhabdomyosarcoma Study-IV: results for patients with nonmetastatic disease. J Clin Oncol. 2001;19(12):3091–102.
18. Hawkins DS, Spunt SL, Skapek SX. Children's Oncology Group's 2013 blueprint for research: soft tissue sarcomas. Pediatr Blood Cancer. 2013;60(6):1001–8.
19. Arndt CA, et al. Vincristine, actinomycin, and cyclophosphamide compared with vincristine, actinomycin, and cyclophosphamide alternating with vincristine, topotecan, and cyclophosphamide for intermediate-risk rhabdomyosarcoma: Children's Oncology Group Study D9803. J Clin Oncol. 2009;27(31):5182–8.
20. Sultan I, Ferrari A. Selecting multimodal therapy for rhabdomyosarcoma. Expert Rev Anticancer Ther. 2010;10(8):1285–301.
21. Weigel BJ, et al. Role of high-dose chemotherapy with hematopoietic stem cell rescue in the treatment of metastatic or recurrent rhabdomyosarcoma. J Pediatr Hematol Oncol. 2001;23(5):272–6.

22. Raney Jr RB, et al. Disease patterns and survival rate in children with metastatic soft-tissue sarcoma. A report from the Intergroup Rhabdomyosarcoma Study (IRS)-I. Cancer. 1988;62(7):1257–66.
23. Koscielniak E, et al. Metastatic rhabdomyosarcoma and histologically similar tumors in childhood: a retrospective European multi-center analysis. Med Pediatr Oncol. 1992;20(3):209–14.
24. Casanova M, Ferrari A, Bisogno G, et al. Vinorelbine and low-dose cyclophosphamide in the treatment of pediatric sarcomas. Pilot study for the upcoming European Rhabdomyosarcoma Protocol. Cancer. 2004;101(7):1664–71.
25. Al-Jumaily U, et al. Improved care of rhabdomyosarcoma in Jordan using less intensive therapy. Pediatr Blood Cancer. 2013;60(1):53–8.
26. Arndt C, et al. Age is a risk factor for chemotherapy-induced hepatopathy with vincristine, dactinomycin, and cyclophosphamide. J Clin Oncol. 2004;22(10):1894–901.
27. Crist W, et al. The Third Intergroup Rhabdomyosarcoma Study. J Clin Oncol. 1995;13(3):610–30.
28. Flamant F, et al. Treatment of non-metastatic rhabdomyosarcomas in childhood and adolescence. Results of the second study of the International Society of Paediatric Oncology: MMT84. Eur J Cancer. 1998;34(7):1050–62.
29. Koscielniak E, et al. Results of treatment for soft tissue sarcoma in childhood and adolescence: a final report of the German Cooperative Soft Tissue Sarcoma Study CWS-86. J Clin Oncol. 1999;17(12):3706–19.
30. Raney RB, et al. Rhabdomyosarcoma and undifferentiated sarcoma in the first two decades of life: a selective review of Intergroup Rhabdomyosarcoma Study Group experience and rationale for Intergroup Rhabdomyosarcoma Study V. J Pediatr Hematol Oncol. 2001;23(4):215–20.
31. Stevens MC, et al. Treatment of nonmetastatic rhabdomyosarcoma in childhood and adolescence: third study of the International Society of Paediatric Oncology—SIOP Malignant Mesenchymal Tumor 89. J Clin Oncol. 2005;23(12):2618–28.
32. Wolden SL, et al. Indications for radiotherapy and chemotherapy after complete resection in rhabdomyosarcoma: A report from the Intergroup Rhabdomyosarcoma Studies I to III. J Clin Oncol. 1999;17(11):3468–75.
33. Terezakis SA, Wharam MD. Radiotherapy for rhabdomyosarcoma: indications and outcome. Clin Oncol (R Coll Radiol). 2013;25(1):27–35.
34. Breneman J, et al. Local control with reduced-dose radiotherapy for low-risk rhabdomyosarcoma: a report from the Children's Oncology Group D9602 study. Int J Radiat Oncol Biol Phys. 2012;83(2):720–6.
35. Eaton BR, et al. Radiation therapy target volume reduction in pediatric rhabdomyosarcoma: implications for patterns of disease recurrence and overall survival. Cancer. 2013;119(8):1578–85.
36. Hays DM, et al. Primary reexcision for patients with 'microscopic residual' tumor following initial excision of sarcomas of trunk and extremity sites. J Pediatr Surg. 1989;24(1):5–10.
37. Raney RB, et al. Results of treatment of fifty-six patients with localized retroperitoneal and pelvic rhabdomyosarcoma: a report from The Intergroup Rhabdomyosarcoma Study-IV, 1991–1997. Pediatr Blood Cancer. 2004;42(7):618–25.
38. Hays DM, et al. Secondary surgical procedures to evaluate primary tumor status in patients with chemotherapy-responsive stage III and IV sarcomas: a report from the Intergroup Rhabdomyosarcoma Study. J Pediatr Surg. 1990;25(10):1100–5.
39. Arndt CA, et al. Significance of persistent mature rhabdomyoblasts in bladder/prostate rhabdomyosarcoma: results from IRS IV. J Pediatr Hematol Oncol. 2006;28(9):563–7.
40. Oberlin O, et al. Treatment of orbital rhabdomyosarcoma: survival and late effects of treatment—results of an international workshop. J Clin Oncol. 2001;19(1):197–204.
41. Lin C, et al. Effect of radiotherapy techniques (IMRT vs. 3D-CRT) on outcome in patients with intermediate-risk rhabdomyosarcoma enrolled in COG D9803–a report from the Children's Oncology Group. Int J Radiat Oncol Biol Phys. 2012;82(5):1764–70.
42. Childs SK, et al. Proton radiotherapy for parameningeal rhabdomyosarcoma: clinical outcomes and late effects. Int J Radiat Oncol Biol Phys. 2012;82(2):635–42.
43. Michalski JM, et al. Influence of radiation therapy parameters on outcome in children treated with radiation therapy for localized parameningeal rhabdomyosarcoma in Intergroup Rhabdomyosarcoma Study Group trials II through IV. Int J Radiat Oncol Biol Phys. 2004;59(4):1027–38.
44. Defachelles AS, et al. Treatment of nonmetastatic cranial parameningeal rhabdomyosarcoma in children younger than 3 years old: results from international society of pediatric oncology studies MMT 89 and 95. J Clin Oncol. 2009;27(8):1310–5.
45. Ferrari A, et al. Is alveolar histotype a prognostic factor in paratesticular rhabdomyosarcoma? The experience of the Italian and German Soft Tissue Sarcoma Cooperative Group. Pediatr Blood Cancer. 2004;42:134–8.
46. Alexander N, Lane S, Hitchcock R. What is the evidence for radical surgery in the management of localized embryonal bladder/prostate rhabdomyosarcoma? Pediatr Blood Cancer. 2012;58(6):833–5.
47. Martelli H, et al. Conservative surgery plus brachytherapy treatment for boys with prostate and/or bladder neck rhabdomyosarcoma: a single team experience. J Pediatr Surg. 2009;44(1):190–6.
48. Ferrari A, Casanova M, Bisogno G, et al. Rhabdomyosarcoma in infants younger than one year

old: a report from the Italian Cooperative Group. Cancer. 2003;97(10):2597–604.
49. Malempati S, et al. Rhabdomyosarcoma in infants younger than 1 year: a report from the Children's Oncology Group. Cancer. 2011;117(15):3493–501.
50. Chisholm JC, et al. Prognostic factors after relapse in nonmetastatic rhabdomyosarcoma: a nomogram to better define patients who can be salvaged with further therapy. J Clin Oncol. 2011;29(10):1319–25.
51. Wood R, et al. Genitourinary rhabdomyosarcoma: lessons from a developing-world series. J Pediatr Surg. 2012;47:2083–6.
52. Hessissen L, et al. Pediatric rhabdomyosarcoma in Morocco. Pediatr Blood Cancer. 2010;54:25–8.
53. Friedrich P, et al. Pediatric sarcoma in Central America: outcomes, challenges, and plans for improvement. Cancer. 2013;119(4):871–9. doi:10.1002/cncr.27816.
54. Badr MA, et al. Epidemiological characteristics and survival studies of rhabdomyosarcoma in East Egypt: a five-year multicenter study. ISRN Oncol. 2012;2012:674523. doi:10.5402/2012/674523. Epub 2012 May 17.
55. Antillon F, et al. Treating pediatric soft tissue sarcomas in a country with limited resources: the experience of the Unidad Nacional de Oncologia Pediatrica in Guatemala. Pediatr Blood Cancer. 2008;51:760–4.
56. Shouman T, El-Kest I, Zaza K, et al. Rhabdomyosarcoma in childhood: a retrospective analysis of 190 patients treated at a single institution. J Egypt Natl Canc Inst. 2005;17(2):67–75.
57. Ferrari A, et al. Symptom interval in children and adolescents with soft tissue sarcomas. Cancer. 2010; 116(1):177–83.
58. Ferrari A, et al. Soft tissue sarcoma across the age spectrum: a population-based study from the Surveillance Epidemiology and End Results database. Pediatr Blood Cancer. 2011;57(6):943–9.
59. WHO classification of tumours. Pathology and genetics. Tumours of soft tissue and bone. In: Fletcher CDM, Unni KK, Mertens F, eds. Lyon: IARC Press; 2002.
60. Chibon F, et al. Validated prediction of clinical outcome in sarcomas and multiple types of cancer on the basis of a gene expression signature related to genome complexity. Nat Med. 2010;16(7):781–7.
61. Spunt SL, et al. Prognostic factors for children and adolescents with surgically resected non-rhabdomyosarcoma soft tissue sarcoma: an analysis of 121 patients treated at St Jude's Children Research Hospital. J Clin Oncol. 1999;17:1219.
62. Spunt SL, et al. Clinical features and outcome of initially unresected nonmetastatic pediatric non rhabdomyosarcoma soft tissue sarcoma. J Clin Oncol. 2002;20:3225–35.
63. Ferrari A, et al. Adult-type soft tissue sarcomas in pediatric age: experience at the Istituto Nazionale Tumori in Milan. J Clin Oncol. 2005;23:4021–30.
64. Ferrari A, et al. Non metastatic unresected pediatric non-rhabdomyosarcoma soft tissue sarcomas: results of a pooled analysis from United States and European groups. Eur J Cancer. 2011;47:724–31.
65. Parham DM, et al. Nonrhabdomyosarcomatous soft tissue sarcomas of the childhood: formulation of a simplified system for grading. Mod Pathol. 1995;8: 705–10.
66. Coindre JM, Terrier P, Bui NB, et al. Prognostic factors in adult patients with locally controlled soft tissue sarcoma. A study of 546 patients from the French Federation of Cancer Centers Sarcoma Group. J Clin Oncol. 1996;14:869–77.
67. Carli M, et al. Malignant peripheral nerve sheath tumours in pediatric age: a report from the Italian and German Soft Tissue Sarcoma Cooperative Group. J Clin Oncol. 2005;23:8422–30.
68. Casanova M, et al. Epithelioid sarcoma in children and adolescents: a report from the Italian Soft Tissue Sarcoma Committee. Cancer. 2006;106:708–17.
69. Bisogno G, et al. Sequential intensified chemotherapy with stem cell rescue for children and adolescents with desmoplastic small round-cell tumor. Bone Marrow Transplant. 2010;45:907–11.
70. Ferrari A, et al. Fibroblastic tumors of intermediate malignancy in childhood. Expert Rev Anticancer Ther. 2013;13(2):225–36.
71. Orbach D, et al. Infantile fibrosarcoma: place of chemotherapy and treatment proposals based on the European experience. J Clin Oncol. 2010;28:318–23.
72. Ferrari A, et al. Neonatal soft tissue sarcomas. Semin Fetal Neonatal Med. 2012;17(4):231–8.
73. Meazza C, et al. Aggressive fibromatosis in children and adolescents: the Italian experience. Cancer. 2010;116:233–40.
74. Ferrari A, et al. Synovial sarcoma in children and adolescents: a critical reappraisal of staging investigations in relation to the rate of metastatic involvement at diagnosis. Eur J Cancer. 2012;48(9):1370–5.
75. Ferrari A, et al. Soft tissue sarcoma of childhood and adolescence: the prognostic role of tumor size in relation to patient body size. J Clin Oncol. 2009;27(3): 371–6.
76. Ferrari A, et al. Adult-type soft tissue sarcomas in paediatric age: a nomogram-based prognostic comparison with adult sarcoma. Eur J Cancer. 2007;43(18):2691–7.
77. Hayes-Jordan A, et al. Nonrhabdomyosarcoma soft tissue sarcomas in children: is age at diagnosis an important variable? J Pediatr Surg. 2000;35:948–54.
78. Ferrari A, et al. New concepts for the treatment of pediatric non-rhabdomyosarcoma soft tissue sarcomas. Expert Rev Anticancer Ther. 2005;5(2): 307–18.
79. Gronchi A, et al. Status of surgical margins and prognosis in adult soft tissue sarcomas of the extremities: a series of 911 consecutive patients treated at a single institution. J Clin Oncol. 2005;23(1):96–104.

80. Ferrari A, et al. Salvage rates and prognostic factors after relapse in children and adolescents with initially localised synovial sarcoma. Eur J Cancer. 2012;48: 3448–55.
81. Pappo AS, et al. Phase II trial of neoadjuvant vincristine, ifosfamide, and doxorubicin with granulocyte colony-stimulating factor support in children and adolescents with advanced-stage nonrhabdomyosarcomatous soft tissue sarcomas: a Pediatric Oncology Group Study. J Clin Oncol. 2005;23:4031–8.
82. Pratt CB, Maurer HM, Gieser P, et al. Treatment of unresectable or metastatic pediatric soft tissue sarcomas with surgery, irradiation, and chemotherapy: a Pediatric Oncology Group Study. Med Pediatr Oncol. 1998;30:201–9.
83. Ferrari A, et al. The role of adjuvant chemotherapy in children and adolescents with surgically resected, high-risk adult-type soft tissue sarcomas. Pediatr Blood Cancer. 2005;45(2):128–34.
84. Pratt CB, et al. Role of adjuvant chemotherapy in the treatment of surgically resected pediatric nonrhabdomyosarcomatous soft tissue sarcomas: a Pediatric Oncology Group Study. J Clin Oncol. 1999;17: 1219–26.
85. Ferrari A. Role of chemotherapy in pediatric nonrhabdomyosarcoma soft-tissue sarcomas. Expert Rev Anticancer Ther. 2008;8:929–38.
86. Frustaci S, et al. Adjuvant chemotherapy for adult soft tissue sarcomas of extremities and girdles: results of the Italian randomized cooperative trial. J Clin Oncol. 2001;19(5):1238–47.
87. Sultan I, et al. Comparing children and adults with synovial sarcoma in the Surveillance, Epidemiology and End Results Program, 1983 to 2005: an analysis of 1268 patients. Cancer. 2009;115:3537–47.
88. Okcu MF, et al. Synovial sarcoma of childhood and adolescence: a multicenter, multivariate analysis of outcome. J Clin Oncol. 2003;21(8):1602–11.
89. Ferrari A, et al. Synovial sarcoma: a retrospective analysis of 271 patients of all ages treated at a single institution. Cancer. 2004;101:627–34.
90. Ferrari A, Bisogno G, Alaggio G, et al. Synovial sarcoma of children and adolescents: the prognostic role of axial sites. Eur J Cancer. 2008;44:1202–9.
91. Brecht IB, et al. Grossly-resected synovial sarcoma treated by the German and Italian Pediatric Soft Tissue Sarcoma Cooperative Group: discussion on the role of adjuvant therapies. Pediatr Blood Cancer. 2006;46(1):11–7.
92. Maki R, et al. Randomized phase II study of gemcitabine and docetaxel compared with gemcitabine alone in patients with metastatic soft tissue sarcomas: results of Sarcoma Alliance for Research Through Collaboration study 002. J Clin Oncol. 2007;5:2755–63.
93. Grosso F, et al. Efficacy of trabectedin (ecteinascidin-743) in advanced pretreated myxoid liposarcomas: a retrospective study. Lancet Oncol. 2007;8: 595–602.
94. Penel N, Bui B, Bay JO, et al. Phase II trial of weekly paclitaxel for unresectable angiosarcoma: the ANGIOTAX Study. J Clin Oncol. 2008;26: 5269–74.
95. Ganjoo K, Jacobs C. Antiangiogenesis agents in the treatment of soft tissue sarcomas. Cancer. 2010;116: 1177–83.
96. Maki RG, D'Adamo DR, Keohan ML, et al. Phase II study of sorafenib in patients with metastatic or recurrent sarcomas. J Clin Oncol. 2009;27:3133–40.
97. Sleijfer S, et al. Pazopanib, a multikinase angiogenesis inhibitor, in patients with relapsed or refractory advanced soft tissue sarcoma: a phase II study from the European Organisation for Research and Treatment of Cancer–Soft Tissue and Bone Sarcoma Group (EORTC study 62043). J Clin Oncol. 2009;27:3126–32.

Bone Tumors

22

Carlos Rodriguez-Galindo, Fulgencio Baez, and Ana Patricia Alcasabas

Malignancies of the bone comprise approximately 6 % of childhood cancer, with an average annual incidence of 8.7 per million children younger than 20 years of age in the United States [1]. The two most common bone malignancies are osteosarcoma and Ewing sarcoma, both present around the second and third decades of life, with overlapping age distribution and presenting signs. However, some distinctive features may help in the differential diagnosis (Table 22.1).

Osteosarcoma

Epidemiology

Osteosarcoma, a malignant neoplasm derived from primitive mesenchymal cells and characterized by the presence of osteoid-producing spindle cell stroma, is the most common malignant bone tumor in the pediatric age group, accounting for approximately 3 % of all cancers in children [2]. The estimated annual incidence in children in the United States is 3.9 cases per one million population among white children and 4.5 per one million population among African-American children [1]. Most osteosarcomas occur during the first 2 decades of life, a period characterized by rapid skeletal growth [3]. Boys are affected more commonly than girls. Several observations support the association between skeletal growth velocity and osteosarcoma. First, patients with osteosarcoma tend to be taller than their counterparts without this disease. Second, osteosarcoma develops at an earlier age in female patients than in male patients, perhaps because of differences in the timing of onset of puberty and the growth spurt [4]. The lack of population-based cancer registries in low- and middle-income countries (LMIC) limits our understanding of the epidemiology of this bone malignancy. Available data suggests that there is rather little geographic and ethnic variation in the incidence of osteosarcoma; however, lowest rates have been observed in Asian populations, and in the United States the incidence is higher in the black population than in whites [5].

C. Rodriguez-Galindo, M.D. (✉)
Dana-Farber/Boston Children's Cancer and Blood Disorders Center and Harvard Medical School, Boston, MA, USA
e-mail: Carlos_Rodriguez-Galindo@dfci.harvard.edu

F. Baez, M.D.
Hospital Infantil Manuel de Jesús Rivera "La Mascota," Managua, Nicaragua

A.P. Alcasabas, M.D.
Philippines General Hospital, Manila, Philippines

Biology

Unlike osteosarcoma in adults, in whom more than 25 % of tumors are associated with preexisting pathologic osseous conditions such as Paget's disease or fibrous dysplasia, most pediatric

D.C. Stefan and C. Rodriguez-Galindo (eds.), *Pediatric Hematology-Oncology in Countries with Limited Resources: A Practical Manual*, DOI 10.1007/978-1-4614-3891-5_22,

Table 22.1 Distinctive features of osteosarcoma and Ewing sarcoma

Characteristic	Osteosarcoma	Ewing sarcoma
Incidence (cases per $10^6 < 20$ years old)	4.8	2.9
Age peak (years)	12–18	5–25
Cell of origin	Osteoblast	Primitive neuroectodermal cell
Biology	Alteration of tumor supresor genes (*TP53*, *RB1*)	Oncogene activation (EWS-FLI1, EWS-ERG, EWS-ATF1)
Bone structure	Metaphysis > diaphysis > flat bones	Flat bones > diaphysis > metaphysis
Primary sites	Lower limbs (78 %) Upper limbs (11 %) Central axis (5 %) Face/skull (3 %)	Central axis (45 %) Lower limbs (30 %) Upper limbs (14 %) Short bones (4 %) Face/skull (3 %)
Treatment	Chemotherapy Surgery No radiation therapy	Chemotherapy Surgery Radiation therapy

osteosarcomas arise spontaneously in areas of bone without any abnormality. Irradiation is the best-characterized etiologic factor contributing to the development of secondary osteosarcoma. Osteosarcoma as a second malignancy is often associated with retinoblastoma; osteosarcoma is the most common malignancy in survivors of retinoblastoma, both in the irradiated and the non-irradiated areas, and it accounts for 25–40 % of all second neoplasms in this population [6]. Half to two-thirds of osteosarcomas occur in the irradiated fields of the skull and face, one-third of tumors develop in the extremities, and less than 10 % in the trunk. Osteosarcoma is also a very frequent malignancy in individuals with germline *TP53* mutations (Li-Fraumeni syndrome) [7] and in patients with REC/helicase-associated disorders (Rothmund-Thomson, Werner, and Bloom syndromes) [8]. Consistent with the association of osteosarcoma with retinoblastoma survivors and Li-Fraumeni syndromes, alterations in components of the cell cycle control system appear to characterize the ontogeny of osteosarcoma. Studies of the retinoblastoma gene (*RB1*) have shown that alterations affect the *RB1* gene in as many as 80 % of cases and that other events, such as *CDK4* alterations, also may result in *RB1* inactivation [9, 10]. Genetically engineered mice based on osteoblast-restricted deletion of p53 and pRb develop short-latency high-grade osteosarcoma that reproduces many of the defining features of human osteosarcoma, including cytogenetic complexity and comparable gene expression signatures, histology, and metastatic behavior [11].

Pathology

Osteosarcoma is characterized by the presence of spindle cell stroma that produces osteoid. Conventional osteosarcoma can be subdivided histologically into three major groups depending on the predominant cell type. Approximately 50 % of tumors are categorized as *osteoblastic*, because the predominant extracellular element is osteoid, whereas 25 % are *chondroblastic*, with a prominent cartilaginous component. Approximately 25 % have a herringbone pattern similar to that observed in fibrosarcoma and are therefore called *fibroblastic*. No significant differences in outcome are apparent among these three histologic subtypes.

Clinical Manifestations

Pain is the most common symptom in children and adolescents with osteosarcoma. Onset of pain often is insidious and usually involves the area affected by tumor. Severe pain of sudden onset commonly is associated with pathologic fracture. Swelling around the affected bone is the

Table 22.2 Diagnostic work-up of bone tumors

Site	Test	Osteosarcoma	Ewing sarcoma
Primary tumor	Plain XR	Yes	Yes
	CT/MRI	Yes[a]	Yes[a]
	Biopsy	Yes	Yes
Distant disease	Plain XR chest	Yes	Yes
	Chest CT	Yes[a]	Yes[a]
	Bone scan	No[b]	Yes[a]
	Bone marrow aspirate and biopsy	No	Yes
Organ function evaluation	Echocardiogram	Yes	Yes
	Audiogram	Yes	No
	Renal function	Yes	Yes
	Liver function	Yes	Yes

[a] Strongly recommended if available
[b] Recommended if multifocal disease is suspected

second most common clinical finding. The tumor may be easily palpable when located in areas such as the anterior surface of the femur but may manifest only as leg edema when occurring in difficult-to-appreciate areas such as the popliteal fossa. A painful limp that increases with weight bearing is the third most common symptom. Systemic signs and symptoms such as fever and weight loss are uncommon. Osteosarcoma most commonly involves the long bones, most tumors occurring around the knee. The most frequent sites of involvement are the distal part of the femur, the proximal portion of the tibia, and the proximal part of the humerus. The axial skeleton, including the pelvis, is rarely affected in children (fewer than 10 % of cases) but more frequently is involved in patients older than 60 years [2, 12]. Overt macroscopic metastatic disease occurs in 20 % of cases and carries a grave prognosis [13]. In countries with limited resources, late diagnosis and difficulties in accessing care result in patients presenting with a higher tumor burden, with large tumors and higher frequency of metastatic disease, often in excess of 40 % [14, 15].

Laboratory and Radiologic Evaluation

Laboratory evaluation often is unrevealing. Elevations of serum lactate dehydrogenase (LDH) and alkaline phosphatase levels are the most common laboratory abnormalities. The latter appears to correlate with osteoblastic activity and has therefore proved useful in monitoring response to therapy [16]. Radiologic evaluation of a patient with osteosarcoma must include assessment of the primary site as well as a search for distant metastatic lesions (Table 22.2) [17]. Plain radiography is the most effective method of detection of bone tumors. Characteristic radiologic findings in osteosarcoma commonly include a metaphyseal permeative lesion with periosteal new bone formation and destruction of preexisting cortical bone. A soft-tissue mass is present in more than 90 % of cases. Other radiologic signs commonly associated with osteosarcoma include cumulus cloud-like density and the presence of Codman's triangle (Fig. 22.1). If available, magnetic resonance imaging (MRI) offers the best estimate of intramedullary tumor extension, joint and vascular involvement, detection of "skip" metastatic lesions, and delineation of the soft-tissue component; this is particularly important if a limb-salvage procedure is considered for local control, but less relevant if an amputation is planned. A baseline chest radiograph should be obtained to search for distant metastatic lesions; however, when possible, a computed tomography (CT) should also be performed at the time of diagnosis for better documentation of metastatic disease. Biopsy of the primary tumor should be done carefully, preferably by the surgeon who will ultimately perform the definitive operation.

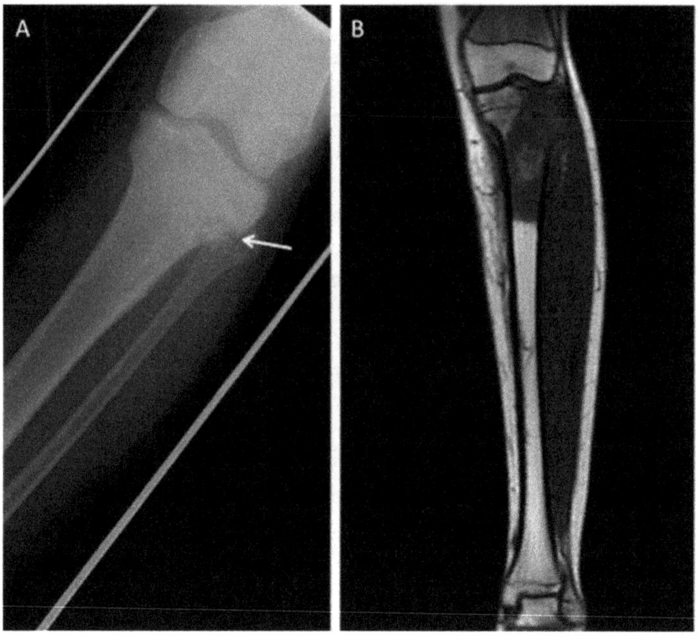

Fig. 22.1 Imaging characteristics of an osteosarcoma of the tibia in a 14-year-old boy. (**a**) Moth eaten, mixed osteolytic and sclerotic appearance is demonstrated involving the proximal tibial metaphysis with cortical destruction (*arrow*) and periosteal reaction along the right lateral aspect of the proximal tibial metaphysis. (**b**) T1-weighted MRI shows low-signal intramedullary lesion extending and destroying the metaphysical cortex

In performance of biopsy of a suspected bone tumor, the following basic principles should be observed: (1) avoidance of transverse incisions, which can make subsequent surgery difficult; (2) avoidance of contamination of multiple compartments and hematoma formation, because successful limb-sparing procedures can be jeopardized; and (3) if feasible, biopsy of the soft-tissue component only.

Osteosarcoma Subtypes

In addition to conventional osteosarcoma, a small proportion of patients present with clinical subtypes that are characterized by distinct clinical, radiologic, and histologic characteristics.

1. *Telangiectatic osteosarcoma* is characterized microscopically by blood-filled spaces divided by septa containing neoplastic sarcomatous cells. Both radiologically and histologically, it is difficult to differentiate from aneurysmal bone cyst. It accounts for less than 4 % of cases of osteosarcoma. Age and anatomic distributions are similar to those in conventional osteosarcoma. On imaging studies, telangiectatic osteosarcoma manifests as a purely lytic lesion with a permeative destructive growth pattern; it usually disrupts the cortex, but with minimal or no periosteal new bone formation, which often is multilayered, in an onionskin pattern. Histologically, telangiectatic osteosarcoma is very hemorrhagic, similar to the gross appearance of aneurysmal bone cysts. Microscopically, this tumor consists of cyst-like spaces divided by septa, which are composed of highly atypical sarcomatous tissue. With appropriate multimodality therapy, the outcome of telangiectatic osteosarcoma is similar to or better than conventional osteosarcoma [18].
2. *Low-grade intramedullary osteosarcoma* is a very rare variant of osteosarcoma, accounting for less than 1 % of cases. Its anatomic distribution is similar to conventional osteosarcoma, with predilection for the distal femur and proximal tibia. In contrast with conventional osteosarcoma, symptoms typically develop over many months or even years before the patient comes to medical attention. Imaging studies usually show a variable pattern of lytic foci and dense areas, poorly demarcated.

Periosteal new bone formation is minimal. Histologically, it shows a predominantly differentiated fibroblastic and osseous component, similar to what is seen in parosteal osteosarcoma. The differential diagnosis is with fibrous dysplasia. Treatment includes a complete resection of the lesion. Incomplete resection invariably results in local recurrence, and dedifferentiation increases with each recurrence.

3. *Surface osteosarcomas* originate and grow predominantly on the surface of the bone, and include the parosteal, periosteal, and high-grade surface osteosarcomas. *Parosteal osteosarcoma* is a low-grade tumor that grows predominantly on the surface of long bones, in an exophytic pattern. Because it is derived from the outer layer of the periosteum, it grows without causing elevation of the periosteum or evidence of periosteal new bone formation. They tend to occur in skeletally mature patients, with diagnosis during the third and fourth decades of life. More than 80 % of these tumors are located in the distal portion of the femoral shaft, in its posterior aspect, within the superior popliteal area. Imaging shows a tumor growing on the surface of the bone, with a broad base, in a mushroom-like fashion. The mass typically is densely mineralized and has lobulated outlines. Microscopically, these tumors are characterized by the presence of a spindle cell fibroblastic component, with variable osteoid production, low mitotic rate, and no atypical features. The treatment is surgical, and a complete resection is mandatory; chemotherapy is not necessary. *Periosteal osteosarcoma* is a low- to intermediate-grade tumor that has a predominantly chondroblastic differentiation. It originates in the deep layer of the periosteum, so its growth is manifested by a separation and elevation of the periosteum from the cortex, causing a prominent periosteal new bone formation. Periosteal osteosarcoma is a tumor of childhood, with a peak incidence during the second decade of life, and it has a female predominance. The usual location is in the long bones of the lower extremity, most commonly the tibia, with an affinity for the diaphysis. The presentation is similar to that with conventional osteosarcoma, with pain and swelling of short duration. Imaging studies show a predominantly fusiform lesion on the surface of a long bone.

Prognostic Factors

The most important adverse prognostic factor in patients with osteosarcoma is the presence of metastatic disease [13]. In addition, primary tumor location is associated with outcome. Children with primary tumors of the tibia and distal femur appear to have a more favorable prognosis than those with axial primary tumors. This finding highlights the importance of complete surgical resection in the management of this malignant disease [13]. For patients with localized disease, factors associated with poor prognosis include measures of tumor burden, such as tumor size, and levels of alkaline phosphatase and LDH [13]. The percentage of tumor necrosis after preoperative chemotherapy is the most consistent and important factor associated with outcome in children and adolescents with localized osteosarcoma. A favorable response (more than 90 % tumor necrosis) correlates with excellent overall survival. Patients who have less than 90 % tumor necrosis are considered poor responders, for whom the prognosis usually is poor [13]. Finally, a proportion of patients with extremity osteosarcoma present with a pathologic fracture, or a pathologic fracture develops after institution of therapy. This has been considered a poor prognostic factor and an indication for immediate amputation. It is possible, however, that with the use of preoperative chemotherapy and judicious use of limb-sparing techniques, a selected group of patients with pathologic fracture may still do well without amputation.

Treatment

Optimal management of osteosarcoma consists of multiple-agent chemotherapy and local control measures, including amputation or limb-sparing surgical procedures. Generally, treatment is initiated with pre-surgery chemotherapy, followed by local control in 6–12 weeks. Before the development of limb-sparing procedures, amputation was the standard surgical method used for curative treatment of osteosarcoma, and it still continues to offer the best local control rates. Limb function after above- or below-the-knee amputation can be reasonably good with an external prosthesis. However, over the past several years, the role of limb-sparing procedures has increased dramatically. As a result of refinements in neoadjuvant chemotherapy, bioengineering, and imaging techniques, it is estimated that as many as 80 % of patients with osteosarcoma in high-income countries (HIC) will eventually be candidates for limb-sparing procedures, which may include vascularized autologous bone grafts, allografts, and endoprostheses. The criteria for limb-sparing procedures include (1) absence of major neurovascular involvement by tumor, (2) feasibility of wide surgical excision to include a normal muscle cuff in all directions and en bloc removal of all biopsy sites, (3) resection of the adjacent joint and capsule, (4) adequate motor reconstruction with regional muscle transfer, and (5) adequate soft-tissue coverage [19]. When these procedures are appropriately performed, the risk of local recurrence is low (less than 5 %) [20]. Long-term functional outcome, however, must be carefully compared with that obtained with amputation alone. Complications of limb-sparing surgery include infection, nonunion, fracture, and unstable joints. In countries with limited resources, options for limb-salvage are limited by the large tumor burden, the lack of infrastructure and trained personnel, and the costs associated with those procedures. However, with the development of centers of excellence and locally grown bioengineering approaches, limb-preserving surgeries are also feasible in LMIC [21–24]. In the development of a limb-salvage program, a very good and careful selection of candidates needs to take place. Local failure rates should be kept under 10 % for a program to be considered effective.

Before the introduction of adjuvant chemotherapy, fatal metastatic disease developed in more than 80 % of patients with osteosarcoma [25]. Currently, the use of systemic chemotherapy in combination with radical surgery of the primary tumor may result in cure rates of 50–70 % for patients with localized disease. Standard treatment includes high-dose methotrexate, Adriamycin (doxorubicin), and cisplatin (MAP regimen) (Fig. 22.2) [26]. One of the major limitations to the implementation of the MAP regimen in LMIC is the use of high-dose methotrexate. Methotrexate was among the first drugs reported to have an antitumor effect in osteosarcoma and it has been a major component of the osteosarcoma treatment ever since [25]. Further, there is evidence that suggests that the pharmacokinetics of this agent may influence outcome, although this influence is minor in the context of more intensive multiagent protocols. However, the role of methotrexate appears to be limited to the administration of high doses (usually 12 g/m^2), because the administration of lower doses appears to have a lesser therapeutic effect. The administration of high-dose methotrexate requires close monitoring of serum levels, which cannot be performed in many institutions, particularly those of developing countries, and extensive supportive measures, including hyperhydration, urine alkalinization, and leucovorin rescue, which must be adjusted to the methotrexate serum levels. The development of acute renal failure, mediated by the precipitation of methotrexate and its metabolites in the renal tubules, is a potentially life-threatening complication. Even among patients receiving all available monitoring and supportive care, severe nephrotoxicity develops in 2 % of them, and the mortality for those patients is 4.4 % [27]. This morbidity can be much worse in LMIC and thus the benefit of the use of high doses of methotrexate should be balanced against the elevated risk of severe morbidity. Studies have shown the possibility of obtaining comparable outcomes without the use of methotrexate, using regimens that maximize exposure to cisplatin and anthracyclines [28]; a simple regimen with six cycles of cisplatin and doxorubicin can cure up to 50 % of patients with localized osteosarcoma, and this seems to be a very good regimen for LMIC [29, 30]. One of the most important prognostic factors in osteosarcoma is the histologic

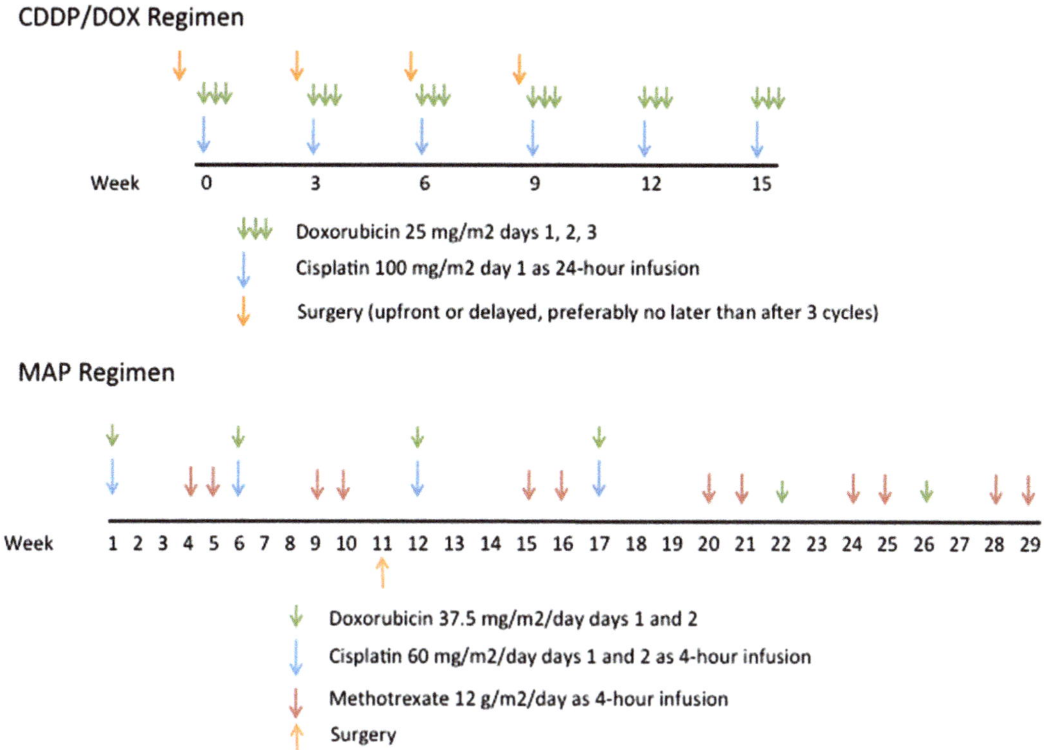

Fig. 22.2 Treatment of osteosarcoma

response to preoperative chemotherapy; this finding has influenced the development of many strategies that have included the modification of postoperative chemotherapy, usually with the addition of ifosfamide and etoposide (MAP-IE regimen) [31]. The impact of such approach is not yet clear; the EURAMOS protocol is currently investigating this through a randomized study.

In countries with limited resources, patients present with more advanced disease and higher metastatic rates; however, studies have shown that with a multidisciplinary approach that integrates aggressive surgery and intensive chemotherapy up to 50 % of patients with localized disease can be cured, usually with regimens that exclude high-dose methotrexate [32–35]. The standard regimen of 6 cycles of cisplatin and doxorubicin appears to be a very feasible approach [30]. The Central American consortium AHOPCA explored further intensification by adding the combination of ifosfamide and etoposide to the cisplatin/doxorubicin backbone regimen; using this approach, the 3-year survival estimates for patients with localized disease that completed therapy was close to 70 % [32]. Refusal and abandonment of therapy is a major cause of therapeutic failure in LMIC, affecting up to 50–60 % of children and thus often exceeding all other causes of failure [36, 37]. For osteosarcoma, most patients abandon early, usually at the time of amputation [15, 32, 33]. For this reason, strategies directed at decreasing treatment refusal and abandonment should be incorporated into the treatment plans for osteosarcoma. The AHOPCA group is currently investigating the impact of upfront amputation versus delayed amputation in the incidence of abandonment.

Approximately 20 % of patients with osteosarcoma in HIC, and up to 40 % in LMIC have clinically detectable metastatic disease at diagnosis, and their outcome usually is very poor [13]. Optimal treatment for these patients entails a very aggressive multimodality approach that combines intensive preoperative and postoperative chemotherapy with resection of both the primary tumor and metastatic lesions. When these guidelines are followed, contemporary protocols that incorporate ifosfamide or the combination of ifosfamide and etoposide, along with high-dose methotrexate, doxorubicin, and cisplatin, may result in 2–5-year progression-free survival rates of 25–45 % [38, 39].

Lung metastases develop in most patients in whom therapy fails. Treatment for this group of patients is mainly surgical; chemotherapy doesn't have a major role in the salvage of patients with recurrent disease. Patients with late recurrences and patients with a small number of pulmonary nodules may be cured with aggressive thoracotomies [40].

Ewing Sarcoma Family of Tumors

Epidemiology

The term *Ewing sarcoma family of tumors* defines a group of small round cell neoplasms of neuroectodermal origin that manifest as a continuum of neurogenic differentiation. On this continuum, Ewing sarcoma of bone represents the least differentiated (most primitive) form of neuroectodermal tumors and peripheral neuroepithelioma represents the most differentiated form. Ewing sarcoma is the second most common malignant bone tumor in children and adolescents (Table 22.1). The estimated incidence among white children younger than 15 years is 2.8 cases per one million population [3]. In the United States, Ewing sarcoma is rare in the nonwhite population. Compared with osteosarcoma, there is considerably more variation in risk between populations for Ewing sarcoma, with particularly low incidence rates in Africa and East and South-East Asia [5, 41, 42].

Tumor Biology

The histogenesis of Ewing sarcoma has been a source of controversy since the first description of the tumor in 1921. The existence of either a mesenchymal stem cell or an early primitive neuroectodermal cell that has retained its ability for multilineage differentiation is the currently accepted hypothesis, and it is now well accepted that the Ewing family of tumors constitute a single group of neurally derived neoplasms that share unique immunocytochemical, cytogenetic, and molecular markers [43, 44]. Nearly all cases of Ewing sarcoma have a reciprocal translocation that involves the *EWS* gene in chromosome 22q12, with genes of the *ETS* family of transcription factors (*FLI1* in chromosome, *ERG* in chromosome 22, or *ETV1* in chromosome 7) [45].

Pathology

Microscopic examination shows that Ewing sarcoma is the prototypical small round blue cell tumor of childhood. Ewing sarcoma is characterized by the presence of a dimorphic pattern of densely packed cells with variable amounts of large clear cytoplasm. Immunohistochemical analysis shows vimentin and CD99 reactivity (Fig. 22.3). The diagnosis can be confirmed with cytogenetic (FISH with *EWS* break-apart probe) or molecular (RT-PCR for the *EWS* fusion transcripts) studies [46]. These techniques are a useful adjunct in differential diagnosis from other soft-tissue small round cell tumors, such as rhabdomyosarcoma.

Clinical Manifestations

Ewing sarcoma commonly manifests during the second decade of life (median age, 13 years) with localized pain and a visible palpable mass [47]. Back pain, extremity weakness, or altered sensation should raise suspicion for the presence of primary or metastatic disease. Systemic manifestations such as fever are more frequent than in osteosarcoma. Ewing sarcoma has a tendency to involve the shaft of long tubular bones, pelvis, and ribs, but almost every bone can be affected. More than 50 % of the tumors arise from axial bones, the pelvis being the most commonly involved (25 %); one-third of the tumors originate in the lower extremities, and less than 10 %

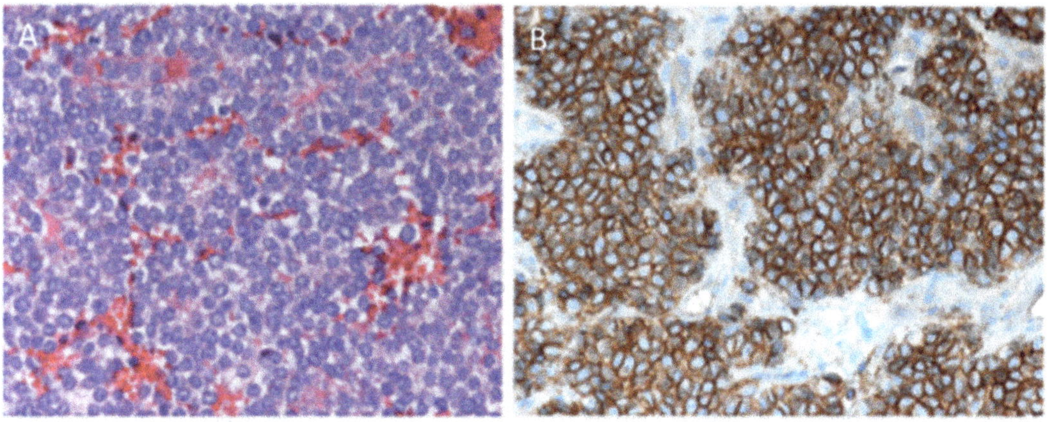

Fig. 22.3 Pathology of Ewing sarcoma typically shows the features of a small round blue cell tumor (**a**) with strong membranous CD99 staining (**b**)

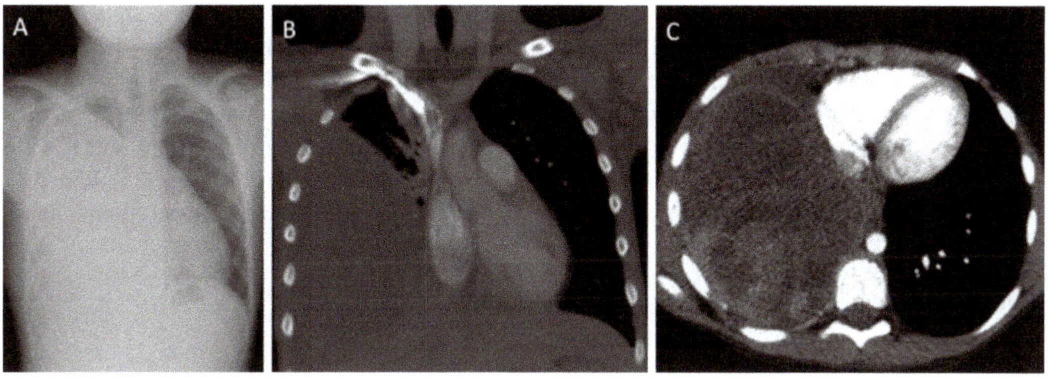

Fig. 22.4 Imaging characteristics of an Ewing sarcoma of the right chest wall in a 11-year-old girl presenting with chest pain and respiratory distress. Plain chest XR shows opacification of the right hemithorax (**a**); coronal (**b**) and sagittal (**c**) computed tomography images reveal a large thoracic mass

in the upper extremities. Approximately 20–25 % of patients with this tumor have metastatic disease when they present for evaluation. The most common sites of metastatic disease are in the lungs, followed by the bones and bone marrow. Metastatic disease appears to be associated with older age and with large tumor or pelvic primaries [48].

Laboratory and Radiologic Evaluation

Patients with suspected Ewing sarcoma should be thoroughly evaluated to define the extent of local disease and the presence of metastatic lesions. In Ewing sarcoma, elevation of erythrocyte sedimentation rate and of serum LDH is not uncommon. Bone marrow aspiration and biopsy should be performed, and evaluation with molecular techniques such as FISH or RT-PCR (if available) may be helpful to identify disease. Important imaging studies are chest radiography, plain radiography of primary and metastatic sites, bone scintigraphy, CT of the chest, and MRI of the primary site (Table 22.2 and Fig. 22.4) [17]. In Ewing sarcoma, plain radiographs typically show a diaphyseal destructive lesion with a laminated periosteal reaction and large soft-tissue mass.

Prognostic Factors

Metastatic disease, older age, large tumor size, and trunk and pelvic primary sites are usually associated with worse outcome [48]. However, with refinement in the multidisciplinary approach to this disease that entails newer and more intensive chemotherapeutic regimens and superior local control measures, some of these classic prognostic factors are being redefined. Although less documented than for osteosarcoma, poor histologic response to chemotherapy may also identify a subgroup of patients with worse prognosis [49, 50]. The most important prognostic factor remains the presence of metastatic disease at diagnosis [48]. Advances in management of Ewing sarcoma have resulted in only very modest improvement in outcome among patients with metastatic lesions. However, even among patients with metastatic disease, heterogeneity is common. With an appropriately intensive treatment that includes bilateral lung irradiation, patients with isolated metastatic lesions in the lung may have a better prognosis, albeit still inferior to that for patients with localized disease [48].

Treatment

Before the introduction of systemic chemotherapy, less than 20 % of children with Ewing sarcoma treated with either surgery or radiation therapy alone were expected to be long-term survivors [51]. In the past 3 decades, major advances have been made in the management of Ewing sarcoma, through a better definition of the risk groups and the basic principles of local and systemic therapy. Different from osteosarcoma, Ewing sarcoma is very radiosensitive, and thus radiation therapy is a key component of the treatment for this malignancy. In the United States, the systemic therapy commonly used includes alternating cycles of vincristine, cyclophosphamide and doxorubicin (VCD) with ifosfamide and etoposide (IE) (Fig. 22.5). With this regimen, along with aggressive local control, more

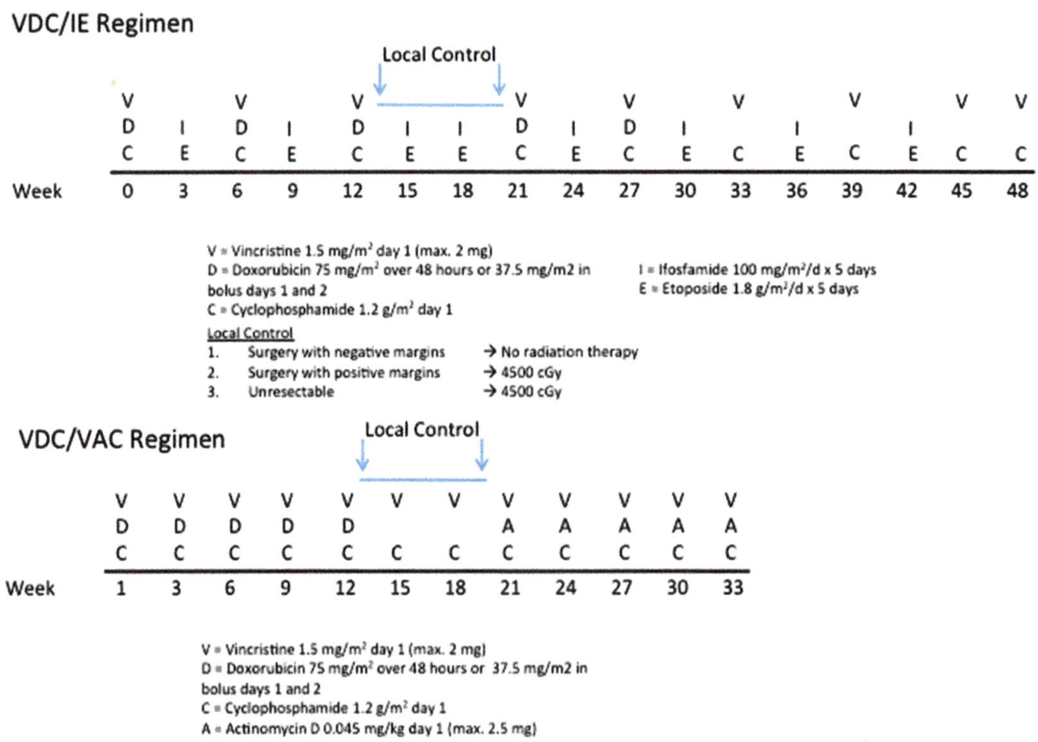

Fig. 22.5 Treatment of Ewing sarcoma

than two-thirds of patients can be cured [52, 53]. In a recently completed randomized study, the Children's Oncology Group compared the administration of the VCD and IE cycles every 3 weeks vs. every 2 weeks, in the regimen known as "dose compression," for patients with localized disease. The administration of chemotherapy every 2 weeks resulted in a significantly better event-free survival (73 % vs. 65 %) [54]. This dose-compressed approach is currently considered the standard of care in the United States. While it cannot be delivered without the use of G-CSF, it is otherwise feasible and doesn't result in more toxicity than the 3-week regimen. The European groups, organized around the EURO-EWING protocol, use the same five drugs, but following a risk-adapted regimen. All patients receive an induction phase with VIDE (vincristine, ifosfamide, doxorubicin, and etoposide), followed by local control, and risk-adapted therapy based on the size of the primary, the response to chemotherapy, and the presence of metastases [55]. Importantly, the use of high doses of alkylating agents (cyclophosphamide and ifosfamide), along with the intensification of topoisomerase II inhibitors (doxorubicin and etoposide), has resulted in high rates (1–5 %) of treatment-related myelodysplastic syndromes and acute myeloid leukemia [56].

There is very limited information on adapted Ewing sarcoma chemotherapeutic regimens in LMIC. While the ideal regimen should include all active agents as explored in the COG and EURO-EWING groups, it is important to note that more than 50 % of patients with localized disease can be cured with a regimen that includes standard therapy with vincristine, doxorubicin, cyclophosphamide, and actinomycin D as documented by the studies performed prior to the introduction of the ifosfamide/etoposide combinations [48, 53]. In this regard, in the presence of severe limitations to care, a regimen maximizing on cyclophosphamide and doxorubicin delivery, and use of actinomycin D after maximum doses of doxorubicin have been achieved, could represent a reasonable approach for patients with localized disease, provided that aggressive local control is performed (Fig. 22.5).

Local control for Ewing sarcoma includes different combinations of surgery and radiation therapy. Usually, local control is implemented within the first 10–12 weeks, after 3–6 cycles of chemotherapy. Advances in systemic therapy by means of incorporation of new drugs and treatment intensification also appear to contribute to better local control [57]. With current multimodality intensive protocols, rates of local recurrence have decreased significantly, and little difference in efficacy has been observed between surgery and radiation therapy for local control [48, 57]. In principle, if the tumor is resectable, surgery is the preferred method. Radiation therapy is used in case of unresectable tumors (usually in axial locations) or after surgery if resection margins are positive. Surgery generally offers slightly better results, with local relapse rates of <10 %, but this observation is biased by the fact that small lesions are more likely to be managed surgically. For unresectable tumors or in case of gross residual disease, recommended doses are 55–60 Gy. Doses of 40–45 Gy are used for microscopic disease. The risk of secondary sarcoma after radiation therapy is not negligible [56]. This risk is dose-dependent, but use of lower doses of radiation therapy has been associated with higher local recurrence rates [57].

While local control for osteosarcoma is relatively easier given its common location in extremities and possibility of amputation, treatment of the primary site in Ewing sarcoma may be more challenging in countries with limited resources. Aggressive surgery is always preferred, particularly considering the common limitations to access to radiation therapy facilities. However, for axial tumors, surgery is often not possible, and identification of a center where radiation therapy could be delivered should be done early in the treatment in order to achieve local control in a timely and effective manner.

Despite improvement, the prognosis for patients with metastatic disease continues to be very poor, and only 20–25 % survive [48]. Patients with metastatic disease limited to the lungs have better prognosis (survival rates up to 40 %) than those with disease in the bones or bone marrow. In general it is recommended that patients with lung disease receive whole lung radiation (15–18 Gy).

References

1. Gurney JG, Swensen AR, Bulterys M: Malignant bone tumors, in Ries LAG SM, Gurney JG (ed): Cancer incidence and survival among children and adolescents: United States SEER Program 1975–1995, NIH Pub, 1999. p. 99–110.
2. Dorfman HD, Czerniak B. Osteosarcoma. In: Dorfman HD, Czerniak B, editors. Bone tumors. St. Louis, MO: Mosby; 1998. p. 128–252.
3. Link MP, Gebhardt MC, Meyers PA: Osteosarcoma in Principles and Practice of Pediatric Oncology Eds Pizzo PA and Poplack DG (ed 5th), Lippincott Williams & Wilkins, 2006 pp. 1074–1115.
4. Glass AG, Fraumeni JF. Epidemiology of bne cancer in children. J Natl Cancer Inst. 1970;44(1):187–99.
5. Parkin D, Kramarova E, Draper G. International incidence of childhood cancer. Cary, NC: International Agency for Research on Cancer; 1998. p. 391.
6. Kleinerman RA, Tucker MA, Tarone RE, et al. Risk of new cancers after radiotherapy in long-term survivors of retinoblastoma: an extended follow-up. J Clin Oncol. 2005;23(10):2272–9.
7. Porter D, Holden S, Steel C, Cohen B, Wallace M, Reid R. A significant proportion of patients with osteosarcoma may belong to Li-Fraumeni cancer families. J Bone Joint Surg Br. 1992;74-B:883–6.
8. Kansara M, Thomas DM. Molecular pathogenesis of osteosarcoma. DNA Cell Biol. 2007;26:1–18.
9. Wadayama B, Toguchida J, Shimizu T, et al. Mutation spectrum of the retinoblastoma gene in osteosarcoma. Cancer Res. 1994;54(11):3042–8.
10. Wei G, Lonardo F, Ueda T, et al. CDK4 gene amplification in osteosarcoma: reciprocal relationship with INK4 gene alterations and mapping of 12q13 amplicons. Int J Cancer. 1999;80(2):199–204.
11. Walkley CR, Qudsi R, Sankaran VG, et al. Conditional mouse osteosarcoma, dependent on p53 loss and potentiated by loss of Rb, mimics the human disease. Genes Dev. 2008;22:1662–76.
12. Bacci G, Pignatti G, Dallari D, et al. Primary chemotherapy and delaye dsurgery (neoadjuvant chemotherapy) for telangiectatic osteogenic sarcoma of the extremities. J Chemother. 1989;1(3):190–6.
13. Bielack SS, Kempf-Bielack B, Delling G, et al. Prognostic factors in high-grade osteosarcoma of the extremities or trunk: an analysis of 1,702 patients treated on neoadjuvant Cooperative Osteosarcoma Study Group Protocols. J Clin Oncol. 2002;20:776–90.
14. Pan K, Zolqarnain A, Chia Y. Delay in treatment of primary malignant and aggressive musculoskeletal tumours. Med J Malaysia. 2006;61:53–6.
15. Friedrich P, Ortiz R, Strait K, et al. Pediatric sarcoma in Central America. Cancer. 2013;119:871–9.
16. Bacci G, Picci P, Ferrari S, et al. Prognostic significance of serum alkaline phosphatase measurements in patients with osteosarcoma treated with adjuvant or neoadjuvant chemotherapy. Cancer. 1993;71(4):1224–30.
17. Fletcher BD. Imaging pediatric bone sarcomas. Diagnosis and treatment-related issues. Radiol Clin North Am. 1997;35(6):1477–94.
18. Bacci G, Bertoni F, Longhi A, et al. Neoadjuvant chemotherapy for high-grade central osteosarcoma of the extremity: histologic response to preoperative chemotherapy correlates with histologic subtype of the tumor. Cancer. 2003;97(12):3068–75.
19. Meyer WH, Malawer MM. Osteosarcoma. Clinical features and evolving surgical and chemotherapeutic strategies. Pediatr Clin North Am. 1991;38(2):317–48.
20. Weeden S, Grimer RJ, Cannon SR, Taminiau AHM, Uscinska BM. The effect of local recurrence on survival in resected osteosarcoma. Eur J Cancer. 2001;37(1):39–46.
21. Pan K, Chan W, Ong G, et al. Limb salvage in osteosarcoma using autoclaved tumor-bearing bone. World J Surg Oncol. 2012;10:105.
22. Agarwal M, Anchan C, Shah M, Puri A, Pai S. Limb salvage surgery for osteosarcoma: effective low-cost treatment. Clin Orthop Relat Res. 2007;459:82–91.
23. Lawal Y, Garba E, Ogirima M, et al. Use of non-vascularized autologous fibula strut graft in the treatment of segmental bone loss. Ann Afr Med. 2011;10:25–8.
24. Haidar R, Sagghieh S, Muwakitt S, et al. Limb salvage surgery for children and adolescents with malignant bone tumors in a developing country. Pediatr Blood Cancer. 2008;51:787–91.
25. Jaffe N, Frei E, Traggis D, Bishop Y. Adjuvant methotrexate and citrovorum-factor treatment of osteogenic sarcoma. N Engl J Med. 1974;291:994–7.
26. Hogendoorn PCW, ESMO/EUROBONET Working Group, et al. Bone sarcomas: ESMO clinical practice guidelines for diagnosis, treatment and follow-up. Ann Oncol. 2010;21:v204–13.
27. Janeway KA, Grier HE. Sequelae of osteosarcoma medical therapy: a review of rare acute toxicities and late effects. Lancet Oncol. 2010;11:670–8.
28. Daw NC, Neel MD, Rao BN, et al. Frontline treatment of localized osteosarcoma without methotrexate. Cancer. 2011;117:2770–8.
29. Bramwell VHC, Burgers M, Sneath R, et al. A comparison of two short intensive adjuvant chemotherapy regimens in operable osteosarcoma of limbs in children and young adults: the first study of the European Osteosarcoma Intergroup. J Clin Oncol. 1992; 10:1579–91.
30. Souhami RL, Craft AW, Van der Eijken JW, et al. Randomised trial of two regimens of chemotherapy in operable osteosarcoma: a study of the European Osteosarcoma Intergroup. Lancet. 1997;350:911–7.
31. Meyers PA, Schwartz CL, Krailo M, et al. Osteosarcoma: a randomized, prospective trial of the addition of ifosfamide and/or muramyl tripeptide to cisplatin, doxorubicin, and high-dose methotrexate. J Clin Oncol. 2005;23(9):2004–11.
32. Ortiz R, Baez F, Valverde P, et al. Pediatric osteosarcoma in low-income countries: experience of the

Central American Association of Pediatric Hematology-Oncology. Pediatr Blood Cancer. 2010; 55:831 (abstract).
33. Wiromrat P, Jetsrisuparb A, Komvilaisak P, Sirichativapee W, Kamsa-ard S, Wiangnon S. Incidence and survival rates among pediatric osteogenic sarcoma cases in Khon Kaen, Thailand, 1985–2010. Asian Pac J Cancer Prev. 2012;13:4281–4.
34. Min D, Lin F, Shen Z, et al. Analysis of prognostic factors in 333 Chinese patients with high-grade osteosarcoma treated by multidisciplinary combined therapy. Asia Pac J Clin Oncol. 2013;9:71–9.
35. Petrilli AS, de Camargo B, Filho VO, et al. Results of the Brazilian Osteosarcoma Treatment Group Studies III and IV: prognostic factors and impact on survival. J Clin Oncol. 2006;24(7):1161–8.
36. Mostert S, Arora RS, Arreola M, et al. Abandonment of treatment for childhood cancer: position statement of a SIOP PODC Working Group. Lancet Oncol. 2011;12:719–20.
37. Bonilla M, Rossell N, Salaverria C, et al. Prevalence and predictors of abandonment of therapy among children with cancer in El Salvador. Int J Cancer. 2009;125:2144–6.
38. Bacci G, Briccoli A, Ferrari S, et al. Neoadjuvant chemotherapy for osteosarcoma of the extremity: long-term results of the Rizzoli's 4th protocol. Eur J Cancer. 2001;37:2030–9.
39. Goorin AM, Harris MB, Bernstein M, et al. Phase II/III trial of etoposide and high-dose ifosfamide in newly diagnosed metastatic osteosarcoma: a Pediatric Oncology Group trial. J Clin Oncol. 2002; 20:426–33.
40. Kempf-Bielack B, Bielack SS, Jürgens H, et al. Osteosarcoma relapse after combined modality therapy: an analysis of unselected patients in the Cooperative Osteosarcoma Study Group (COSS). J Clin Oncol. 2005;23:559–68.
41. Stiller CA. International patterns of cancer incidence in adolescents. Cancer Treat Rev. 2007;33:631–45.
42. Settakorn J, Lekawanvijit S, Arpornchayanon O, et al. Spectrum of bone tumors in Chiang Mai University Hospital, Thailand according to WHO classification 2002: a study of 1,001 cases. J Med Assoc Thai. 2006;89:780–7.
43. Dehner LP. Primitive neuroectodermal tumor and Ewing's sarcoma. Am J Surg Pathol. 1993; 17:1–13.
44. de Alava E, Gerald WL. Molecular biology of the Ewing's sarcoma/primitive neuroectodermal tumor family. J Clin Oncol. 2000;18(1):204–13.
45. Delattre O, Zucman J, Melot T, et al. The Ewing family of tumors: a subgroup of small-round-cell tumors defined by specific chimeric transcripts. N Engl J Med. 1994;331:294–9.
46. Hill DA, O'Sullivan MJ, Zhu X, et al. Practical application of molecular genetic testing as an aid to the surgical pathologic diagnosis of sarcomas: a prospective study. Am J Surg Pathol. 2002;26(8):965–77.
47. Widhe B, Widhe T. Initial symptoms and clinical features in osteosarcoma and Ewing sarcoma. J Bone Joint Surg Am. 2000;82(5):667–74.
48. Rodriguez-Galindo C, Liu T, Krasin MJ, et al. Analysis of prognostic factors in Ewing sarcoma family of tumors: review of St. Jude Children's Research Hospital studies. Cancer. 2007;110(2):375–84.
49. Picci P, Bohling T, Bacci G, et al. Chemotherapy-induced tumor necrosis as a prognostic factor in localized Ewing's sarcoma of the extremities. J Clin Oncol. 1997;15(4):1553–9.
50. Paulussen M, Ahrens S, Dunst J, et al. Localized Ewing tumor of bone: final results of the Cooperative Ewing's Sarcoma Study CESS-86. J Clin Oncol. 2001;19:1818–29.
51. Zucker JM, Henry-Amar M, Sarrazin D, Blache R, Patte C, Schweisguth O. Intensive systemic chemotherapy in localized Ewing's sarcoma in childhood. A historical trial. Cancer. 1983;52(3):415–23.
52. Granowetter L, Womer R, Devidas M, et al. Dose-intensified compared with standard chemotherapy for nonmetastatic Ewing sarcoma family of tumors: a Children's Oncology Group Study. J Clin Oncol. 2009;27:2536–41.
53. Grier HE, Krailo MD, Tarbell NJ, et al. Addition of ifosfamide and etoposide to standard chemotherapy for Ewing's sarcoma and primitive neuroectodermal tumor of bone. N Engl J Med. 2003;348(8):694–701.
54. Womer RB, West DC, Krailo MD, et al. Randomized controlled trial of interval-compressed chemotherapy for the treatment of localized Ewing sarcoma: a report from the Children's Oncology Group. J Clin Oncol. 2012;30(33):4148–54.
55. Juergens C, Weston C, Lewis I, et al. Safety assessment of intensive induction with vincristine, ifosfamide, doxorubicin, and etoposide (VIDE) in the treatment of Ewing tumors in the EURO-E.W.I.N.G. 99 clinical trial. Pediatr Blood Cancer. 2006; 47:22–9.
56. Navid F, Billups C, Liu T, Krasin MJ, Rodriguez-Galindo C. Second cancers in patients with the Ewing sarcoma family of tumours. Eur J Cancer. 2008;44:983–91.
57. Rodriguez-Galindo C, Navid F, Liu T, Billups CA, Rao BN, Krasin MJ. Prognostic factors for local and distant control in Ewing sarcoma family of tumors. Ann Oncol. 2008;19:814–20.

23 Neuroblastoma

Soad Fuentes Alabí and Nehal S. Parikh

Epidemiology in Developing Countries

Neuroblastoma is an embryonic tumor of the autonomic nervous system, originating from the incomplete development of the precursor cell tissue in the neural crest. Neuroblastoma belongs to a group of "small round blue cell tumors" in children, within a family of tumors that includes the neuroblastoma (NB), Ganglioneuroblastoma (GNB), and ganglioneuroma (GN). Other similar-appearing tumors on H&E immunostaining are Ewing sarcoma, lymphoma, soft tissue sarcoma, and other neuroectodermal tumors. Neuroblastoma is primarily a disease of childhood with a median age of 17 months; 90 % of cases are diagnosed by 6 years of age [6]. Neuroblastoma is the most common extracranial solid tumor in childhood with a prevalence of 1 case per 7,000 live births. Although the incidence of neuroblastoma appears to be consistent in the developed countries, the reported rates in the resource-limited countries are lower [2, 7]. It is unclear if the lower incidence is due to under-reporting or truly a reflection of lower incidence pattern due to genetic or environmental influences. Additionally, despite reports of occupational influence in development of neuroblastoma, there has been lack of consistent studies to suggest that environmental influences significantly impact its outcomes [8].

S.F. Alabí, M.D.
Hospital Nacional de Niños Benjamín Bloom, San Salvador, El Salvador

N.S. Parikh, M.D. (✉)
Connecticut Children's Medical Center, 282 Washington Street, Suite 2J, Hartford, CT 06106, USA
e-mail: nparikh@ccmckids.org

Biology of Neuroblastoma

Neuroblastoma tumors reflect varying degrees of maturity, ranging from dense undifferentiated cells with large nuclei and a small cytoplasm (undifferentiated or poorly differentiated neuroblastoma) to well differentiated cells with abundant neuropil, mature ganglion cells, and Schwann cells (ganglioneuroma). Those tumors that have a spectrum of differentiation that lies in between the two are considered ganglioneuroblastomas [9]. In 1999, Shimada and colleagues developed a classification system for neuroblastic tumors in childhood, categorizing tumors as favorable or unfavorable histology, based on the degree of differentiation, content of stromal Schwann cells origin, mitotic karyorrhexis index (MKI), and age at diagnosis [10]. Further modification to the Shimada classification resulted in an International Neuroblastoma Pathology Classification (INPC) system [11].

Established prognostic markers in neuroblastoma such as stage of disease, age of the patient, *MYCN* gene amplification, DNA ploidy, and

D.C. Stefan and C. Rodriguez-Galindo (eds.), *Pediatric Hematology-Oncology in Countries with Limited Resources: A Practical Manual*, DOI 10.1007/978-1-4614-3891-5_23,

histological classification based on Shimada have facilitated risk stratification and treatment assignment [1, 4, 5]. Additional impact on prognosis has been noted in tumors with gain of chromosome 17q, loss of the chromosome 14q, and loss of the chromosome 11q [5, 12].

The amplification of the *MYCN* on chromosome 2q24, first described in 1983, was one of the first genetic abnormalities that correlated with prognostic implications in pediatric oncology. Currently, *MYCN* is routinely used in clinical practice for assignment of therapy intensity [13]. The definition of the *MYCN* amplification has been defined as greater than fourfold increase in *MYCN* signals as compared to reference signals. *MYCN* amplification is found in 30–40 % of stages 3 and 4 of neuroblastoma and in only 5 % of the stages 1, 2, or 4S neuroblastoma. Some infants with disseminated disease in a specific metastatic pattern without *MYC* amplification have excellent survival with minimal or no treatment [14]. Stage, age, histological category, grade of tumor differentiation, the status of the *MYCN* oncogene, chromosome 11q status, and DNA ploidy were the most highly statistically significant and clinically relevant factors. A new staging system (INRG Staging System) based on clinical criteria and tumor imaging has been proposed by the International Neuroblastoma Risk Group (INRG) Task Force. The optimal age cut-off was determined to be between 15 and 19 months, as 18 months was cut-off selected for the INRG classification system. Sixteen pretreatment groups were defined on the basis of clinical criteria and statistically significantly different EFS of the cohort stratified by the INRG criteria. Patients with 5-year EFS more than 85 %, more than 75 % to ≤85 %, ≥50 % to ≤75 %, or less than 50 % were classified as very low risk, low risk, intermediate risk, or high risk, respectively [15].

The content of DNA is also a useful prognostic indicator in neuroblastoma. The DNA index (DI), where 1 is equivalent to diploid content of DNA, can be measured by flow cytometric or by cytogenetic analysis [16]. Early research identified prognostic implication of the DNA ploidy in neuroblastoma and has since been used for the stratification of treatments in many European and North American trials [16].

The allelic loss of 1p36 has been observed in 25–35 % of neuroblastomas and has been shown to be significantly associated as a marker of aggressive disease and *MYCN [*17, 18]. Reports have shown that 1p status independently affects outcome in patients with low and intermediate risk [19]. The deletion of 1p36 is currently being used for the stratification of treatment in clinical trials including US and German led trials [20].

More recently, loss of heterozygosity at chromosome 11q has been shown to affect prognosis, seen in 35–45 % of neuroblastoma. The deletion of 11q in regions of 11q23 has been detected in 15–20 % of neuroblastoma at the time of diagnosis [20]. Loss of heterozygosity at 11q23 is associated with characteristics of advanced disease stage, with unfavorable biology and older children and is inversely correlated to the amplification of *MYCN* [21]. The neuroblastoma cohorts with loss of heterozygosity of 11q and the presence of *MYCN* amplification appear to represent two different molecular subgroups of aggressive neuroblastoma. Activating somatic mutations of the *ALK* gene were recently identified in approximately 8 % of neuroblastomas [21, 22]; its implications on prognosis and specific activating mutations that impact outcome is actively being evaluated [23].

Clinical Manifestations

The clinical manifestations of neuroblastoma are as diverse as the sites of presentation. The presenting symptoms depend on the site of tumor origination and any areas of metastatic disease. The majority of these tumors are located in the abdomen (65 %), with the remaining tumors seen in thoracic, cervical, and pelvic region. In a small group of patients (approximately 1 %), the origin of the tumor cannot be accurately determined [24]. Cervical or high-level thoracic tumors frequently present with Horner syndrome (ptosis, miosis, and exophthalmos [24] (Fig. 23.1). Mediastinal tumors may result in respiratory distress although those found in the lower mediastinum may be asymptomatic and discovered incidentally on routine radiographs obtained for unassociated medical reasons (Fig. 23.2).

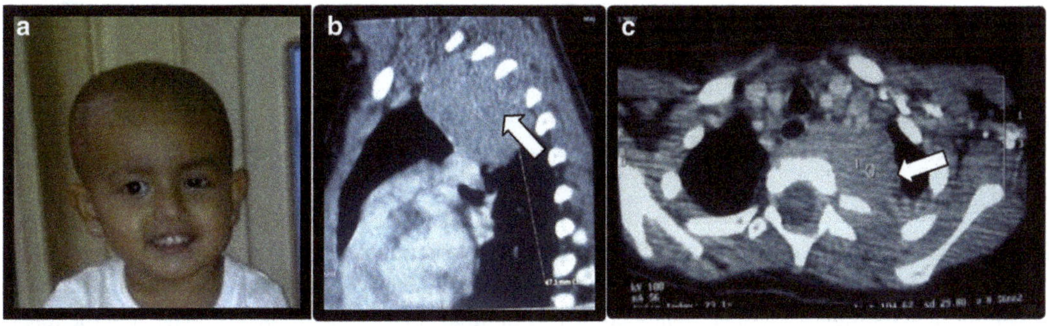

Fig. 23.1 Clinical presentations of neuroblastoma. (**a**) Evidence of left-sided ptosis in a child with high-level thoracic tumor. This tumor frequently present with Horner's syndrome (ptosis, miosis, and exophthalmos). (**b**) High thoracic neuroblastic tumors seen on computed tomography (CT scan). (**c**) Lower thoracic tumors surrounding the airway and likely intraspinal extension noted.

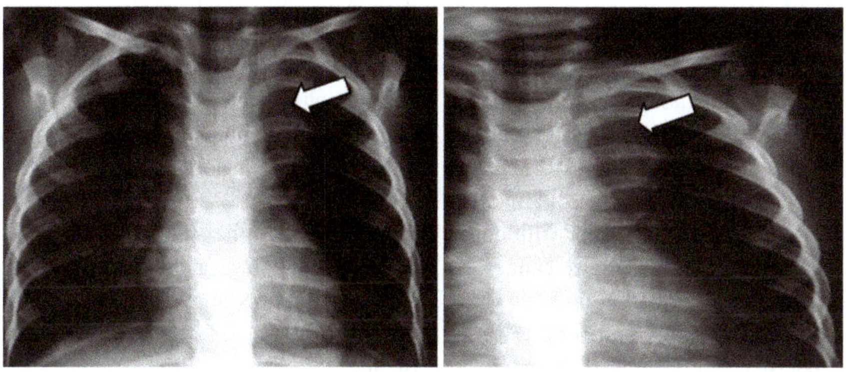

Fig. 23.2 Mediastinal tumors may results in respiratory distress, although those found in the lower mediastinum may be asymptomatic and discovered incidentally on routine radiographs obtained for unassociated medical reasons

The majority of children with neuroblastoma present with disseminated disease at diagnosis, with metastasis to bone marrow, bone, liver, lymph nodes, and less frequently lungs and central nervous system [25, 26]. Disseminated disease is usually associated with nonspecific symptoms, including fever, pallor, and anorexia and bone pain with subsequent changes in mood and refusal to ambulate. Disseminated neuroblastoma may present with several classic signs, such as infiltration of periorbital bone with proptosis and ecchymosis. A small group of infants with stage 4S may present with multiple bluish, painless, subcutaneous nodular lesions. Occasionally, these infants have massive hepatomegaly leading to coagulopathy, respiratory compromise, and renal insufficiency [27].

Tumor extension and growth within the foramen of the vertebrae with spinal compression are seen in approximately 5–15 % of young children with paraspinal tumors, resulting in symptomatic weakness, paralysis, bowel and/or bladder dysfunction, and radicular pain [28].

There have been two reported paraneoplastic syndromes associated with neuroblastoma. Opsoclonus-myoclonus is characterized by rapid multi-directional movements of the eyes (opsoclonus), muscle twitching/jerking (myoclonus), and thalamic ataxia and occurs in 1–2 % of the patients [29]. The exact mechanism of this autoimmune reaction and the reasons for its association with severe neurological sequelae is unknown. Another paraneoplastic syndrome is VIP syndrome; the tumors can secrete intestinal peptide vaso-active (VIP), which leads to chronic diarrhea, failure to thrive, hypokalemia, and dehydration. The VIP-secreting tumors are often ganglioneuroblastoma or ganglioneuroma and have an overall favorable prognosis [30].

Diagnostic Evaluation

A careful and thorough physical examination is critical; blood pressure for hypertension, complete neurologic examination to detect Horner's syndrome, symptoms of spinal cord compression or abnormal movements such as opsoclonus, myoclonus, or ataxia to indicate OMS, skin nodules, or hepatomegaly for 4s disease, and proptosis to indicate a high-risk patient with orbital metastasis, thoracic, abdominal, or pelvic mass. Baseline laboratory studies should include CBC with differential and platelet, liver function tests, creatinine, serum LDH, ferritin, and urinalysis [29, 31]. The diagnosis of neuroblastoma requires the involvement of pathologists who are familiar with childhood tumors. Some neuroblastomas cannot be distinguished from other small round blue cell tumors of childhood, such as lymphomas, primitive neuroectodermal tumors, and rhabdomyosarcomas, using conventional light microscopy and routine H&E staining. Evidence for sympathetic neuronal differentiation may be demonstrated by immunohistochemistry, or by finding elevated levels of urine catecholamine metabolites, such as vanillylmandelic acid (VMA) or homovanillic acid (HVA), although 5–10 % of neuroblastomas do not secrete catecholamines [32].

Surgical Procedure

Surgical management of a child with suspected neuroblastoma should be thoroughly reviewed and discussed with the pediatric oncology team prior to taking the child to the operating room. In general, a limited initial open biopsy to obtain an adequate specimen for diagnostic and analysis of available prognostic markers should be considered [33]. Extensive upfront surgical resection and surgical laminectomy should be limited as this may result in delay in appropriate chemotherapy and potentially result in avoidable surgical complications [34].

Evaluation of the Bone Marrow

Disseminated disease is predictive and prognostic of poor outcome in children with neuroblastoma. Its accurate and sensitive assessment can facilitate optimal treatment decisions. The International Neuroblastoma Risk Group (INRG) Task Force has defined standardized methods for the determination of minimal disease by immunocytology and quantitative reverse transcriptase-polymerase chain reaction using disialoganglioside GD2 and tyrosine hydroxylase mRNA, respectively. One of the most common sites of metastasis in high-risk neuroblastoma is the bone marrow. Due to the heterogeneity of the bone marrow infiltration, it is critical to obtain multiple biopsies to detect neuroblastoma clusters. Unfortunately, the cytological and histological techniques lack sensitivity and standardization. Recently, the INRG group published its consensus criteria for the detection of neuroblastoma cells in bone marrow, peripheral blood (PB), and peripheral blood stem cells [35]. The objective of the International Risk Group Classification (INRG) is to develop standardized procedures to ensure the consistency of the results and allow comparisons between institutions.

Radiological Procedures

Treatment for children with neuroblastoma is guided by appropriate disease staging at time of initial diagnosis. Therefore, clinical staging should include:

1. CT/MRI of the primary and metastatic sites.
2. Bone scan.
3. I^{123} metaiodobenzylguanidine (MIBG) (preferable over bone scan) or positron emission tomography (PET) scan.

CT Scan/MRI

CT scan and/or MRI of the chest, abdomen, and pelvis are considered the standard modalities for evaluation of solid tumor malignancies in children; additional areas of imaging may be guided based on presentation.

MRI is most effective in the detection of tumor extension into the epidural or leptomeninges and may provide a better definition of tumor extent for surgical planning. There has been an increased trend and preference for use of MRI, in an effort to limit the potential risks of secondary malignancies from radiation exposures of CT scans.

Metalodobenzylguanidine and Positron Emission Tomography

The MIBG scan is a very sensitive and specific imaging modality for neuroendocrine tumors, particularly neuroblastomas. This scan aids in detection of primary and metastatic sites of neuroblastoma and response to therapy. Current data suggest that ^{123}I-MIBG scan is preferred to the ^{131}I-MIBG and Tc-99 bone scan, because of greater sensitivity, improved image quality, fewer days of review, and lower risk of toxicity to the thyroid gland. The PET scan measures the metabolic activity through the absorption of 2-(fluorine-18)-fluoro-2-deoxy-D-glucose ($^{18F-FDG}$), which is directly proportional to the amount of disease and cell proliferation. A recent study showed that the PET and MIBG have relative sensitivity for neuroblastoma tumors, with $^{18F-FDG}$ PET suggesting benefit in lower stage patients. ^{123}I-MIBG continues to be the gold standard for imaging in all patients, including advanced stage [36].

A disadvantage of the PET is its inability to visualize lesions in the cranial vault and may have lower sensitivity for bony lesions in comparison to MIBG scans [36]. PET scan can help especially in the management and diagnosis of MIBG-negative neuroblastoma.

Alternate Imaging

In the absence of advanced technologies for radiographic imaging, it would be advisable to obtain a Tc-99 bone scan and/or skeletal survey (if Tc-99 bone scan is unavailable).

Pathology and Molecular Evaluations

The biopsy specimen must be handled with conditions that allow for relative sterility. The specimen should be fresh and not fixed in formalin. Genetic and molecular studies require at least 100 mg tissue. Specimens can be divided into following manner for appropriate diagnostic evaluations:

1. Ten imprints without fixing with remainder fixed in formalin.
2. Specimen in sterile culture medium, for DNA cytometry and cytogenetic.
3. Three and four specimens are frozen and kept in liquid N2.

Fixed specimens can be evaluated for a structural study. A trained pathologist with experience in childhood solid tumors is critical to appropriate processing of tissue and selection of critical diagnostic immunohistochemical testing on the tumor specimen. Histological classification using the International Neuroblastoma Pathology Committee (INPC) guidelines will help guide risk stratification, using tumor category, MKI, and degree of differentiation [37]. Distinguishing neuroblastoma tumors from other small round blue cell tumors can be made using immunohistochemistry if the urine catecholamine is negative or unavailable [38].

Pathology report should include the following data:

- Histologic category.
- Histologic subtype.
- MKI in the category of neuroblastoma (Fig. 23.3).
- Other data of interest such as the presence of calcification.
- Potential involvement of lymph nodes and adjacent organs.
- Results of the special studies.
- Determination of the prognostic group according to the INPC histology favorable or unfavorable [39].

The histological data obtained in a metastasis should correlate with the primary tumor and should be indicated in the report. On the contrary, after chemo treatments and/or radiotherapy

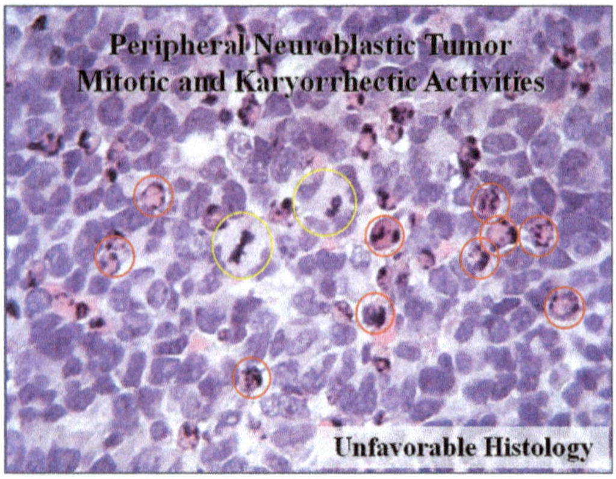

Fig. 23.3 The *mitosis-karyorrhexis index* (MKI) is defined as the number of tumor cells in mitosis and in the process of karyorrhexis. The index is defined this way so that mitotic activity and karyorrhexis can be assessed in relation to the cellularity of the tumor, rather than in relation to the number of high-power microscopic fields (HPFs)

histology varies greatly from area to area and there are frequent areas of necrosis and calcification; this is not relevant for prognostic assessment. Occasionally, the diagnosis of neuroblastoma may be challenging on a simple H&E staining, especially for the undifferentiated histology. The differential diagnosis should include lymphomas and leukemias, soft tissue sarcomas, and PNET/Ewing. Immunohistochemistry staining can be utilized to help guide appropriate diagnosis and management [38].

Cytogenetic and Molecular Studies

MYC-N amplification analysis: A fresh tumor tissue is required to determine *MYCN* amplification or chromosomal aberrations. Detection is based on fluorescence in situ hybridization (FISH) testing, real-time quantitative PCR assay, or a southern blot (Fig. 23.4).

Tumor cell ploidy analysis: A flow cytometric analysis on fresh tumor cell suspension is required to assess DNA index. DNA index, when available, is a useful marker of prognostic significance in infants and toddlers, with loss of utility in older children with advance disease [40].

Other Molecular Analyses

In neuroblastoma, several nonrandom genomic alterations have been described to be closely associated with distinct phenotypes of the disease [41]. Recently, loss of 11q has been reported to be highly correlated with an adverse outcome [20, 42] and has thus been proposed as a stratifying prognostic marker in the INRG classification system [15]. As 11q CNA and *MYCN* amplification are inversely correlated in neuroblastoma, these two genomic alterations have been suggested to delineate molecularly distinct subgroups [43, 44]. In contrast, the majority of favorable neuroblastomas lack structural genomic aberrations but show numerical variations of whole chromosomes [45, 46]. In neuroblastoma, loss of large genomic regions at 11q occurs in approximately 30 % of the tumors and is associated with an unfavorable clinical outcome [45].

Disease Risk Assignment

European and North American cooperative groups have selected various factors to define the risk in patients with neuroblastoma, but these have not been uniform, for example: The International Society of Pediatric Oncology Europe Neuroblastoma Group (SIOPEN) uses age, image-defined surgical risk factor (IDRF), and *MYCN* status for risk assignment in local/regional tumors, on the other hand, the Children's Oncology Group (COG) uses age, postsurgical stage, *MYCN* status, DNA ploidy, loss of heterozygosity at 11q, 1p, and histology [1, 47]. Estimated 5-year survival rates for patients with non-high-risk and high-risk neuroblastoma are 90 and 50 %, respectively. Recent clinical trials have shown excellent outcomes with reduced therapy for non-high-risk disease. For patients with high-risk neuroblastoma treated with chemo radiotherapy, surgery, and stem cell transplantation, the addition of anti-disialoganglioside GD2 immunotherapy plus cytokines improves survival. Upcoming trials will study the incorporation of targeted radionuclide therapy prior to myeloablative chemotherapy into high-risk treatment [48].

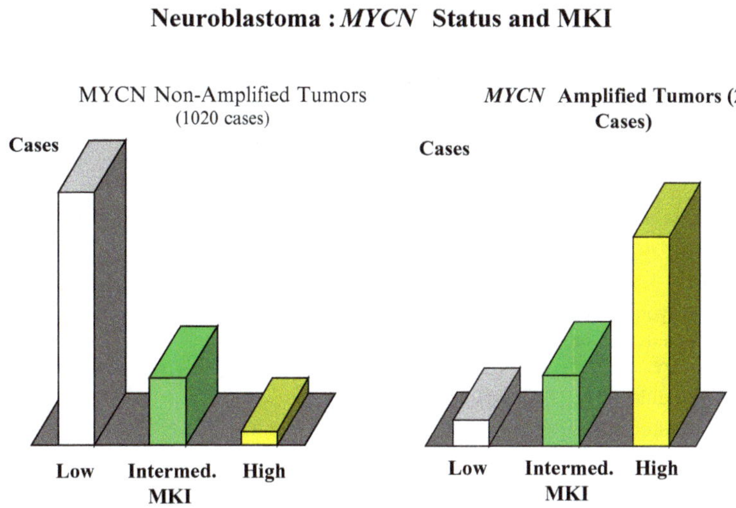

Fig. 23.4 The definition of the *MYCN* amplification has been defined as greater than fourfold increase in *MYCN* signals as compared to reference signals. *MYCN* amplification is found in a 30–40 % of stages 3 and 4 of neuroblastoma and in only 5 % of the stages 1, 2, or 4S neuroblastoma

A new staging system (INRG) was developed for neuroblastoma risk assignment and stratification of patients at the time of diagnosis and prior to initiating treatment (Table 23.1). This staging incorporates the extension of local, regional disease as the presence or absence of image-defined presurgical risk in L1 and L2 tumors; disseminated disease is categorized as M stage, with the exception of Ms stage, which defines the presence of metastatic disease limited to the skin, liver, bone marrow without commitment to the cortical bone, in children between the ages of 0–18 months with small primary tumors. Additional evaluations that have been recommended are molecular diagnostic tests in the tumor tissue, bone marrow analysis, and radiographic imaging [15] (Table 23.2.). Because the treatment effect of tumor excision is an inherent part of the INSS, the prognostic value of specific stages within INRGSS and INSS cannot be directly compared. The INRGSS differs from INSS in four important ways. First, it is based on preoperative imaging and image-defined risk factors (IDRFs), not surgicopathologic findings. Second, the midline is not included in the staging criteria of the INRGSS. Third, lymph node status is not included in the staging of localized disease. Fourth, whereas INSS stage 4S has an upper age limit of 12 months, the Task Force decided to extend the age group for stage MS to patients younger than 18 months. The INRGSS is a preoperative staging system that has been developed specifically for the INRG classification system. The extent of disease is determined by the presence or absence of IDRFs and/or metastatic tumor at the time of diagnosis, before any treatment. Use of this pretreatment staging system and the INRG classification system will facilitate the ability to compare results of risk-based clinical trials conducted in different regions of the world, and thereby, provide insight into optimal treatment strategies for patients with neuroblastic tumors [49].

In the resource-limited countries (RLC), there are significant limitations in the diagnosis of neuroblastoma. The majority of the centers in these countries do not have the resources to obtain all the biological and genetic data that is suggested for a complete treatment stratification and therapy assignment. Therefore, a modified stratification is typically considered based on resource availability with current use of the INSS system.

Table 23.1 International Neuroblastoma Risk Group (INRG) Staging System (INRGSS)

INRG	Age (month)	Histologic category	Degree of differentiation of the tumor	N-MYC	Aberration of the 11q	Ploidy	Pretreatment risk group
L1/L2	Mature GN or mix GN						A very low
L1	Any with exception mature GN or mix GNB			N/A			B very low
				Amp			K High
L2	<18	Anyone except mature GN or mixed GNB		N/A	No		D Low
					Yes		G Intermediate
	>18	Nodular GN	Differentiated	N/A	No		E Low
		Neuroblastoma			Yes		
				N/A			H Intermediate
			Poorly differentiated or undifferentiated	Amp			N High
M	<18			N/A		Hyperploidy	F Low
	<12 months			N/A		Ploidy	I Intermediate
	12 months <18			N/A		Ploidy	J Intermediate
	<18			Amp			O High
	<18						P High
MS	<18			N/A	No		C Very low
					Yes		Q High
				Amp			R High

Source: J Clin Oncol. 2009 Jan 10;27(2):298–303. doi: 10.1200/JCO.2008.16.6876. Epub 2008 Dec 1

Table 23.2 Descriptions of new INRG tumor stages

Tumor stage	Description
L1	Localized tumor not involving vital structures, as defined by the list of IDRFs, and confined to one body compartment
L2	Local-regional tumor with presence of one or more IDRFs
M	Distant metastatic disease (except stage MS tumor)
MS	Metastatic disease in children younger than 18 months, with metastases confined to skin, liver, and/or bone morrow

Source: Monclair T, Brodeur GM, Ambros PF, et al. The International Neuroblastoma Risk Group (INRG) staging system: an INRG Task Force report. J Clin Oncol 2009;27(2):298–303

Complete definitions of these stages are cited in the text

IDRFs image-defined risk factors

Prognostic Considerations

The Age of Presentation

Analysis of the COG and INRG data shows that age has a strong predictive value as a variable for the risk stratification. The effect of age at the time of diagnosis in the 5-year survival is profound; patients with 4S disease (7–10 % of neuroblastoma) have a more favorable outcome than other patients with metastatic neuroblastoma, often demonstrating spontaneous maturation and regression. Estimated survival rates of 70–90 % have been reported, and these tumors are usually associated with favorable biologic features. Recently, the INRG developed consensus guidelines for a modified staging system based on clinical and radiologic criteria. The INRG increased the upper limit of age from 12 to 18 months for 4S disease (now designated Ms), defined as metastases limited to skin, liver, and bone marrow (<10 %) without cortical bone involvement and either L1 or L2 stage tumors, including large unresectable primary tumors that cross the midline [50]. Children with ages from 1 to 4 years old has shown an OS >68 %, ages 5–9 years old is 52 %, and 10–14 years old is 66 % [23, 47].

Histological Classification

The INPC involves the evaluation of tumor specimens obtained prior to the treatment with respect to the degree of development and maturation, the presence of neuroblastic stroma, and the rate of mitosis-karyorrhexis [31]. These histological parameters are used to define favorable and unfavorable characteristics. Several studies have confirmed the prognostic significance of this classification system and other related systems that employ similar strategies [51] (Table 23.3).

MYC-N amplification: Numerous studies have shown that MYC-N amplification is the most critical assessment in guiding treatment strategies and outcomes. This impact is most significantly noted in guiding treatment for all stage 3 and 4 and 45 NB patients less than 18 months, [51]. Children >18 months with stage 4 NB would generally be treated based on high-risk protocol and therefore less critical for therapeutic guidance [64].

Tumor cell ploidy: DNA index has been shown to be a strong predictor of outcome in infants and toddlers with metastatic disease and those with stage 4S disease [47]. The prognostic impact in other patients is less apparent in a multivariate analysis.

Table 23.3 International Neuroblastoma Pathology Classification

Category and subtype	Prognostic group
Neuroblastoma (Schwannian stroma-poor)	
Undifferentiated, poorly differentiated	Differentiating FH and UH subgroups, based on the combination of age, grade of neuroblastic differentiation, and MKI class
Ganglioneuroblastoma, intermixed (Schwannian stroma-rich)	FH
Ganglioneuroma (Schwannian stroma-dominant)	FH
Maturing	
Mature	
Ganglioneuroblastoma, nodular (Schwannian stroma-rich/stroma-dominant and stroma-poor)	UH[a]

Source: Shimada H, Umehara S, Monobe Y, Hachitanda Y, Nakagawa A, Goto S, et al. International Neuroblastoma Pathology Classification for prognostic evaluation of patients with peripheral neuroblastic tumors: a report from the Children's Cancer Group. Cancer. 2001;92(9): 2451–61

FH favorable histology, *UH* unfavorable histology, *MKI* mitosis-karyorrhexis index

[a]Tumors in this category were classified into an unfavorable histology group according to the International Neuroblastoma Pathology Classification. However, two prognostic subsets, i.e., favorable and unfavorable, are distinguished based on the results of our recent study

Additional Serum Markers: LDH, Ferritin, Neuron-Specific Enolase

Ferritin, neuron-specific enolase (NSE), and lactate dehydrogenase (LDH), are commonly assessed in children suspected to have neuroblastoma. The univariate prognostic benefit that has been suggested in numerous studies has been less obvious in multivariate analysis of large cohorts, especially in the setting of established independent prognostic factors such as age, MYC-N amplification, and stage of disease, histology, and cell ploidy.

LDH values above 1,500 U/dL in stage 4 patients were associated with a worse outcome, independent of age and stage. LDH levels >1,500 U/dL also suggested correlation with *MYCN* amplification, and therefore, may serve as a useful surrogate for *MYCN* amplification. This relationship has yet to be evaluated in a clinical trial. Similarly, NSE levels >200 ng/mL positively associated with a worse outcome only in stage 4 patients without *MYCN* amplification, thus limiting their utility in patient risk stratification. The ferritin >142 ng/mL has also been shown to have prognostic implications [52]. In resources-limited countries, it is therefore imperative to continue to utilize the previously accepted standard risk classification based on INSS, until advanced diagnostic resources are readily available.

Staging

International Neuroblastoma Staging System (INSS): International criteria for a common neuroblastoma staging system were first described in 1988 and subsequently revised in 1993. The INSS is a surgicopathologic staging system that depends on the completeness of resection of the primary tumor, assessment of ipsilateral and contralateral lymph nodes, and the relation of a primary tumor to the midline (Table 23.4). Although INSS has been shown to have prognostic relevance, there have been some difficulties with its widespread use. The expertise and aggressiveness of the surgeon max influence tumor staging, and lymph node sampling, extent of disease resection [53]. The INSS combines certain features of the previously used POG and CCG systems and has identified distinct prognostic groups. Based on preliminary experience, there was a need for modifications and clarifications in the INSS and International Neuroblastoma Response Criteria (INRC). A meeting was held to review experience with the INSS and INRC and to revise or clarify the language and intent of the originally proposed criteria. Substantial changes included a redefinition of the midline, restrictions on age and bone marrow involvement for stage 4S, and the recommendation that MIBG scanning be implemented for evaluating the extent of disease. Other modifications and clarifications of the INSS and INRC are presented. In addition, the criteria for the diagnosis of neuroblastoma were modified. Finally, proposals were made for the development of risk groups that incorporate both clinical and biologic features in the prediction of prognosis. The biologic features that were deemed important to evaluate prospectively included serum ferritin, NSE, and lactic dehydrogenase (LDH); tumor histology; tumor-cell DNA content; assessment of *MYCN* copy number; assessment of 1p deletion by cytogenetic or molecular methods [31].

Table 23.4 International Neuroblastoma Staging System

1	Localized tumor with complete gross excision, with or without microscopic residual disease; representative ipsilateral lymph nodes negative for tumor microscopically (nodes attached to and removed with primary tumor may be positive)
2A	Localized tumor with incomplete gross excision; representative ipsilateral nonadherent lymph nodes negative for tumor microscopically
2B	Localized tumor with or without complete gross excision, with ipsilateral nonadherent lymph nodes positive for tumor. Enlarged contralateral lymph nodes must be negative microscopically
3	Unresectable unilateral tumor infiltrating across the midline,[a] with or without regional lymph node involvement; or localized unilateral tumor with contralateral regional lymph node involvement; or midline tumor with bilateral extension by infiltration (unresectable) or by lymph node involvement
4	Any primary tumor with dissemination to distant lymph nodes, bone marrow, bone, liver, skin, and/or other organs (except as defined for stage 4[S])
4S	Localized primary tumor (as defined for stage 1 and 2[A], or 2[B]), with dissemination limited to skin, liver, and/or bone marrow[b] (limited to infants <1 year of age)

Adapted from [31].

The MIBG scan (if performed) should be negative in the marrow

[a]The midline is defined as the vertebral column. Tumors originating on one side and crossing the midline must infiltrate to or beyond the opposite side of the vertebral column

Marrow involvement in stage 4(S) should be minimal, that is, <10 % of total nucleated cells identified as malignant on bone marrow biopsy or on marrow aspirate. More extensive marrow involvement would be considered stage

Treatment Assignment Based on Risk Group Stratification

In the developing countries, neuroblastoma tumor treatment and risk assignment still remains a challenge; greater than 50 % of children with neuroblastoma succumb to the disease. Resource limitations impact our ability to adequately diagnose, risk stratify, and provide effective therapies to cure this disease. In an effort to improve the outcomes, we need to develop a consistent strategy that encompasses resource availability in each setting to help guide appropriate therapies. Until this approach is available, each center should attempt to direct care based on INSSs [53].

Low-Risk Neuroblastoma

Patients with low-risk disease have an excellent outcome with >95 % survival rates at 3 years. The low-risk category includes children with stage 1 disease, those with stage 2A/2B, *MYCN-non-amplified* disease and greater than 50 % tumor resection, and infants (age less than 1 year) with stage 4s, *MYCN*-non-amplified, favorable histology, and hyperdiploid tumors [53]. Patients, who have undergone >50 % surgical resection, can be monitored every 3 months with ultrasound for the first year and then every 6 months until 3 years after diagnosis. Infants with asymptomatic stage 4s disease can be monitored without the need for surgical resection as greater than 50 % of patients have spontaneous tumor regression. Most patients do not require additional chemotherapy and/or radiation, and these treatment modalities should be reserved for disease recurrence [54].

Intermediate-Risk Disease

Intermediate-risk therapy stratification is guided by patient's age, stage, and biological characteristics of the tumor. Baker and colleagues showed that moderate de-intensification of therapy while maintaining survival is feasible [33]. The outcome after reduced chemotherapy for intermediate-risk neuroblastoma showed that 3-year overall survival for the entire group was 96 %; survival was 98 % for those with favorable biological features, and 93 % for those with unfavorable features [33]. The INRG classification table outlines appropriate treatment assignments (Table 23.1).

The most recent COG protocol (ANBL0531) utilized advanced molecular diagnostics to further intensify therapy in patients who did not have biologically unfavorable segmental chromosomal abnormalities (Table 23.5).

Recent intermediate-risk studies have shown that aggressive surgery and radiation therapy can be avoided in most patients [54]. Therefore, surgical resection should be focused on tumor debulking without increasing risk of surgical complications which may results in significant morbidities and mortalities. Radiation therapy should be provided for intermediate-risk group patients who have refractory disease or local recurrences [55], while maintaining similar outcome. The overall surgical goal in intermediate-risk patients is to perform the most complete tumor resection possible, consistent with preservation of full organ and neurologic function. This may necessitate leaving residual disease adherent to critical anatomic structures. If a primary tumor is judged by the surgeon to be unresectable, a diagnostic biopsy is generally obtained and chemotherapy initiated. Delayed surgery is performed after the prescribed number of cycles, as dictated by the group assignment. A reduction in surgical therapy is being evaluated for infants with 4S disease as it is not suggested that they undergo resection of their primary tumor [54].

High-Risk Neuroblastoma

Patients with high-risk neuroblastoma are defined as all patients older than 1.5 years with stage 4 disease and those with stage 3 diseases and unfavorable histology. It has also been shown that stage 4 disease patients, age 12–18 months with unfavorable histology and diploid tumors, tend to have poorer response to therapy. Tumors with

Table 23.5 Children's Oncology Group (COG) neuroblastoma low-, intermediate-, and high-risk group assignment schema used for COG-9641 and COG-A3961 studies[a]

INSS stage	Age	MYCN status	INPC classification	DNA ploidy[b]	Risk group
1	0–21 y	Any	Any	Any	Low
2A/2B[c]	<365 d	Any	Any	Any	Low
	≥365 d–21 y	Nonamplified	Any	–	Low
	≥365 d–21 y	Amplified	Favorable	–	Low
	≥365 d–21 y	Amplified	Unfavorable	–	High
3[d]	<365 d	Nonamplified	Any	Any	Intermediate
	<365 d	Amplified	Any	Any	High
	≥365 d–21 y	Nonamplified	Favorable	–	Intermediate
	≥365 d–21 y	Nonamplified	Unfavorable	–	High
	≥365 d–21 y	Amplified	Any	–	High
4[d]	<548 d	Nonamplified	Any	Any	Intermediate
	<365 d	Amplified	Any	Any	High
	≥548 d–21 y	Any	Any	–	High
4S[e]	<365 d	Nonamplified	Favorable	>1	Low
	<365 d	Nonamplified	Any	=1	Intermediate
	<365 d	Nonamplified	Unfavorable	Any	Intermediate
	<365 d	Amplified	Any	Any	High

Source: Park JR, Bagatell R, London WB, Maris JM, Cohn SL, Mattay KM, et al. Children's Oncology Group's 2013 blueprint for research: neuroblastoma. Pediatr. Blood Cancer. June, 2013; 60(6):985–93

INPC International Neuroblastoma Pathologic Classification, *INSS* International Neuroblastoma Staging System

[a]The COG-9641 and COG-A3961 trials established the current standard of care for neuroblastoma patients in terms of risk group assignment and treatment strategies

[b]DNA ploidy: DNA index (DI) > 1 is favorable, = 1 is unfavorable; hypodiploid tumors (with DI < 1) will be treated as a tumor with a DI > 1 (DI < 1 [hypodiploid] to be considered favorable ploidy)

[c]INSS stage 2A/2B symptomatic patients with spinal cord compression, neurologic deficits, or other symptoms should be treated with immediate chemotherapy for four cycles

[d]INSS stage 3 or stage 4 patients with clinical symptoms as listed above should receive immediate chemotherapy

[e]INSS stage 4S infants with favorable biology and clinical symptoms should be treated with immediate chemotherapy until asymptomatic (2–4 cycles). Clinical symptoms include respiratory distress with or without hepatomegaly or cord compression and neurologic deficit or inferior vena cava compression and renal ischemia; or genitourinary obstruction; or gastrointestinal obstruction and vomiting; or coagulopathy with significant clinical hemorrhage unresponsive to replacement therapy

MYCN amplification have consistently been shown to lead to poor outcomes; therefore, patients of any age and any stage (except stage 1) with *MYCN*-amplified tumors should be classified as high risk. Numerous studies have shown correlation with elevated LDH and poorer outcomes. These serum markers lose their statistical significance in the presence of LOH and *MYCN* biological markers [56]. High-risk neuroblastoma should be treated with multimodal therapy, including surgery, radiotherapy, chemotherapy, autologous hematopoietic stem cell transplant, and biological/immunological therapy. Induction therapy entails time and dose-intensive chemotherapy with goal of complete or very good partial response at the end of induction phase of therapy. Recent data suggests that end-of-induction response based on the Curie scoring system is highly correlative to outcome [53]. The North American approach to induction therapy is based on the N7 Memorial Sloan-Kettering Cancer Center induction regimen with modification of first two cycles to minimize toxicities, while maintaining similar outcomes (ANBL02P1) [57]. The most successful approach to date for treating high-risk neuroblastoma patients has included intensive induction chemotherapy, myeloablative consolidation therapy with stem cell rescue, and targeted therapy for minimal residual [57]. The induction regimen from the COG ANBL02P1 study demonstrates tolerability and feasibility of delivering a dose-intensive topotecan and cyclophosphamide regimen to newly diagnosed patients with high-risk neuroblastoma [58]. The first two cycles of therapy entail cyclophosphamide and topotecan, followed by alternating cyclophosphamide, doxorubicin, and vincristine, and cisplatin and etoposide.

The European-based SIOPEN regimen has similar end of induction outcomes with use of intensively timed Rapid COJEC regimen, which entails cisplatin (C), vincristine (O), carboplatin (J), etoposide (E), and cyclophosphamide (C). Despite similar end of induction outcomes, these studies have not been compared in a randomized controlled trial. Additionally, the Rapid COJEC regimen has relatively higher risk of infectious complications [59].

The role of surgery in the management of children with high-risk neuroblastoma is controversial. Several reports have suggested that patients with INSS stage 3 or 4 disease that undergo gross total resection of their primary tumor and loco regional disease experience improved local tumor control and increased overall survival [60]; however, other reports have differed in their analysis. Despite the uncertainty of the role of surgery, the COG high-risk protocol currently recommends attempting gross total resection of the primary tumor and loco regional disease in patients with high-risk neuroblastoma. Most children undergo surgery after the completion of the fourth or fifth cycle of induction chemotherapy, given that tumor volume reduction plateaus after the second or third cycle [60].

Patients with a good end of induction response should undergo a high-dose myeloablative autologous bone marrow transplant, followed by radiation therapy. Numerous studies have shown that high-dose myeloablative therapy with stem cell rescue improves outcome in children with high-risk therapy [59]. However, there is some controversy regarding the optimal conditioning regimen [61]. The SIOPEN group recently completed their trial showing an improved outcome with use of Busulfan/Melphalan conditioning regimen compared to the COG's conditioning regimen, cisplatin, etoposide, and melphalan. Currently it is unclear, which regimen is superior, as the induction regimen was different with the two groups. COG's current study is evaluating the use of Busulfan/Melphalan in a pilot study using the ANBL0532 induction regimen [48]. Recently, Children's Oncology Group protocol (ANBL0532) evaluated single vs. tandem autologous stem cell transplant and boost radiation to the residual tumor volume. Patients who have achieved a complete response at primary tumor site at the end of induction therapy, should receive 21.6 Gy to the site of primary loco regional disease while areas with gross residual disease should be treated with an additional boost of 14.4 Gy (36-Gy total). Sites of persistent active metastatic disease prior to stem cell transplantation (i.e., positive sites on metaiodobenzylguanidine [MIBG] or those that do not show diminished enhancement on serial bone scans) should be irradiated at the same time and with the same dose as the primary site [55, 62].

Maintenance therapy is aimed towards targeting the minimal residual disease. 13-*cis* retinoic acid has been shown to help residual neuroblastoma cells differentiate and thereby improving outcomes when used in the minimal residual disease setting [27]. The therapy entails 6 monthly 14-day cycles. Recently, Children's Oncology Group showed that outcome for children with high-risk neuroblastoma was improved with addition of immunotherapy using chimerical ch14.18 directed against neuroblastoma tumor antigen GD2, combined with cytokines (IL-2) and granulocyte-macrophage colony stimulating factor (GMCSF) [63]. However, these therapies are not typically available in the resource-limited settings at this time [57].

Follow-Up Studies for Monitoring Disease Activity

The surveillance studies during and immediately after treatment are capable of detecting asymptomatic and unsuspected relapses in a substantial group of patients. These studies are the most reliable test to detect disease activity.

- *Urinary and serum catecholamines*: More than 90 % of patients show at least one elevation of the serum catecholamine, dopamine, adrenaline, or noradrenalin and/or its metabolites, urinary homovanillic acid and vanyilmandelic acid. These levels decrease with tumor regression and in many cases increase with the progression of the tumor. It should be noted that persistence of urine catecholamines in isolation may not definitively identify disease recurrence as these catecholamines may be elevated with ganglioneuroblastoma and ganglioneuroma.
- *Radiographic imaging*: The radiographic modalities such as computerized tomography (CT) scan or magnetic resonance imaging (MRI) are commonly used for upfront disease staging and ongoing monitoring of disease activity. Due to the recent concerns of increased risk of secondary malignancies, there has been a trend towards greater use of MRI, when possible. ^{99m}Tc-bone scan has also been utilized for assessing of metastatic bone lesions. A more sensitive and specific alternative in resource-rich countries is the use of I-123 or I-131 MIBG scan or (or FDG-PET if MIBG unavailable or negative).
- *Bone marrow analysis*: One of the most common sites of metastases in the high-risk neuroblastoma is spread to the bone marrow. Due to the patchy and often heterogeneous bone marrow involvement, it is suggested that a bilateral bone marrow aspirate and biopsy be done for analysis. A simple H&E can be done to analyze for metastatic disease. If bone marrow tissue is used to make the primary diagnosis of neuroblastoma, additional immunohistochemistry staining should be done to accurately diagnose neuroblastoma.

Recurrent Neuroblastoma

High-risk neuroblastoma continues to be a challenge and has a recurrence rate of >50 % despite intensive upfront therapies, including autologous bone marrow transplantation. Time to first relapse is a significant predictor of death after relapse; the risk of death is higher for patients who relapse between 6 and 18 months after diagnosis than it is for patients who relapse more than 18 months from diagnosis. Stratification of relapsed patients with neuroblastoma according to the timing of first relapse, age, stage, and *MYCN* status is important in retrieval study designs, especially for patients with stage 3 or 4 *MYCN* amplified tumors [64]. Patients who relapse after having undergone high-risk therapy could be offered irinotecan/temozolomide or cyclophosphamide/topotecan, although the response rates to these therapies for high-risk patients remain <30 % [65].

(131)I-metaiodobenzylguanidine (MIBG) is specifically taken up in neuroblastoma, with a response rate of 20–37 % in relapsed disease. Nonradioactive carrier MIBG molecules inhibit uptake of (131)I-MIBG, theoretically resulting in less tumor radiation and increased risk of cardiovascular toxicity. There has been some success with the use of therapeutic MIBG therapy, but this is not commonly available in resource-limited settings [66]. In developing countries any recurrence in patients initially classified as high risk signifies a very poor prognosis, and palliative care regimen should be strongly considered. Oral etoposide or cyclophosphamide can be considered as a palliative care regimen to aid with life prolongation.

Prognosis

The risk of relapse is based on age at diagnosis; INSS stage, *MYCN* status, and time from diagnosis to first relapse, and are therefore are significant prognostic factors for postrelapse survival [64]. With the current therapeutic stratification in patients with neuroblastoma, prognosis of these patients has improved over last 30 years. In patients treated for low-risk and intermediate-risk disease in the developed countries, the overall survival rates are >97 % and 87 %, respectively. Patients with high-risk disease continue to have a poorer outcome, with 40–50 % overall survival, currently [58]. There is significant need for advancement in the care of children with neuroblastoma, especially in the resource-limited setting.

Limitations in Resource-Limited Settings

Despite progress made in the care of children with neuroblastoma in many developed countries, the challenges remain in resource-limited settings. The challenges are not only due to diagnostic and treatment capabilities but also due to limited supportive measures such as availability of antibiotics, blood product support, oncology-trained medical support staff, intensive care unit, infection control, and patient living conditions. Each of these limitations, among many others, compounds the difficulties that are inherently apparent to the providers caring for children with neuroblastoma in these settings. Although these challenges cannot be remedied by any simple measure, a diligent and focused approach to care delivery will help guide progress. The international community and subcommittee of SIOP, Pediatric Oncology in developing countries (PODC), is leading a strong effort to help address some of these challenges. The PODC is spearheading efforts to develop series of treatment guidelines for each pediatric cancer, outlining appropriate diagnostic and treatment strategies that may be suitable based on the institutional setting and resource availability. These guidelines will also help institutions navigate in the safest approach to intensifying therapies and assessing their own resource capabilities to providing the more intensified care.

References

1. Øra I, Eggert A. Progress in treatment and risk stratification of neuroblastoma: impact on future clinical and basic research. Semin Cancer Biol. 2011;21(4):217–28.
2. Parkin DM, Stiller CA, Draper GJ, Bieber CA. The international incidence of childhood cancer. Int J Cancer. 1988;42(4):511–20.
3. Evans AE, D'Angio GJ, Randolph J. A proposed staging for children with neuroblastoma. Children's Cancer Study Group A. Cancer. 1971;27(2):374–8.
4. Brodeur GM, Seeger RC, Barrett A, Castleberry RP, D'Angio G, De Bernardi B, et al. International criteria for diagnosis, staging and response to treatment in patients with neuroblastoma. Prog Clin Biol Res. 1988;271:509–24.
5. Ambros PF, Ambros IM, Brodeur GM, Haber M, Khan J, Nakagawara A, et al. International consensus for neuroblastoma molecular diagnostics: report from the International Neuroblastoma Risk Group (INRG) Biology Committee. Br J Cancer. 2009;100(9):1471–82.
6. Pizzo PA, Poplack DG, editors. Principles and practice of pediatric oncology. 6th ed. Philadelphia: Lippincott Williams & Wilkins; 2010.
7. Stiller CA, Parkin DM. International variations in the incidence of neuroblastoma. Int J Cancer. 1992;52(4):538–43.
8. Olshan AF, Smith J, Cook MN, Grufferman S, Pollock BH, Stram DO, et al. Hormone and fertility drug use and the risk of neuroblastoma: a report from the Children's Cancer Group and the Pediatric Oncology Group. Am J Epidemiol. 1999;150(9):930–8.
9. Shimada H, Ambros IM, Dehner LP, Hata J, Joshi VV, Roald B. Terminology and morphologic criteria of neuroblastic tumors: recommendations by the International Neuroblastoma Pathology Committee. Cancer. 1999;86(2):349–63.
10. Shimada H, Ambros IM, Dehner LP, Hata J, Joshi VV, Roald B, et al. The International Neuroblastoma Pathology Classification (the Shimada system). Cancer. 1999;86(2):364–72.
11. Triche TJ. Neuroblastoma—biology confronts nosology. Arch Pathol Lab Med. 1986;110(11):994–6.
12. Canete A, Gerrard M, Rubie H, Castel V, Di Cataldo A, Munzer C, et al. Poor survival for infants with MYCN-amplified metastatic neuroblastoma despite intensified treatment: the International Society of Pediatric Oncology European Neuroblastoma Experience. J Clin Oncol. 2009;27(7):1014–9.
13. Brodeur GM, Seeger RC, Schwab M, Varmus HE, Bishop JM. Amplification of N-myc in untreated human neuroblastomas correlates with advanced disease stage. Science. 1984;224(4653):1121–4.
14. De Bernardi B, Gerrard M, Boni L, Rubie H, Cañete A, Di Cataldo A, et al. Excellent outcome with reduced treatment for infants with disseminated neuroblastoma without MYCN gene amplification. J Clin Oncol. 2009;27(7):1034–40.
15. Cohn SL, Pearson ADJ, London WB, Monclair T, Ambros PF, Brodeur GM, et al. The International Neuroblastoma Risk Group (INRG) classification system: an INRG Task Force report. J Clin Oncol. 2009;27(2):289–97.
16. Goldsby RE, Matthay KK. Neuroblastoma: evolving therapies for a disease with many faces. Paediatr Drugs. 2004;6(2):107–22.
17. Maris JM, Weiss MJ, Guo C, Gerbing RB, Stram DO, White PS, et al. Loss of heterozygosity at 1p36 independently predicts for disease progression but not decreased overall survival probability in neuroblastoma patients: a Children's Cancer Group study. J Clin Oncol. 2000;18(9):1888–99.
18. Streutker CJ, Thorner P, Fabricius N, Weitzman S, Zielenska M. Telomerase activity as a prognostic factor in neuroblastomas. Pediatr Dev Pathol. 2001; 4(1):62–7.

19. Ambros PF, Ambros IM, Kerbl R, Luegmayr A, Rumpler S, Ladenstein R, et al. Intratumoural heterogeneity of 1p deletions and MYCN amplification in neuroblastomas. Med Pediatr Oncol. 2001;36(1):1–4.
20. Attiyeh EF, London WB, Mossé YP, Wang Q, Winter C, Khazi D, et al. Chromosome 1p and 11q deletions and outcome in neuroblastoma. N Engl J Med. 2005;353(21):2243–53.
21. George RE, Sanda T, Hanna M, Fröhling S, Luther II W, Zhang J, et al. Activating mutations in ALK provide a therapeutic target in neuroblastoma. Nature. 2008;455(7215):975–8.
22. Azarova AM, Gautam G, George RE. Emerging importance of ALK in neuroblastoma. Semin Cancer Biol. 2011;21(4):267–75.
23. Yamamoto K, Hayashi Y, Hanada R, Kikuchi A, Ichikawa M, Tanimura M, et al. Mass screening and age-specific incidence of neuroblastoma in Saitama Prefecture, Japan. J Clin Oncol. 1995;13(8):2033–8.
24. Mahoney NR, Liu GT, Menacker SJ, Wilson MC, Hogarty MD, Maris JM. Pediatric Horner syndrome: etiologies and roles of imaging and urine studies to detect neuroblastoma and other responsible mass lesions. Am J Ophthalmol. 2006;142(4):651–9.
25. DuBois SG, Kalika Y, Lukens JN, Brodeur GM, Seeger RC, Atkinson JB, et al. Metastatic sites in stage IV and IVS neuroblastoma correlate with age, tumor biology, and survival. J Pediatr Hematol Oncol. 1999;21(3):181–9.
26. Castleberry RP. Neuroblastoma. Eur J Cancer. 1997; 33(9):1430–7. discussion 1437–8.
27. Hsu LL, Evans AE, D'Angio GJ. Hepatomegaly in neuroblastoma stage 4s: criteria for treatment of the vulnerable neonate. Med Pediatr Oncol. 1996;27(6):521–8.
28. De Bernardi B, Balwierz W, Bejent J, Cohn SL, Garrè ML, Iehara T, et al. Epidural compression in neuroblastoma: diagnostic and therapeutic aspects. Cancer Lett. 2005;228(1–2):283–99.
29. Matthay KK, Blaes F, Hero B, Plantaz D, De Alarcon P, Mitchell WG, et al. Opsoclonus myoclonus syndrome in neuroblastoma a report from a workshop on the dancing eyes syndrome at the advances in neuroblastoma meeting in Genoa, Italy, 2004. Cancer Lett. 2005;228(1–2):275–82.
30. Bourdeaut F, de Carli E, Timsit S, Coze C, Chastagner P, Sarnacki S, et al. VIP hypersecretion as primary or secondary syndrome in neuroblastoma: a retrospective study by the Société Française des Cancers de l'Enfant (SFCE). Pediatr Blood Cancer. 2009;52(5):585–90.
31. Brodeur GM, Pritchard J, Berthold F, Carlsen NL, Castel V, Castelberry RP, et al. Revisions of the international criteria for neuroblastoma diagnosis, staging, and response to treatment. J Clin Oncol. 1993; 11(8):1466–77.
32. Laug WE, Siegel SE, Shaw KN, Landing B, Baptista J, Gutenstein M. Initial urinary catecholamine metabolite concentrations and prognosis in neuroblastoma. Pediatrics. 1978;62(1):77–83.
33. Baker DL, Schmidt ML, Cohn SL, Maris JM, London WB, Buxton A, et al. Outcome after reduced chemotherapy for intermediate-risk neuroblastoma. N Engl J Med. 2010;363(14):1313–23.
34. Strother DR, London WB, Schmidt ML, Brodeur GM, Shimada H, Thorner P, et al. Outcome after surgery alone or with restricted use of chemotherapy for patients with low-risk neuroblastoma: results of Children's Oncology Group study P9641. J Clin Oncol. 2012;30(15):1842–8.
35. Beiske K, Burchill SA, Cheung IY, Hiyama E, Seeger RC, Cohn SL, et al. Consensus criteria for sensitive detection of minimal neuroblastoma cells in bone marrow, blood and stem cell preparations by immunocytology and QRT-PCR: recommendations by the International Neuroblastoma Risk Group Task Force. Br J Cancer. 2009;100(10):1627–37.
36. Taggart DR, Han MM, Quach A, Groshen S, Ye W, Villablanca JG, et al. Comparison of iodine-123 metaiodobenzylguanidine (MIBG) scan and [18F]fluorodeoxyglucose positron emission tomography to evaluate response after iodine-131 MIBG therapy for relapsed neuroblastoma. J Clin Oncol. 2009;27(32):5343–9.
37. Shimada H, Umehara S, Monobe Y, Hachitanda Y, Nakagawa A, Goto S, et al. International Neuroblastoma Pathology Classification for prognostic evaluation of patients with peripheral neuroblastic tumors: a report from the Children's Cancer Group. Cancer. 2001;92(9):2451–61.
38. Sebire NJ, Gibson S, Rampling D, Williams S, Malone M, Ramsay AD. Immunohistochemical findings in embryonal small round cell tumors with molecular diagnostic confirmation. Appl Immunohistochem Mol Morphol. 2005;13(1):1–5.
39. Peuchmaur M, d'Amore ESG, Joshi VV, Hata J, Roald B, Dehner LP, et al. Revision of the International Neuroblastoma Pathology Classification: confirmation of favorable and unfavorable prognostic subsets in ganglioneuroblastoma, nodular. Cancer. 2003; 98(10):2274–81.
40. Schleiermacher G, Michon J, Ribeiro A, Pierron G, Mosseri V, Rubie H, et al. Segmental chromosomal alterations lead to a higher risk of relapse in infants with MYCN-non-amplified localised unresectable/disseminated neuroblastoma (a SIOPEN collaborative study). Br J Cancer. 2011;105(12):1940–8.
41. Fischer M, Bauer T, Oberthür A, Hero B, Theissen J, Ehrich M, et al. Integrated genomic profiling identifies two distinct molecular subtypes with divergent outcome in neuroblastoma with loss of chromosome 11q. Oncogene. 2010;29(6):865–75.
42. Spitz R, Hero B, Ernestus K, Berthold F. FISH analyses for alterations in chromosomes 1, 2, 3, and 11 define high-risk groups in neuroblastoma. Med Pediatr Oncol. 2003;41(1):30–5.
43. Brodeur GM. Neuroblastoma—clinical applications of molecular parameters. Brain Pathol. 1990;1(1): 47–54.
44. Bilke S, Chen Q-R, Whiteford CC, Khan J. Detection of low level genomic alterations by comparative genomic hybridization based on cDNA micro-arrays. Bioinformatics. 2005;21(7):1138–45.

45. Spitz R, Hero B, Simon T, Berthold F. Loss in chromosome 11q identifies tumors with increased risk for metastatic relapses in localized and 4S neuroblastoma. Clin Cancer Res. 2006;12(11 Pt 1):3368–73.
46. Janoueix-Lerosey I, Schleiermacher G, Michels E, Mosseri V, Ribeiro A, Lequin D, et al. Overall genomic pattern is a predictor of outcome in neuroblastoma. J Clin Oncol. 2009;27(7):1026–33.
47. Katzenstein HM, Bowman LC, Brodeur GM, Thorner PS, Joshi VV, Smith EI, et al. Prognostic significance of age, MYCN oncogene amplification, tumor cell ploidy, and histology in 110 infants with stage D(S) neuroblastoma: the pediatric oncology group experience–a pediatric oncology group study. J Clin Oncol. 1998;16(6):2007–17.
48. Park JR, Bagatell R, London WB, Maris JM, Cohn SL, Mattay KM, et al. Children's Oncology Group's 2013 blueprint for research: neuroblastoma. Pediatr Blood Cancer. 2013;60(6):985–93.
49. Monclair T, Brodeur GM, Ambros PF, Brisse HJ, Cecchetto G, Holmes K, et al. The International Neuroblastoma Risk Group (INRG) staging system: an INRG Task Force report. J Clin Oncol. 2009;27(2):298–303.
50. Taggart DR, London WB, Schmidt ML, DuBois SG, Monclair TF, Nakagawara A, et al. Prognostic value of the stage 4S metastatic pattern and tumor biology in patients with metastatic neuroblastoma diagnosed between birth and 18 months of age. J Clin Oncol. 2011;29(33):4358–64.
51. Goto S, Umehara S, Gerbing RB, Stram DO, Brodeur GM, Seeger RC, et al. Histopathology (International Neuroblastoma Pathology Classification) and MYCN status in patients with peripheral neuroblastic tumors: a report from the Children's Cancer Group. Cancer. 2001;92(10):2699–708.
52. Cangemi G, Reggiardo G, Barco S, Barbagallo L, Conte M, D'Angelo P, et al. Prognostic value of ferritin, neuron-specific enolase, lactate dehydrogenase, and urinary and plasmatic catecholamine metabolites in children with neuroblastoma. Onco Targets Ther. 2012;5:417–23.
53. Davidoff AM. Neuroblastoma. Semin Pediatr Surg. 2012;21(1):2–14.
54. Perez CA, Matthay KK, Atkinson JB, Seeger RC, Shimada H, Haase GM, et al. Biologic variables in the outcome of stages I and II neuroblastoma treated with surgery as primary therapy: a Children's Cancer Group study. J Clin Oncol. 2000;18(1):18–26.
55. Simon T, Hero B, Bongartz R, Schmidt M, Müller RP, Berthold F. Intensified external-beam radiation therapy improves the outcome of stage 4 neuroblastoma in children>1 year with residual local disease. Strahlenther Onkol. 2006;182(7):389–94.
56. Volchenboum SL, Cohn SL. Progress in defining and treating high-risk neuroblastoma: lessons from the bench and bedside. J Clin Oncol. 2009;27(7):1003–4.
57. Cheung NK, Kushner BH, LaQuaglia M, Kramer K, Gollamudi S, Heller G, et al. N7: a novel multimodality therapy of high risk neuroblastoma (NB) in children diagnosed over 1 year of age. Med Pediatr Oncol. 2001;36(1):227–30.
58. Park JR, Scott JR, Stewart CF, London WB, Naranjo A, Santana VM, et al. Pilot induction regimen incorporating pharmacokinetically guided topotecan for treatment of newly diagnosed high-risk neuroblastoma: a Children's Oncology Group study. J Clin Oncol. 2011;29(33):4351–7.
59. Ladenstein R, Valteau-Couanet D, Brock P, Yaniv I, Castel V, Laureys G, et al. Randomized Trial of prophylactic granulocyte colony-stimulating factor during rapid COJEC induction in pediatric patients with high-risk neuroblastoma: the European HR-NBL1/SIOPEN study. J Clin Oncol. 2010;28(21):3516–24.
60. Moon S-B, Park K-W, Jung S-E, Youn W-J. Neuroblastoma: treatment outcome after incomplete resection of primary tumors. Pediatr Surg Int. 2009;25(9):789–93.
61. Matthay KK, Villablanca JG, Seeger RC, Stram DO, Harris RE, Ramsay NK, et al. Treatment of high-risk neuroblastoma with intensive chemotherapy, radiotherapy, autologous bone marrow transplantation, and 13-cis-retinoic acid. Children's Cancer Group. N Engl J Med. 1999;341(16):1165–73.
62. Laprie A, Michon J, Hartmann O, Munzer C, Leclair M-D, Coze C, et al. High-dose chemotherapy followed by locoregional irradiation improves the outcome of patients with international neuroblastoma staging system stage II and III neuroblastoma with MYCN amplification. Cancer. 2004;101(5):1081–9.
63. Yu AL, Gilman AL, Ozkaynak MF, London WB, Kreissman SG, Chen HX, et al. Anti-GD2 antibody with GM-CSF, interleukin-2, and isotretinoin for neuroblastoma. N Engl J Med. 2010;363(14):1324–34.
64. London WB, Castel V, Monclair T, Ambros PF, Pearson ADJ, Cohn SL, et al. Clinical and biologic features predictive of survival after relapse of neuroblastoma: a report from the International Neuroblastoma Risk Group project. J Clin Oncol. 2011;29(24):3286–92.
65. Bagatell R, London WB, Wagner LM, Voss SD, Stewart CF, Maris JM, et al. Phase II study of irinotecan and temozolomide in children with relapsed or refractory neuroblastoma: a Children's Oncology Group study. J Clin Oncol. 2011;29(2):208–13.
66. Matthay KK, Weiss B, Villablanca JG, Maris JM, Yanik GA, Dubois SG, Stubbs J, Groshen S, Tsao-Wei D, Hawkins R, Jackson H, Goodarzian F, Daldrup-Link H, Panigrahy A, Towbin A, Shimada H, Barrett J, Lafrance N, Babich J. Dose escalation study of no-carrier-added 131I-metaiodobenzylguanidine for relapsed or refractory neuroblastoma: new approaches to neuroblastoma therapy consortium trial. J Nucl Med. 2012;53(7):1155–63.

Nephroblastoma

24

Jean-Jacques Atteby Yao, Norbert Graf, and Gordan M. Vujanic

Introduction

Nephroblastoma or Wilms tumor (named after the German surgeon Max Wilms who in 1899 reported a series of renal tumors in children suggesting that they all represent one tumor with different histological patterns) is the most common malignant renal tumor in children. Other renal tumors of childhood include mesoblastic nephroma (4–5 %), clear cell sarcoma of the kidney (CCSK) (3–4 %), rhabdoid tumor of the kidney (RTK) (2 %), renal cell carcinomas (3 %), and other very rare tumors [1].

Nephroblastoma represents about 7–8 % of all childhood cancers in Europe [1]. In Africa rates are not well known but hospital statistics place it in the second place after Burkitt's lymphoma [2]. In some areas of Africa nephroblastoma is recognized as the most common malignant tumor in children [3].

Over the last few decades a very significant progress has been made in the treatment of the disease with a cure rate of about 90 % in Europe and Northern America [4], making it one of the most treatable malignant tumors in children.

J.-J.A. Yao (✉)
Département of MERE-ENFANT,
UFR SM Univresité Cocody/Abidjan RCI,
Abidjan, Republique de Cote d'Ivoire
e-mail: attebyjj@yahoo.fr

N. Graf, M.D.
Department of Pediatric Oncology and Oncology,
Saarland University, Homburg 66421, Germany

G.M. Vujanic, M.D.
School of Medicine Cardiff University, Cardiff, UK

Definition

Nephroblastoma is a malignant embryonal tumor of the kidney that develops from nephrogenic tissue and it mimics embryonic stages of the renal development. It is by far the most common malignant renal tumor of childhood, representing about 85 % of renal tumors at this age group [5].

Epidemiology

Nephroblastoma occurs mainly in young children with the median age at presentation 3–5 years, and 98 % of cases in children under 10 years of age [1]. It is uncommon in neonates and is exceptionally rare in adults. The incidence is lower among Asians, but higher among African-Americans [1]. Girls are slightly more affected than boys [1], and it occurs equally in both kidneys. Most cases are unilateral and unicentric, but in 8–10 % of cases tumor presents as bilateral disease [6] (Fig. 24.1).

In 90 % of cases nephroblastoma is sporadic, but in 10 % of cases it is associated with congenital anomalies and syndromes [7] (Table 24.1).

Molecular genetic studies of these syndromes led to identification of *WT1* gene on the chromosome

D.C. Stefan and C. Rodriguez-Galindo (eds.), *Pediatric Hematology-Oncology in Countries with Limited Resources: A Practical Manual*, DOI 10.1007/978-1-4614-3891-5_24,

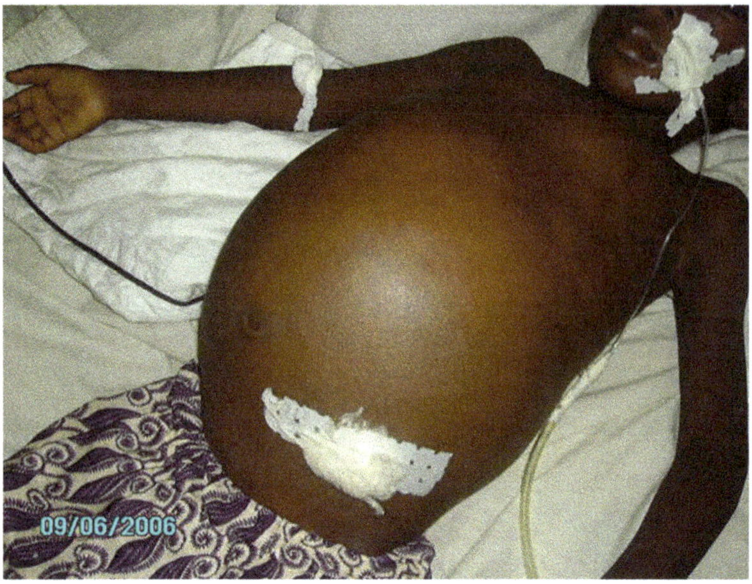

Fig. 24.1 Bilateral nephroblastoma in a 7 year old boy with pulmonary distress

Table 24.1 The most common congenital anomalies and syndromes associated with nephroblastoma

Cryptorchidism
Hypospadia
Pseudohermaphroditism
Hemihypertrophy
Beckwith–Wiedemann syndrome
WAGR (Wilms, aniridia, genital anomalies, retardation) syndrome
Denys–Drash syndrome
Frasier syndrome
Perlman syndrome

11p13, and it is likely that the second gene, *WT2*, is located close to it, on the chromosome 11p15 [8]. However, only about 1 % of WTs are familial.

Diagnosis

Clinical Features

Wilms tumor is usually detected incidentally as a large abdominal mass by the patient's parents or during a physical examination performed for other medical reasons. The mass is usually painless, hard, smooth, and confined to the flank or one side of the abdomen. Other symptoms and signs that may occur include abdominal pain (in approximately 30 % of patients), hematuria (12–25 % of patients), and hypertension (25 % of cases) [1]. No serum markers to diagnose the tumor are used in clinical practice.

Clinical Examination

Once the child is diagnosed with a large abdominal mass, further investigations are needed in order to reach the diagnosis. During the initial clinical examination one should look for possible anomalies associated with nephroblastoma (Fig. 24.2).

It is important to prevent any abdominal trauma by temporarily prohibiting risky activities (jump-bike) and to refer the child as soon as possible to a team specialized in the management of childhood tumors.

This team will confirm the diagnosis by imaging and will complete the staging.

Imaging Studies

There is no laboratory test that can be done in order to diagnose nephroblastoma. Urinary catecholamine metabolites are performed in the dif-

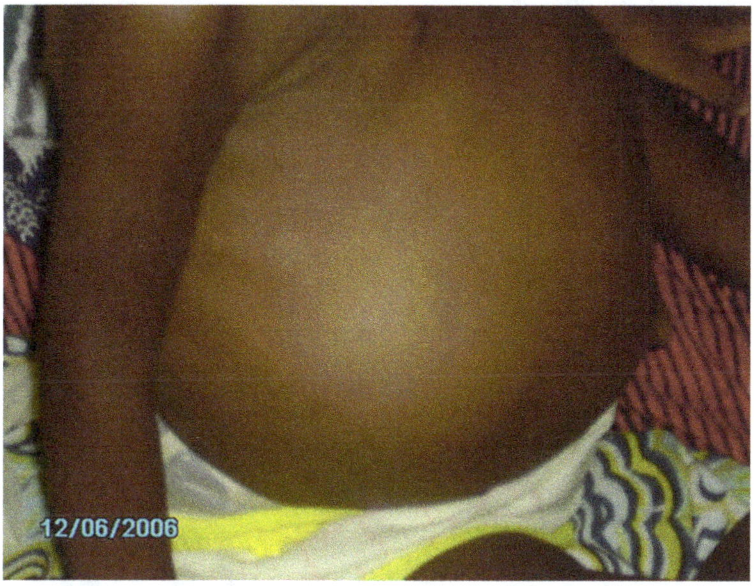

Fig. 24.2 Massive nephroblastoma of the right kidney in a 15 months old girl

ferential diagnosis of neuroblastoma; they are normal in nephroblastoma. The preoperative diagnosis of nephroblastoma is based on imaging studies [9] including:

- Abdominal ultrasound
- Abdominal computed tomography (CT)
- Intravenous urography (IVU)
- Abdominal magnetic resonance imaging (MRI)

Abdominal Ultrasound Scan

Abdominal ultrasound scan is adequate for reaching the diagnosis of nephroblastoma in 90 % of cases and it is the first imaging study to be done in any child presenting with an abdominal mass. The tumor is hyperechoic and often shows areas of necrosis. It is important to assess the location of tumor in the kidney and to measure tumor in three dimensions as it is important for assessment of the response to preoperative chemotherapy. Other things that one should look for are the presence of any vascular thrombi, lymphadenopathy, contralateral kidney, and possible hepatic metastases [9].

Abdominal CT Scan

CT scan is only used when the diagnosis is difficult [9] such as in cases when some extrarenal tumors invade the kidney (especially neuroblastoma), in cases of suspected tumor rupture (to assess its extent and intraperitoneal rupture), and in cases of contralateral lesions and suspected liver metastases. A series of images in a child with a nephroblastoma are presented in Fig. 24.3.

Intravenous Urography

This test may be useful when the diagnosis is uncertain. It may show the urinary tract opacification observed in a Wilms tumor (kidney tumor syndrome) with disruption of normal pyelocalyceal architecture that appears stretched, distorted, and amputated. In 5–10 % of cases, the kidney does not show up or excrete very low contrast agent. So it is recommended to increase the dose of contrast agent if the kidney function is normal and also perform a later x-ray.

Abdominal MRI

MRI may aid in the diagnosis of thrombus of the vena cava and it allows verify the possibility of rupture within or behind the peritoneum. Finally, MRI can assess if the other kidney is involved [9].

Differential Diagnosis

Imaging studies are helpful in the differential diagnosis of other tumors, cystic malformations,

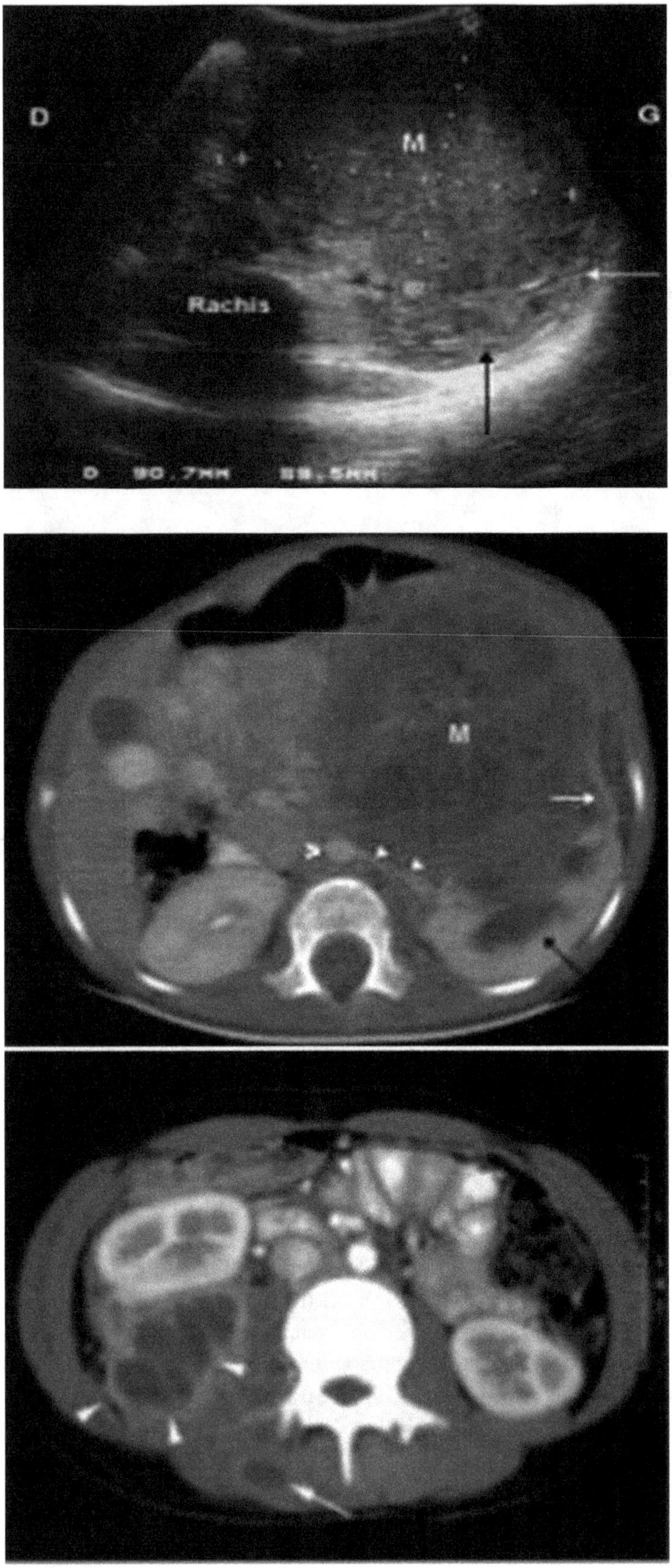

Fig. 24.3 Radiology nephroblastoma

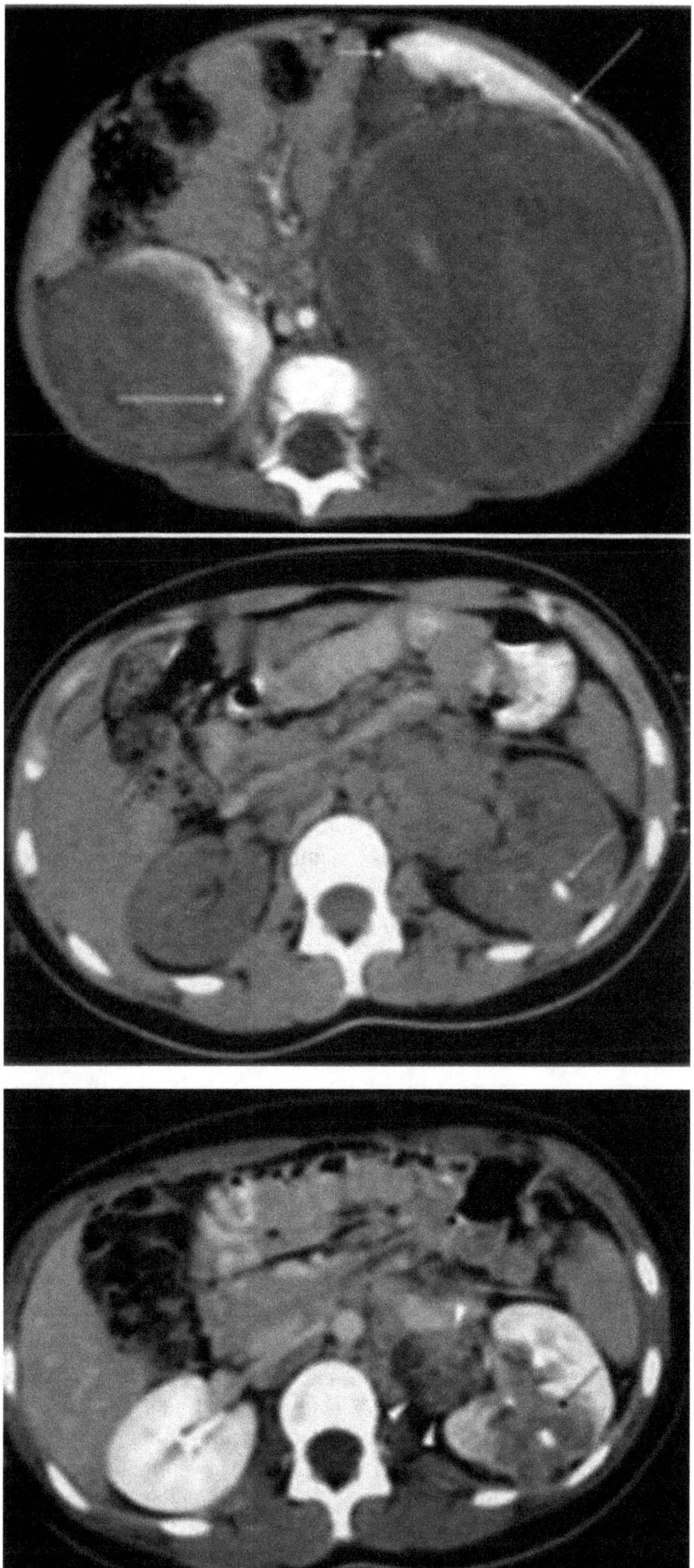

Fig. 24.3 (continued)

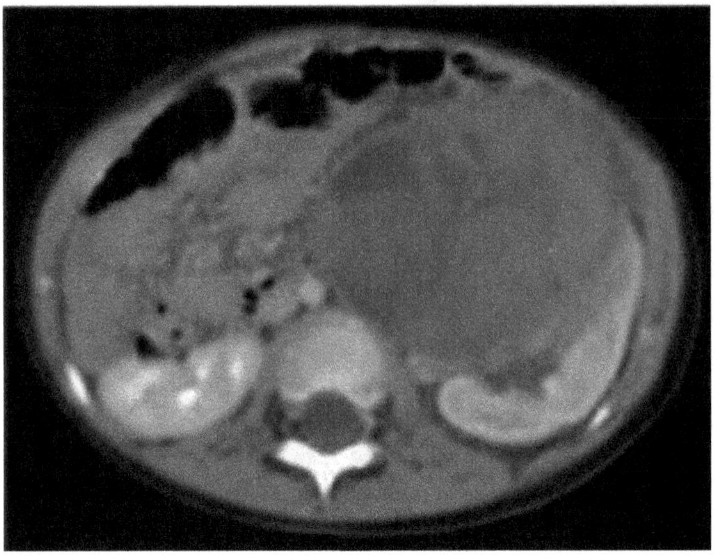

Fig. 24.3 (continued)

and hydronephrosis. In the differential diagnosis other retroperitoneal solid masses that should be considered include:

- Abscess of the kidney (infectious syndrome).
- Renal localization of Burkitt's lymphoma.
- Other retroperitoneal extrarenal tumors in particular neuroblastoma (imposing determination of urinary metabolites, catecholamines), hepatoblastoma, and germ cell tumor (teratoma) which may require measurements of serum level of alpha feto-protein and beta HCG.

Pathology

Gross Pathology

Wilms tumor is usually a large, grossly distorting tumor of the kidney located anywhere within the organ, and very rarely may be even extrarenal. The average weight is about 500 g (300 g after preoperative chemotherapy), but it may range from 60 g to 6.5 kg [5]. The tumor is usually single or rarely multifocal, heterogeneous, often with solid and soft areas due to hemorrhage and/or necrosis, especially in cases treated with preoperative chemotherapy when it may also show a prominent cystic pattern. It may invade renal pelvis, which explains hematuria. Renal vein may be occupied by a tumor thrombus that sometimes grows into the inferior vena cava and reaches the right atrium. Regional lymph nodes are often bulky but are invaded by a tumor only in 15 % of cases [5].

Primarily operated Wilms tumor is a fragile tumor that can rupture and bleed easily and disseminate in the retroperitoneum. If surgery is done following preoperative chemotherapy, tumor's capsule is much thicker reducing a risk of intraoperative ruptures.

Microscopy

Nephroblastoma is typically composed of different histological components including blastemal, epithelial, and stromal elements which may be represented in any proportion [5, 10]. If none of these components is predominant, tumor is subclassified as triphasic or mixed type, but biphasic or even monophasic type is not rare. The blastemal component may show numerous patterns, and the epithelial and stromal components may show different lines and different degrees of differentiation resulting in innumerable histological patterns. The epithelial component may show primitive epithelial structures such as rosettes, poorly to moderately differentiated tubules, or well-differentiated glomeruli structures. The stromal component may contain a hypocellular, primitive stroma, or a well-differentiated stroma

Table 24.2 The COG and SIOP histological classifications of renal tumors of childhood

COG	SIOP
	Low risk
Mesoblastic nephroma	Mesoblastic nephroma
Cystic partially differentiated nephroblastoma (CPDN)	CPDN
	Completely necrotic type
Favorable histology	*Intermediate risk*
Mixed	Mixed type
Epithelial predominant	Epithelial type
Stromal predominant	Stromal type
Blastemal predominant	Regressive type
	Focal anaplasia
Unfavorable histology	*High risk*
Focal and diffuse anaplasia	Diffuse anaplasia
	Blastemal type
Clear cell sarcoma of kidney (CCSK)	CCSK
Rhabdoid tumor of kidney (RTK)	RTK

with rhabdomyoblastic differentiation, fat and cartilage. Each tumor component may exhibit anaplasia (found in 5–8 % of nephroblastomas) which is defined as the presence of enlarged, atypical, multipolar mitoses, nuclear enlargement, and hyperchromasia. Anaplasia is further classified as focal and diffuse. Preoperative chemotherapy destroys tumor's components and changes its histological features making histological subclassification more challenging [11]. Histological criteria in the International Society of Pediatric Oncology (SIOP) and Children's Oncology Group (COG) classifications differ and should be applied according to preoperative treatment (i.e., if no preoperative chemotherapy was given, the COG criteria should be used [5]; if preoperative chemotherapy was given, the SIOP criteria should be applied) [11]. In both classifications, tumors are stratified into three prognostic groups [5, 12] (Table 24.2).

Staging

Staging criteria slightly differ between the SIOP [11] and the COG (formerly NWTS—Wilms Tumor National Study Group) (Table 24.3).

Table 24.3 Staging criteria developed by the SIOP 2001 Trial

Stage I	Tumor is limited to the kidney and is completely excised. The capsule is intact; no tumor rupture; completely excised
Stage II	Tumor infiltrates the renal sinus or extends beyond the tumor capsule, into the perirenal fat but is completely excised
Stage III	Tumor excision incomplete; tumor rupture (pre- or intraoperative); regional lymph nodes contain tumor; open ("wedge") biopsy
Stage IV	Distant metastases (lungs, liver, bone, lymph nodes beyond the abdominopelvic region)
Stage V	Bilateral renal involvement at diagnosis (each side has to be staged separately)

The full staging of the patient requires the imaging/ultrasonographic studies in search for lung metastases which are by far the most frequent, whereas other sites like bone are a more common metastatic site for CCSK. The contralateral kidney should always be checked in order to exclude bilateral disease.

Treatment

There are two internationally accepted protocols used in treatment of nephroblastoma:

- SIOP protocol which uses preoperative chemotherapy followed by postoperative chemotherapy and radiotherapy (if necessary) [13, 14].
- COG protocol which recommends primary surgery followed by further chemotherapy and radiotherapy, if necessary.

In both protocols, there is a small group of patients who are not treated with any postoperative chemotherapy. In the SIOP, it is the patients with stage I completely necrotic nephroblastoma [15], and in the COG it is the patients younger than 24 months of age, with tumors under 550 g in weight, with favorable (non-anaplastic) histology, and stage I disease (with examined lymph nodes) [16].

The SIOP approach with preoperative chemotherapy makes tumors smaller and better encapsulated, reducing a risk of pre- or intraoperative rupture [17–19]. Preoperative therapy is given if a tumor shows typical clinical and imaging features of nephroblastoma, with no histological diagnosis. Postoperative treatment is based on histological subclassification and stage of a tumor [12, 13].

Surgery

A transverse laparotomy incision with subcostal incision is the preferred approach. The exploration begins with the contralateral kidney to ensure the absence of contralateral tumor. An examination of the abdominal cavity, liver, and lymph nodes needs to be done. Any suspicious lesion should be biopsied. Then we proceed with ligation of the first renal vessels reached starting from the artery. Careful examination of the inferior vena cava and renal vein in search of an invasion of the wall and a thrombus is then made. Total nephro-ureterectomy is made by cutting the ureter as low as possible. At all costs the tumor rupture should be avoided as it leads to very aggressive postoperative treatment. Sample of the para-aortic lymph node should be systematically taken even if they appear normal in size. On the other hand, para-aortic lymphadenectomy is not recommended but indicated if they are enlarged.

Before sending the specimen to pathologist, the surgeon should mark the points where there are adhesions or suspected invasions.

Surgery is necessarily selective and individualized in bilateral forms: remove as much as possible the entire tumor tissue or suspected tumor, leaving the maximum healthy renal parenchyma and taking the minimum risk: lumpectomy, partial nephrectomy of the less involved side, or one side total nephrectomy.

Partial nephrectomy is recommended in unilateral forms of small tumors that show regression after preoperative chemotherapy and are located at the poles of a kidney.

Chemotherapy

According to the SIOP protocol, a 2-drug (vincristine and adriamycin D) preoperative chemotherapy is given for 4 weeks for unilateral, localized tumors. Stage IV tumors at diagnosis are treated with 3-drug preoperative chemotherapy (actinomycin D, vincristine, and doxorubicin) for 6 weeks. Postoperative treatment depends on histological subclassification and stage of the tumor [13] (Table 24.4).

Table 24.4 The SIOP postoperative treatment of localized unilateral WT

Risk group	Stage	Postoperative treatment
Low risk	I	No further treatment
	II	N/A (does not exist)
	III	AV (27 weeks)
Intermediate risk	I	AV (4 weeks)
	II	AV (27 weeks)
	III	AV (27 weeks) + RT
High risk	I	AVD (27 weeks)
	II	VP16-Carbo-Cyclo-Dox (34 weeks)
	III	VP16-Carbo-Cyclo-Dox (34 weeks) + RT

A actinomycin D, *V* vincristine, *D* doxorubicin, *Carbo* carboplatin, *VP16* etoposide, *Cyclo* cyclophosphamide, *RT* radiotherapy

The COG postoperative treatment is based on more criteria, including tumor histology, tumor stage, patient age, tumor weight, and molecular markers (loss of heterozygosity at 1p and 16q). On the basis of these criteria, patients are stratified into five risk categories including very low risk, low risk, standard risk, higher-risk favorable histology, and high risk [20].

Some drugs used in nephroblastoma treatment which emerged more recently include ifosfamide (alkylating agent, often effective but with toxicity, especially renal and neurological), etoposide (remarkably effective in nephroblastoma treatment, but with the side effect in the etiology of a variety of secondary leukemias), and carboplatin (efficient, but shows renal toxicity).

Radiotherapy

Radiotherapy is reserved only for advanced stages (3 and 4) and is given in association with prolonged chemotherapy according to the protocols. Radiotherapy is given locally to the renal bed or the whole abdomen (tumor rupture) or to distant metastases (pulmonary) [21].

Conclusions

Nephroblastoma is a tumor which prognosis has been markedly improved over the last few decades due to chemotherapy and multidisciplinary care. It is a tumor relatively easy to diagnose, requiring minimal laboratory and imaging investigations, and, when treated in early stages, has an excellent prognosis [22].

Preoperative chemotherapy has advantages for reducing large tumors, making them safe to operate on and in children with severe malnutrition or associated infections.

An awareness program including nephroblastoma will help in the early recognition of the disease.

Practical Notes for Nephroblastoma in Developing Countries

1. Consider nephroblastoma in an apparently healthy child below the age of 5 who presents with an abdominal mass
2. Look for anomalies and syndromes known to be associated with nephroblastoma
3. Keep laboratory investigations to minimum (electrolytes, blood count, viral tests; consider checking catecholamines to exclude neuroblastoma)
4. In most cases an abdominal ultrasound will be sufficient to make the diagnosis (requires tumor's dimensions and assessment of inferior vena cava involvement)
5. Ask for chest x-rays to exclude lung metastases
6. If available, ask for CT scans of abdomen and chest to obtain more information
7. Do not ask/perform a biopsy (upgrades the tumor to stage 3) and also do not puncture
8. Restart chemotherapy (if required) not later than 10 days after surgery
9. Regular meetings (weekly) with the interdisciplinary team (surgeon, pathologist, pediatric oncologist, social worker, dietician, psychologist, etc.)
10. A strong relationship should be build between the medical team, the child, and the family

References

1. Birch JM, Breslow N. Epidemiologic features of Wilms tumor. Hematol Oncol Clin North Am. 1995;9:1157–78.
2. Stefan DC, Nortje SH, Forman D. Distribution of childhood cancers in Sub-Saharan Africa. 34th International Association of Cancer Registries (IACR) Conference, Cork, Ireland, 17–19 Sept 2012.
3. Stefan DC. Stones DK, Poole JE, Kruger M, Vujanic G. Treatment of nephroblastoma in Africa: which one and at what cost? 44th Congress of the International Society of Paediatric Oncology (SIOP), London, UK, (5–8 October 2012). Pediatr Blood Cancer. 2012;59(6):1060 (PH036).
4. de Kraker J, Prichard-Jones K. Treatment of Wilms tumor: an international perspective. J Clin Oncol. 2005;23:3156–7.
5. Murphy WM, Grignon DJ, Perlman EJ. Kidney tumors in children. In: Tumors of the kidney, bladder, and urinary structures. In: Atlas of tumor pathology, 4th Series, Fascicle 1. Washington, DC: Armed Forces Institute of Pathology; 2004. p. 1–47.
6. Coppes MJ, de Kraker J, Van Dijken PJ, et al. Bilateral Wilms' tumor: long-term survival and some epidemiological features. J Clin Oncol. 1989;7:310–5.
7. Scott RH, Stiller CA, Walker L, Rahman N. Syndromes and constitutional chromosomal abnormalities associated with Wilms syndrome. J Med Genet. 2006;43:705–15.
8. Pritchard-Jones K, Vujanic GM. Recent developments in the molecular pathology of paediatric renal tumours. Open Pathol J. 2010;4:32–9.
9. Brisse HJ, Smets AM, Kaste SC, Owens CM. Imaging in unilateral Wilms tumour. Pediatr Radiol. 2008;38:18–29.
10. Vujanic GM. Renal tumours of childhood: an overview. Diagn Histopathol. 2009;15:501–9.
11. Vujanic GM, Sandstedt B. The pathology of nephroblastoma: the SIOP approach. J Clin Pathol. 2010;63:102–9.
12. Vujanic GM, Sandstedt B, Harms D, Kelsey A, Leuschner I, de Kraker J. Revised International Society of Paediatric Oncology (SIOP) working classification of renal tumors of childhood. Med Pediatr Oncol. 2001;38:79–82.
13. Graf N, Tournade M-F, de Kraker J. The role of preoperative chemotherapy in the management of Wilms' tumor. Urol Clin North Am. 2000; 27:443–54.
14. D'Angio GJ. Pre- or postoperative therapy for Wilms' tumor? J Clin Oncol. 2008;26:4055–7.
15. Boccon-Gibod L, Rey A, Sandstedt B, et al. Complete necrosis induced by preoperative chemotherapy in Wilms' tumor as an indicator of low risk: report of the International Society of Paediatric Oncology (SIOP) Wilms' tumor trial and study 9. Med Pediatr Oncol. 2000;34:183–90.

16. Green DM, Breslow NE, Beckwith JB, Ritchey ML, Shamberger RC, et al. Treatment with nephrectomy only for small, stage I/favourable histology Wilms' tumor: a report from the National Wilms' Tumor Study Group. J Clin Oncol. 2001;19:3719–24.
17. Fuchs J, Kienecker K, Furtwangler R, Warman SW, Burger D, Thurhoff JW, Graf N. Surgical aspects in the treatment of patients with unilateral Wilms tumor: a report from the SIOP 93-10/GPOH. Ann Surg. 2009;249:666–71.
18. Godzinski J, Tournade MF, de Krakere J, et al. Rarity of surgical complications after postchemotherapy nephrectomy for nephroblastoma. Experience of the International Society of Pediatric Oncology. Eur J Pediatr Surg. 1998;8:83–6.
19. Ritchey ML, Shamberger RC, Haase G, Horwitz J, Bergemann T, Breslow NE. Surgical complications after primary nephrectomy for Wilms' tumor: report from the National Wilms' Tumor Study Group. J Am Coll Surg. 2001;192:63–8.
20. Gratias EJ, Dome JS. Current and emerging chemotherapy treatment strategies for Wilms tumor in North America. Paediatr Drugs. 2008;10:115–24.
21. Paulino AC, Wen BC, Brown CK, et al. Late effects in children treated with radiation therapy for Wilms' tumor. Int J Radiat Oncol Biol Phys. 2000; 46:1239–46.
22. Kastle SC, Dome JS, Babyn PS, et al. Wilms tumour: prognostic factors, staging, therapy and late effects. Pediatr Radiol. 2008;38:2–17.

Paediatric Neuro-Oncology

25

Nisreen Amayiri and Eric Bouffet

Introduction

Great disparities exist in the care of children with cancer around the world. It is estimated that more than 80 % of all paediatric cancers occur in countries with limited resources and most disparities are related to differences in health care resources and organization of health care systems [1]. However, in addition to economic barriers, other issues may limit the quality of care delivered to this vulnerable population. In this chapter, we will review the challenges associated with the management of central nervous system tumours in the paediatric population in countries with limited resources and will provide some suggestions and recommendations based on recent successful experiences.

N. Amayiri, M.D.
King Hussein Cancer Center,
202 Queen Rania Al Abdullah Street, P.O Box1269,
Al-Jubeiha, Amman 11941, Jordan
e-mail: namayiri@khcc.jo

E. Bouffet, M.D. (✉)
Hospital for Sick Children, 555 University Avenue,
Toronto, ON, Canada M5G 1X8
e-mail: Eric.bouffet@sickkids.ca

Incidence of CNS Tumours in Countries with Limited Resources

There are only few reports on childhood brain tumours in countries with limited resources. Most publications represent single institution experiences rather than collaborative studies [2–4]. The incidence of childhood brain tumours is difficult to estimate in these countries due to the lack of population-based cancer registries [5, 6]. There are indeed numerous obstacles for the implementation of cancer registries in developing countries. Many of these countries face general problems of poverty, which make cancer diagnosis, treatment and compliance a low priority. In addition, some low-income countries have large shifts in population due to wars, migration, or rapid changes in incidence of birth or death, which result in inaccurate age-specific population estimates [6, 7]. Infection and malnutrition are major causes of death in children from developing countries, thus cancer treatment gets little attention from health care authorities. Due to the complexity of the care of paediatric brain tumour patients, even when epidemiologic studies are available, these patients are often not included [8, 9]. However, proper cancer registries would be the first step to appreciate the extent of the problem in order to implement cancer programs. Registries may also help to identify unique genetic or environmental risks, and allow proper

D.C. Stefan and C. Rodriguez-Galindo (eds.), *Pediatric Hematology-Oncology in Countries with Limited Resources: A Practical Manual*, DOI 10.1007/978-1-4614-3891-5_25,

and timely intervention to improve detection and outcome [6, 7].

Available data suggest a low incidence of CNS tumour in countries with limited resources. While the incidence of brain tumour in the CBTRUS (Central Brain Tumor Registry of the United States) was 4.92 per 100,000 person–years for children less than 15 years during the period 2004–2008 [10]; Manoharan et al. reported an incidence of 0.9 per 100,000 in the Delhi Population Based Cancer Registry (PBCR) for the period 2003–2007 [11]. Whether this lower incidence is real or related to other factors is unknown. One common proposed cause of lower reported incidence of childhood cancer in general in low-income countries is the high mortality rate in young children (under the age of 5 years) that may lead to early death before the child develops cancer. However, there is no statistical reason that this high rate of premature death should influence the overall incidence of childhood cancer. Using data from the International Agency for Cancer Research (IARC), Howard et al. reported a close correlation between the reported incidence of childhood leukemia and the mean annual per capita gross national income [6]. There is no similar study for childhood brain tumours. However, it is very likely that in many low-income countries, children with brain tumour die before diagnosis.

Delay in the Diagnosis of CNS Tumours

Despite advances in neuro-imaging, timely diagnosis of CNS tumours remains a problem in high-income countries [12]. There are no specific studies that have analyzed differences in the delay to diagnosis of CNS tumours between high- and low-income countries. However, the issue of late diagnosis of CNS tumours is obvious for neurosurgeons and oncologists who practice in these countries. Beyond the usual challenges of non-specific symptoms such as vomiting, failure to thrive, hypoactivity, headaches or visual disturbance that are usual factors involved in delayed diagnosis [13], access to neuro-imaging facilities is the main obstacle that patients and families face. The limited number of CT or MRI scans, long waiting lists, particularly when sedation is needed, and in many places the prohibitive cost of these tests are amongst the many reasons that delay or prevent the diagnosis of brain tumour in children in these countries. In most places, the imaging study will be limited to the brain and it is exceptional to have preoperative imaging of the spine when a malignant brain tumour such as medulloblastoma is suspected. Once a brain tumour is diagnosed on imaging, then confirmation of the correct diagnosis would mean a referral to a specialized centre able to take care of these children. Most developing countries lack these centres whether due to unavailability of experienced staff or shortage of equipment [14]; and even when they have one, families from rural areas often face difficulties to access these specialized centres due to financial costs and difficulties in transportation, which will also complicate future compliance during treatment and follow-up.

Cultural Barriers

Confronted with the initial symptoms of a brain tumour, some families tend to seek help from local “healers” or use of complementary and alternative medicine. As a result, this may affect the natural history of the disease and delay the diagnosis of cancer even more [15, 16]. A classical example is the delay to diagnose optic pathways gliomas, and the incidence of blindness associated with this condition, which is much higher in countries with limited resources.

Cancer is a condition that relates to fate, myths and beliefs. In the context of the diagnosis of brain tumour, some families may refuse to be referred to a Cancer Centre because of the risk of marginalization and stigmatization associated with this condition. Cancer-related stigma and myths may also cause families to abandon treatment [17]. Belief that cancer equates death or stigmatism from the diagnosis or its related disability, whether physical or mental will also influence parental of family decisions.

Because the social stigmata of cancer can be so powerful, social barriers must be fully understood before any improved strategy is implemented in low-income countries. Some cultural choices, like treating boys over girls, may affect incidence, survival and mortality data of cancer in some cultural contexts [18]. Other social factors are critical, such as financial and transportation difficulties that have been identified as major sources of abandonment of treatment [19].

Management of Paediatric Brain Tumours in Countries with Limited Resources

Neurosurgery

With a few exceptions, neurosurgical management is generally the first step in the treatment of paediatric brain tumours. Neurosurgeons in low-income countries are overloaded with work and neurosurgical units are generally understaffed [20]. Neurosurgery in these countries faces two main challenges, i.e. quality and quantity in both resources and qualified personnel [14]. The World Health Organization African Subcommittee conducted a survey on African neurosurgical services in the late 1990s. This survey reported a ratio of one African neurosurgeon per 1,352,000 individuals compared to 1/121,000 in Europe and 1/81,000 in North America [21]. Similar figures are described in the South Asian continent. In addition, there are a limited number of neurosurgeons with a paediatric expertise in low-income countries and thus, general neurosurgeons, when available, are expected to operate on children. In such conditions, specific knowledge of the principles of paediatric neuro-oncology is important and unfortunately many general neurosurgeons are not familiar with this specialty. As a result, in most places, surgical intervention is limited to the insertion of a ventriculo-peritoneal shunt when evidence of hydrocephalus is present on the preoperative imaging study. Attempt at complete or near-complete surgical resection is not a common practice, and surgery is usually limited to a biopsy to allow histological diagnosis. Unfortunately, less than gross total resection greatly impacts survival of children with brain tumour like ependymoma or/and would upgrade risk status for some other tumours like medulloblastoma [22, 23]. Neuronavigation and the use of intraoperative microscope are known to facilitate surgery and to improve tumour resection; however, these equipments are scarce in low-income countries, or available in selected private practices, and trained neurosurgeons with the expertise to use these techniques are limited [24]. A recurrent challenge in this context is the management of children who underwent incomplete tumour resection. Most often, neurosurgeons consider that there is no role for further surgery and they refer the child to radiation oncologists or paediatric oncologists for adjuvant treatment. While local oncologists are often unsuccessful in trying to convince referring neurosurgeons to proceed to second look surgery in the context of an incomplete resection, telemedicine experiences that involve a contact between neurosurgeons appear to offer a unique opportunity to discuss such technical issues and to optimize the quality of surgical management [25].

Post-operative intensive care with good monitoring of intracranial pressure, fluids and electrolyte balance is crucial when caring with brain tumour patients especially when hormonal problems are expected like in craniopharyngioma surgery. The lack of such specialized multidisciplinary care will increase perioperative morbidity and mortality.

Neuropathology

Experienced pathologists able to differentiate subtypes of paediatric neurological tumours are absent in many developing countries. The lack of trained personal and inadequate technical equipment is therefore limiting the possibility to achieve a timely and accurate diagnosis in many places. Often, clinicians are faced with long turnover times—sometimes exceeding 1 month—before a diagnosis is proposed [26]. Availability of some important staining techniques may also compromise the possibility to accurately identify tumour types. A classical example is the availability of the BAF47 staining [27]. This staining that has now become part of the standard battery of immunohistochemical staining performed in the context of embryonal tumours of the central nervous system. In this context, collaboration between neuropathologists is critical. In a report on a telemedicine twinning experience in paediatric neuro-oncology between two multidisciplinary programs, the most common recommendation was a review of the neuropathology, which in resulted several cases in a change in the initial diagnosis or in the grading of the tumour with significant consequences in terms of subsequent management [25]. However, a number of factors are limiting this practice that would greatly benefit paediatric neuro-oncology programs in countries with limited resources. In this context, it is likely that a significant number of children are treated without an adequate diagnosis.

Radiation and Radiotherapy Services

Radiation therapy is a critical component of treatment of many central nervous system tumours in children; however, limited radiotherapy machines and personnel make them available only at large centres with long waiting lists [8]. There is evidence that delay in starting radiotherapy has a negative impact on survival in medulloblastoma [28] and there is no doubt that the extent of neurological recovery will be closely dependent on the time to initiate radiation in patients with diffuse pontine glioma patients.

Radiation indications, treatment volumes and doses are determined by tumour histology, extent of disease, anticipated pattern of spread and expected pattern of failure. In malignant CNS tumours, such as medulloblastoma and ependymoma, excellent survival rates have been reported, particularly in patients with average risk features (complete resection and absence of metastatic disease) [29, 30]. Survival rates are above 90 % in patients with germinoma, regardless of metastatic stage, with a combination of chemotherapy and radiation [31]. However, access to radiation oncology services is a prerequisite for successful outcome and the number of radiotherapy machines available in most countries with limited resources is the main barrier to optimal patient care. It is clear that paediatric neuro-oncology programs cannot be developed or implemented in countries, which have no radiation oncology services. A survey of radiotherapy equipments in Africa conducted in 1998 reported that 9/56 countries had no radiotherapy at all, 24 had orthovoltage facilities only, and 2/3 of the Megavoltage equipments available in the continent were located in two countries (Egypt and South Africa) [32]. The supply of radiation equipments available in the continent represented at that time 18 % of the estimated needs. As a consequence, access to radiation is a major issue in most countries with limited resources, and delay in initiation of radiation treatment is a common problem. In several places, paediatric oncologists are trying to overcome this problem by designing protocols that offer post-operative chemotherapy prior to radiation, in particular for medulloblastoma patients. Although this is not an ideal option, this approach may help prevent early recurrence or dissemination following initial surgery. Another limiting factor in the management is the number of well-qualified personnel with an expertise in CNS radiation techniques, and more specifically in paediatrics. Craniospinal radiotherapy (CSI), which is commonly used in the management of medulloblastoma patients, is one of the most complex radiotherapy techniques and evidence from several medulloblastoma trials has suggested that the quality of CSI impacts on outcome [33]. Some groups have started to address specific issues related to the availability of radiation machines. In particular, a group in Cairo has run a randomized trial that has shown similar survival between patients with diffuse intrinsic pontine glioma (DIPG) treated with normal fractionation (30 sessions at 1.8 Gy each) and hypofractionation (13 sessions of 3 Gy each) [34]. The results of this trial may benefit DIPG patients in countries that face limitations in the access to radiation services. Ideally, the radiotherapeutic management of children with CNS tumour in countries with limited resources would benefit from a central referral system that would review and validate indications and facilitate timely access to the most appropriate equipment. Hopefully, cooperative groups and support groups will be able to advocate for the development of such process.

Paediatric Neuro-Oncologists

Dedicated paediatric oncologists interested in neuro-oncology are few. In the absence of oncologists with specific training in paediatric neuro-oncology, treatment may lean more toward the use of radiation rather than chemotherapy. This is particularly the case in the management of low-grade tumours such as low-grade gliomas of the optic pathways, of the brainstem or of the spinal cord that can be managed with low dose chemotherapy in most situations [35–37]. Absence of properly designed chemotherapy protocols suitable for developing countries, the intermittent supply of chemotherapeutic drugs and the absence of well-trained nurses would also affect the medical management of childhood brain tumours in these conditions.

Multidisciplinary Meetings

In paediatric neuro-oncology, there is a critical need for interaction between disciplines such as neurosurgery, neuroradiology, neuropathology, radiation oncology and oncology. Optimization of cancer treatment depends on careful orchestration of the different treatment modalities in order to provide patients with maximal benefit. Discussions amongst team members will allow organizing the treatment plan for each specific patients [38]. Multidisciplinary meetings are part of the standard of care in many institutions in high-income countries and some jurisdictions, including France and the UK have required for each newly diagnosed paediatric neuro-oncology patient review of the case and the agreement on a treatment plan by a multidisciplinary team of experts. Implementation of multidisciplinary neuro-oncology programs in countries with limited resources is slow. Most physicians in low-income countries still work in silo and are not convinced of the benefit of a dialog between team members, particularly with physicians outside their area of expertise. The role of the paediatric oncologist in this context is critical, even when patients may not require chemotherapy. Multidisciplinary meetings should involve all team members with no exception, in order to discuss every aspect of the care of the patient. In this context, the presence of neuroradiologists, pathologists, neurosurgeons, oncologists and radiation oncologists at these meetings is critical.

Most Common Paediatric Brain Tumours and Management in the Context of Countries with Limited Resources (Table 25.1)

The diversity of paediatric brain tumours is huge and there are no formal guidelines for the management of these tumours in countries with limited resources. A working group in the International Society of Paediatric Oncology is currently developing guidelines for the management of paediatric brain tumours in countries with limited resources. However, the management is primarily dependent on the resources available locally, in particular in terms of neurosurgical and radiation oncology equipments and this will significantly influence the application of these proposed recommendations.

1. Low-grade gliomas

   Low-grade gliomas are the most common brain tumour in the paediatric age group. Most paediatric low-grade gliomas are pilocytic (grade 1). In this category, cerebellar astrocytomas are the prototype of the so-called surgical tumours and complete resection is curative. When resection is incomplete, a wait and watch approach is recommended and repeat surgery is only performed in case of progression of residual tumour [39].

   When the tumour is located in an unresectable location such as the optic pathway or the brainstem (although a subset of these tumour

Table 25.1 The most common diagnoses and treatment options in high income countries

Diagnosis	Location	Standard treatment	Options	Outcome in high-income countries	Prognostic factors
Low-grade glioma in surgical areas	All sites	Surgery	None	Excellent (95–100 % survival)	Extent of resection
Unresectable low-grade glioma	Optic pathways hypothalamus other sites may include thalamus, brainstem, and spinal cord. Disseminated low-grade gliomas	Chemotherapy (children <10) Chemotherapy or Radiation (children >10)	– Conformal radiation in younger children – Chemotherapy as a first option regardless of age	85–90 % at 10 years	– Age (more aggressive in children under the age of 1) – Response to chemotherapy – NF (better prognosis)
Ependymoma	All sites	Surgery + focal radiation	– Chemotherapy to delay irradiation in young children – Chemotherapy + second look surgery before radiation in the case of incomplete resection	70 % at 5 years in case of complete resection (30 % if resection is incomplete)	– Extent of resection
Diffuse brainstem glioma	Brainstem	Focal radiation	Innovative approaches in addition to radiation	Poor. Median survival time: 9 months	– Younger age (less than 4 or 3 years old) is associated with longer survival time
Medulloblastoma in children >3 years old	Posterior fossa	Surgery + craniospinal irradiation + chemotherapy	– Concomitant chemo-radiotherapy (high risk patients) – High dose chemotherapy following radiation (high risk patients) – Reduced dose irradiation (average risk patients)	50–80 %	– Extent of disease (metastasis) – Extent of resections

Medulloblastoma in infants and children <3 years old	Posterior fossa	Surgery followed by chemotherapy without radiation	– Chemotherapy followed by delayed irradiation – Chemotherapy and focal irradiation (average risk patients) – High dose chemotherapy ± radiation	20–40 %	– Extent of disease – Extent of resection – Nodular (desmoplastic histology, associated with excellent outcome with post-operative chemotherapy only, no radiation)
High-grade glioma	All sites	Surgery + focal radiation + chemotherapy	– Concomitant chemo and radiotherapy	20–40 %	– Extent of resection – P53 status (poor outcome if positive)
Germ cell tumours (germinoma)	Suprasellar-pineal	Surgery (biopsy) + chemotherapy + radiation (ventricular)	Craniospinal radiation only	90–95 %	– None
Germ cell tumours (non-germinomatous germ cell tumours)	Suprasellar-pineal	Surgery (optional: diagnosis can be done on markers —HCG and AFP). Chemotherapy + focal or craniospinal radiation	High dose chemotherapy in poor responders to treatment	70 %	– Response to treatment

The definition of standard treatment is generally based on the best reported results. However, although some treatment approaches remain labelled "current standard", alternatives are being developed either to improve survival rates or to minimize late effects of radiation, especially in younger children. The feasibility of these approaches in countries with limited resources remains to be demonstrated are amenable to complete or subtotal resection), non-surgical treatment may be considered, based on the risk associated with tumour progression. Chemotherapy is the treatment of choice, with several potential options [37]. The combination of vincristine and carboplatin is a standard regimen worldwide [40]; however, other protocols have shown benefit (such as TPCV—a combination of thioguanine, procarbazine, lomustine and vincristine [41]—the etoposide-cisplatin [42] combination, or single agent vinblastine [43] or vinorelbine [44] amongst others). The response rate to chemotherapy varies from 30 to 70 %. However, most children will eventually show progression and will require further treatment. Recent reports have suggested that multiple lines of chemotherapy allow avoidance of radiation [45]. Still, the management of children with unresectable low-grade gliomas is challenging and the respective role of chemotherapy and focal radiation is currently unsettled, particularly in children who show progression after a first line of chemotherapy.

2. Medulloblastoma

   Most common malignant brain tumour in the paediatric age group, medulloblastoma is often not diagnosed in countries with limited resources, as children essentially succumb before diagnosis. When the tumour is identified on imaging, treatment should ideally include surgery followed by craniospinal radiation and chemotherapy, depending of the resources available. Ideally patients should have a complete preoperative staging prior to surgery, including MRI scan of the brain and the spine. If this radiological assessment does not show evidence of dissemination, maximum resection should be attempted, as extent of resection has a significant impact on survival [22]. In children with disseminated disease, the impact of resection is less obvious. Radiation should include the craniospinal axis with a boost to the posterior fossa or the tumour bed. The dose to the posterior fossa depends on the initial staging: children with no evidence of dissemination (no evidence of metastatic disease on initial imaging, and no evidence of CSF involvement on CSF cytology performed at least 10 days after surgical resection), the recommendation is a dose f 23.4 Gy to the craniospinal axis in 13 fractions and a posterior fossa or (better) a tumour bed boost of 30.6 Gy is recommended [29]. For patients with incomplete resection (residue >1.5 cm in diameter) or patients with metastatic disease, a dose of 36 Gy in 20 fractions with a boost of 18 Gy to the posterior fossa/tumour bed is recommended [46]. Numerous chemotherapy protocols could be used. The current template used by the SIOP committee is a combination of etoposide and cisplatin for three courses, followed by a combination of cyclophospamide and vincristine for three courses.

3. Ependymoma

   Ependymoma accounts for around 10 % of paediatric CNS tumours. More than 90 % occur in the brain; two thirds of them in the posterior fossa [23]. Clinical presentation depends on the site of the tumour.

   The histological grading of ependymoma and its correlation with outcome is still a matter of controversies. So far, the treatment of ependymoma is essentially identical, regardless of the histological grading (i.e. grade 2 or grade 3). The most widely accepted prognostic factor is the degree of surgical resection with complete resection associated with a better prognosis (70–80 % overall survival) at 5 years with gross total resection compared to 30 % with subtotal/partial resection [38]. Therefore the role of the surgeons is critical and second look surgery is recommended in case of incomplete resection. The role of chemotherapy is still unclear in this disease [47]. There is some suggestion that chemotherapy may facilitate a second resection when residual tumour is present after initial resection. In any case, radiation is a critical component of the post-operative treatment. Modern techniques of radiation allow the delivery of high dose radiation in small volumes without significant impact on neurocognitive outcome. In this context, current protocols in high-income countries consider focal radiation at a dose of

54–59.4 Gy in 1.8 G fractions since the age of 1 [30]. When conformal or stereotactic radiation is not available, chemotherapy may be an alternative in infants and young children under the age of 3 [48, 49]. However, the results of a post-operative chemotherapy-only approach are essentially disappointing.

Guidelines regarding the management of other tumour types are provided in Table 25.1. However, these are essentially based on the experience reported in high-income countries. The relevance and the feasibility of these recommendations in countries with limited resources remain to be demonstrated.

Treatment Side Effects

During the course of treatment, children with brain tumours are prone to many challenges whether related to their original disease or to the applied treatment protocols. They may require physical and occupational rehabilitation, mental and psychosocial support and reintegration programs in schools and community to allow them to be functionally productive in the future. When present, visual impairment as well as hearing deficits needs to be assessed, and patients should be directed to specific facilities that will help them to deal with these handicaps. These are generally not a priority in low-income countries and physicians should be aware that the use of ototoxic medications, for example, can lead to irreversible hearing loss and the need of usually unaffordable correcting devises.

Many children will also need hormonal supplementation after brain irradiation [50]. Availability of regular endocrine testing and daily administration of hormone replacement, like growth hormone, may be challenging in countries with limited resources. In reality, most children with CNS tumours are very early lost to follow-up in countries with limited resources. A recent international survey showed that the number of aftercare program in countries with limited resources was limited [51]. It is clear that well-designed programs for assessment of aftercare morbidities are difficult to implement in this context.

Palliative Care

Owing to the delayed diagnosis, many children with brain tumour diagnosed in countries with limited resources present with advanced disease and very often in this context, supportive care and palliative treatment would be the most appropriate option. In addition, a number of paediatric brain tumours have a poor prognosis, such as high-grade glioma, DIPG or atypical teratoid rhabdoid tumours. It is expected that in such context, a majority of patients will eventually succumb to their disease. Pain control and proper palliative care interventions would be important at this stage. Low-income countries are particularly lacking such services [52, 53] and families often perceive palliative care as an abandonment of treatment. Other issues are critical such as access to appropriate pain medications. There is an obvious need to develop palliative care guidelines that address the need of the paediatric brain tumour population in these countries and that also take into account local or regional specificities, in particular social, cultural or religious contexts. A recent work conducted in families of children diagnosed with DIPG in Jordan suggested that it is possible to address palliative care issues at an early stage and this approach can facilitate the implementation of end of life decisions [54].

Twinning Programs

In the face of the many challenges associated with the management of childhood brain tumour in countries with limited resources, efforts have been developed to implement neuro-oncology programs through twinning initiatives. Such initiatives have shown success in the management of childhood leukemia and have demonstrated that proven treatment regimens can be adapted for use in countries with limited resources [55]. Although the multidisciplinary care in neuro-oncology requires specific attention, successful twinning initiatives have been described with significant impact on management and outcomes [56, 57].

Conclusion

The concept of paediatric neuro-oncology is still at its infancy in countries with limited resources. Appropriate neuro-imaging facilities, neurosurgical units, radiation equipment and paediatric oncology services are prerequisites for the implementation of such programs. A number of programs have been recently implemented, often in the context of twinning initiatives.

References

1. Ribeiro RC, Steliarova-Foucher E, Magrath I, Lemerle J, Eden T, Forget C, et al. Baseline status of paediatric oncology care in ten low-income or mid-income countries receiving My Child Matters support: a descriptive study. Lancet Oncol. 2008;9(8):721–9. Epub 2008/08/02.
2. Asirvatham JR, Deepti AN, Chyne R, Prasad MS, Chacko AG, Rajshekhar V, et al. Pediatric tumors of the central nervous system: a retrospective study of 1,043 cases from a tertiary care center in South India. Childs Nerv Syst. 2011;27(8):1257–63. Epub 2011/02/24.
3. Ahmed N, Bhurgri Y, Sadiq S, Shakoor KA. Pediatric brain tumours at a tertiary care hospital in Karachi. Asian Pac J Cancer Prev. 2007;8(3):399–404. Epub 2007/12/28.
4. Katchy KC, Mallik AA, Al-Nashmi NM, Joseph E, Alexander S, Al-Ramadan A. Intracranial tumors in Kuwait: a 15-year survey. J Neurooncol. 2011;104(1):271–7. Epub 2010/12/08.
5. Curado MP, Voti L, Sortino-Rachou AM. Cancer registration data and quality indicators in low and middle income countries: their interpretation and potential use for the improvement of cancer care. Cancer Causes Control. 2009;20(5):751–6. Epub 2008/12/30.
6. Howard SC, Metzger ML, Wilimas JA, Quintana Y, Pui CH, Robison LL, et al. Childhood cancer epidemiology in low-income countries. Cancer. 2008;112(3):461–72. Epub 2007/12/12.
7. Valsecchi MG, Steliarova-Foucher E. Cancer registration in developing countries: luxury or necessity? Lancet Oncol. 2008;9(2):159–67. Epub 2008/02/02.
8. Al-Hadad SA, Al-Jadiry MF, Al-Darraji AF, Al-Saeed RM, Al-Badr SF, Ghali HH. Reality of pediatric cancer in Iraq. J Pediatr Hematol Oncol. 2011;33 Suppl 2:S154–6. Epub 2011/10/05.
9. Usmani GN. Pediatric oncology in the third world. Curr Opin Pediatr. 2001;13(1):1–9. Epub 2001/02/15.
10. Dolecek TA, Propp JM, Stroup NE, Kruchko C. CBTRUS statistical report: primary brain and central nervous system tumors diagnosed in the United States in 2005–2009. Neuro Oncol. 2012;14 Suppl 5:v1–49. Epub 2012/11/01.
11. Manoharan N, Julka PK, Rath GK. Descriptive epidemiology of primary brain and CNS tumors in Delhi, 2003–2007. Asian Pac J Cancer Prev. 2012;13(2):637–40. Epub 2012/04/25.
12. Wilne S, Collier J, Kennedy C, Koller K, Grundy R, Walker D. Presentation of childhood CNS tumours: a systematic review and meta-analysis. Lancet Oncol. 2007;8(8):685–95. Epub 2007/07/24.
13. Dang-Tan T, Franco EL. Diagnosis delays in childhood cancer: a review. Cancer. 2007;110(4):703–13. Epub 2007/07/11.
14. El-Fiki M. African neurosurgery, the 21st-century challenge. World Neurosurg. 2010;73(4):254–8. Epub 2010/09/21.
15. Ariffin H, Abdullah WA, de Bruyne J, Lee CL, Peng LH. Belief in traditional healers amongst Malaysian parents of children with cancer. J Trop Pediatr. 1997;43(6):375–6. Epub 1998/02/26.
16. Hamidah A, Rustam ZA, Tamil AM, Zarina LA, Zulkifli ZS, Jamal R. Prevalence and parental perceptions of complementary and alternative medicine use by children with cancer in a multi-ethnic Southeast Asian population. Pediatr Blood Cancer. 2009;52(1):70–4. Epub 2008/10/22.
17. Daher M. Cultural beliefs and values in cancer patients. Ann Oncol. 2012;23 Suppl 3:66–9. Epub 2012/06/01.
18. Bhopal SS, Mann KD, Pearce MS. Registration of cancer in girls remains lower than expected in countries with low/middle incomes and low female education rates. Br J Cancer. 2012;107(1):183–8. Epub 2012/05/12.
19. Mostert S, Arora RS, Arreola M, Bagai P, Friedrich P, Gupta S, et al. Abandonment of treatment for childhood cancer: position statement of a SIOP PODC Working Group. Lancet Oncol. 2011;12(8):719–20. Epub 2011/07/02.
20. Nadkarni TD, Goel A, Pandya SK. Neurosurgery in India. J Postgrad Med. 2002;48(4):332–5. Epub 2003/02/07.
21. El Khamlichi A. African neurosurgery: current situation, priorities, and needs. Neurosurgery. 2001;48(6):1344–7. Epub 2001/06/01.
22. Zeltzer PM, Boyett JM, Finlay JL, Albright AL, Rorke LB, Milstein JM, et al. Metastasis stage, adjuvant treatment, and residual tumor are prognostic factors for medulloblastoma in children: conclusions from the Children's Cancer Group 921 randomized phase III study. J Clin Oncol. 1999;17(3):832–45.
23. Bouffet E, Perilongo G, Canete A, Massimino M. Intracranial ependymomas in children: a critical review of prognostic factors and a plea for cooperation. Med Pediatr Oncol. 1998;30(6):319–29; discussion 29–31.
24. Dwarakanath S, Suri A, Sharma BS, Mahapatra AK. Neuronavigation in a developing country: a pilot study of efficacy and limitations in intracranial surgery. Neurol India. 2007;55(2):111–6. Epub 2007/06/15.

25. Qaddoumi I, Mansour A, Musharbash A, Drake J, Swaidan M, Tihan T, et al. Impact of telemedicine on pediatric neuro-oncology in a developing country: the Jordanian-Canadian experience. Pediatr Blood Cancer. 2007;48(1):39–43.
26. Berezowska S, Tomoka T, Kamiza S, Milner Jr DA, Langer R. Surgical pathology in sub-Saharan Africa–volunteering in Malawi. Virchows Arch. 2012;460(4):363–70. Epub 2012/03/13.
27. Judkins AR. Immunohistochemistry of INI1 expression: a new tool for old challenges in CNS and soft tissue pathology. Adv Anat Pathol. 2007;14(5):335–9. Epub 2007/08/25.
28. Lannering B, Rutkowski S, Doz F, Pizer B, Gustafsson G, Navajas A, et al. Hyperfractionated versus conventional radiotherapy followed by chemotherapy in standard-risk medulloblastoma: results from the randomized multicenter HIT-SIOP PNET 4 trial. J Clin Oncol. 2012;30(26):3187–93. Epub 2012/08/02.
29. Packer RJ, Gajjar A, Vezina G, Rorke-Adams L, Burger PC, Robertson PL, et al. Phase III study of craniospinal radiation therapy followed by adjuvant chemotherapy for newly diagnosed average-risk medulloblastoma. J Clin Oncol. 2006;24(25):4202–8.
30. Merchant TE, Li C, Xiong X, Kun LE, Boop FA, Sanford RA. Conformal radiotherapy after surgery for paediatric ependymoma: a prospective study. Lancet Oncol. 2009;10(3):258–66. Epub 2009/03/11.
31. Bouffet E, Baranzelli MC, Patte C, Portas M, Edan C, Chastagner P, et al. Combined treatment modality for intracranial germinomas: results of a multicentre SFOP experience. Societe Francaise d'Oncologie Pediatrique. Br J Cancer. 1999;79(7–8):1199–204.
32. Levin CV, El Gueddari B, Meghzifene A. Radiation therapy in Africa: distribution and equipment. Radiother Oncol. 1999;52(1):79–84. Epub 1999/11/30.
33. Carrie C, Alapetite C, Mere P, Aimard L, Pons A, Kolodie H, et al. Quality control of radiotherapeutic treatment of medulloblastoma in a multicentric study: the contribution of radiotherapy technique to tumour relapse. The French Medulloblastoma Group. Radiother Oncol. 1992;24(2):77–81. Epub 1992/06/01.
34. Zaghloul M, Ahmed S, Eldebaway E, Mousa A, Amin A, Elkhateeb N, et al. Hypofractionated radiotherapy for pediatric diffuse intrinsic pontine glioma (DIPG): a prospective controled randomized trial. Neuro Oncol. 2012:i26.
35. Ronghe M, Hargrave D, Bartels U, Tabori U, Vaidya S, Chandler C, et al. Vincristine and carboplatin chemotherapy for unresectable and/or recurrent low-grade astrocytoma of the brainstem. Pediatr Blood Cancer. 2010;55(3):471–7. Epub 2010/06/11.
36. Scheinemann K, Bartels U, Huang A, Hawkins C, Kulkarni AV, Bouffet E, et al. Survival and functional outcome of childhood spinal cord low-grade gliomas. Clinical article. J Neurosurg Pediatr. 2009;4(3):254–61. Epub 2009/09/24.
37. Reddy AT, Packer RJ. Chemotherapy for low-grade gliomas. Childs Nerv Syst. 1999;15(10):506–13. Epub 1999/11/07.
38. Pollack IF. Multidisciplinary management of childhood brain tumors: a review of outcomes, recent advances, and challenges. J Neurosurg Pediatr. 2011;8(2):135–48. Epub 2011/08/03.
39. Sievert AJ, Fisher MJ. Pediatric low-grade gliomas. J Child Neurol. 2009;24(11):1397–408. Epub 2009/10/21.
40. Packer RJ, Ater J, Allen J, Phillips P, Geyer R, Nicholson HS, et al. Carboplatin and vincristine chemotherapy for children with newly diagnosed progressive low-grade gliomas. J Neurosurg. 1997;86(5):747–54.
41. Prados MD, Edwards MS, Rabbitt J, Lamborn K, Davis RL, Levin VA. Treatment of pediatric low-grade gliomas with a nitrosourea-based multiagent chemotherapy regimen. J Neurooncol. 1997;32(3):235–41.
42. Massimino M, Spreafico F, Cefalo G, Riccardi R, Tesoro-Tess JD, Gandola L, et al. High response rate to cisplatin/etoposide regimen in childhood low-grade glioma. J Clin Oncol. 2002;20(20):4209–16.
43. Bouffet E, Jakacki R, Goldman S, Hargrave D, Hawkins C, Shroff M, et al. Phase II study of weekly vinblastine in recurrent or refractory pediatric low-grade glioma. J Clin Oncol. 2012;30(12):1358–63. Epub 2012/03/07.
44. Cappellano AM, Bouffet E, Silva F, Paiva P, Alves M, Cavalheiro S, et al. Vinorelbine in progressive unresectable low-grade glioma in children. J Clin Oncol. 2011;29(15S):591.
45. Scheinemann K, Bartels U, Tsangaris E, Hawkins C, Huang A, Dirks P, et al. Feasibility and efficacy of repeated chemotherapy for progressive pediatric low-grade gliomas. Pediatr Blood Cancer. 2011;57(1):84–8. Epub 2010/12/03.
46. Jakacki RI, Burger PC, Zhou T, Holmes EJ, Kocak M, Onar A, et al. Outcome of children with metastatic medulloblastoma treated with carboplatin during craniospinal radiotherapy: a Children's Oncology Group Phase I/II study. J Clin Oncol. 2012;30(21):2648–53. Epub 2012/06/06.
47. Souweidane MM, Bouffet E, Finlay J. The role of chemotherapy in newly diagnosed ependymoma of childhood. Pediatr Neurosurg. 1998;28(5):273–8.
48. Grundy RG, Wilne SA, Weston CL, Robinson K, Lashford LS, Ironside J, et al. Primary postoperative chemotherapy without radiotherapy for intracranial ependymoma in children: the UKCCSG/SIOP prospective study. Lancet Oncol. 2007;8(8):696–705.
49. Grill J, Pascal C, Chantal K. Childhood ependymoma: a systematic review of treatment options and strategies. Paediatr Drugs. 2003;5(8):533–43. Epub 2003/08/05.
50. Laughton SJ, Merchant TE, Sklar CA, Kun LE, Fouladi M, Broniscer A, et al. Endocrine outcomes for children with embryonal brain tumors after risk-adapted craniospinal and conformal primary-site irradiation and high-dose chemotherapy with stem-cell rescue on the SJMB-96 trial. J Clin Oncol. 2008;26(7):1112–8. Epub 2008/03/04.

51. Qaddoumi I, Unal E, Diez B, Kebudi R, Quintana Y, Bouffet E, et al. Web-based survey of resources for treatment and long-term follow-up for children with brain tumors in developing countries. Childs Nerv Syst. 2011;27(11):1957–61. Epub 2011/05/18.
52. Koshy RC, Rhodes D, Devi S, Grossman SA. Cancer pain management in developing countries: a mosaic of complex issues resulting in inadequate analgesia. Support Care Cancer. 1998;6(5):430–7. Epub 1998/10/17.
53. Delgado E, Barfield RC, Baker JN, Hinds PS, Yang J, Nambayan A, et al. Availability of palliative care services for children with cancer in economically diverse regions of the world. Eur J Cancer. 2010;46(12):2260–6. Epub 2010/06/15.
54. Qaddoumi I, Ezam N, Swaidan M, Jaradat I, Mansour A, Abuirmeileh N, et al. Diffuse pontine glioma in Jordan and impact of up-front prognosis disclosure with parents and families. J Child Neurol. 2009;24(4):460–5. Epub 2008/12/17.
55. Howard SC, Pedrosa M, Lins M, Pedrosa A, Pui CH, Ribeiro RC, et al. Establishment of a pediatric oncology program and outcomes of childhood acute lymphoblastic leukemia in a resource-poor area. JAMA. 2004;291(20):2471–5. Epub 2004/05/27.
56. Qaddoumi I, Musharbash A, Elayyan M, Mansour A, Al-Hussaini M, Drake J, et al. Closing the survival gap: implementation of medulloblastoma protocols in a low-income country through a twinning program. Int J Cancer. 2008;122(6):1203–6. Epub 2007/11/07.
57. Baskin JL, Lezcano E, Kim BS, Figueredo D, Lassaletta A, Perez-Martinez A, et al. Management of children with brain tumors in Paraguay. Neuro Oncol. 2013;15(2):235–41. Epub 2012/12/01.

HIV and Malignancy in Children 26

Joyce Balagadde-Kambugu, Jackson Orem, and Daniela Cristina Stefan

Abbreviations

ABV	Adriamycin bleomycin and vincristine
ACTG	AIDS Clinical Trial Group
AIDS	Acquired immune deficiency syndrome
ALL	Acute lymphoblastic leukaemia
ALT	Alanine transaminase
AML	Acute myeloid leukaemia
AZT	Azidothymidine
BL	Burkitt's lymphoma
BV	Bleomycin and vincristine
CBC	Complete blood count
CDC	Centers for Disease Control
CNS	Central nervous system
CSF	Cerebrospinal fluid
CT	Computed tomography
CXR	Chest X-ray
DLBCL	Diffuse large B cell lymphoma
DNA	Deoxyribonucleic acid
EBNA	Epstein–Barr nuclear antigen
EBV	Epstein–Barr virus
FBC	Full blood count
FDA	United States Food and Drug Administration (USFDA)
GI	Gastrointestinal
GIT	Gastrointestinal
HAART	Highly active antiretroviral therapy
HHV8	Human herpesvirus type 8
HIV	Human immunodeficiency virus
HIV-HL	HIV-associated Hodgkin lymphoma
HIV-NHL	HIV-associated non-Hodgkin lymphoma
HIVRM	Human immunodeficiency virus related malignancy
HIV-Tat	Human immunodeficiency virus trans-activator of transcription
HL	Hodgkin lymphoma
HRM	Human immunodeficiency virus related malignancy
IL	Interleukin
IRIS	Immune reconstitution inflammatory syndrome
KS	Kaposi's sarcoma
KSHV	Kaposi's sarcoma-associated herpes virus
LD	Lymphocyte depletion
LDH	Lactate dehydrogenase
LFT	Liver functions tests
LMP	Latent membrane protein
MC	Mixed cellularity
MMPS	Matrix metalloproteinases
NFkB	Nuclear factor kappa-light-chain-enhancer of activated B cells
NHL	Non-Hodgkin lymphoma

J. Balagadde-Kambugu, M.B. Ch.B., M.Med(Pead)., M.Phil. • J. Orem, M.B., Ch.B., M.Med(Med). (✉)
Uganda Cancer Institute, Kampala, Uganda
e-mail: jorem@mucwru.or.ug

D.C. Stefan, M.D., Ph.D.
Department of Paediatrics and Child Health, Stellenbosch University & Tygerberg Hospital, Tygerberg, South Africa

D.C. Stefan and C. Rodriguez-Galindo (eds.), *Pediatric Hematology-Oncology in Countries with Limited Resources: A Practical Manual*, DOI 10.1007/978-1-4614-3891-5_26,

NNRTI	Non-nucleoside reverse-transcriptase inhibitor
PCNSL	Primary central nervous system lymphoma
PI	Protease inhibitor
RFT	Renal function tests
RS	Reed Sternberg cell
TB	Tuberculosis
TNF	Tumour necrosis factors
VEGF	Vascular endothelial growth factor
WHO	World Health Organization

Background

The risk of developing cancer is elevated in persons infected with the human immunodeficiency virus (HIV) as a result of their impaired immunity. Further, the diagnosis and treatment of incidental cancers in this population is difficult due to the HIV infection itself as well as its co-morbidities such as TB. Cancers that occur in the setting of HIV infection are called HIV-related malignancies (HIVRM) and they have infectious aetiology: human herpes virus type 8 (HHV8) associated with Kaposi sarcoma, Epstein Barr Virus (EBV) associated with Burkitt lymphoma, human papilloma virus in the cervical cancer, etc. HIV-related malignancies are further subdivided into AIDS-defining and HIV-associated malignancies.

In children there are two AIDS-defining malignancies: Kaposi sarcoma (KS) and B-cell Lymphoma (including primary CNS lymphoma [PCNSL]). They are so described because they occur most frequently when the CD4 count/CD4 percentage is very low and hence are considered sufficient to signify progression to the advanced stage of HIV infection (AIDS). Thus, they fall in stage IV of the current World Health Organization (WHO) staging of paediatric HIV disease and category C of the CDC staging system. The HIV-associated malignancies include leiomyosarcoma and Hodgkin lymphoma (HL). Leiomyosarcoma falls into category B of the CDC staging system of paediatric HIV disease, but is not listed by the WHO staging system. HL is not listed by either of the two staging systems of paediatric HIV disease.

With the emergence of the HIV pandemic the incidence of certain cancers in the population increased. This increase was largely due to markedly elevated risk of the AIDS-defining malignancies, KS and Non-Hodgkin lymphoma (NHL) [1–4].

Since the introduction of highly active antiretroviral therapy (HAART), patients with HIV infection are living longer, with improved immune function and a reduced risk of developing AIDS. Along with improved viral control, there has been a substantial change in the landscape of malignancies occurring in the setting of HIV in the developed world. AIDS-defining cancers such as KS and NHL have declined, while HIV-associated malignancies like HL have remained stable or have increased in incidence [5, 6].

It is difficult to state that this pattern has been clearly observed in Africa where the greatest numbers of persons with HIVRM are likely to be. However, it is reasonable to expect that the incidence of AIDS-defining malignancies though still high has shown a decline even in Africa following the advent of HAART.

In general, HIVRM occur much less frequently in paediatric patients compared with adults [7]. Corresponding paediatric analyses have not yet been performed; however, anecdotal reports and logical comparison suggest similar trends, despite differences in presumed interaction between HIV and malignancies in children as compared to adults.

Kaposi Sarcoma (KS)

Kaposi sarcoma (KS) was noted in the early 1980s and became the first AIDS-defining illness. Since, with the development of antiretroviral therapy (ART), KS has again become a rare disease in resource-rich settings, especially in paediatric patients. However, KS remains the second most frequent HIV-related malignancy (HRM) and most common HRM in sub-Saharan Africa where HIV is most prevalent and human herpesvirus-8 (HHV-8) endemic [8].

Kaposi sarcoma is a mesenchymal tumour involving blood and lymphatic vessels of multifactorial origin. There are four recognized clinical variants of the disease including classic, endemic, iatrogenic and epidemic KS. Classic KS is a rare and mild form of the disease first described in 1872 by the Hungarian dermatologist Moritz Kaposi as a vascular tumour affecting the lower extremities of elderly men of Mediterranean, east European, or Jewish heritage. Endemic or African KS is a variant of disease affecting HIV seronegative children and adults in some areas in sub-Saharan Africa. Iatrogenic KS is associated with use of immunosuppressant drugs, and in patients with autoimmune disorders, inflammatory conditions or solid organ transplantation. Epidemic or AIDS-associated KS is a more aggressive form of this disorder. It more commonly occurs in the context of advanced immunosuppression even though it may develop throughout the entire spectrum of HIV disease [9]. Further discussion of the former three clinical variants of KS is beyond the scope of this chapter.

Epidemic KS

Aetiopathogenesis

The current belief is that the initiation and progression of KS is a confluence of viral oncogenesis by human herpesvirus-8 (HHV8) also known as Kaposi's sarcoma-associated virus (KSHV), and cytokine-induced growth factor together with some form of immune compromise (Fig. 26.1).

It is now known that the pathogenesis of all clinical variants of KS involves infection with KSHV, a deoxyribonucleic acid (DNA) virus first isolated by Chang et al. in 1994 from the KS lesions of an AIDS patient. It has also been established that although necessary, KSHV by itself is not sufficient for initiation and progression of KS. In HIV-seropositive patients it is postulated that HIV-mediated immune suppression/dysregulation promotes T-helper type-1 cytokines such

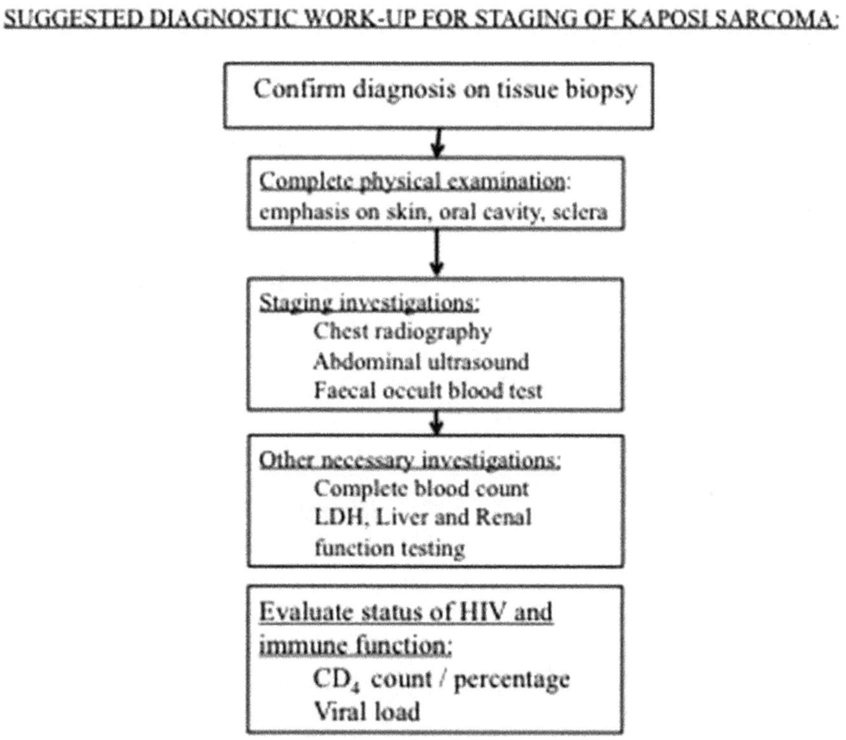

Fig. 26.1 Suggested diagnostic work-up for staging of Kaposi sarcoma

as TNF-alpha, Interleukin-1b (IL-1b) and IL-6. Production and release of HIV-Tat protein from HIV-infected cells further contribute to release of proinflammatory cytokines, vascular endothelial growth factor (VEGFs) and matrix metalloproteinases (MMPS), which all together facilitate the proliferation of endothelial cells and development of KS. HIV-Tat protein and chronic inflammation also mediate reactivation and replication of latent KSHV, promoting expression of viral gene products implicated in angiogenesis [9, 10].

KSHV Seroprevalence and Mode of Transmission

The seroprevalence of KSHV among the general population varies geographically. The precise mode of its transmission though not clearly understood is believed to include vertical, horizontal through sex or oral shedding, blood transfusion and injection drug use, as well as solid organ or bone marrow transplantation [11]. In areas where KSHV infection is endemic the infection is thought to be acquired in childhood from seropositive family members and seroprevalence rates increase with age reaching as high as 80 %.

Natural Course of HHV8 Infection in Children

In immunocompetent children, HHV8 may be associated with a febrile maculopapular skin rash while in HIV-infected older children a transient angiolymphoid hyperplasia occurs as part of the HHV8 seroconversion syndrome. In children it is believed that KS is a manifestation of primary infection, whereas in older children KS occurs after primary infection.

Clinical Features

Epidemic KS has a wide spectrum of presentation ranging from minimal disease that is discovered incidentally on a routine clinic visit to aggressive growth with significant morbidity and mortality. In general the presentation may be classified into lymphadenopathic, cutaneous, mucosal, visceral and other [9, 11].

Lymphadenopathic KS

This is the most common presentation of disease in children. It tends to occur in younger children with relatively higher CD4 counts likely owing to recent HHV8 infection with a rapid progression to malignancy (since the virus is tropic for lymph nodes during seroconversion) [12]. Lymph node involvement may be the sole presentation of disease. Massive lymph node enlargement and lymphoedema may develop.

Cutaneous KS

Cutaneous lesions vary in size characteristics and number ranging from a small number of isolated lesions to widespread cutaneous involvement. The lesions may be small sub-centimeter macular/popular or large confluent nodules 10 cm or larger in the widest diameter. They are dark, almost black in dark/olive skinned patients and if chronic may appear violaceous and hairy. In some patients they may be arranged linearly and symmetrically along skin tension lines, while in others they are randomly distributed. When large they may become painful otherwise they are usually painless and non-pruritic. There may be associated woody edema. Plaque-like lesions may also occur. These lesions are similar to nodules but are more extensive locally, suggesting the coalescence of multiple nodules. The plaque-like lesions occur on the thighs, calves or soles of the feet and may be exophytic and fungating with breakdown of overlying skin. The lesions are often complicated with lymphoedema, which may occur as a relatively isolated finding and may be out of proportion to the extent of visible cutaneous disease. Plaque-like lesions may ulcerate, bleed or become a focus for secondary bacterial infection.

Mucosal Disease

Disease involving the oral cavity may be the initial presentation of KS. Oral lesions range from flat, red to violet papules to exophytic, ulcerative nodules. Lesions most commonly occur on the palate, oropharynx and gingival, but may involve any part of the mucosal surface including the tongue, tonsillar pillars and floor of the mouth, pharynx or trachea. These lesions may become painful, bleed or ulcerate if traumatized during normal chewing. They may become secondarily infected. When bulky they may interfere with nutrition and speech.

Laryngeal involvement may occur, the most common site being the epiglottis. Presenting symptoms of laryngeal KS may include pain, bleeding, dysphagia speech abnormalities and airway compromise. Indeed laryngeal KS must be excluded when a suspicious lesion in an HIV-infected patient is seen, as it is associated with severe bleeding, airway obstruction and death.

KS involving the sclera is commonly missed. In the early stages of disease it may appear as painless conjunctival injection particularly at the canthi of the eyes and is commonly treated as conjunctivitis. Red or purplish nodular lesions may also be seen involving the tarsal conjuctiva.

Visceral Presentation

- Pulmonary involvement

Pulmonary KS must be excluded in the evaluation of HIV-infected patients with respiratory symptoms or abnormal chest X-ray (CXR) findings, especially in the presence of cutaneous KS. Pulmonary involvement usually occurs as a late manifestation of HIV disease, although it may occur at any stage of HIV. Almost all intra-thoracic structures may be involved in this disease including the tracheobronchial tree, pulmonary parenchyma and pleura. The lymph nodes may also be involved. Common presenting symptoms of pulmonary KS include cough, haemoptysis and shortness of breath, pleuritic chest pain and fever. Physical examination may be normal or non-specific with the presence of crackles or wheeze related to the involvement of the upper respiratory tract.

- Gastrointestinal involvement

GI involvement may occur in the absence of cutaneous disease and many patients with GI KS remain asymptomatic. Patients with GI lesions may present with nausea, vomiting, abdominal pain, weight loss, upper and lower GI bleeding or intestinal obstruction.

- Other organs

KS may involve other organs as well including the heart and pericardium, kidneys, urogenital tract and bone marrow. Involvement of the brain and intraorbital structures is rare likely owing to their lack of lymphatics.

KS Histology and Diagnosis

The diagnosis must be proven on tissue biopsy. Microscopic features of KS include an abundance of proliferating mononuclear inflammatory and spindle cells, ill-defined vascular channels, haemorrhage and oedema.

Initial work-up for staging epidemic KS involves a complete physical examination that includes evaluation of the skin, oral cavity and sclera to determine extent of mucocutaneous involvement.

Staging investigations will establish the presence of visceral involvement and include a Chest X-ray, Abdominal Ultrasound scan and faecal occult blood test.

Other necessary investigations include: a CBC, CD4 count/percentage, HIV viral load if possible, LDH, RFTs and LFTs (Fig. 26.1).

Staging and Prognosis of Epidemic KS

The outlook for HAART-naïve patients with epidemic KS is influenced at least as much by the presence of other AIDS-related problems as it is by the spread of KS. Thus, staging of epidemic KS also considers factors such as how much the

Table 26.1 ACTG staging system for Kaposi sarcoma

Parameter	Good risk (all of the following symptoms)	Poor risk (any of the following symptoms)
Tumour bulk	Confined to the skin and/or lymphnodes and/or minimal oral disease (non-nodular KS confined to the palate)	Tumour-associated oedema or ulceration
		Extensive oral KS
		Gastrointestinal KS
		KS in other non-nodal viscera
Immune status	CD4 count >200	CD4 count <200
	CD4 percentage>15 %	CD4 percentage <15 %
Severity of illness	No history of opportunistic infection or thrush	History of opportunistic infection and/or thrush
	No B symptoms[a]	B symptoms[a] present
	Karnofsky Performance status >70[b]	Karnofsky Performance Status <70
		Other HIV-related illness (e.g. neurologic disease, lymphoma)

[a]Unexplained fever, night sweats, involuntary weight loss (>10 %) or diarrhoea persisting longer than 2 weeks
[b]Patient is up and about most of the time and able to care of himself

immune system is damaged and the presence of AIDS-related infections [11]. In 1988, the AIDS Clinical Trial Group (ACTG) of the National Cancer Institute of Health developed a system that divides patients into good and poor risk groups based on three parameters and it considers three factors:

- The extent of the tumour (abbreviated T)
- The status of the immune system (I), as measured by the number of certain cells (CD4) or in the case of children less than 5 years, the CD4 percentage present in the blood
- The extent of involvement within the body of systemic illness (S)

Under each of these major headings, there are two subgroups identified by either a zero (0 or good risk) or a 1 (poor risk) (Table 26.1).

The current prognostic indicators for the staging of epidemic KS, proposed by Nasti et al., include tumour extension (T) and HIV-related systemic illness (S) resulting in good and poor survival depending on the combination of prognostic markers [13]. Patients with a combination of advanced disease and constitutional symptoms (T_1S_1) have the worst prognosis, while those with minimal disease (T_0S_0) had the best prognosis with the other patients (T_0S_1, T_1S_0) falling in between these extremes.

From his work the following tentative recommendations were made with regard to treatment of epidemic KS (Table 26.2).

Table 26.2 Recommended staging system for Kaposi sarcoma peadiatric HIV

Severity of AIDS-KS	Management approach
T_0S_0 (focal disease in the absence of systemic illness)	Watchful waiting, consideration of CD4 count, viral load and active opportunistic infections prior to HAART initiation
T_0S_1 (Early but mildly symptomatic KS, e.g. minimal cutaneous disease)	HAART ± local therapy
T_1S_0 (Early progressive AIDS-KS)	HAART
T_1S_1 disease	HAART + chemotherapy
Extensive disfiguring skin lesions	
Widespread symptomatic cutaneous disease + edema	
Rapidly progressive disease	
Symptomatic visceral involvement	
Obstructive or painful oropharyngeal disease	
Inadequate response to HAART alone	
IRIS-associated KS	

Treatment

Due to resource limitations and lack of evidence-based guidelines, practice in sub-Saharan Africa for paediatric KS is variable.

Management of epidemic KS is not aimed at cure rather it aims at palliation and control of KS progression and HAART is an integral component of this process.

HAART is the mainstay of treatment because the resultant immune restoration may be sufficient to induce remission. ART should be started promptly prior to referral to a paediatric oncology unit for staging and definitive management.

ART should be given to HIV-infected children, but there is no evidence to indicate whether ARTs should be started before, at the same time or after chemotherapy. It is also not determined if chemotherapy should be given to limited KS.

It is important to note that the advent of HAART has somewhat affected the prognostic significance of the ACTG staging system [13]. It was observed that patients on HAART who develop KS have less severe forms of disease compared to HAART-naïve patients at the time of KS diagnosis; i.e. severity of immunosuppression reflected in CD4 count is not an independent prognostic indicator for staging epidemic KS. HAART may be NNRTI or PI based. Although protease inhibitors are thought to have specific antiangiogenic effects, the choice of HAART regimen does not appear to influence protection against epidemic KS.

Local Therapy

Local therapy is safe, easy to administer and 1 for limited, asymptomatic mucocutaneous lesions of epidemic KS. It may also be considered when HAART is unavailable; response to HAART is less than optimal or as a palliative measure in patients with rapidly progressive mucocutaneous lesions causing pain, aesthetic concerns or interference with function. The local therapies available include

- Cryotherapy with liquid nitrogen for focal skin lesions.
- Surgical excision for focal superficial mucocutaneous lesions.
- Sclerotherapy.
- Intralesional therapy with vincristine or vinblastine. The procedure is painful and there may be necrosis if healthy tissue is injected; however, the effect lasts about 4 months. Other intralesional agents include bleomycin or alpha interferon. It is usually not recommended in children.
- Radiotherapy is effective management of local or regional KS causing pain, bleeding or oedema, but it is not always available in all developing countries and if it is available it usually is not a priority for the treatment of KS in children.
- Laser ablation therapy has been used particularly in lesions affecting the face or oral cavity.
- Topical therapy with 0.1 % alitretinoin, imiquimod 5 % cream. The alitretinoin gel must be applied two to five times daily as tolerated and therapeutic response may take up to 3 months to be registered. It is also expensive and may be accompanied by skin reactions.

Systemic Therapy

- Chemotherapy

The main drugs used in the treatment of KS in children are the following: vincristine, bleomycin, doxorubicin, etoposide, cyclophosphamide and paclitaxel.

The protocols described in the literature include monotherapy with vincristine, 2 drugs (most used are the vincristine and bleomycin), or 3 drugs (adding anthracycline—doxorubicin) (Table 26.3).

Adult guidelines recommend first-line liposomal doxorubicin, an expensive chemotherapeutic agent not readily available or sustainable in resource-limited settings, not approved as a first-line agent by the United States Food and Drug Administration (FDA), and yet to be approved by the FDA for paediatric patients [14, 15].

No evidence is available on the use of liposomal doxorubicin in paediatric HIV-associated KS. Therefore, alternative, more available and less expensive primary regimens consisting of adriamycin, bleomycin and vincristine (ABV) are utilized in resource-limited settings [12, 16].

Table 26.3 Protocols

Single agent regimens (Monotherapy)
Oral:Etoposide 100 mg/m^2 po three times a week (may be increased to 200 mg/m^2)—not recommended
Intravenous: Vincristine 1.5 mg/m^2 weekly for 3 weeks (six courses)
Two agent regimens
Vincristine 1.5 mg/m^2 IV and bleomycin 15 iu/m^2 IV or IM weekly every 3 weeks (6 courses)
Three agent regimens
ABV
Day 1 and 15 doxorubicin 25 mg/m^2 IV in 50 mL 5 % DW over 30 min; bleomycin 10 iu/m^2 IV in 0.9 % saline over 15 min; vinblastine 6 mg/m^2 IV bolus (4–6 courses)
Single doses of vincristine or actinomycin should not exceed 2 mg; Cumulative doses of doxorubicin should not exceed 300 mg/m^2
When anthracyclines are given, a baseline echocardiogram should be done and repeated after a total cumulative dose of 200 mg/m^2
A: Adriamycin (doxorubicin); B, bleomycin; V, vincristine; Vinblastine can be replaced with vincristine at a dose of 1.5 g/m^2

Adult evidence is equivocal whether ABV or BV is inferior to liposomal doxorubicin, especially with ART [14].

Other drugs used in the treatment of KS but with less good results are represented by etoposide and cyclophosphamide.

- Immune modulators: The example here is interferon alpha 2b which has both antiviral and antiangiogenic effects and has been shown to have dose-dependent efficacy in treatment of epidemic KS.
- Experimental and targeted therapies include antiherpes therapy (ganciclovir, foscarnet), angiogenic inhibitors like thalidomide, VEGF inhibitors Tyrosine kinase inhibitors and MMPs.

For the relapsed KS, Paclitaxel is the drug of choice. However, the evidence from the literature remains limited and the drug remains expensive and not yet fully accepted for use in children.

KS Immune Reconstitution Inflammatory Syndrome

In some HIV-infected children KS develops within a few weeks of commencing HAART contrary to the expectation that HAART should cause a decline in the incidence and severity of epidemic KS. This paradoxical exacerbation of opportunistic infections such as KS despite immunologic recovery and favourable virologic response with HAART is known as Immune Reconstitution Inflammatory Syndrome (IRIS). The management of IRIS-associated KS generally does not involve interruption of HAART, but may necessitate additional modes of therapy. KS IRIS has been reported in adult patients following initiation of ART [17, 18].

Reports from Mozambique and South Africa suggest that KS IRIS occurs in 10–11.8 % of adult patients. It is associated with a baseline haemoglobin concentration of less than 10 g/dL and a low CD4 count [17]. Typically there is clinical deterioration with fever, swelling, and pain at the site of lesions—the so-called "KS flare" [19].

HIV-Associated B-Cell Non-Hodgkin Lymphoma

There is an increased incidence of high-grade B-cell NHL among HIV-infected children with a relative risk of NHL in this population, 1,200-fold higher than in non-HIV-infected children. These tumours arise because of failure of their immune system to eradicate the lymphocytes latently infected with EBV. This virus is known to cause malignant transformation of lymphocytes that harbour it by causing unrestricted proliferation. Burkitt's lymphoma (BL) is now a well-described prototype of EBV's lymphomagenesis.

First described in children in equatorial Africa by Denis Burkitt in 1958, BL is a highly proliferative B-cell tumour that includes three variants: endemic (affecting children in equatorial Africa and New Guinea), sporadic (children and young adults throughout the world) and immunodeficiency related (primarily in association with HIV infection). In all variants constitutive activation of the c-myc oncogene on chromosome 14 through its translocation from this locus into one of the immunoglobulin loci on chromosome 8, 2, or 22 is clearly the key factor in the oncogenesis of Burkitt lymphoma. In those patients co-infected with EBV, the Epstein Barr Nuclear

Antigen (EBNA-1), a viral protein required for the replication and maintenance of the latent viral episomal DNA, is found consistently in BL cells. The presence of latent EBV in BL cells has been shown to promote genetic instability, suggesting a mechanism by which latent EBV could contribute to genetic alterations required for the development of BL. In addition, some latent EBV transcription patterns found in BL produce viral proteins that are likely to protect BL cells from apoptosis induced by deregulated c-myc expression. Given the strong apoptotic effects of overexpressed c-myc, the role of EBV in some cases of BL could therefore consist of protecting BL cells against this side effect of c-*MYC* translocation [20, 21].

Diffuse large B cell lymphoma (DLBCL) is the most commonly occurring B cell NHL among HIV-infected children in whom it tends to be more indolent. Other histological forms of B-NHL include Burkitt's lymphoma, immunoblastic lymphoma and PCNSL [22].

Clinical Presentation

While abdominal lymphadenopathy is still the most common presentation of HIV-related B-NHLs, extranodal disease occurs relatively more frequently among this population compared to HIV-negative children and involves sites such as the CNS, bone marrow, sinuses, adrenal gland, heart, lungs and mediastinum. Disease tends to be aggressive and the children will commonly present with advanced disease (CNS, bone marrow).

Diagnosis and Investigations

Diagnosis is made by biopsy and histology of the suspicious mass by whatever means appropriate (lymphnode excision, ultrasound-guided biopsy, bone marrow biopsy, etc.) following which the child should be referred to the oncology unit for appropriate management.

Appropriate baseline investigations in a child in whom this diagnosis is suspected will include lactate dehydrogenase (LDH) that will be raised in the presence of a normal alanine transaminase (ALT) (thus ruling out liver dysfunction), and a raised Uric acid level. Additionally the FBC may be abnormal with one or more cell lines depressed suggesting bone marrow involvement. A CXR should be done looking for mediastinal or hilar adenopathy, and an abdominal ultrasound scan to look for abdominal lymphadenopathy.

In the HAART-naïve child with generalized lymphadenopathy, persistent generalized lymphadenopathy (WHO stage 1 of paediatric HIV disease) is an important consideration that should be entertained before one undertakes tissue biopsy of a child with this presentation. If the LDH and uric acid are normal, and TB has been ruled out, it is reasonable to initiate HAART and adopt a watchful waiting approach. If, on the other hand, generalized lymphadenopathy occurs in a child already established on HAART, the diagnosis of B-NHL must be pursued aggressively; a lymph node biopsy (not fine needle aspirate) must be taken off for histology.

Pancytopaenia in the HIV-infected child should raise the suspicion of leukaemia (ALL or AML) or importantly, lymphoma (like a stage IV Burkitt's) alongside the diverse differential diagnosis of this condition. The peripheral smear may contain blasts and the LDH and uric acid will be elevated. If leukaemia is suspected, a bone marrow should be done and it will reveal the characteristic features of leukaemia, while it will be non-specific in other causes of pancytopaenia in the HIV-infected child.

Children with B-NHL should have the status of their immune function established by obtaining a baseline CD4 count percentage and viral load (Fig. 26.2).

Management Considerations

If HAART has not been initiated, it should as soon as possible since immune reconstitution is important for the optimal response of these cancers to chemotherapy. Adherence to the instituted HAART cannot be over-emphasized for the same reasons, thus adherence counselling must form an integral component of the management plan of these children. The regimen instituted should not contain azidothymidine (AZT) as it is known to

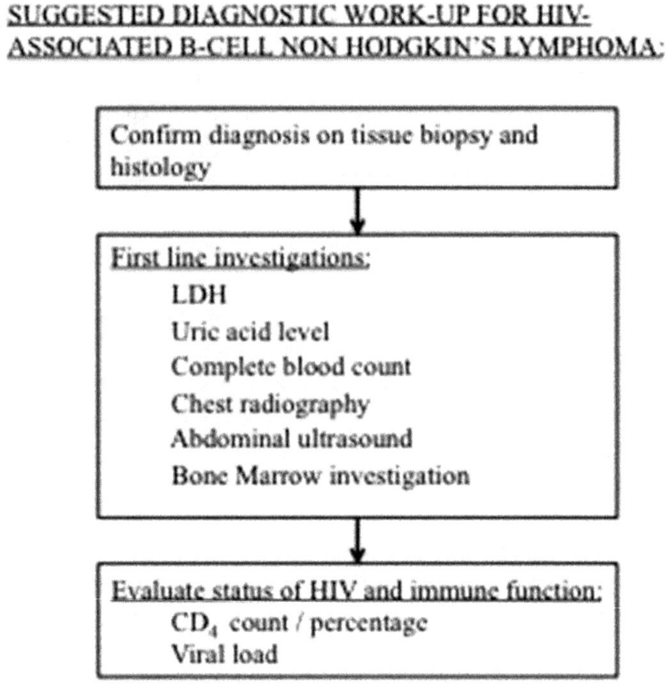

Fig. 26.2 Suggested diagnostic work-up for HIV-associated B-cell Non-Hodgkin lymphoma

cause marrow suppression and would thus exacerbate chemotherapy-induced cytopenias or confound optimal evaluation and management of the child once chemotherapy is instituted.

Beware starting HIV-infected children in whom B-NHL is suspected on glucocorticoids for whatever reason before a diagnosis has been established, as these tumours are exquisitely steroid-sensitive. Not only would this jeopardize making the diagnosis, but it may also precipitate life-threatening tumour lysis.

A big source of management dilemmas in evaluation and management of HIV-infected children with malignancy especially lymphomas is TB. This is largely because both TB and malignancy share a similar symptom profile (lymphadenopathy, fevers, weight loss, profuse night sweats). While children on chemotherapy are at higher risk for development of TB, and TB may masquerade as malignancy, in HIV-negative children the two almost never occur simultaneously in the same patient. Not true for the HIV-infected children in whom the two can and do occur in the same child and the definitive diagnosis of one does not necessarily rule out the other. Children with both should be started on both HAART and antiTB medication as soon as possible. Moreover, the risk of TB IRIS is lower in this population and is outweighed by the risk of TB progression with consequent delays in chemotherapy administration.

Further abdominal masses that could be TB or malignancy should not presumptively be treated as TB in the absence of a *positive tuberculin skin* test even though HIV-infected children are likely to have a negative tuberculin skin test because of their anergy. The increased likelihood of a false negative test does not absolve the clinician of his responsibility to insist on a "cumbersome" tissue biopsy (by ultrasound guidance or otherwise) before instituting antiTB therapy and missing the probable diagnosis of a lymphoma.

Primary CNS Lymphomas

PCNSL occur almost exclusively in HIV-infected children and have been reported to make up to 20 % of AIDS-related lymphomas in some studies [23, 24]. They tend to be cerebral but in rare cases they may spread through the cerebrospinal fluid (CSF) to cause spinal metastases. They mainly present with features of raised intracranial pressure such as headaches and vomiting. Additionally they present with convulsions, ataxia, gait disturbances and neuropsychiatric symptoms.

In a child who fits this symptomatic profile neuroimaging should be carried out. PCNSL will constitute one of the differential diagnoses alongside infectious entities such as toxoplasmosis, cerebral abscess and progressive multifocal leukoencephalopathy. The decision to biopsy suspicious lesions will require combined efforts of an oncologist, a surgeon, infectious diseases specialist and a radiologist. Main stay of treatment is steroids, high doze methotrexate and, in older children, radiotherapy [25]. Due to diagnostic challenges in developing countries probably most cases of PCNSL are missed.

HIV-Associated Hodgkin lymphoma (HIV-HL)

The epidemiologic and pathologic pattern of HIV-HL is distinct from that observed in HIV-negative patients. There is a tenfold increased risk of developing HL in HIV-infected patients compared to the general population. This risk remains high despite HAART which improves immunity and decreases opportunistic infections [26, 27].

One of the theories advanced to explain this paradox is that the Reed Sternberg cells (RS) produce several growth factors that increase the influx of CD4 cells and inflammatory cells, which in turn provide proliferation signals for the RS neoplastic cells. On the other hand, in the case of severe immune suppression, leading to an unfavourable milieu, the progression of RS neoplastic cells can be compromised [26].

Further, EBV has been isolated from almost all tissues of HIV-HL and appears to play a greater role in HIV-HL than in the general population. HIV-associated immune suppression is a state that permits the unchecked and uncontrolled proliferation of EBV infection. One of the EBV-transforming proteins-latent membrane protein 1 (LMP-1) expressed in virtually all HIV-HL patients represents the principal mechanism for constitutive nuclear factor NFkB activity, which confers apoptosis-resistant phenotype to the RS cells [20].

HIV-HL is pathologically distinct from HL in HIV-negative patients in that it is characterized by the high incidence of unfavourable histological subtypes of mixed cellularity (MC) and lymphocyte depletion (LD). The greater proportion of MC and LD subtypes appeared related to severe immune compromise in HIV.

HIV-HL is characterized by advanced disease at presentation with frequent involvement of extranodal sites (bone marrow, liver spleen) and increased occurrence of systemic "B" symptoms (fever, night sweats and/or weight loss >10 % of the normal body weight) [26, 27]. The diagnostic and management challenges in HIV-NHL, especially in resource-constrained settings, are quite similar to HIV-NHL and have already been elaborated on above.

In well-resourced countries outcome of treatment of HIV-HL in the post-HAART era has greatly improved owing to the improved control of HIV infection, immune status and performance status allowing for administration of full doze intensive regimens, and the less aggressive presentation of HL. In sub-Saharan Africa, however, where there is a significant burden of HIV/AIDS and where most of the patients are HAART-naive, overall survival likely remains less favourable than in HIV-negative patients.

Leiomyosarcoma

Leiomyosarcomas are the second most common malignancies seen in HIV-infected children in the developed world [22]. The relative risk that these smooth muscle lesions will develop in an HIV-infected child compared with an HIV-infected child is 10,000. In the setting of HIV infection this tumour appears to be associated with EBV infection [28]. In these children most lesions have been found in various anatomical locations including the gastrointestinal tract, liver spleen, lung and CNS. The pulmonary lesions are often visible as nodules on chest CT, whereas the GI tumours present with evidence of obstruction, abdominal pain and blood y diarrhoea. The course of disease is highly variable with indolent tumours (more likely leiomyomas) that probably do not necessitate intervention in some children and very aggressive, disseminated tumours in others.

Incidental Malignancies

The spectrum of incidental malignancies is similar to that in HIV-negative children. The incidence of childhood malignancy is relatively stable overtime; however, given that the prevalence of HIV among children is expected to increase over time especially with the advent of HAART and therefore increased survival of HIV-infected children, the incidence of incidental malignancies is also expected to rise with time.

The need to establish the HIV serology of children with malignancy cannot be overemphasized as immunosuppression may complicate treatment, resulting in increased toxicity and causing interruptions, which could compromise outcome. Knowing the HIV serostatus for instance may require that chemotherapy be modified. Further, many children with malignancy will be exposed to blood products and the small risk of HIV transmission mandates documentation of HIV status at diagnosis.

Outcomes of Treatment of HIV-Infected Children with Cancer

The prognosis of children infected with HIV has increased dramatically over the last decade and it is expected now that children who are positive will lead a normal and long life.

The survival in children diagnosed with cancer has also increased dramatically especially in developed countries reaching now an overall survival of more than 80 %. Unfortunately the overall survival of children with cancer in most resource-limited countries remains low due to a multitude of factors involving late presentation, lack of drugs and investigations, cost, complexity of associated diseases and co-morbidities.

In this context, the outcomes of cancer treatment in this population of HIV-positive children are much improved for children who have access to HAART, with an estimated 5-year overall survival for the South African cohort of 45.2 % for Burkitt's lymphoma, 67.4 % for Kaposi's sarcoma and 69.6 % for incidental malignancy. These results are still inferior to those for HIV-negative children, where estimated 5-year overall survival for Burkitt's lymphoma usually exceeds 80 % [25].

A more recent South African study showed an overall survival rate after treatment of 52.6 % for HIV-positive and -negative children together [29]. While this figure is much lower than the 79–82 % survival reported from countries like USA, UK or Canada, it is close to published figures from China (55.7 %) and compares favourably with the 40 % survival recorded in India [30, 31].

The comparison of crude survival figures of the same South African study between the two groups analysed (HIV-positive versus HIV-negative) found a slightly lower rate for the HIV-positive children than for HIV-negative. The most significant finding was the percentage of children who died due to the toxicity of the treatment and which was almost 60 times greater in the series with HIV than in the one without HIV: 11.9 % versus 0.2 % respectively (Fisher's exact test, two-tailed $p<0.0001$) [29]. Children with HIV and cancer require special adapted protocols associated with an increased effort in monitoring their complications in order to increase their survival.

Practical guidelines in the management of children with HIV and malignancies are included in Table 26.4.

Conclusions

Much progress has been already achieved worldwide in the treatment of HIV infection in the paediatric population as well as in the treatment of cancer in children.

Table 26.4 Practical notes: HIV and malignancy in children

Disclose the details and prognosis of malignancy to parents and children able to comprehend the diagnosis
Involve social worker with all new children diagnosed with a malignancy (supportive role for child and parents)
Children not yet on HAART:
Evaluate parent insight and lifelong commitment for initiation of HAART
Arrange counselling session pre-initiation of HAART
Identify primary caregiver and treatment supporter
Assist with disclosure to family members and friends
Baseline investigations to be done before initiation of HAART: Viral load and CD_4, Liver function tests, Renal function tests
Calculate dosage for HAART on last/recent weight
Test both parents and other children for HIV and eligibility for HAART
Children already on HAART:
Confirm treatment compliance; ask to see current drugs and process of administration
Evaluate HIV viral suppression and CD_4 count
Confirm appropriate HAART regimen and recalculate dosage on last/recent weight
Test both parents and other children for HIV and eligibility for HAART
Involve infectious disease specialist if available
It is important to evaluate the nutritional state pre-initiation of chemotherapy (higher risk of treatment toxicity and death in malnourished children)
Involve dietician services to evaluate and support nutrition and prescribe appropriate diet supplementation
Screen for associated co-morbidities before initiating chemotherapy (geographically dependant, e.g. Pulmonary Tuberculosis, Malaria, Parasitic infestations and Schistosomiasis)
Take pictures of visible lesions to compare progress of treatment on follow-up
Consider overall cost of chemotherapy regimen before initiation of treatment/Guarantee availability of chemotherapy for the duration of treatment
Apply for Social Support Grant and Disability Grant where appropriate
Confirm transport arrangements for future follow-up visits and support where needed
Ask parents to bring all medication to follow-up visits to continually evaluate compliance
Emphasize the importance of non-treatment interruption in HAART for children and parents
If possible chemotherapy should be given on weekdays and not weekends (when trained staff available)
Check the neutrophil count (or total white cell count) before administering chemotherapy, should be $>1\times10^9$/L and platelets $>100\times10^9$/L
Delay chemotherapy if child has fever, until such time as the infection is under control and patient stable (follow completely the protocol)
Remember to monitor urine output as well as intake, BP and other vital signs when the chemotherapy commences
Make sure you have supportive drugs needed before chemotherapy commences, i.e. anti-emetics, allopurinol, IVI fluids, etc.
Make sure you have adequate supplies of chemotherapy and rescue medications to complete all the cycles
Check the surface area, weight before each chemotherapy cycle, make sure of the dose to be given (per m^2 or per kilogram), recalculate if unsure or dose seems inappropriate
Check the chemotherapy dose together with another colleague or nurse
Make sure you know how to give chemotherapy, i.e. IVI push, infusion, mixes with what fluids, what other supportive measures needed
Chemotherapy should be mixed by an experienced person (physician/pharmacist/nurse) in a separate area with a laminar flow unit if available, if not then an extractor hood above mixing surface (the person mixing chemotherapy should be fully trained, have clothed appropriately or follow safety measures)
For new patients, even with abnormal blood counts or those who are critically ill, the chemotherapy is commenced with appropriate supportive measures
Vincristine causes a fatal encephalopathy if given via the intra-thecal route. Always make sure that the intra-thecal medication is given at a different time to the vincristine
If possible, share drugs between patients; this will decrease costs to the hospital, parents or the supplier of the medication
Develop protocol sheets that are easy to understand and sign off the medication as it is given
Cost of treatment should be guaranteed when treatment starts

Despite the fact that the survival remains low in the treatment of childhood cancer in resource-limited countries, an increased awareness in the early diagnosis, combined with special adapted protocols and monitoring of complications of the treatment of the immunosuppressed patients, will increase the chances of survival of the HIV-positive children with cancer.

References

1. Engels EA, Biggar RJ, Hall HI, et al. Cancer risk in people infected with human immunodeficiency virus in the United States. Int J Cancer. 2008;123:187–94.
2. Cairncross LL, Davidson A, Millar AJ, Pillay K. Kaposi sarcoma in children with HIV: a clinical series from Red Cross Children's Hospital. J Pediatr Surg. 2009;44:373–6.
3. Clifford GM, Polesel J, Rickenbach M, et al. Cancer risk in the Swiss HIV Cohort Study: associations with immunodeficiency, smoking, and highly active antiretroviral therapy. J Natl Cancer Inst. 2005;97:425–32.
4. Orem J, Otieno MW, Remick SC. AIDS-associated cancer in developing nations. Curr Opin Oncol. 2004;16:468–76.
5. Shiels MS, Pfeiffer RM, Gail MH, et al. Cancer burden in the HIV-infected population in the United States. J Natl Cancer Inst. 2011;103:753–62.
6. Powles T, Robinson D, Stebbing J, et al. Highly active antiretroviral therapy and the incidence of non-AIDS-defining cancers in people with HIV infection. J Clin Oncol. 2009;27:884–90.
7. Granovsky MO, Mueller BU, Nicholson HS, Rosenberg PS, Rabkin CS. Cancer in human immunodeficiency virus-infected children: a case series from the Children's Cancer Group and the National Cancer Institute. J Clin Oncol. 1998;16:1729–35.
8. Martellotta F, Berretta M, Vaccher E, Schioppa O, Zanet E, Tirelli U. AIDS-related Kaposi's sarcoma: state of the art and therapeutic strategies. Curr HIV Res. 2009;7:634–8.
9. Hengge UR, Ruzicka T, Tyring SK, et al. Update on Kaposi's sarcoma and other HHV8 associated diseases. Part 1: epidemiology, environmental predispositions, clinical manifestations, and therapy. Lancet Infect Dis. 2002;2:281–92.
10. Ganem D. KSHV and the pathogenesis of Kaposi sarcoma: listening to human biology and medicine. J Clin Invest. 2010;120:939–49.
11. Fatahzadeh M. Kaposi sarcoma: review and medical management update. Oral Surg Oral Med Oral Pathol Oral Radiol. 2012;113:2–16.
12. Gantt S, Kakuru A, Wald A, et al. Clinical presentation and outcome of epidemic Kaposi sarcoma in Ugandan children. Pediatr Blood Cancer. 2010;54:670–4.
13. Nasti G, Talamini R, Antinori A, et al. AIDS-related Kaposi's Sarcoma: evaluation of potential new prognostic factors and assessment of the AIDS Clinical Trial Group Staging System in the Haart Era–the Italian Cooperative Group on AIDS and Tumors and the Italian Cohort of Patients Naive From Antiretrovirals. J Clin Oncol. 2003;21:2876–82.
14. Di Lorenzo G, Konstantinopoulos PA, Pantanowitz L, Di Trolio R, De Placido S, Dezube BJ. Management of AIDS-related Kaposi's sarcoma. Lancet Oncol. 2007;8:167–76.
15. Cooley T, Henry D, Tonda M, Sun S, O'Connell M, Rackoff W. A randomized, double-blind study of pegylated liposomal doxorubicin for the treatment of AIDS-related Kaposi's sarcoma. Oncologist. 2007;12:114–23.
16. Stefan DC, Stones D, Wainwright L, Newton R. Kaposi sarcoma in South African children. Pediatr Blood Cancer. 2011;56(3):392–6.
17. Letang E, Almeida JM, Miró JM, et al. Predictors of immune reconstitution inflammatory syndrome-associated with Kaposi sarcoma in Mozambique: a prospective study. J Acquir Immune Defic Syndr. 2010;53:589–97.
18. Bower M, Nelson M, Young AM, et al. Immune reconstitution inflammatory syndrome associated with Kaposi's sarcoma. J Clin Oncol. 2005;23:5224–8.
19. Murdoch DM, Venter WD, Feldman C, Van Rie A. Incidence and risk factors for the immune reconstitution inflammatory syndrome in HIV patients in South Africa: a prospective study. AIDS. 2008;22:601–10.
20. Rezk SA, Weiss LM. Epstein-Barr virus-associated lymphoproliferative disorders. Hum Pathol. 2007;38:1293–304.
21. Carbone A, Cesarman E, Spina M, Gloghini A, Schulz TF. HIV-associated lymphomas and gamma-herpes viruses. Blood. 2009;113:1213–24.
22. Mueller BU. Cancers in children infected with the human immunodeficiency virus. Oncologist. 1999;4:309–17.
23. Biggar RJ, Frisch M, Goedert JJ. Risk of cancer in children with AIDS. AIDS-Cancer Match Registry Study Group. JAMA. 2000;284:205–9.
24. Caselli D, Klersy C, de Martino M, et al. Human immunodeficiency virus-related cancer in children: incidence and treatment outcome–report of the Italian Register. J Clin Oncol. 2000;18:3854–61.
25. Davidson A, Eley B. HIV and childhood cancer. CME. 2010;28:337–42.
26. Spina M, Carbone A, Gloghini A, Serraino D, Berretta M, Tirelli U. Hodgkin's disease in patients with HIV infection. Adv Hematol. 2011, Article ID 402682, 7 pages, 2011. doi:10.1155/2011/402682.
27. Jacobson CA, Abramson JS. HIV-associated Hodgkin's lymphoma: prognosis and therapy in the era of cART. Adv Hematol. 2012;2012:507257.
28. McClain KL, Leach CT, Jenson HB, et al. Association of Epstein-Barr virus with leiomyosarcomas in children with AIDS. N Engl J Med. 1995;332:12–8.

29. Stefan DC, Stones D. Children with cancer and HIV infection: what is different about them? J Pediatr Hematol Oncol. 2013;35(5) doi:10.1097/MPH.0b013e3182913e6a [Epub ahead of print]
30. Bao PP, Zheng Y, Wu CX, et al. Population-based survival for childhood cancer patients diagnosed during 2002–2005 in Shanghai, China. Pediatr Blood Cancer. 2012;59:657–61.
31. Basta NO, James PW, Gomez-Pozo B, Craft AW, McNally RJ. Survival from childhood cancer in northern England, 1968–2005. Br J Cancer. 2011; 105:1402–8.

27 Hematopoietic Stem Cell Transplant

Julia Palma and Cristián Sotomayor

Introduction

Countries with limited resources are a very heterogeneous group regarding epidemiology, health system organization, health services access, health insurance, income, and economic development [1]. Thus, local experience of a hematopoietic stem cell transplant unit in a specific country with limited resources may not reflect the difficulties seen elsewhere but can rather be seen as a compass to trace your own path.

Chile is a nation of approximately 17 million people where approximately 500 new cases of pediatric cancer are diagnosed yearly. In 1988, Chilean pediatric oncologists founded a cooperative group termed PINDA (Programa Infantil Nacional de DrogascAntineoplasicas) introducing national protocols available to all children with cancer among the country. Treatment protocols were based on American and European studies and result in overall 5-year event-free survival (EFS) rates of about 65 ± 5 %, comparable to that of other countries [2–5]. In 1997, hematopoietic stem cell transplantation (HSCT) was not available for pediatric patients within the public system. To develop HSCT, PINDA initiated an international collaborative program with St. Jude Children's Research Hospital in Memphis, Tennessee, the United States of America. The first objective was to train physicians and nurses on pediatric HSCT and then to develop a transplantation unit. HSCT unit was developed at the Luis Calvo Mackenna Hospital (LCMH), a large pediatric hospital with experience in complex patients. A section of the Oncology ward was refurbished according to national and international standards to host the new unit. Following a detailed cost study, the Chilean Ministry of Health approved budgeting HSCT for an increasing number of patients per year. Patients are selected for transplantation following presentation to a PINDA HSCT committee that meets on a monthly basis and assures representation of patients throughout the country. Soon after the unit activity started in 1999, charity foundations supported the housing of out of town families solving a mayor problem in a country with long distances.

Our initial experience was published in 2006 [6], then we reported our results with new diagnostic techniques [7, 8] and with stem cell collecting protocols [9]. We faced the lack of information regarding best treatment for locally prevalent diseases, so we looked forward to collaborate with regional experts within South America [10]. Through the years we gain expertise in the management of complex patients [11, 12] and we felt confident enough to expand the program to offer transplants from alternative

J. Palma, M.D. (✉) • C. Sotomayor, M.D.
Bone Marrow Transplant Unit, Hospital Dr. Luis Calvo Mackenna, Antonio Varas 360, Providencia, Santiago de Chile, Chile
e-mail: jpalmab@vtr.net

D.C. Stefan and C. Rodriguez-Galindo (eds.), *Pediatric Hematology-Oncology in Countries with Limited Resources: A Practical Manual*, DOI 10.1007/978-1-4614-3891-5_27,

donors such as unrelated cord blood (UCB) and haploidentical (HI) donors [13]. This is a mayor issue for us since our population corresponds to an ethnic minority [14], not well represented in international registries [15]. Periodic review of our local conditions has permitted up to date supportive care [16–19].

The pediatric-transplanted patients represent a high-risk population for many chronic conditions [20] so a follow-up clinic was established from the inception of the unit.

Local and national authorities are constantly demanding us reports on our ongoing results. In order to maintain their support (political, organizational, and economical) it has been very important for us to go step by step and show that we are able to achieve one goal before dealing with new challenges.

Accreditation Requirements for an HSCT Unit

International agencies, such as the Foundation for the Accreditation of Cellular Therapy (FACT) and the Joint Accreditation Committee International Society for Cellular Therapy—European Group for Blood and Marrow Transplantation (JACIE), have agreed on minimum standards to assure quality treatment for HSCT patients. Since improved clinical results are achieved in accredited programs, an accreditation process is absolutely necessary and must be a prerequisite for any program [21–23].

To achieve and to accredit international standards is expensive [24], challenging, and not always seen as feasible by hospitals in limited resource countries [25]. Physicians face many pitfalls due to the lack of support from local health authorities.

For HSCT programs in limited resource countries to operate according to these standards, international cooperation is needed. Experienced teams within other limited resource countries or from well-resourced countries may act as twinning programs, or partners and help less experienced teams to reach the required level.

HSCT Unit Requirements

Many guidelines define the requirements of infrastructure, personnel, and associated support units needed for an HSCT program to function in a proper manner [21]. All efforts must be made in order to fulfill those standards when a new transplant program is set up.

Clinical units must have single patient rooms, positive air pressure and flow from the room to an external space, high efficiency particulate air (HEPA) filter use, over 12 air changes per hour, and minimal leakage in order to establish a protective environment (PE) [26–29]. There is strong evidence that allogeneic transplants must be performed exclusively under PE conditions. Even if there is no evidence that autologous transplant requires a PE, we strongly suggest that any transplant in a newly developed HSCT program is performed in a PE facility. The personnel must have experience in critically ill pediatric patient management and at least one of the attending physicians must have experience in transplanted pediatric patient care, as well as specific laboratory procedures. A physician should be available 24 h per day and specialized nursing care should be provided 24 h a day. All personnel should participate regularly in HSCT training activities [21].

Supportive care should include easy access to pediatric subspecialist evaluation including cardiology, endocrinology, gastroenterology, infectious diseases, nephrology, neurology, palliative care, pathology, psychiatry, pulmonology, radiology, radiotherapy, surgery, transfusion medicine, and others if required. Critical care beds should be readily available [21].

Collection and processing facilities must be built or refurbished and organized according to standards that assure safety for the personnel and patients.

HSCT Donor Types and Sources

Hematopoietic stem cells (HSCs) can be obtained from different sources and donors.

The HSCT donor type can be autologous (patient's own cells) or allogeneic (from a different person). Allogeneic donors can be relatives, usually siblings, or unrelated donors. Syngeneic transplant refers to a transplant from an identical twin.

Human leukocytes antigen (HLA) is the major histocompatibility complex in humans and, through its class I (ABC) and class II (DP, DQ, and DR) molecules, plays a pivotal role in immunological recognition of the self and immunological reaction against foreign antigens and tumor cells [30]. Transplant donors are further classified according to the donor–recipient HLA matching as match or mismatch donors.

The HLA matching criteria and cell dose required are different depending on the source and donor type (see Table 27.1). When the donor and the recipient share less than 9/10 HLA genes they are classified as HI donors.

The available sources of HSCs are bone marrow, peripheral blood, and cord blood. HSCs from peripheral blood are used for all autologous transplants; they are collected through apheresis after receiving chemotherapy and granulocyte colony stimulating factor (G-CSF).

Bone marrow is the main source for allogeneic transplants in children. Peripheral blood might be utilized in some allogeneic procedures; in such cases donors are stimulated with G-CSF (10 μg/kg for 7–10 days). When an HI donor is used most of the time ex vivo graft manipulation is required such as rosetting or immune magnetic cell selection. Recently protocols without manipulation have been reported but this technique is still under investigation in adult trials and should be performed only by experienced teams [31].

Cord blood is safely collected at birth and does not require any treatment or special procedure to the donor. Collection, transportation, storage, and distribution of cord blood are very standardized procedures that need to fulfill many safety measures. Cord blood is a very attractive HSC source since banked units are readily available and less strict HLA matching is required [32].

Table 27.1 Hematopoietic stem cell transplant classification according to donor type, stem cell source, HLA matching, and cell dose

Allogeneic donor type	Source	HLA matching and cell dose
Sibling	Peripheral blood	Match sibling donor: 6/6, 8/8 or 10/10
		Mismatch sibling donor: over 8/10
	Bone marrow	Haploidentical: less than 9/10 and over 10×10^6 CD34 cells/recipient weight in kg
	Cord blood	Match sibling cord: 6/6 eventually 5/6
		Cell dose equal or over 2.5×10^7 TNC/recipient kg
Relative	Peripheral blood	Match family donor:10/10
		Mismatch family donor: over 8/10
	Bone marrow	Haploidentical: less than 9/10 and over 10×10^6 CD34 cells/recipient weight in kg
	Cord blood	Usually 6/6 eventually 5/6 cell dose not defined, suggested equal or over 3×10^7 TNC/recipient weight in kg
Unrelated	Peripheral blood	Match unrelated donor 10/10 or 12/12
	Bone marrow	
	Cord blood	Match unrelated cord: 6/6 or 5/6 for oncological patients 6/6 for non-oncological patients and cell dose equal or over 3×10^7 TNC/recipient's weight in kg
		Mismatch unrelated cord: 4/6 for oncological patients, 5/6 for non-oncological patients and cell dose equal or over 5×10^7 TNC/recipient weight in kg

Table 27.2 Relative comparison between different types of donor regarding access and clinical outcomes

Donor	Speed of access	Relative cost	Risk to donor	Speed of engraftment	Graft failure	GvHD
MSD	Immediate	Low	Low	Moderate	Low	Low
MFaD	Immediate	Intermediate	Low	Moderate	Low	Moderate
MUD	3–4 months	High	Low	Moderate	Low	High
UCB	2–3 weeks	High	None	Slow	Moderate	Moderate
Haplo	Immediate	Intermediate to high	Low	Fast	Moderate to high	High to low

GvHD graft versus host disease, *MSD* match sibling donor, *MFaD* match family donor, *MUD* match unrelated, *UCB* banked unrelated cord blood, *Haplo* haploidentical donor

Costs are a main issue for developing countries. There are great controversies worldwide on cord blood banking best policy; this is beyond the objective of this chapter [33–35]. We concur with the American Academy of Pediatrics and Netcord and we encourage public cord blood banking and directed donation and discourage banking for family or autologous use [36, 37].

There are differences in outcome between the different donor types, sources used, as well as the extent of HLA matching; see Table 27.2.

The main selection criterion for a transplant donor is HLA matching. Other criteria include blood group, CMV status, sex, weight difference, and transplantation urgency [38–41].

HSCT Indications

HSCT indication guidelines by international institutions, such as the European Group for Blood and Marrow Transplant (EBMT) [42] and the American Society for Blood and Marrow Transplantation [43, 44], are easily available and should be the base for local HSCT indications. Biological, economical and social issues, as well as health service conditions and outcomes differ widely from one country to the other so indications in a well-resourced country may not be sensible in a limited resource country. Isolated published case reports or clinical trials from well-resourced countries do not necessarily constitute standard indications for HSCT. At the beginning of an HSCT program, standard of care indication for HSCT should be performed mainly with autologous and related allogeneic grafts. Once standard of care HSCT is mastered, non-routine HSCT could be performed in a few instances, i.e., HI in children with Primary Immune Deficiency and UCB transplants in patients with very high-risk acute lymphoblastic leukemia (ALL) without a family donor. Worldwide populations are ethnically diverse and HLA differs widely; on the other hand cord blood banks and donor registries are located mainly in Western Europe and North America, that's why population from countries with different ethnic background is not well represented in those registries. Only recently cord blood banks and donor registries are becoming available in other globe regions [45–50], but they face many difficulties [51] and most of them are not accredited [52]. At our program as in others, only 20 % of children have a suitable match sibling donor (MSD), and our population is not well represented in the registries and sometime we don't find any donor even in the cord blood banks; using an HI donor and reduced-intensity conditioning (RIC) regimen for high-risk pediatric leukemia and non-oncological diseases, although difficult, has been proven feasible in limited resource settings [53].

We strongly recommend constituting an HSCT medical committee with representatives from the HSCT unit and the referring centers. Such a committee may review indications and should discuss all cases and establish patients' priority taking into account only medical conditions.

HSCT is a very dynamic field and indications for the procedure are always changing; thus periodic review is mandatory. Our indications have been changing every 5 years approximately; as an example present indications for acute leukemias are summarized in Table 27.3.

Table 27.3 Hematopoietic stem cell transplant indication at the PINDA group

	MSD	MFaD	CB MD	MMD
Acute lymphoblastic leukemia in first complete remission (ALL CR 1)				
Hypodiploidy (≤44 chromosomes)	+	+	+	–
PPR + Over 25 % blast in the BM by day 15 of treatment and/or MRD > 10 %	+	+	+	–
PPR + T-ALL	+	+	+	–
PPR + PRO-B ALL	+	+	+	–
PPR + WBC ≥ 100,000/mL	+	+	+	–
No remission by day 33 of induction therapy	+	+	+	+
Acute lymphoblastic leukemia Ph (+) in first complete remission (ALL CR 1)				
Any t(9;22) with MRD (+) according to				
MRD(+) ≥ 0.05 % (at the end of procol IB/pre HR1)	+	+	+	+
MRD(+) 0.005–0.05 % (at the end of protocol IB/pre HR1) any value of MRD POST HR3	+	+	+	+
Infant acute lymphoblastic leukemia in first complete remission (ALL CR 1)				
High-risk infant ALL at diagnosis, >6 months of age + MLL gene rearrangement + WBC ≥300,000 or PPR	+	+	+	–
Intermediate-risk infant ALL at diagnosis (fails at least 1 high-risk criteria) and pre OCTADA(D) MRD $\geq 10^{-4}$	+	+	+	–
Acute lymphoblastic leukemia in second and third remission (ALL CR2 and CR3)				
Any relapse for t(9;22) (+) ALL	+	+	+	+
Very early BM or combined relapse, before 18 months of diagnosis (S4)	+	+	+	+
Early or late BM relapse with T-immune phenotype (S4)	+	+	+	+
Early or late combined relapse with T-immune phenotype (S4)	+	+	+	+
Early BM relapse, non-T, between 18 years 30 months of the diagnosis or before 6 months of the end the treatment (S3)	+	+	+	+
Late BM or combined relapse non-T-immune phenotype, after 30 months of the diagnosis, with no response after F2 (S2B)	+	+	+	–
Early combined relapse, between 18 years 30 months of the diagnosis, non-T, with response after F2 (S2B)	+	+	+	–
Late BM, non-T, with >10.000 blasts in PB (S2C)	+	+	+	–
Bilateral isolated testes relapse, early or very early, before 30 months of the diagnosis (S2D)	+	+	+	–
Early CNS relapse, T-immune phenotype, before 30 months of the diagnosis (S2D)	+	+	+	–
Isolated CNS relapse, no T, before 18 months of the diagnosis, any age (S2D)	+	+	+	–
Isolated CNS relapse, no T, before 30 months of the diagnosis (S2D)	+	+	+	–
ALL in 3CR, only patients whose first relapse was at an extramedullary side	+	+	+	+

Relapse timing: *BM* bone marrow, *PB* peripheral blood; *Very early*: <18 months of the first diagnosis, *Early*: >18 months of the first diagnosis and <6 months after finishing therapy, *Late*: >6 months after finishing therapy. ALL acute lymphoblastic leukemia, PPR poor prednisolone responder

Pre-transplant Evaluation

In order to perform a safe procedure, a comprehensive pre-transplant evaluation must be done in a systematic manner and include a proper patient clinical history, details of disease status, thorough physical examination of the recipient and donor, blood biochemical studies, baseline immune status, assessment of infection risk, and evaluation of social service, mental health, and dental services [54, 55]. Patients and donors might require special investigations according to risks of specific transplant procedures; see Table 27.4.

Consensus on medical and psychological contraindications in pediatrics has not been reached and must be defined locally. Table 27.5 represents contraindications used at our unit.

Table 27.4 Pre-transplant evaluation at the LCMH BMT

	Auto	MSD/MFD	Haplo/CB
Organ function status			
CBC	x	x	x
Coagulation tests	x	x	x
Blood group (AB0 and Rh)	x	x	x
Bone marrow smear	x	x	x
Blood biochemistry[a]	x	x	x
β-CGH	x	x	x
Urine test	x	x	x
Infection assessment			
Toxoplasma gondii (IgG)	x	x	x
Toxocara canis (IgG)	x	x	x
Tripanosoma cruzeii (IgG)	x	x	x
Hepatitis A virus (IgM)	x	x	x
CMV (IgG and IgM)	x	x	x
VEB (IgG and IgM)	x	x	x
Herpes simplex type I and II (IgG and IgM)	x	x	x
Total antibodies hepatitis B virus	x	x	x
Anticore antibodies hepatitis B virus	x	x	x
Superficial antigen hepatitis B virus	x	x	x
Hepatitis C virus	x	x	x
Treponema pallidum test (VDRL)	x	x	x
HIV I and II (ELISA)	x	x	x
HTLV I and II (ELISA)	x	x	x
Galactomanan			x
Adenovirus (qualitative PCR)			x
VEB (quantitative PCR)			x
CMV (quantitative PCR)			x
Immune status			
Inmunoglobulins G, A, M	x	x	x
Lymphocytes subpopulations (flow cytometry)	x	x	x
Pre-transplant chimerism	x	x	x
Cross-match		x	x
HLA antibodies specificity		x	x
Subspecialist evaluations			
Cardiologist: EKG and heart US	x	x	x
Pulmonologist: chest X-ray and lung functional test	x	x	x
Nutrition: weight, height, nutrition status	x	x	x
Otorhinolaringology: audiometry and paranasal X-ray	x	x	x
Psychosocial assessment: psychologist, social worker	x	x	x
Anaesthesiologist	x	x	x
Transfusional medicine	x	x	x
Infectious disease	x	x	x

Autologous autologous transplant, *MSD/MFaD* transplant from a match sibling donor or a match family donor, *CB* transplant from a cord blood, *Haplo* haploidentical transplant

[a]Blood chemistry include: electrolytes, vein gases, creatinine, transaminases (ALAT/ASAT,GGT), lactate dehydrogenase, alkaline phosphatase, bilirubin, glicemia, calcium, phosphorus, magnesium, ferritin

Table 27.5 Absolute medical contraindications for transplantation

1. Karnofsky index less than 70 % or Lansky index less than 60 %
2. Bilirubin over 3 mg/dL and transaminases over 500 U/mL (ASAT or ALAT)
3. Creatinine over two times the normal value
4. Left ventricular fraction < 45 %
5. Pulmonary function test: forced vital capacity less than 60 % for age and/or pulse oximetry less than 93 % with FiO_2 21 %
6. Serious psychiatric disease, not allowing long-term hospitalization
7. Active infectious disease

Conditioning Regimens

Conditioning regimens are very heterogeneous and depend on the HSC source, the patient diagnosis, and pre-transplant complications. The classical objectives of conditioning are (1) destroy any remaining tumoral cells, (2) produce enough immunosuppression to avoid graft rejection, and (3) "to generate the space" within the receptor bone marrow to let the transplanted HSC to grow. There are two major groups of conditioning regimens: (1) myeloablative where high doses of chemotherapy with or without radiotherapy are given and (2) no myeloablative where a combination of lower dose chemotherapy with or without radiotherapy and/or biological agents produces intense immunosuppression and minor organ damage. Myeloablative conditioning is always used in autologous transplantation. Allogeneic transplant can be performed with either myeloablative or no myeloablative conditioning. We recommend to start with standard myeloablative conditioning before starting more unusual non-myeloablative conditioning associated with less known complications. In Table 27.6 we summarize our local conditioning protocols.

HSCT Controversies

Pediatric HSCT is accepted as a well-documented treatment for many diseases; however, it remains ethically controversial. It is associated with significant morbidity and mortality, so it poses ethical dilemmas to the patients, parents, and health care team [56]. In most limited resource countries it is the most expensive medical procedure and thus many more dilemmas exist regarding to whom, when, and how to provide this treatment. The cost of MSD transplant at LCMH was $50,000, and the cost of an autologous transplant was $25,000. Costs included pre-transplant evaluation in recipients and donors, complete hospitalization, and 1 or 2 years clinical follow-up for autologous and allogeneic MSD transplants, respectively.

There is evidence from well-resourced countries that it is an economically viable treatment [57], but no data is available from limited resource countries.

Follow-up Evaluation

A proposed post-transplant evaluation is shown in Table 27.7. It includes chimerism and immune reconstitution studies in all patients.

Conclusion

A pediatric HSCT program in a public hospital of a developing country is feasible. Of great importance to a successful program is the prior existence of an organized pediatric referral network. This allows a relatively uniform primary treatment for all patients and appropriate evaluation of children at the HSCT selection committee. Transplant personnel should receive adequate training before the onset of the clinical work. Collaboration with recognized HSCT units is strongly advised. The benefits of such an agreement will reach beyond the establishment of an HSCT program. Transplant units must meet current international standards. This can be done either remodeling an existing ward or building a new facility (Table 27.8).

We emphasize that the most important measure to prevent infections is hand washing. Effective 24 h nursing care plays a major role in a successful program as well as supportive services and a long-term patient follow-up. Due to budgeting restrictions in developing countries it

Table 27.6 Local conditioning protocols

	HSCT type	Condition	Conditioning regimen Chemotherapy	Radiotherapy
Malignancies	Autologous	Lymphoma	BEAM	
		AML	Bu and Cy	
		Neuroblastoma	Me + Bu	
	MSD	AML >3 years old	Cy	Total body irradiation (TBI) 12 Gy twice daily × 3 days
		AML <3 years old	Cy and Bu	
		ALL	Cy and Bu and Et	
		CML	Cy and Bu	
		MDS	Cy and Bu	
Benign conditions	MSD	Severe AA	Cy 120–200 mg/kg over 4 days and ATG	OR total nodal irradiation (TNI) 7 Gy instead of ATG
		SCID	Bu and Cy with or without ATG	
		Chediak Higashi syndrome in accelerated phase	Bu and Cy and Et	
		Fanconi anemia	Cy (20 mg/kg)	TNI 5 Gy
		Kostmann disease, osteopetrosis, and Blackfan Diamond anemia	Bu and Cy	
Any	HI		RIC regimen: fludarabine, thiotepa, melphalan, ATG, rituximab, methylprednisolone	TNI 7 Gy

Abbreviations and doses unless otherwise specified:
BEAM: BCNU = 300–600 mg/m^2 (1×); Et (etoposide) = 100–200 mg/m^2 (4×); Cytarabine: 200–400 mg/m^2 (4×); Melphalan = 140 mg/m^2 (1×)
Bu (busulfan) = 16 mg/kg daily (4×), Cy (cyclophosphamide) = 120 mg/kg daily (2×), Me (melphalan) = 140 mg/m^2, Et (etoposide) = 30 mg/kg on day-6, ATG = antithymocyte globulin
AML acute myeloid leukemia, *ALL* acute lymphocytic leukemia, *CML* chronic myeloid leukemia, *MDS* myelodysplastic syndrome, *AA* aplastic anemia, *SCID* severe combined immunodeficiency

Table 27.7 Post-transplant follow-up and subspecialist evaluation

HSCT clinical outpatient[a]	Weekly until day +60 post-HSCT
	Twice month until day + 90 post-HSCT[b]
	Monthly until 1 year post-HSCT
1-Year post-HSCT	Spirometry and pulmonologist evaluation
	Ecocardiography and cardiologist evaluation
	Endocrinologist evaluation
	Ophthalmologist evaluation
	Odontologist evaluation
	Gynecologist evaluation
Chimerism	Day +21 and/or +28, then +90, +180, and +365 post-HSCT
Immune reconstitution	Day +90, +180, and +365 post-HSCT

HSCT hematopoietic stem cell transplantation
[a] include physical examination, viral surveillance, hematological and metabolic laboratory tests
[b] CMV antigenemia or PCR weekly until day +100 post-HSCT

Table 27.8 Tips for starting a new HSCT Unit

Summary of practical guidelines when establishing a new HSCT program
1. To have preestablished pre-transplant treatment protocols within a network
2. Seek sustainable funding
(a) Government coverage and NGO
(b) Leadership: social, politics, and private company
3. Establish twinning program or partnership with an experienced HSCT unit
(a) All new staff members should receive HSCT training
(b) At least one team physician must have experience in managing pediatric transplant patients
4. Design transplantation in patient unit according to international standards
(a) Single rooms, positive air pressure and laminar flow, HEPA filters, over 12 air changes per hour, etc.
5. Ensure international accreditation requirements are met
6. Ensure meticulous infection prevention measures
(a) Hand washing, barrier nursing, infection surveillance program, etc.
7. Establish HSCT committee with monthly meetings
(a) Establish local HSCT indications and contraindications and review regularly
8. Ensure availability of pediatric subspecialist services and intensive care beds
(a) Other supportive services must also be available, e.g., social services, psychology, physiotherapy, blood bank
9. Establish working relationship with local laboratories
(a) All required special investigation tests should be available
10. Comprehensive pre-transplant evaluations should be performed
(a) Include psychosocial evaluation
11. All pharmacological agents must be available, as well as radiotherapy
12. Establish long-term follow-up HSCT clinic
13. Regular critical review of results and progress
(a) Publish reports of experience
14. Once standard HSCT has been mastered, endeavour to also master more complex HSCT

is important to maximize cost-effectiveness. Information in the HSCT scientific literature is biased to well-resourced countries reality; experiences of centers in limited resourced countries are oddly reported, thus; we encourage teams and medical journals to publish papers from these centers to learn from them and to have a proper picture on difficulties and clever solutions on common problems in HSCT.

Periodic analysis of infection, mortality, and morbidity must be done to assure good quality treatment and after mastering standard HSCT, a program should expand and learn how to perform higher-risk transplants.

References

1. Goss PE, Lee BL, Badovinac-Crnjevic T, Strasser-Weippl K, Chavarri-Guerra Y, Louis JS, et al. Planning cancer control in Latin America and the Caribbean. Lancet Oncol. 2013;14(5):391–436. doi:10.1016/S1470-2045(13)70048-2.
2. Campbell M, Salgado C, Quintana J, Becker A, Vargas L, Cabrera ME, et al. Improved outcome for acute lymphoblastic leukemia in children of a developing country: results of the Chilean National Trial PINDA 87. Med Pediatr Oncol. 1999;33(2):88–94.
3. Villarroel M, Tordecilla J, Salgado C, Luo X, Messen S, Rayo Y, et al. Multimodal therapy for children and adolescents with Ewing sarcoma: results of the First National Chilean Trial (1986-1991). Med Pediatr Oncol. 1997;29(3):190–6.
4. Santolaya ME, Alvarez AM, Becker A, Cofre J, Enriquez N, O'Ryan M, et al. Prospective, multicenter evaluation of risk factors associated with invasive bacterial infection in children with cancer, neutropenia, and fever. J Clin Oncol. 2001;19(14):3415–21.
5. Santolaya ME, Alvarez AM, Aviles CL, Becker A, Cofre J, Enriquez N, et al. Prospective evaluation of a model of prediction of invasive bacterial infection risk among children with cancer, fever, and neutropenia. Clin Infect Dis. 2002;35(6):678–83.
6. Palma J, Mosso C, Paris C, Campbell M, Tong X, et al. Establishment of a pediatric HSCT program in a public hospital in Chile. Pediatr Blood Cancer. 2006;46:803.
7. Farfán M, Torres JP, Vergara A, Donoso G, Alba A, Paris C, et al. Comparison of real-time polymerase chain reaction and antigenemia assay to detect cyto-

megalovirus in pediatric transplants. Rev Chilena Infectol. 2011;28(2):113–7.
8. Schmidt N, Palma J, King A, Santolaya ME. C reactive protein and procalcitonin levels for the diagnosis of invasive bacterial infections in allogenic hematopoietic stem cell transplantation recipients. Rev Med Chil. 2007;135(8):982–9.
9. Anguita-Compagnon AT, Dibarrart MT, Palma J, Paredes L, Mosso C, Montalva R, et al. Mobilization and collection of peripheral blood stem cells: guidelines for blood volume to process, based on CD34-positive blood cell count in adults and children. Transplant Proc. 2010;42:339–44.
10. Palma J, Sasso DF, Dufort G, Koop K, Sampor C, Diez B, et al. Successful treatment of metastatic retinoblastoma with high-dose chemotherapy and autologous stem cell rescue in South America. Bone Marrow Transplant. 2012;47(4):522–7. doi:10.1038/bmt.2011.108. Epub 2011 May 23.
11. Palma J, Catalán P, Mardones P, Santolaya ME. Mycobacterium tuberculosis infection in a pediatric patient who underwent a hematopoietic stem cell transplant. Rev Chilena Infectol. 2013;30(2):202–5.
12. Paris C, Palma J, Kopp K, Santolaya ME, Zepeda AJ. Cytomegalovirus infection in children undergoing hematopoietic stem cell transplantation in Chile. Pediatr Blood Cancer. 2009;53(3):453–8.
13. Palma J, Salas L, Carrión F, Sotomayor C, Catalán P, Paris C, Turner V, Jorquera H, Handgretinger R, Rivera GK. Haploidentical stem cell transplantation for children with high-risk leukemia. Pediatr Blood Cancer. 2012;59(5):895–901.
14. Dilioglou S, Embrey CE, Fernandez-Vina M, Turner EV. Alleles and haplotypes of a Chilean population. Hum Immunol. 2007;68:S69 (abstract 108-P).
15. Barriga F, Wietstruck MA. Search for unrelated donor umbilical cord blood units for allogeneic stem cell transplantation: results in two time periods. Transplant Proc. 2007;39(3):629–30.
16. Payá E, Noemí I, Tassara R, Catalán P, Avilés CL. Prophylaxis against Toxoplasma gondii disease in pediatric and adult patients undergoing solid organ and hematopoietic stem cells transplantation. Rev Chilena Infectol. 2012;29 Suppl 1:S37–9.
17. Catalán P, Alba A. Prophylaxis against Epstein Barr disease in pediatric and adult patients undergoing solid organ and hematopoietic stem cells transplantation. Rev Chilena Infectol. 2012;29 Suppl 1:S29–31.
18. Álvarez AM, Catalán P, Alba A, Zubleta M. Prophylaxis against respiratory viral disease in pediatric and adult patients undergoing solid organ and hematopoietic stem cells transplantation. Rev Chilena Infectol. 2012;29 Suppl 1:S33–6.
19. Benítez R, Noemí I, Tassara R, Catalán P, Avilés CL. Prophylaxis against Chagas disease in pediatric and adult patients undergoing solid organ and hematopoietic stem cells transplantation. Rev Chilena Infectol. 2012;29 Suppl 1:S41–3.
20. Paris C, Yates L, Lama P, Zepeda AJ, Gutiérrez D, Palma J. Evaluation of metabolic syndrome after hematopoietic stem cell transplantation in children and adolescents. Pediatr Blood Cancer. 2012;59(2):306–10.
21. Keever-Taylor C, Warkentin P, Pamphilon D; Cellular Therapy Standards Committee Leadership; FACT Accreditation Office and JACIE Accreditation Office International standards for cellular therapy product collection, processing, and administration. Fifth Edition Version 5.2. 2012.
22. Caunday O, Agulles O, McGrath E, Empereur F, Stoltz JF, Chabannon C. Implementation of JACIE accreditation results in the establishment of new indicators that unevenly monitor processes contributing to the delivery of hematopoietic SCT. Bone Marrow Transplant. 2013;48(4):604–9. doi:10.1038/bmt.2012.181.
23. Chabannon C, Pamphilon D, Vermylen C, Gratwohl A, Niederwieser D, McGrath E, et al. JACIE celebrates its 10-year anniversary with the demonstration of improved clinical outcome. Cytotherapy. 2011;13(6):765–6.
24. Apperley J. Just another cost increasing exercise (JACIE)? Bone Marrow Transplant. 2004;34(10):835–8.
25. Zahnd D, Leibundgut K, Zenhäusern R, Pabst T, Fontana S, Schneider R, Tobler A, Zwicky C. Implementation of the JACIE standards for a haematopoietic progenitor cell transplantation programme: a cost analysis. Bone Marrow Transplant. 2004;34(10):847–53.
26. Sehulster LM, Chinn RYW, Arduino MJ, Carpenter J, Donlan R, et al. Guidelines for environmental infection control in health-care facilities. Recommendations from CDC and the Healthcare Infection Control Practices Advisory Committee (HICPAC). Chicago, IL: American Society for Healthcare Engineering/American Hospital Association; 2004.
27. Siegel JD, Rhinehart E, Jackson M, Chiarello L; Healthcare Infection Control Practices Advisory Committee. 2007 Guideline for isolation precautions: preventing transmission of infectious agents in healthcare settings. 2007. http://www.cdc.gov/ncidod/dhqp/pdf/isolation2007.pdf
28. Dykewicz C. Hospital infection control in hematopoietic stem cell transplant recipients. Emerg Infect Dis. 2001;7(2):263–7.
29. Centers for Disease Control and Prevention. Guidelines for preventing opportunistic infections among hematopoietic stem cell transplant recipients: recommendations of CDC, the Infectious Disease Society of America, and the American Society of Blood and Marrow Transplantation. MMWR Recomm Rep. 2000;49(RR-10):1–125. CE1-7.
30. Speiser DE, Tiercy JM, Rufer N, et al. High resolution HLA matching associated with decreased mortality after unrelated bone marrow transplantation. Blood. 1996;87:4455–62.
31. Luznik L, O'Donnell PV, Fuchs EJ. Post-transplantation cyclophosphamide for tolerance induction in HLA-haploidentical bone marrow transplantation. Semin Oncol. 2012;39(6):683–93.
32. Peters C, Cornish JM, Parikh SH, Kurtzberg J. Stem cell source and outcome after hematopoietic stem cell transplantation (HSCT) in children and adolescents with acute leukemia. Pediatr Clin North Am. 2010;57(1):27–46.

33. O'Connor MA, Samuel G, Jordens CF, Kerridge IH. Umbilical cord blood banking: beyond the public-private divide. J Law Med. 2012;19(3):512–6.
34. Machin LL, Brown N, McLeod D. Giving to receive? The right to donate in umbilical cord blood banking for stem cell therapies. Health Policy. 2012;104(3):296–303.
35. Petrini C. Ethical issues in umbilical cord blood banking: a comparative analysis of documents from national and international institutions. Transfusion. 2013;53(4):902–10.
36. Gluckman E, Ruggeri A, Rocha V, Baudoux E, Boo M, Kurtzberg J, et al.; Eurocord, Netcord, World Marrow Donor Association and National Marrow Donor Program. Family-directed umbilical cord blood banking. Haematologica. 2011;96(11):1700–7.
37. American Academy of Pediatrics Section on Hematology/Oncology, American Academy of Pediatrics Section on Allergy/Immunology, Lubin BH, Shearer WT. Cord blood banking for potential future transplantation. Pediatrics. 2007;119(1):165–70.
38. Bosi A, Bartolozzi B. Safety of bone marrow stem cell donation: a review. Transplant Proc. 2010;42(6):2192–4.
39. Hough R, Cooper N, Veys P. Allogeneic haemopoietic stem cell transplantation in children: what alternative donor should we choose when no matched sibling is available? Br J Haematol. 2009;147(5):593–613.
40. Shaw BE, Veys P, Pagliuca A, Addada J, Cook G, Craddock CF, et al. Recommendations for a standard UK approach to incorporating umbilical cord blood into clinical transplantation practice: conditioning protocols and donor selection algorithms. Bone Marrow Transplant. 2009;44(1):7–12.
41. Spellman SR, Eapen M, Logan BR, Mueller C, Rubinstein P, et al.; National Marrow Donor Program; Center for International Blood and Marrow Transplant Research. A perspective on the selection of unrelated donors and cord blood units for transplantation. Blood. 2012;120(2):259–65.
42. Ljungman P, Bregni M, Brune M, Cornelissen J, de Witte T, Dini G, et al.; European Group for Blood and Marrow Transplantation. Allogeneic and autologous transplantation for haematological diseases, solid tumours and immune disorders: current practice in Europe 2009. Bone Marrow Transplant. 2010;45(2):219–34.
43. American Society for Blood and Marrow Transplantation. The role of cytotoxic therapy with hematopoietic stem cell transplantation in the therapy of acute myeloid leukemia in children. Biol Blood Marrow Transplant. 2007;13:500–1.
44. American Society for Blood and Marrow Transplantation. The role of cytotoxic therapy with hematopoietic stem cell transplantation in the treatment of acute lymphoblastic leukemia in children. Biol Blood Marrow Transplant. 2006;12:370–1.
45. Liu J, He J, Chen S, Qin F, Wang F, Xu G, et al. Cord blood banking and transplantation in China: a ten years experience of a single public bank. Transfus Med Hemother. 2012;39(1):23–7.
46. Gan G, Teh A, Chan L, Cheong S, Chang K, Ibrahim H. Bone marrow and stem cell transplantation: Malaysian experience. Bone Marrow Transplant. 2008;42 Suppl 1:S103–5.
47. Novelo-Garza B, Limon-Flores A, Guerra-Marquez A, Luna-Bautista F, Juan-Shum L, Montero I, et al. Establishing a cord blood banking and transplantation program in Mexico: a single institution experience. Transfusion. 2008;48(2):228–36.
48. Lange A, Dera-Joachimiak D, Madej S, Polak M, Koscinska K, Pietraszek E, et al. Activity of the National Polish Bone Marrow Donor Registry—analysis of the matching process successfully completed with hematopoietic stem cell transplantation. Transplant Proc. 2010;42(8):3316–8.
49. Lee TD. Marrow donor registry and cord blood bank in Taiwan. Int J Hematol. 2002;76 Suppl 1:312–4. PubMed PMID: 12430871.
50. Ayas M, Al-Seraihi A, Al-Jefri A, Al-Ahmari A, Al-Mahr M, Al-Ghonaium A, et al. Unrelated cord blood transplantation in pediatric patients: a report from Saudi Arabia. Bone Marrow Transplant. 2010;45(8):1281–6.
51. Jangi S. Problems of creating bone marrow donor registries in emerging economies. BMJ. 2013;346:f2976.
52. http://www.factwebsite.org/CordSearch.aspx?&type=CordBloodBank&country=&state=
53. Dufort G, Pisano S, Incoronato A, Castiglioni M, Carracedo M, Pagés C, et al. Feasibility and outcome of haploidentical SCT in pediatric high-risk hematologic malignancies and Fanconi anemia in Uruguay. Bone Marrow Transplant. 2012;47(5):663–8.
54. Sacchi N, Costeas P, Hartwell L, Hurley CK, Raffoux C, Rosenmayr A, et al.; Quality Assurance and Clinical Working Groups of the World Marrow Donor Association. Haematopoietic stem cell donor registries: World Marrow Donor Association recommendations for evaluation of donor health. Bone Marrow Transplant. 2008;42:9–14.
55. Foster LW, McLellan L, Rybicki L, Tyler T, Bolwell BJ. Ethical reasoning about patient eligibility in allogeneic BMT based on psychosocial criteria. Bone Marrow Transplant. 2009;44(9):607–12.
56. Bendorf A, Kerridge IH. Ethical issues in bone marrow transplantation in children. J Paediatr Child Health. 2011;47(9):614–9.
57. Matthes-Martin S, Pötschger U, Barr R, Martin M, Boztug H, Klingebiel T, Attarbaschi A, Eibler W, Mann G. Costs and cost-effectiveness of allogeneic stem cell transplantation in children are predictable. Biol Blood Marrow Transplant. 2012;18(10):1533–9.

Index

D.C. Stefan and C. Rodriguez-Galindo (eds.), *Pediatric Hematology-Oncology in Countries with Limited Resources: A Practical Manual*, DOI 10.1007/978-1-4614-3891-5,

R

T

U

V

W

Y

CPSIA information can be obtained
at www.ICGtesting.com
Printed in the USA
LVHW020142220819
628463LV00003B/81/P

9 781461 438908